Clinical Wisdom and Interventions
in Acute and Critical Care

Patricia Benner, RN, PhD, FAAN, is a Professor Emerita of Nursing in the Department of Social and Behavioral Sciences Nursing at the University of California, San Francisco (UCSF). She is a Fellow in the American Academy of Nursing and an Honorary Fellow in the Royal College of Nursing, United Kingdom. She is the author of *From Novice to Expert: Excellence and Power in Clinical Nursing Practice*, which has been translated into 10 languages and provides the background for this research; has coauthored with Judith Wrubel in *The Primacy of Caring, Stress and Coping in Health and Illness*; *Expertise in Nursing Practice: Caring, Clinical Judgment and Ethics* with Christine Tanner and Catherine Chesla; and The Carnegie Foundation for the Advancement of Teaching National Nursing Education Study entitled, *Educating Nurses: A Call for Radical Transformation* (Benner, Sutphen, Leonard, & Day, 2010). Dr. Benner coedited *Interpretive Phenomenology in Health Care Research* (Chan, Brykczynski, Malone, & Benner, 2010). Dr. Benner is currently conducting research on clinical knowledge and experiential learning of nurses caring for wounded warriors in combat zones with Dr. Patricia Kelley and colleagues from the Federal Tri-Service Research Program.

Patricia Hooper Kyriakidis, RN, PhD, is a consultant and researcher at Practice Solutions, Inc., in Nashville, Tennessee. As a consultant, she educates and consults on the development of expertise, educational, and administrative conditions that support practice development, understanding practice using interpretative methods, and professional recognition programs. In her research, she examines clinical knowledge development, clinical judgment, and the clinical, administrative, and educational conditions that support or impede the development of practice. Her clinical, educational, and research publications are in journals such as *Advanced Practice Nursing Quarterly, Clinical Nurse Specialist, Critical Care Nurse, Critical Care Nursing Clinics of North America, and Journal of Cardiovascular Nursing*. She is currently working with Dr. Joan Vitello-Cicciu on an interpretive study that examines the effects of applying Benner's research implications on the clinical and ethical development of new nurses over their first 2 years in practice.

Daphne Stannard, RN, PhD, CCRN, CCNS, FCCM, is the Associate Chief Nurse Researcher and Perianesthesia Clinical Nurse Specialist at UCSF Medical Center. She is a member of the American Association of Critical-Care Nurses, American Society of Anesthesiologists, American Society of Perianesthesia Nurses, Association of Perioperative Registered Nurses, National Association of Clinical Nurse Specialists, Sigma Theta Tau, Society of Critical Care Medicine, and the Western Institute of Nursing. With Drs. Benner and Hooper Kyriakidis, she is co-recipient of the AJN Book of the Year Award and Media of the Year Awards. She has contributed 13 peer-reviewed journal articles, 9 book chapters, and co-edited the recently published text, *Perianesthesia Nursing Care: A Bedside Guide to Safe Recovery*.

Clinical Wisdom and Interventions in Acute and Critical Care

A Thinking-in-Action Approach

Second Edition

Patricia Benner, RN, PhD, FAAN
Patricia Hooper Kyriakidis, RN, PhD
Daphne Stannard, RN, PhD, CCRN, CCNS, FCCM

SPRINGER PUBLISHING COMPANY
NEW YORK

Springer Publishing Company, LLC
11 West 42nd Street
New York, NY 10036
www.springerpub.com

Acquisitions Editor: Allan Graubard
Senior Production Editor: Diane Davis
Cover Design: Steven Pisano
Composition: Absolute Service, Inc., Project Manager, Gil Rafanan

ISBN: 978-0-8261-0573-8
E-book ISBN: 978-0-8261-0574-5

11 12 13 14/ 5 4 3 2 1

The author and the publisher of this work have made every effort to use sources believed to be reliable to provide information that is accurate and compatible with the standards generally accepted at the time of publication. Because medical science is continually advancing, our knowledge base continues to expand. Therefore, as new information becomes available, changes in procedures become necessary. We recommend that the reader always consult current research and specific institutional policies before performing any clinical procedure. The author and publisher shall not be liable for any special, consequential, or exemplary damages resulting, in whole or in part, from the readers' use of, or reliance on, the information contained in this book. The publisher has no responsibility for the persistence or accuracy of URLs for external or third-party Internet Web sites referred to in this publication and does not guarantee that any content on such Web sites is, or will remain, accurate or appropriate.

Library of Congress Cataloging-in-Publication Data

Benner, Patricia E.
  Clinical wisdom and interventions in acute and critical care : a thinking-in-action approach / Patricia Benner, Patricia Hooper Kyriakidis, Daphne Stannard. — 2nd ed.
    p. ; cm.
  Rev. ed. of: Clinical wisdom and interventions in critical care / Patricia Benner, Patricia Hooper Kyriakidis, Daphne Stannard.
  Includes bibliographical references and index.
  ISBN 978-0-8261-0573-8 — ISBN 978-0-8261-0574-5 (e-book)
  I. Hooper-Kyriakidis, Patricia Lee. II. Stannard, Daphne. III. Benner, Patricia E. Clinical wisdom and interventions in critical care. IV. Title.
  [DNLM: 1. Critical Care—methods. 2. Nursing Care—methods. 3. Critical Illness—nursing. WY 154]
  RT120.I5B46 2011
  616.02'8—dc22
                    2010044600

Special discounts on bulk quantities of our books are available to corporations, professional associations, pharmaceutical companies, health care organizations, and other qualifying groups.

If you are interested in a custom book, including chapters from more than one of our titles, we can provide that service as well.

For details, please contact:
Special Sales Department, Springer Publishing Company, LLC
11 West 42nd Street, 15th Floor, New York, NY 10036-8002
Phone: 877-687-7476 or 212-431-4370; Fax: 212-941-7842
Email: sales@springerpub.com

Printed in the United States of America by Hamilton.

Contents

Foreword

This new edition of *Clinical Wisdom* is intended for undergraduate and graduate nursing students who are learning critical care, for educators teaching clinical reasoning, and for those seeking to improve systems of care and leadership in clinical practice. However, the concepts laid out in this book will resonate with all who confront the complex and demanding business of clinical reasoning and action in dynamic patient care situations. This is not an ordinary, well-done, and accurate text on critical and acute care nursing; it is, instead, a lavishly detailed guide to the essence of becoming an expert nurse.

The approach is grounded on the findings of ethnographic studies of critical and acute care nurses building on the substantial previous work of Patricia Benner and the other authors. Different in its construction from most nursing or medical texts, it takes advantage of the depth of detail and intrigue found in "nurse stories." Every chapter is replete with real-life incidents used to illustrate the complex ideas and ambiguities inherent in caring for the critically ill and their families. Nurses and doctors and other health care professionals have always told stories to articulate and explain their work. As a historian, I find these stories invaluable in comprehending the day-to-day practices of those who care for the sick. This book weaves the stories told by caregivers and learners into the authors' framework for understanding nursing knowledge and practice. Arguing that "expert critical care nurses are always dwelling in meaningful stories . . . [to help them in] keep[ing] an up-to-the-minute clinical and human grasp of the significance of the situation" (p. 14), the authors illustrate "thinking-in-action" and "reasoning-in-transition" by embedding the concepts in real time, in context, and with all the complications likely to be found in real practice situations.

This text does not simplify or reduce critical care to principles in an attempt to make it easier to learn. Instead, the book provides an amazingly whole picture enabling the learner to visualize what critical care is really like and to comprehend the expectations placed on critical care nurses. A good example is Chapter 9, "Facing Death: End-of-Life Care and Decision Making." Here the text and the nurse stories illustrate how the illness experience cannot be seen as a series of decisions built on one another. Instead, in any illness, the patient's understanding of the illness, caregivers' understanding, and family understanding all unfold unevenly over time. In this sense, learning expert practice is a search for knowing how to go ahead with imperfect knowledge. When patients are dying, critical care nurses must reframe their imagination of the right care for the patient from curative action to palliative action. The author directly confronts the difficulties caregivers face in being the persons who actually withhold care or intervene. Death in critical care situations is underdiscussed; this excellent chapter goes a long way to improve that insufficiency.

This book richly illustrates the larger concepts of clinical grasp and inquiry and clinical forethought, devoting two chapters to ways or styles of practice found and described by expert nurses. Following chapters are built on nine domains of practice organized around common clinical goals and concerns. Each chapter includes a summary of the intent of the text to guide the learner.

Although there are three authors, the transitions are remarkably smooth and the text is easily readable. I believe many clinicians and educators will read this book for interest, whether they practice or teach in critical care or not. The text is also written clearly enough to be accessible to informed lay readers. Any medical reporter who wants to understand how caregivers think and work and what happens in critical care would benefit from reading it.

Perhaps, the most important accomplishment of this text is its insistence on incorporating all the elements of critical care: clinical reasoning and thinking ahead, caregiving to patients and families, ethical and moral issues, dealing with breakdown and technological hazard, communication and negotiating among all participants, teaching and coaching, and understanding the linkages between the larger systems and the individual patient. Moreover, the text repeatedly reveals the limitation of relying on taxonomies, simple categorization, or protocols as a way to convey understanding of, or even to actually practice critical care. Instead, the authors insist that, to get the best answer, experts must create "the best account of the clinical situation under the circumstances of uncertainty" (p. 5). The marriage of a narrative understanding of the specific situation with reflection allows the caregiver to use scientific knowledge melded and suffused by the time, place, and conditions of care, which, in turn, leads to clinical wisdom.

I believe this outstanding book will secure a place on most educators' and expert clinicians' bookshelves. Every once in a while a better book comes along; this is one of those times.

Joan E. Lynaugh, PhD, RN, FAAN
Professor Emerita, University of Pennsylvania School of Nursing
Philadelphia, Pennsylvania

Foreword II

In 1999, as editor of *Canadian Journal of Nursing Research* (CJNR), I received a copy of *Clinical Wisdom and Interventions in Critical Care: A Thinking-in-Action Approach* for review. The title intrigued me. It was the first time I had seen the use in nursing of such phrases as *clinical wisdom* and *thinking-in-action* rather than the more familiar *clinical understanding* or *reflection-on-action*. Then I noted that Patricia Benner was its first author. I was familiar with Dr. Benner's previous books and her many writings and had developed a deep and abiding respect for the quality of her scholarship. And so, it was with great anticipation that I picked up the book and began to read.

I was not disappointed. Even today, almost 11 years later, I can still recall my excitement as I read each chapter. I knew then that the groundbreaking book I was holding would lead to new understandings of how nurses nursed. What Benner, Hooper Kyriakidis, and Stannard had captured was the essence of nursing and the thinking behind clinical judgment and decision making. They had detailed with great clarity the work of nurses: the thinking and decision-making processes involved in clinical judgment, the nature of moral and ethical comportment, and what caring looks like in the practice world of critical care. The authors had also captured—through compelling stories, observations, vignettes, and nurses' narratives—the complexities involved in nursing acts that had gone unnoticed, unrecognized, and underappreciated. They had put words to actions and described processes in precise terms that had previously eluded description. Moreover, they had discovered the power of the narrative to express in vivid detail the moment-to-moment, day-to-day acts of nursing. In this book, interpretative phenomenology found a champion as a valid methodology for generating knowledge about nursing phenomena—and brought credibility to this approach because of the rigor of scholarship involved.

At the time, I believed that this would be an important book for clinicians, educators, and even administrators. During the intervening years, I found myself returning to this book regularly, using it as a resource for different purposes. It continued to speak to me, and with each reread, I uncovered new layers of meaning. It was thought provoking, relevant, and instructional. The messages it contained were timely and timeless. Thus, I was intrigued to learn of a second edition and curious as to what new insights these authors had discovered during the intervening decade.

The new edition takes into account the changing circumstances and context of the health care system and reflects the development of nursing. Much has transpired during the past decade. As the authors point out, the boundaries between the acute and critical care health care systems have blurred, and many hospitals are offering multiple layers of critical care from stable critical to intensively critical. In short, many of our tertiary care hospitals are critical care facilities, both fast-paced and demanding. They require skilled and wise nurses to deal with high levels of uncertainty, ambiguity, unpredictable clinical situations, rapidly unfolding clinical trajectories, and complex patient situations. Nursing is carried out in challenging practice environments that are in flux, which require attending to the needs of and demands from many people including other nurses, physicians, and staff. All this is happening in an environment that is ever more reliant on sophisticated technology to identify, solve, and manage problems. The pressures and stresses that nurses experience day after day are palpable. Within this context, the nurse's role is to keep the patients at the center of care—getting to know them as a person, recognizing their unique ways of responding to insults, and advocating for them to provide care that is grounded in understanding, knowledge, and wisdom.

The term *clinical wisdom* continues to intrigue me. What differentiates *clinical wisdom* from *clinical understanding* or *clinical knowledge*? Belenky, Clinchy, Goldberger, and Tarule (1986) in their now classic book, *Women's Ways of Knowing*, provide some insights. Understanding involves some familiarity and acquaintance with the person or a task. On the other hand, knowledge goes beyond mere understanding. It includes understanding and an intimacy that can only be achieved through developing a connection with the person or task by empathy or seeing the situation through a different lens other than one's own. The most developed knower is passionate and a connected participator. Wisdom moves the process of knowing further along. As the saying goes, "Knowledge has a way of coming and going whereas wisdom tends to stick around" (Baird, 2000). *Clinical wisdom*, as Benner, Hooper Kyriakidis, and Stannard have shown, emerges when nurses become passionate knowers and transform understanding and knowledge into clinical wisdom. It is expressed in maxims and principles derived from understanding and intimate knowledge of clinical practice. It is at the heart of nurses' ethical and moral comportment that ultimately defines nursing excellence. Throughout the book, we are privileged to have access to nurses' clinical wisdom and how it is acquired. In the process, we come to appreciate the wisdom of these authors.

As with the first edition, Benner and her colleagues continue to make the invisible visible and the inaccessible accessible. They articulate and label the processes underlying clinical judgment and clinical decision making. With exquisite, in-depth precision, they describe the habits of thought and action in the nine domains of nursing practice. They include what happens during moment-to-moment clinical assessments and judgments and everyday skillful ways of practicing. They shed light on what goes on in nurses' heads. They help us enter the nurses' world of interpretive decision making: the importance of perceptual acuity and attunement, selecting what is salient, being open, and moving from universal knowledge of evidence-based research to how general population knowledge applies to a specific patient. The authors uncover and discover the thinking of reflecting-in-action and reflecting-on-action. They teach us the importance of sustained curiosity for the detective work of nursing—to understand and solve puzzles. This book illustrates how nurses learn patterns of patient responses by comparing incidences between and within situations, and thus, developing knowledge that can be generalized. They have succeeded in helping us, their readers, understand the intricacies and complexities of thinking-in-action through the narrative by getting nurses to tell stories.

Nurses' rich and detailed narratives, which form the core of each chapter, give this book its texture and depth, and place it in a class of its own. Each story is compelling, more so than any television script with its main plot and subplots and array of characters. Here, nurses are given voice. They speak of the scope of their practice and the nature of their work. We experience nursing as frontline health care workers do—the challenges they grapple with, the dilemmas and the ambiguities they face, their angst, disappointments, failures, and triumphs. We enter the practice world of nursing and learn from what nurses have learned.

The stories and how the authors present them illustrate graphically the central role that nurses play in safeguarding patients from harm, making sure that patients' wants and needs are heard, preserving patients' dignity, serving as patient and family advocates, and rescuing patients from near misses caused by inexperienced doctors, other nurses, and so forth. The stories also capture the power that nurses have in the health care system because they are with patients 24/7. They explain why nurses are the glue that makes and keeps the health care system working. They illustrate the depth and breadth of knowledge that skilled nurses need to do their job and why nursing requires individuals who are smart, strong, savvy, and sophisticated to deal with crises, dramas, plots, and subplots that require their constant attention. These stories remain, revealing and teaching us long after the page is turned and the chapter completed. They also serve double duty. As they inform about nursing, illustrating clinical wisdom and thinking-in-action, they are excellent teaching tools for learning to nurse.

Each story has been selected for a purpose and followed by a commentary. Benner, Hooper Kyriakidis, and Stannard are superb teachers. They draw our attention to what is salient and compelling about a story. They use the story to help link formal knowledge to practical knowledge, thereby integrating theory and practice. The authors uncover clinical wisdom and in clear, unambiguous language make theoretical concepts come alive in the practice world. They then offer new insights by interpreting the stories through different lenses, drawing on knowledge from diverse disciplines—such as philosophy, sociology, psychology—to add depth and understanding to nurses' work. They then suggest ways of being and doing, as well as identify maxims and principles to serve as a framework for moral and ethical caring. Although all chapters follow this structure, Chapter 8, "Preventing Hazards in a Technological Environment" and Chapter 9, "Facing Death: End-of-Life Care and Decision Making" are excellent illustrations of this approach.

This edition goes beyond the first edition, incorporating pedagogical approaches to assist inexperienced nurses develop expertise in practice through situated and experiential learning. It integrates the insights from Benner, Stuphen, Leonard, and Day's (2010) work on educating nurses for the future and takes their insights from classroom to the clinical setting, focusing on nurses' needs for lifelong learning, with pedagogical strategies woven into each chapter. The importance of educating is underscored with the addition of "Chapter 13, Educational Strategies and Implications." In a significant way, this book ties the threads of Benner's career quest for understanding, uncovering, and describing what constitutes expert, ethical, and caring practice—what it is, how it happens, what experiences help to develop it. This journey began 36 years ago in Benner's groundbreaking work that documented the stages of clinical competence and skill acquisition in her classic book, *From Novice to Expert* (Benner, 1984), and expanded on in *Expertise in Nursing Practice* (Benner, Tanner & Chesla, 1996, 2009). This current book, the second edition, represents an integration of more than 40 years of experience and insights that Benner has gained with different collaborators.

This book is one from which all nurses can learn—students and new nurses who are first learning to nurse, nurses who want to become advanced practitioners, and seasoned clinicians. All nurses need to develop a sense of salience—recognize what is most urgent or significant as they identify and then define the problems. The process is complex as it involves perception and engagement skills. Every situation is charged with emotion that, in turn, affects perceptions, thoughts, and subsequently judgments. However, it is the recognition and the development of salience that is the heart of clinical grasp (understanding). It is the bedrock of sound clinical decision making.

Benner and her colleagues make a compelling case for using the narrative as an educational strategy and teaching tool. They believe that clinical learning is experienced as a story. It is by nurses' own stories and listening to (in this case, reading) the narratives of other nurses that inexperienced, as well as experienced, nurses can develop their expertise. It is in the telling of and reflecting on stories of practice that nurses learn about clinical issues, issues that can be generalized from a particular patient and situation to a different population and another setting. Stories help nurses learn how to identify and articulate best nursing practices, practice situation-responsive nursing, uncover moral struggles, and come to appreciate how vision and imaginings help them to see possibilities and recognize opportunities. They argue against the use of classificatory systems, prescriptive lists, evidence-based protocols and the like, as these approaches are not designed to capture the patient's and family's experiences. The current use of such systems is a "one-size-fits-all" approach, when, in effect, professional nursing requires—no it demands—a situation-responsive approach that respects the uniqueness of each patient and family, their situation, history, experience, and circumstance.

With the first edition of *Clinical Wisdom and Interventions in Critical Care*, Benner, Hooper Kyriakidis, and Stannard left their footprint. With this second edition, they have left an even deeper footprint. They have given us the knowledge, language, methods, and tools for developing expertise in clinical practice. Now, we need to heed their wisdom and follow their footsteps to help nurses fulfill their social contract of caring for patients and families with knowledge and compassion.

Laurie N. Gottlieb, RN, PhD
Professor
Flora Madeline Shaw Chair of Nursing
Editor, CJNR
Nurse–scholar in residence, Jewish General Hospital
McGill University, School of Nursing
Montreal, Canada

REFERENCES

Baird, D. (2000). *A thousand paths to wisdom*. London: MQ Publications.

Belenky, M. F., Clinchy, B. M., Goldberger, N. R., & Tarule, J. M. (1986). *Women's ways of knowing: The development of self, voice, and mind*. New York, NY: Basic Books.

Benner, P. (1984). *From novice to expert: Excellence and power in clinical nursing practice*. Menlo Park, CA: Addison-Wesley.

Benner, P., Stuphen, M., Leonard, V., & Day, L. (2010). *Educating nurses: A call for radical transformation*. San Francisco, CA: Jossey-Bass.

Benner, P., Tanner, C. A., & Chesla, C. A. (1996). *Expertise in nursing practice: Caring, clinical judgment, and ethics*. New York, NY: Springer Publishing Company.

Benner, P., Tanner, C. A., & Chesla, C. A. (2009). *Expertise in nursing practice: Caring, clinical judgment, and ethics* (2nd ed.). New York, NY: Springer Publishing Company.

Preface

This book presents a way of thinking about clinical inquiry, reasoning, judgment, and experiential learning in clinical practice. It is about human expertise and wisdom in the practice of nursing. This work gives language to clinical and moral imagination and multiple domains of excellent practice. We hope that nurses will read the articulation of key domains of acute and critical care and will have the spontaneous response: "You have put into words what I have always known in my practice but had not expressed." Experiential learning in practice is a way of knowing and developing clinical knowledge in its own right and clinicians always know more in their practice than they can put into words (Polanyi, 1958/1962). Nurses develop a tacit, yet demonstrable knowledge learned in their practice over time that may not yet be articulated well in theory and that might not yet be fully explained in science (Gallagher, 2009; Hooper, 1995; Polanyi, 1958/1962; Sunvisson, Haberman, Weiss, & Benner, 2009). Part of the reason for this "hidden knowledge" or undisclosed knowledge in practice is the culmination of many comparisons of whole clinical situations where clinicians add to their perceptual acuity, their clinical practical wisdom, skillful clinical reasoning through patient changes, tacit knowledge, and their abilities to make qualitative distinctions in particular clinical situations. This allows for nurses (and other expert clinicians) to recognize early warnings to changes in patients' condition (Benner, 2000) and think-in-action in clinical practice. In sum, we hope that readers will experience a sense of self-discovery about clinical wisdom in nursing. Although this study is about critical care and acute care nursing practice, it is centrally about nursing knowledge and practice. In that regard, nurses, along with the clinicians they practice with, will find points of mutual entry and meaning, including the interprofessional and intraprofessional contrasts discussed.

This work presents the aspects of clinical understanding and reasoning not captured in static formal models that have been traditionally used to teach decision making. It is based on the premise drawn in Benner, Tanner, and Chesla (2009) that there is an eclipse of clinical judgment and reasoning in formal decision-making models based on probability assessments at particular points in time. It was argued in *Expertise in Nursing Practice* (Benner et al., 2009) that clinical reasoning involves reasoning about a particular patient across time and that the gains and losses in understanding of the patient's changing condition creates the clinician's understanding of the situation. In moving from Point A to Point B, expert clinicians take into account the gains and losses in understandings and meanings inherent in the sequencing of patient changes. Much of clinical judgment and understanding of the patient's condition is based on understanding actual trends and trajectories in the patient's condition. Such thinking-in-action and reasoning-in-transition about particular patients requires an agent-centered understanding of ethical and clinical reasoning.

Clinical reasoning is a form of practical reasoning. The nurse is situated in particular clinical situations, makes sense of them (Gallagher, 2009; Lave & Wenger, 1991; Weick, 2009) and acts. In the Carnegie National Study of Nursing Education (Benner et al., 2010), it was found that nursing faculty and nursing students alike conflated clinical reasoning and critical thinking. Critical reflective thinking is *necessary* for all kinds of professional clinicians; however, it is not sufficient for clinicians because critical thinking cannot replace situated clinical reasoning across time about particular patients. For example, in a situation of resuscitating patients, the advanced cardiac life support (ACLS) algorithms and standard practices are adjusted, when needed, according to the patient's particular clinical situation and responses. There is no time to reexamine the ACLS algorithms from the ground up at the point of resuscitation except in relation to a particular patient's sensitivities or intolerance to particular medications (known in advance or discovered during the crisis). In a crisis, one thinks in action and engages in the best clinical problem solving about the particular patient in the moment. One does not typically have time to stand back and think critically and reflectively about the event until the crisis is over. Clinical reasoning *uses* science and theory about well-established standards of good practice. Critical thinking is required for practice breakdown situations, and where the received standards of practice need to be questioned and reexamined based on new knowledge and science. For example, taking care of new patient populations with new clinical characteristics, such as returning wounded warriors, requires both critical thinking and creative clinical imagination. Nurses practice more effectively when they use multiple forms of reasoning as the situation calls for different approaches and frames of reference (Benner et al., 2010).

Wise ethical and clinical judgments require the ongoing thinking-in-action and patient and family relationships with nurses and physicians. The matching of patient findings against a predefined template or the application of artificial intelligence can provide decision support, but can never replace the engaged clinical and ethical reasoning of the clinician whose judgment is shaped by the context of the situation.

Few workers in artificial intelligence would disagree with this statement, yet much of our educational materials are developed as if the clinician makes clinical and ethical judgments in the same way that would be derived from decision analysis techniques (Dreyfus, 1992). We view this work as a necessary complementary approach to teaching clinical judgment and critical thinking because it depicts the logic of practice (Bourdieu, 1990) that expert clinicians use (Benner et al., 2009). Additionally, it demonstrates how clinical practice and clinical judgment in nursing and medicine will always require clinician- and patient/family-centered reasoning about the particular across time more than abstract decision-making models, no matter how useful these models may be. For example, when using aggregated scientific evidence about best practices (i.e., evidence-based practice), the clinician is still required to judiciously decide on interventions with the particularity of the patient in mind and judiciously and critically evaluate scientific evidence.

Since the work from *Novice to Expert* (Benner, 1984), the author has been engaged in dialogue with nurse educators about the implications of the Dreyfus model of skill acquisition for clinical teaching and learning (Dreyfus & Dreyfus, 1986). *Expertise in Nursing Practice* (Benner et al., 2009) pointed to many of the educational implications presented in this work. However, in this book, we seek to illustrate the educational implications by providing a thick description of nurses' thinking-in-action and reasoning-in-transition. The book provides a window to central areas of experiential learning required for the development of expertise in nursing practice. Throughout the book, numerous and varied suggestions and examples are provided to assist in the development of nurses toward expertise. Because there is a considerable gap between the patient care demand for expert reasoning and judgment and the availability of expert nurses to provide that level of care

(Burritt & Steckel, 2009), we have highlighted various practical ways of situated teaching and coaching at the bedside where experiential learning is optimal.

Clinicians manage the limits of short-term memory and the enormous array of information available at any point in time by focusing on the most relevant findings, changes, or issues at hand (a sense of salience gained directly from clinical experience). The expert's judgment is always situated. Consequently, *identifying* the most relevant problem(s) is crucial for good priority setting and good clinical judgment. In teaching the nursing process (an adapted version of the scientific problem-solving process), the focus is on the problem-solving process, rather than first defining the problem. Little attention is given to identifying the most salient or relevant problem(s) or concerns. However, it is from situating one's thinking-in-action and problem solving on the most salient issue(s) at hand that the expert nurse develops a strategy for information management and action. We believe that providing a description of clinical judgment and thinking-in-action in this situated way, more closely simulates how clinicians think and act in practice. As such, we describe two pervasive habits of thought and action in Chapters 2 and 3, clinical grasp and clinical forethought, and then nine domains of practice, our "strong clinical situations," in Chapters 4 through 12. These descriptions will assist learners and teachers and can also help leaders better create environments that support the demands of good practice. The "strong clinical situations" or domains of clinical nursing practice include the "telos" or aims of practice; that is, the "in order to do *X* and accomplish *Y* for the sake of scientific evidence of best practice and/or for the sake of patient/family concerns and preferences for treatment." Practice is always situated in actual particular situations that can be captured only dimly and relatively in context-free abstractions and formal theory.

The specific medications used in clinical situations presented here must not be considered "the best" or "lasting approaches." We *do not* intend the reader to slavishly follow concrete actions and therapies used in particular clinical situations because practice standards, new medications, and clinical evidence about interventions are constantly changing. What *can* be taken from the situated examples are clear: the nurse's grasp of the situation, his or her clinical forethought, critical and creative thinking, skilled know-how, and concerns and aims of the patient/family and health care team. The examples should be read imaginatively, with the readers rehearsing what they might do in similar situations. None of the situations are "ideal." They are based on the situated possibilities of nurses working with real colleagues, patients, and families. Certainly, this kind of treatment is most useful for the student nurse and clinician who want to enrich the clinical imagination they possess.

We found that the original inductively generated articulation of domains of practice held as we reviewed 271 new exemplars from across specialties. We chose new exemplars as necessary: when updating a previously used exemplar or when the new exemplar added new insights. Some practices current 11 years ago when *Clinical Wisdom* was first published have since become obsolete or dramatically altered. We sought to replace all such exemplars. However, if the point of the exemplar was primarily about the nurse's creativity and response to a difficult situation and one that offered rich insights, we kept that exemplar while updating particulars. Because practice changes rapidly, there is no way to keep an account of any practice up to the minute. As Weick (2009) points out, the organization is "impermanent." We did highlight stories that were timeless, in terms of the challenges they presented to the nurse, and that demonstrated expert nursing practice at the time. Thirty years from now, this work may well be used as a "historical account" of clinical nursing practice circa 2010.

WHO MIGHT BE INTERESTED IN THIS WORK

First, practicing critical and acute care nurses and nursing students (undergraduate and graduate) who are preparing to work with acutely or chronically critically ill patients and families are the readers for whom this work was designed. This work organizes the major domains of nursing practice for acute and critically ill patients. The domains include the purposes and ends of nursing practice as well as instantiating excellent communication, caring practices, and relational skills. The examples provide a guide for experiential learning and presents many firsthand reports, which will aid students' own experiential learning. The book helps faculty bridge the practice–education gap and the separation of classroom teaching and the clinical. The book is also designed for nurse educators who are teaching acute and critical care nursing practice, clinical reasoning and critical thinking, and clinical judgment in nursing practice. Preceptors, nurse educators in hospitals, and advanced practice nurses will find many practical approaches for helping beginning clinicians, as well as strategies for helping competent clinicians to move to proficient and expert stages of practice.

This book is also designed for advanced practice nurses, nursing managers and administrators, clinical leaders, and those interested in developing or revising organizational systems or information infrastructures for nursing practice. Chapter 11 describes the frontline system design and repair done daily by expert nurses, and Chapter 12 presents a view of leadership based on directing and shaping excellent clinical practice. This chapter captures the ways that those who design, develop, and repair care delivery systems must understand, the links between excellent nursing practice, and good outcomes, and this frontline description provides the first step in that process. Means and patient outcomes are linked in the narratives to better understand how good patient outcomes are created. Chapter 13 presents pedagogical implications and uses of this work, both in schools of nursing and in practice settings.

We believe that this book can also be useful to physicians entering practice, because it gives realistic descriptions of the practical realities in acute and critical care practice. We also believe that less experienced physicians may find descriptions of the habits and domains helpful, because of the similarities in skilled know-how that every clinician must develop to become expert. It can provide many practical directions about cross-disciplinary and cross-experiential level communication. We challenge the physician reader to notice the many positive examples of physician practice and teaching among the instances, where nurses describe making a case to physicians or describe nurse–physician conflict and collaboration. The difficult communications, as well as the successful ones, are described in the hope of improving communication and collaboration between nurses and physicians.

Finally, we believe that contemporary debates and discussions of biomedical ethics would be furthered by including the practice-based approach to teaching ethical and clinical reasoning presented in this book. This work richly demonstrates how ethical and clinical reasoning are linked and articulates notions of good embedded in the clinical practice of nursing and medicine. In this way, this book offers a needed voice for ethics directed by the quest for good practice—everyday ethical comportment rather than a focus on dilemma or practice breakdown ethics. The work offers insights about the role of emotion in moral perception, discernment, action, and relationship. The exemplars demonstrate the ethics of vulnerability, care, and responsibility (Martinsen, 2006) as well as the multifaceted ethics of patient/family advocacy. The work is in the Aristotelian tradition, but takes up relational ethics in the tradition of Kierkegaard (Dreyfus, Dreyfus, &

Benner, 1996; Rubin, 2009) and Løgstrup (1997). Following the work of Taylor (Benner et al., 1996; Rubin, 2009; Taylor, 1985a, 1985b, 1989, 1993), the book illustrates how the method of making qualitative distinctions and reasoning-in-transition are central to ethical and clinical reasoning. We hope that this work will improve the development of expert practice in students and practicing clinicians, enrich the educational strategies that educators embrace to integrate knowledge acquisition and situated *use* (Eraut, 1994) into practice, and strengthen situated coaching and learning in authentic contexts. This work delineates clearer ways that administrators need to support development of expert clinical knowledge in practice settings and ways that administrators and clinicians need to seek out the clinical wisdom of strong clinical leaders to better inform decisions that affect clinical practice.

REFERENCES

Benner, P. (1984). *From novice to expert: Excellence and power in clinical nursing practice.* Menlo Park, CA: Addison-Wesley.

Benner, P. (2000). *From novice to expert: Excellence and power in clinical nursing practice, Commemorative Edition.* Menlo Park, CA: Addison-Wesley.

Benner, P., Sutphen, M., Leonard, V., & Day, L. (2010). *Educating nurses: A call for radical transformation.* San Francisco, CA: Jossey-Bass.

Benner, P., Tanner, C. A., & Chesla, C. A. (1996). *Expertise in nursing practice: Caring, clinical judgment, and ethics.* New York, NY: Springer Publishing Company.

Benner, P., Tanner, C. A., & Chesla, C. A. (2009). *Expertise in nursing practice: Caring, clinical judgment, and ethics* (2nd edition). New York, NY: Springer Publishing Company.

Bourdieu, P. (1990). *The logic of practice.* Stanford, CA: Stanford University Press.

Burritt, J., & Steckel, C. (2009). Supporting the learning curve for contemporary nursing practice. *Journal of Nursing Administration, 39*(11), 479–484.

Chan, G., Brykczynski, K., Malone, R. E., & Benner, P. (2010). *Interpretive phenomenology in health care research: Studying social practice, lifeworlds, and embodiment.* Indianapolis, IN: Sigma Theta Tau International.

Dreyfus, H. L. (1992). *What computers still can't do: A critique of artificial reason.* Cambridge, MA: MIT.

Dreyfus, H. L., & Dreyfus, S. E. (1986). *Mind over machine: The power of human intuition and expertise in the era of the computer.* New York, NY: Free Press.

Dreyfus, H. L., Dreyfus, S. E., & Benner, P. (1996). Implications of the phenomenology of expertise for teaching and learning everyday skillful ethical comportment. In P. Benner, C. Tanner, & C. Chesla (Eds.), *Expertise in nursing practice: Caring, clinical judgment, and ethics* (pp. 258–279). New York, NY: Springer Publishing Company.

Eraut, M. (1994). *Developing professional knowledge and competence.* Philadelphia, PA: Falmer Press, Taylor and Francis, Inc.

Gallagher, S. (2009). Philosophical antecedents of situated cognition. In P. Robbins & M. Aydede (Eds.), *The Cambridge handbook of situated cognition* (pp. 35–52). Cambridge, MA: Cambridge University Press.

Hooper, P. L. (1995). *Expert titration of multiple vasoactive drugs in post-cardiac surgical patients: An interpretive study of clinical judgment and perceptual acuity.* Doctoral dissertation, University of California at San Francisco, San Francisco School of Nursing.

Lave, J. & Wenger, E. (1991). *Situated learning: Legitimate peripheral participation.* New York, NY: Cambridge University Press.

Løgstrup, K. E. (1997). *The ethical demand.* Notre Dame, IN: University of Notre Dame Press.

Martinsen, K. (2006). Nurse–philosopher makes a serious case for COMPASSION as a primary value. Retrieved June 5, 2010, from http://www.publicchristian.com/?p=423

Polanyi, M. (1958/1962). *Personal knowledge: Towards a post-critical philosophy*. London, England: Routledge.

Rubin, J. (2009). Impediments to the development of clinical knowledge and ethical judgment in critical care nursing. In P. Benner, C. A. Tanner, & C. A. Chesla (Eds.), *Expertise in nursing practice: Caring, clinical judgment, and ethics* (pp. 171–198). New York, NY: Springer Publishing Company.

Sunvisson, H., Haberman, B., Weiss, S., & Benner, P. (2009). Augmenting the Cartesian medical discourse with an understanding of the person's lifeworld, lived body, life story, and social identity. *Nursing Philosophy, 10*, 241–252.

Taylor, C. (1985a). *Human agency and language: Philosophical papers 1*. (Vol. 1). Cambridge, MA: Cambridge University Press.

Taylor, C. (1985b). *Philosophy and the human sciences: Philosophical papers II*. (Vol. 2). Cambridge, MA: Cambridge University Press.

Taylor, C. (1989). *Sources of the self: The making of the modern identity*. Cambridge, MA: Harvard University Press.

Taylor, C. (1993). *The quality of life*. Oxford, UK: Clarendon.

Weick, K. (2009). *Making sense of the organization: Volume 2: The impermanent organization*. West Sussex, UK: John Wiley & Sons.

Acknowledgments

First, we want to acknowledge the 205 staff and advanced practice nurses who participated in this work and the many nurse managers, charge nurses, and administrators who facilitated data collection by arranging for rooms and by allowing the extensive participant observation involved in the original research project that generated the first edition of *Clinical Wisdom*, and the work of Patricia Hooper Kyriakidis who collected more than 271 new exemplars that we drew on for the second edition. We sincerely thank the many nurse contributors for sharing their stories. When we included contributed stories, outside of the original research, we chose to use the nurses' names, and took extra precautions to ensure the confidentiality of patient information by not revealing the work setting. We changed many of the identifying details of the story. The nurse contributors, each of whom is expert in his or her specialty, include: Elizabeth Allee, Laura Alter, Beth Baldwin, Mary Anne Bennett, Anne Benson, Katherine Cameron, Julia Chappo, Jackie Cunningham, Corinne Cyr Pryor, Girish Dang, Tracy Hegg Davis, Michael DeMello, Emily Dever, Andrea Edmands, Patricia Ferencz, Laurie Foran, Suzan Foy, Tammy Freehling, Susan Gagne-Rego, Kathy Giannelli, Jennifer Harley, Barbara Hidde, Sandra Kennedy, Sally Kerchner, Luigina Maniscalco, Lisa Mayer, Nancy McClorey, Rosemary Melton, Mary Nottingham, Lucille Raia, Clara Reagan, Paula Reiss, Debra Richards, Cynthia Rogers, Judy Rumensky, Lisa Salines, Carol Samuels, Amanda Savage, Brenda Silvia, Stacey Steuerwald, Priscilla Stoddard, Janice Vincent, and Robin Watson. We appreciate Martina Skibola, a senior student nurse, who contributed a paradigm case. We would also like to thank the American Association of Critical-Care Nurses who supported this work and enabled us to interview advanced practice nurses at one of the National Teaching Institutes. We also want to gratefully acknowledge the Helene Fuld Health Trust for their continuing support and generous contribution. Additionally, the influence and contributions of the Phase One Team (*Expertise in Nursing Practice*), particularly Christine Tanner and Catherine Chesla, are greatly appreciated. This work would not have been possible without them.

Many doctoral and master's students at the University of California, San Francisco also contributed to this work. Jan Boller, Lisa Day, Maria Gudmundsdottir, Colleen O'Leary Kelly, Lori Madden, and Kay Ramsdell assisted with data collection and coding. Additionally, Dr. Sara Weiss assisted with interviews and participant observations, Dr. Weiss and Dr. Joe Merighi helped coach and mentor doctoral students during the data collection process and assisted with the coding of the data. We also had able staff assistance from Dr. Weiss and Dr. Merighi, as well as Andrew Brosnan, Loretta Brady-Visser, Pam Ellingson, Margarita Klein, and Lori Madden.

Numerous nurses (staff nurses, advanced practice nurses, managers, educators, researchers, and students), physicians, and others helped us to further refine our thoughts by carefully reviewing chapters. We would especially like to thank the following individuals for their careful review and thoughtful comments: Pat and Tom Ahrens, Mary Jane Barnes, Richard Benner, Jan Boller, David Boyd, Catherine Chesla, Marianne Chulay,

Deborah Cline, Maria Connolly, Dorothy Corona, Lisa Day, Yoshimi Fukuoka, Chris Kinavey, Erick Kyriakidis, Claudia Ladwig, Lori Madden, Ruth Malone, Joe Merighi, Kathleen McCauley, Beau Simon, Carey Simon, Sara Weiss, and Fay Wright. We would also like to gratefully acknowledge the enormous amount of time and effort Joan Vitello-Cicciu put into reviewing the entire book. In this second edition, we greatly appreciate the expert clinical wisdom and consultation of nurses and physicians who reviewed and assisted us in updating clinical interventions: Corinne Cyr Pryor, Tracy Hegg Davis, Joan Dorr, Andrea Edmands, Brooke Hooper, Michael Hooper, Erick Kyriakidis, Sharon Levine, Lisa McKibban, and Amanda Savage.

The core research team, Patricia Benner, Patricia Hooper Kyriakidis, and Daphne Stannard, each has primary responsibility for the first and final drafts of certain chapters. Therefore, questions should be directed to Patricia Benner for Chapters 1, 3, 6, 9, 10, and 11; Patricia Hooper Kyriakidis for Chapters 2, 4, 5, 12, and 13; and Daphne Stannard for Chapters 7 and 8 and Appendix A. Patricia Benner and Patricia Hooper Kyriakidis edited and approved the final drafts of all the chapters and appendices of this second edition of the work.

Our families were steadfast in their support. Special thanks to Richard, John, and Lindsay Benner; to Erick, Annie, and Seth Kyriakidis; and to Beau and Dylan Simon for their love, encouragement, and unwavering patience. Last but not the least, we appreciate the skill, diligence, and keen eye of Brandee Woleslagle Blank for the final formatting, corrections, and copyediting of this work.

Abbreviations

ABBREVIATIONS OF CLINICAL UNITS

CCU	coronary care unit
CVICU	cardiovascular intensive care unit
ED	emergency department
eICU	electronic intensive care unit
ICN	intensive care nursery
ICU	intensive care unit
L&D	labor and delivery
Medsurg	medical surgical
MICU	medical intensive care unit
OR	operating room
PACU	postanesthesia care unit
Peds	pediatrics
PICU	pediatric intensive care unit
Rehab	rehabilitation
SCN	special care nursery
SICU	surgical intensive care unit

COMMON MEDICAL ABBREVIATIONS USED IN CRITICAL CARE

A-fib	atrial fibrillation
A-line or **Art Line**	arterial line
ABC	airway, breathing, circulation
ABG	arterial blood gas
ACLS or **ALS**	advanced cardiac life support
APN	advanced practice nurse
ARDS	adult respiratory distress syndrome
Bicarb	sodium bicarbonate
Biox	pulse oximeter
BLS	basic life support
BP	blood pressure
BPD	bronchopulmonary dysplasia
Bronch	bronchoscopy
CA	cancer
CABG	coronary artery bypass graft (surgery)
CBC	complete blood count
CHF	congestive heart failure
CNS	clinical nurse specialist

CO_2	carbon dioxide
COAG	coagulation times
COPD	chronic obstructive pulmonary disease
CPAP	continuous positive airway pressure
CPR	cardiopulmonary resuscitation
Cric	cricothyrotomy
CRNA	certified registered nurse anesthetist
CSF	cerebrospinal fluid
C-section	Caesarian section (C/S is also used)
CVP	central venous pressure
CVVH	continuous veno-venous hemofiltration
CXR	chest x-ray
Defib	defibrillation
DEX	glucometer DEX
DIC	disseminated intravascular coagulopathy
DNAR	do not attempt to resuscitate
DNR	do not resuscitate
Dopa	dopamine
DT	delirium tremors
Echo	echocardiogram
ECMO	extracorporeal membrane oxygenation
EKG	electrocardiogram
EMT	emergency medical technician
Epi	epinephrine
ET tube	endotracheal tube (ETT is also used)
$ETCO_2$	end tidal CO_2
FFP	fresh frozen plasma
FiO_2	fraction of inspired O_2
Gases	refers to arterial blood gases
GI	gastrointestinal
HIPAA	Health Insurance Portability and Accountability Act
HR	heart rate
IABP	intra-aortic balloon pump
ICP	intracranial pressure
I:E ratio	inspiratory-to-expiratory ratio
IMV	intermittent mandatory ventilation
INT	interviewer
INT notes	interviewer notes
I&O	intake/output
iSTAT	bloodwork
IV	intravenous
K^+	potassium
KCl	potassium chloride
KUB	kidney-ureter-bladder
Levo	levophed
Lytes	electrolytes
MAP	mean arterial pressure

Meds	medications
Mets	metastasis
MI	myocardial infarction
Mics per kilo	micrograms per kilogram
MSOF	multisystem organ failure
MUGA	multigated acquisition
Neo	neosynephrine
Neuro	neurologic
NG tube	nasogastric tube
Nitro	nitroglycerin
NP	nurse practitioner
NPO	nothing by mouth
NS	normal saline
O_2	oxygen
PA line	pulmonary artery line
$PaCO_2$	partial pressure of CO_2 in arterial blood
PaO_2	partial pressure of O_2 in arterial blood
PCWP	pulmonary capillary wedge pressure
PEEP	positive end expiratory pressure
PIP	peak inspiratory pressure
Pneumo	pneumothorax
PRBC	packed red blood cells
PRN	as needed
PT	prothrombin time
PTT	partial thromboplastin time
Pulse Ox	pulse oximeter
PVC	premature ventricular contraction
RDS	respiratory distress syndrome
Resus	resuscitation
RT	respiratory therapist
SaO_2	saturation of arterial O_2
Sat or **sats**	oxygen saturation
SvO_2	mixed venous oxygen saturation
SVR	systemic vascular resistance
TBI	traumatic brain injury
TPA	tissue plasminogen activator
TPN	total parenteral nutrition
Trach	tracheostomy
VAD	ventricular assist device
Vent	ventilator or ventilated
V-fib	ventricular fibrillation
VSD	ventricular septal defect
V-tach	ventricular tachycardia (**VT** is also used)

1

Thinking-in-Action and Reasoning-in-Transition: An Overview

*C*ritical and acute care nursing practice is intellectually and emotionally challenging, requiring quick judgments and responses to life-threatening conditions where little margin for error exists. Developing expertise in acute and critical care practice requires experiential learning under pressure and "thinking-in-action" (thinking linked with action in ongoing situations). In the past it was easier to separate acute, non-urgent care and critical care. However, the boundaries between acute and critical care have shrunk as hospital days have shrunk, and hospitals now offer multiple layers of critical care, from stable critical to intensively critical. There are few descriptions of expert critical and acute care nursing practice (Benner, Tanner & Chesla, 2009). The discovery and development of instantaneous therapies (eg., hemodynamic monitoring and management) and patient–response based therapies occurred in critical care areas, but the astute levels of clinical judgment required for these "titration" modes of therapy are found throughout the hospital. With the exception of Hooper Kyriakidis' work (1995), we have few descriptions of the clinical judgment and craft required for instantaneous patient-response based therapies such as the titration of multiple vasoactive medications, ongoing monitoring and evaluation of anti-arrhythmic drugs, and signs and symptoms of toxicity, drug reactions and adverse interactions). We have protocols, procedural accounts, and descriptive—though sparse—accounts of the skillful use of the technology and science of critical care nursing practice, but the nature of excellent acute and critical care nursing practice continues to change rapidly (Day, 2009).

The first edition of this work focused on critical care in transport, in-hospital, emergency department and peri-anesthesia nursing. But shorter hospital stays and increasing complexity in acute as well as critical care, trauma, transport and peri-anesthesia have blurred many of the boundaries of where critical care patients are cared for, so this second edition focuses on all critical and acute care provided in acute care hospitals. It is still true to say that we know more in practice than we can account for in our theories (Polanyi, 1958/1962). The articulation of judgment and craft is difficult because critical care occurs in multiple settings and is complex indeed: interventions are instantaneous, highly context-dependent, and interpretable primarily in terms of the immediate clinical history (trajectories and trends) of events, interventions, patient responses, and problems.

To better understand clinical judgment, interventions, and the link between the two, we have conducted a naturalistic, descriptive ethnography of critical and acute care nursing practice with a range of beginning to expert nurses, including advanced practice nurses. We have focused on the intents and the content of clinical situations articulated in this work. In this respect, this document may be considered a descriptive account of some of the major critical issues and clinical distinctions that confront critical and acute care nurses in caring for patients and their families. By describing thinking-in-action, we hope to guide clinical learning and make clinical judgment and clinical knowledge development more visible. Any complex practice depends on both extensive *acquisition* of knowledge, and the *situated use* of knowledge in practice (Eraut, 1994; Benner, Sutphen, Leonard & Day, 2009). Thus, we also aim to illustrate what state-of-the-art integrative teaching must include in preparing student nurses and those staff nurses developing in practice to perform well in acute, trauma and critical care settings based upon the ability to use knowledge in particular clinical situations. Nurses, as knowledge workers, can no longer afford to separate the nursing, natural and social sciences and humanities from the use of knowledge in specific clinical situations. It is no longer pedagogically sound for nurse educators to focus on elements, abstract concepts without pointing to the ways that knowledge must be integrated and used in practice. Nursing students and beginner nurses need to learn simpler aspects of situations before moving on to understand the whole complex, unfolding clinical situation. Recognizing the nature of the clinical situation is at the heart of good clinical reasoning and interventions. We present clinical reasoning as a form of practical reasoning, i.e. situated historical reasoning through transitions in the patient's condition, and/or the clinician's understanding (Taylor, 1993; Benner, 1994).

In Table 1.1, we have identified two habits of thought and action and nine domains of nursing practice that uncover aspects of clinical judgment, clinical knowledge development, and the everyday skillful comportment of acute and critical care nurses. The habits of thought and action refer to styles of practice, thought, and action that constitute typical approaches, while the domains of practice can be thought of as strong situations in that they are organized by common clinical goals and concerns.

TABLE 1.1

Habits of Thought and Action and Domains of Practice in Acute and Critical Care Nursing Practice

Habits of Thought and Action

▨ Clinical grasp and clinical inquiry: Problem identification and clinical problem solving

▨ Clinical forethought: Anticipating and preventing potential problems

Domains of Practice

▨ Diagnosing and managing life-sustaining physiologic functions in acutely ill and unstable patients

▨ The skilled know-how of managing a crisis

▨ Providing comfort measures for the critically and acutely ill

▨ Caring for patients' families

▨ Preventing hazards in a technological environment

▨ Facing death: End-of-life care and decision making

▨ Making a case: Communicating clinical assessments and improving teamwork

▨ Patient safety: Monitoring quality, preventing and managing breakdown

▨ The skilled know-how of clinical and moral leadership and the coaching and mentoring of others

In the next two chapters, we present two pervasive habits of thought and action: clinical grasp and clinical forethought. In Chapter 2, engaged thinking-in-action and reasoning-in-transitions are emphasized as the orienting modes of thinking when identifying relevant clinical problems. In Chapter 3, clinical forethought is presented as a habit of thought that structures engaged thinking and action. The domains of practice overlap and occur simultaneously, but each domain can become central in directing the nurse's attention and work, sometimes capturing high priority while other times necessarily receding into the background. Taken together, these domains demonstrate how being situated in a particular clinical situation guides clinical judgment, thinking, and action. As Bourdieu (1990) points out, recognition of the nature of the situation is central to the logic of practice. In all the domains of practice, reasoning-in-transition and engaged thinking-in-action are the hallmarks of clinical judgment in practice. A loss of understanding or sense of disquietude, puzzlement, or even confusion prompts problem search and reasoning-in-transition, characteristic of ethical and clinical reasoning in actual practice. The anticipation of likely events structures the nurse's preparedness and shapes thinking-in-action.

In this book, we describe the nature of engaged ethical and clinical reasoning. Engaged reasoning requires skillful involvement by the clinician in the situation. In order to grasp the nature of particular clinical situations, inexperienced nurses experientially learn to pay attention to what is most and least salient in open-ended clinical situations. One of the signature pedagogies of nursing education is to coach students and developing nurses to recognize what is most important and least important in actual situation (Benner, Sutphen, Leonard, & Day, 2010). By using narrative accounts, interview excerpts of actual clinical situations and observational accounts of nurses in practice, we focus on what is most salient in the situation and on the thinking-in-action required by rapidly changing clinical situations. By thinking-in-action, we mean the patterns and habits of thought and actions directly tied to responding to patients and families and to the nature of the situation, such as staff availability, other urgent demands on nurses and other members of the health care team. We are interested in the <u>craft</u> of the expert clinician, and craft is best taught when one is actually engaged in the demands of an ongoing situation. This is what Lave and Wenger (1991) mean by situated learning. We have used all levels of practice to articulate the everyday knowledge work of critical care nurses because sometimes the issues of expert practice show up in the ways a learner reaches for a higher level of practice. We focus on stage of skill acquisition in the companion book, *Expertise in Nursing: Caring, Ethics and Clinical Judgment* 2nd Edition (Benner, Tanner & Chesla, 2009). Expert practice is often made more visible in accounts of breakdown (situations that did not go well), because what is missing or the failed good practice becomes more evident. The intent, the failed notion of good, or the failed standard of excellence becomes visible by its absence. But we also draw on examples of successful, well-executed practice, situations that nurses identified as outstanding practice and where the evidence in the descriptive narrative supports their claim.

We advise against using the particular "facts" of the exemplar in terms of interventions or medications used, as state of the art or best practices because it is impossible to present the most up to date or region specific therapies and thinking about particular clinical situations in retrospective accounts of actions taken in particular situations. Rather, we believe that these exemplars are appropriately used to stimulate clinical and moral imagination, and rehearse imaginatively for responding quickly and thinking in action with the current best knowledge available. We are focusing on the craft, situatedness and engaged thinking-in-action rather than particular protocols or the current evidence-based practices. So this approach does not supplant nor replace evidence-based use of knowledge in particular situations. These exemplars allow the nursing student or staff nurse to see family resemblances to the situations presented in their own practice and in response develop moral and clinical imagination about how to act.

The thinking we refer to may not be reflective at the moment of the nurse's engaged thinking-in action, but the written exemplars freeze the moment and allow the reader to reflect on the situation. We intend to illustrate engaged thinking-in-action of practicing nurses upon which their reflection, after the fact, is based. We ask our readers to imaginatively place themselves in the situations described in the narratives so that they may sense the risk and ambiguity and create their own engaged thinking-in-action responses to the clinical examples presented. These clinical narratives all demonstrate particularity or the historical unfolding of clinical situations of particular patients. There is something both singular and universal in the clinical situations we have chosen (Logstrup, 1995). We contend that clinical thinking requires more than placing information into discrete categories. Logstrup (1995) refers to information sorting and categorizing as subsumption or subsuming things into categories. According to Logstrup, sorting/assigning things or events to general categories is a form of rational calculation and classification rather than productive thinking:

> Application and subsumption are unproductive processes. They presuppose understanding and cognition but are themselves neither understanding or cognition, only perhaps a control upon them... We are inclined to denigrate knowledge to subsumption... This has its place. We cannot help doing so nor can we manage without it. Only, in the meantime, we have abandoned cognition [thinking] in a productive sense. Subsumption is not cognition but an application of what we have come to know, an application in which we test whether our cognition was correct (pp. 140-141).

Many students come away from formal education imagining that knowledge production is mere vocabulary mastery and classification of bits of knowledge. Formal professional education fails when the emphasis is primarily learning *about* nursing rather than learning how to take up nursing practice...i.e., how to be a nurse. Experiential clinical learning and situated coaching are central to the *formation* of the nurse's skills, perceptual acuities, knowledge and relational qualities required in nursing practice. By formation we imagine a dynamic process that is required in order to be an expert nurse, therapist, dancer, social worker, teacher. We do not adopt a rigid form or engage in mindless conformity (Benner, Sutphen, Leonard & Day, 2010; Benner, In Press).

Presentations of taxonomies—such as nursing diagnoses and nursing interventions—as useful as they are for codifying and retrieving information are not the same thing as being able to actively think about the issues and clinical conditions to which they refer. They cannot provide the productive thinking and imagination for access to a patient or family whose disease and illness experience have been classified (See Bowker & Star, 1999). Learning only classifications and information systems used to organize and retrieve nursing knowledge would be to learn only about nursing rather than learning to be a nurse.

This work provides an educational planning document to assist nurses in developing expert clinical practice. Since the point is to examine contextually embedded know-how, we ask the reader to think reflectively about the context of the stories. We believe that this work will assist nurses to move from competent to proficient levels of practice. But it can also be a guide for beginning nurses, because it creates a way to understand and guide experiential learning. This book provides examples of "live" first person experience-near accounts of unfolding cases in actual practice, and thus can help nurse educators develop new integrative teaching strategies that integrate knowledge acquisition and knowledge use, the clinical and the classroom and vice a versa. This book cannot substitute for technical procedural accounts required by students and beginners, nor the scientific research that must be continually developed and critically evaluated in order for clinicians to keep abreast of the current state of the science. Educational strategies and implications are more fully described in Chapter 13.

BACKGROUND OF THE WORK

This work is an extension of the articulation work begun in *Expertise in Nursing Practice* (Benner, Tanner & Chesla, 1996) and *From Novice to Expert* (Benner, 1984). By articulation, we mean describing, illustrating, and giving language to taken-for-granted areas of practical wisdom, skilled know-how, and notions of good practice. This book provides a "thick" ethnographic account of excellent critical care nursing practice (Geertz, 1987). By "thick" we mean that we have tried to capture the significance of the events described and not just strategic goals. We have tried to stay true to the clinical mode of knowing that is open-ended, historical, and that must keep track of what has been tried, what responses the patient and family have shown, and what is expected next. Expert practice is characterized by stories of recognizing a turn in the patient and family—a recognition of changing relevance—and responding to it. Observational interviews and clinical narratives are used to illustrate these domains of practice. The storyteller tells the story in terms of the significance and chronology of experience. While reading the clinical narratives in this book, the reader can ask questions about how the meaning of the story is revealed: Why was this the "beginning" of the story? Why were these issues and details included? Why did the story begin or end where it did? Whose account is missing in the story? What is left out? Reading the stories reflectively is good practice for reflecting on and learning from practice. Placing oneself in the story is also a good rehearsal for practice and can stretch one's clinical imagination and ability to allow the situation to call forth knowledge.

Scientific reasoning or formal criterial reasoning seeks certitude. Scientific problem solving is set up to yield absolute "yes" and "no" judgments. While acute critical care nursing requires exacting judgments, their situated clinical judgments cannot be as certain or predicted and controlled to the degree that scientific experiments can. Learning to develop the best account of a clinical situation in order to make the best clinical judgment under circumstances of uncertainty is an interpretive process (Benner, 1994c; Hooper, 1995; Benner, Tanner & Chesla, 2009). The best account of the clinical situation under the circumstances of uncertainty will yield the best judgment. Certitude, while sought, is seldom achieved in actual practice. Snap judgments, tunnel vision, over generalization, and fixation on certain problems to the exclusion of others are all possible sources of poor judgment. The clinical learner always runs the risk of over-generalizing past experiential learning and thus mis-applying prior learning. We recommend that nurses keep a record of instances of strong learning or paradigm cases that teach something new or make a clinical pattern recognizable. Reflecting on one's narrative reasoning can reveal new insights and understanding, but also faulty logic such as tunnel vision or snap judgments.

SAMPLE AND METHODS

This study was begun as a part of the Expertise in Nursing Practice study funded by the Helene Fuld Foundation from 1990 to 1996. This work includes an extension to the original data set of small group interviews with 130 critical care units in eight different hospitals and observations and individual interviews with a sub-sample of 48 of these nurses. From this original study we developed an ethnography of the practice of critical care nurses, but the practice was changing rapidly in the wake of the wide spread introduction of managed care and a privatized market model of healthcare. The boundaries of critical care nursing were changing. We were once again funded by the Helene Fuld Foundation to extend our data collection (1996-1997) to include other critical care areas (including emergency departments, flight nursing, home health, the operating room, and post-anesthesia care units) and enlarge our sample of advanced practice nurses. We were already far along in our thick description of the practice of critical care nurses when the second phase of data collection began, so our inquiry was guided by filling out areas where we had already discovered puzzles or gaps in our understanding.

Five aims that structured data collection and analysis during Phase 1 and Phase 2 included:

1. To delineate the practical knowledge embedded in expert practice
2. To describe the nature of skill acquisition in critical care nursing practice
3. To identify institutional impediments and resources for the development of expertise in nursing practice
4. To begin to identify educational strategies that encourage the development of expertise (Benner, Tanner & Chesla, 2009).
5. To articulate the nature of knowledge and interventions in critical care.

While Phases 1 and 2 represent two separate studies (see Tables 1.2 and 1.3), the qualitative texts from both studies were combined for this book (see Table 1.4). In developing

TABLE 1.2
Experience in Years by Group (N = 130)

	Advanced Beginner			Intermediate			Experienced			Proficient		
	Mean	SD	Md	Mean	SD	Md	Mean	SD	Md	Mean	SD	Md
Years since basic nursing education	.8	.7	.5	5.4	5.3	4.2	12.1	4.3	11.8	12.8	4.7	11.6
Years since BSN	.7	.4	.5	4.3	2.8	3.9	10.2	4.7	9.5	8.0	5.8	9.0
Years in current unit	.5	.3	.4	2.1	.8	1.9	7.5	4.0	7.0	7.6	4.6	7.0

Note: BSN = Bachelor of science in nursing; SD = standard deviation; Md = median. Table from *Expertise in Nursing Practice: Caring, Clinical Judgment, and Ethics* (p. 373), by P. Benner, C. A. Tanner, & C. Chesla, 1996, New York: Springer. Copyright 1996 by Springer Publishing Company.

TABLE 1.3

Experience in Years by Group

	Nurse (N = 43)			Advanced Practice Nurse (N = 32)		
	Mean	SD	Median	Mean	SD	Median
Years in critical care	14.47	6.92	14.00	13.19	7.66	14.50
Years in nursing	16.30	7.07	16.00	17.28	5.74	17.50

Note: SD = standard deviation

this second edition, we have gathered new, more recent expert exemplars in most cases from across clinical specialties (see Table 1.5). In this updating process, we stuck with our original domains of practice, since we were not conducting a new open ended research study. We added nuances and new insights in our interpretation. Since the first edition of this book, and the writing of the second edition of *Expertise in Nursing Practice* (Benner, Tanner & Chesla, 2009), we have further recognized in the literature and in our narratives,

TABLE 1.4

Phases 1 and 2: Nursing Unit by Group

Units	Nurse (N = 173)		Advanced Practice Nurse (N = 32)*		Total (N = 205)*	
	n	%	n	%	n	%
Burn ICU	4	2.3	0	0	4	2.0
Cardiac/Coronary ICU	25	14.5	6	18.8	31	15.1
Cardiovascular surgery ICU	0	0	5	15.6	5	2.4
Emergency department	6	3.5	3	9.4	9	4.4
Medical/Surgical ICU	20	11.6	5	15.6	25	12.2
Medical ICU	16	9.2	3	9.4	19	9.3
Surgical ICU	22	12.7	2	6.3	24	11.7
Neurological/Neurosurgical ICU	4	2.3	1	3.1	5	2.4
Respiratory ICU	0	0	1	3.1	1	0.5
Helicopter trauma	6	3.5	0	0	6	2.9
Trauma ICU	0	0	6	18.8	6	2.9
Neonatal ICU	32	18.5	1	3.1	33	16.1
Pediatric ICU	10	5.8	3	9.4	13	6.3
Operating room	7	4.0	1	3.1	8	3.9
Postanesthesia care unit	4	2.3	2	6.3	6	2.9
Subacute/Intermediate	0	0	4	12.5	4	2.0
Home care	0	0	3	9.4	3	1.5
HIV/AIDS outpatient Clinic	0	0	2	6.3	2	1.0
Non-ICU ward units	7	4.0	0	0	7	3.4
Other	10	5.8	0	0	10	4.9

*Percentage totals do not add up to 100% because many advanced practice nurses work in more than one unit.

ICU = intensive care unit

TABLE 1.5
Acute and Critical Care Exemplars From Across Specialties

Specialty	Nurse (N = 104)*		Exemplars (N = 271)*	
	n	%	*n*	%
Ambulatory care	1	1.0	2	0.7
Anesthetists, Nurse*	2	1.9	2	0.7
Bone marrow transplant	1	1.0	1	0.4
Cardiac catheterization laboratory	1	1.0	3	1.1
Day surgery	2	1.9	4	1.5
eICU, Electronic ICU	1	1.0	4	1.5
Emergency department	8	7.7	19	7.0
Hematology–Oncology clinic	3	2.9	9	3.3
High-risk delivery	1	1.0	2	0.7
Hospice	1	1.0	5	1.8
ICU, Neonatal	2	1.9	3	1.1
ICU, Pediatric*	3	2.9	3	1.1
ICU, Pediatric neurological	1	1.0	2	0.7
ICU, Adult*	9	8.7	25	9.2
ICU, Burn/Trauma	1	1.0	1	0.4
ICU, Neurological/Neurosurgical	1	1.0	1	0.4
Labor and Delivery/OB	4	3.8	10	3.7
Lactation	1	1.0	3	1.1
Maternity/Nursery	4	3.8	12	4.4
Medical	7	6.7	12	4.4
Medical surgical	4	3.8	13	4.8
Medical surgical, Pediatric	3	2.9	9	3.3
Nursery, Special care	3	2.9	8	3.0
Oncology	3	2.9	22	8.1
Oncology clinic	2	1.9	10	3.7
Operating room	6	5.8	8	3.0
PACU	5	4.8	15	5.5
Pain clinic	1	1.0	9	3.3
Pediatric emergency transport	1	1.0	2	0.7
Pediatric hematology oncology*	2	1.9	4	1.5
Pediatric medicine	1	1.0	1	0.4
Prenatal clinic	1	1.0	1	0.4
Psychiatric, Locked	1	1.0	4	1.5
Outpatient, Cardiac rehabilitation	1	1.0	3	1.1
Rehabilitation	1	1.0	1	0.4
Radiation oncology clinic	3	2.9	13	4.8

(Continued)

TABLE 1.5

Acute and Critical Care Exemplars From Across Specialties *(Continued)*

Specialty	Nurse (N = 104)*		Exemplars (N = 271)*	
	n	%	*n*	%
Student	1	1.0	1	0.4
Surgical	1	1.0	1	0.4
Telemetry	7	6.7	18	6.6
Wound care*	2	1.9	4	1.5
Wounded warrior	1	1.0	1	0.4

*Percentage totals do not add up to 100% because many advanced practice nurses work in more than one unit.

eICU = electronic intensive care unit; ICU = intensive care unit; PACU = postanesthesia care unit.

the role of skill of engagement in nursing expertise, and will focus more on articulation of skills of involvement and impediments to engaging in particular clinical situation and the patient's lifeworld concerns (Sunvisson, Habermann, Weiss, & Benner, 2009).

The study in general was also enriched by the doctoral research studies conducted by Patricia Hooper (1995) and Daphne Stannard (1997). While we have not specifically drawn on the data from either of these two doctoral dissertation studies, it is appropriate to acknowledge that the understandings gained in these two separate doctoral studies, to be published in other arenas, added to the understandings in this study. These two doctoral studies operated frequently as points of discussion and sources of insight. This 2nd edition draws on additional doctoral research, Lisa Day (1999), Marilyn Oakes Greenspan (2007), Lori Rodriguez (2007) and Susan McNiesh, (2008). We leave the original data collection sample descriptions because this research was the bases for the domains of practice, now further articulated in this Second Edition.

THE SKILLS OF EXPERT CLINICAL COMPORTMENT, THINKING, AND JUDGMENT

Multiple aspects of clinical judgment and skillful comportment are highlighted in each of the domains of practice. Here we highlight the following nine aspects of being and thinking like a nurse: 1); developing a sense of salience 2) situated learning and integrating knowledge acquisition and knowledge use 3) engaged reasoning-in-transition 4) skilled know-how; 5) response-based practice; 6) agency; 7) perceptual acuity and interpersonal engagement with patients; and 8) integrating clinical and ethical reasoning and finally, 9) developing clinical imagination. These critical aspects of clinical judgment and expert comportment are described in order to guide active reflection on each of the clinical situations in the domains of practice described and illustrated in the following chapters. We believe that this approach to active reflection on practice captures the nature of expert clinical judgment and comportment better than diagnosis and treatment models of clinical judgment (Benner, Tanner & Chesla, 2009). Listing diagnoses and matching interventions are static models that are better suited for information categorization and retrieval than as models for the dynamic reasoning in expert practice. The approach we are presenting is close to Schon's notion of artistry in practice. Schon's two influential works *The Reflective Practitioner* (1987) and *Educating the Reflective Practitioner* (1991), point to the limits of the rational-technical model for learning to become an expert practitioner:

> From the perspective of technical rationality, "thinking like a [nurse]" must be thought to consist in rule-governed inquiry. The competent practitioner is seen as following rules for data gathering, inference, and hypothesis testing, which allow him to make clear connections between presenting situations and the body of professional knowledge, where such connections initially are not already explicit. The currently popular "expert systems," in clinical medicine as in other fields, are attempts to make explicit the information bases, rules, and procedures by which professional knowledge is applied to particular problematic cases (Kassirer & Gory, 1970).
>
> Within this framework, there is little room for professional artistry, except as a matter of style grafted onto technical expertise. One might recognize the existence of professional artists capable of making sense of unique or uncertain situations, but there is no way to talk sensibly about their artistry—except, perhaps, to say that they are following rules that they have not yet made explicit (Schon, 1991, p. 34-35).

Schon goes on to say that the artist (expert) makes up new rules on the spot. We differ with Schon on this point and claim that experts are following tacit knowledge and deep background understanding from prior whole cases (Dreyfus & Dreyfus, 1986). We think the artist is engaged in productive engaged thinking-in-action based upon a narrative understanding of the situation, rather than rule-governed thinking. It will, however, take the rest of this book to illustrate what we mean by engaged thinking-in-action. We have chosen the term engaged thinking-in-action rather than Schon's (1987) phrase "reflection-in-action", because "thinking" conveys the innovative and productive nature of the clinician's active thinking <u>in</u> ongoing situations. Reflection connotes stepping back or being outside the situation. Both are important for developing clinical knowledge. The practitioner's skills of involvement and quality of engagement with the situation and the person determine what can disclosed, noticed, and attended to in the situation. We will use narratives and observational interviews to demonstrate engaged thinking-in-action and reasoning-in-transition. Both engaged thinking-in-action and reasoning-in-transition are examples of practical reasoning (Taylor, 1993; Sullivan & Rosin, 2008).

While this work is based on a large representative sample of critical care nurses from multiple settings, we do not use the term "expert" to indicate that a particular nurse is expert in every aspect of practice. "Expert" is also not used to refer to a specific role such as an advanced practice nurse. Expertise is found in the practice of experienced clinicians and advanced practice nurses. We have designated the advanced practice nurses in the interviews because their roles are typically distinct from staff nurses. Much of the non-clinical work is necessarily left out of this book. We have focused on the clinical aspect of the roles and, in order to demonstrate thinking-in-action about particular strong situations, we could not include all possible strong situations. For example, we have not systematically described the teaching-coaching function of clinicians as a separate domain, yet it shows up repeatedly in the nurses' narratives. We hope that this book will stimulate other acute and critical care nurses to extend the articulation of expert knowledge in critical care.

Unwittingly, teaching-learning strategies have typically emphasized either process <u>or</u> content. The goal in this work is to link process and content as they occur in clinical and ethical reasoning. We hope to convey engaged reasoning and demonstrate strategies for reflecting on practice that facilitate experiential learning. We ask the learner to actively imagine being a part of the clinical episodes presented. Mirroring the sense of risk and imagining possible responses helps one to remember the salient issues in the clinical problems presented. Such an engaged rehearsal can enlarge the reader's own clinical and often moral imagination. Experiential learning does not occur without active participation nor is it guaranteed by the mere passage of time. Experiential learning always requires engagement in the situation and involves learning something new, a "turning around" of preconceptions, recognition of patterns, or sensing something disquieting or puzzling that generates a problem search (Benner, 1984/2000; Gadamer, 1975/1960). The process of experiential learning generates a narrative memory of the content, as well as the related clinical and ethical issues and one's emotional sense of the situation that are significant in the instances where they were learned. Narrative memory can then assist a developing nurse to more skillfully act in similar future situations.

The authors, representing three different generations of critical care nurses, and reflecting on our own practice, as well as those we have studied, agree that critical care nurses manage an enormous amount of continuous physiological data from patients, adjust instantaneous therapies in relation to that data, and additionally sustain essential caring practices. The technology of critical care units rivals cockpits of large modern aircraft. If one considered all of this information as just data points, then artificial intelligence systems would be used to try to formally correlate the data using algorithms. However, even the smartest, fastest artificial intelligence system would run into what artificial intelligence workers call the "frame problem" and philosophers call the "limits of formalism" (Dreyfus, 1992; Dreyfus & Dreyfus, 1986), because computers use artificial intelligence programs to build up an analysis of the situation, element by element, with no background understanding that orders and interprets the data in relation to the "whole picture."

How does one teach such a practice well? We can attest to being mentored into the practice by other critical care nurses, physicians, and other members of the healthcare team. And we can attest to what is left out by mere rational-technical accounts of critical care practice (e.g., traditional textbooks). This work presents a narrative approach to learning acute and critical care nursing practice complete with the moral visions and possibilities of the best of nursing practice. We have left in flaws as very real reminders of the dangerousness of acute and critical care. This work is not about teaching isolated techniques, indeed many of the techniques were becoming obsolete even as we described them. Rather it is about the knowledge work, the thinking-in-action, required in nursing practice.

The Carnegie Foundation for the Advancement of Teaching National Study of Nursing Education was just completed (Benner, Sutphen, Leonard & Day, 2009). This influential study was nested in the larger program of research conducted by the Carnegie Foundation for the Advancement of Teaching to celebrate approximately 100 years after the influential Carnegie study of medicine "The Flexner Report." The professions studied were clergy, engineers, lawyers, physicians and nurses. All the studies examined how the different professions taught the three essential apprenticeship of professional education:

1. The cognitive apprenticeship of science, technology, theory, and literature, the knowledge essential for a knowledgeable, self-improving professional practitioner.

2. The practice apprenticeship of learning how to use knowledge and engage in the situated skilled-know-how of the practitioner, and engage in practical reasoning as well as formal scientific reasoning.
3. The third apprenticeship is that of formation and ethical comportment, engaging in practice that embodies the notions of the good in the particular professional practice.

This recently published national study of nursing education has influenced the writing of this second edition, In this edition of Clinical Wisdom, we try to draw out the pedagogical implications of the expert practice described and examined in this book.

DEVELOPING A SENSE OF SALIENCE

In any complex practice, the practitioner must develop a rich experiential base in order to enter under-determined or ambiguous situations with a sense of salience; that is, recognize what is most urgent or significant. Recognizing what stands out as relevant guides the nurse's thinking, reasoning, judgment and possible interventions. The lack of a sense of salience is at the heart of the problem of the inexperienced learner of any practice. All things can stand out as relevant, or equally important. This is true in sports as well. In learning tennis, the player must come to recognize salient positions and styles of their opponent which informs one where to move and what to anticipate. The novice is given guidelines and rules about what to pay attention to until they get a sense of commonly occurring situations in clinical practice. These explicit guidelines and rules focus their attention and thinking and thereby limit their ability to be flexible, and attend to changing aspects of the situation that they may not have deliberately planned for or thought about. This is why situated coaching (having a more skillful clinician coach the learner while in the midst of a changing clinical situation) is so important to the learner. The clinical teacher fills in the learner's experiential gaps, usually after first assessing the learner's grasp of the situation.

SITUATED LEARNING: INTEGRATING KNOWLEDGE ACQUISITION AND KNOWLEDGE USE

While it is impossible to completely spell out and integrate all aspects of the use of science, nursing theory, and humanities, it remains a powerful pedagogical strategy to point to the clinical use of natural, human and nursing science knowledge being presented in classes. The limits of formalism prevents pointing out all possible relevant clinical uses of knowledge, but even a small range of clinical implications for nursing knowledge presented in the classroom can improve students ability to integrate science and clinical practice knowledge.

Western academia has elevated the teaching and learning of *abstract* knowledge and theory, considering any knowledge use as simply an application of the abstract knowledge or principles. This position overlooks the productive thinking required to use abstract knowledge in practical situations.

Acquiring knowledge and using knowledge are distinct for the beginning student who is not yet familiar enough with clinical practice to imagine the situations where knowledge might be relevant (Eraut, 1994). Situated learning in simulation, skills labs and clinical practice are central for students to learn how to use knowledge. However, the journey of connected learning must begin in the classroom, where the imaginative teacher refers to relevant human situations or clinical conditions where knowledge must be drawn on and taken up by the clinician in actual clinical situations. Lave and Wenger (1991) point out the social nature and situatedness of learning. We lose sight of this when we imagine that formal abstract concepts will automatically be perceived in actual situations where and when this knowledge is relevant. A simple template or "application" model of how knowledge is used and taken up leaves out skills of discernment and situation recognition. Knowledge is socially distributed, and lodged in practice communities and practice situations (Lave and Wenger, 1991). This is why active learning in actual or simulated clinical situations is so central to learning any complex practice. Because a simulated situation draws on imaginative knowledge use, it also requires understanding the nature of the clinical situation and the feasible practice goals for that situation. Sullivan and Rosin (2008) have called for a new agenda in higher education so that practical reasoning (for nurses and physicians, this means clinical reasoning) is taught in addition to formal analytical models of decision making and thinking.

ENGAGED REASONING-IN-TRANSITION

Clinical reasoning requires reasoning-in-transition (or reasoning about the changes in a situation) about *particular* patients and families. Engaged reasoning-in-transition refers to practical reasoning in an evolving or open-ended clinical situation. Practical reasoning moves one's understanding to a better or clearer understanding and resolves contradiction or confusion. Moving through a transition from a poorer to a better understanding is error-reducing, enlarges one's sense of possibility, or clarifies limits (Taylor, 1989; 1993; Benner, 1994c). For instance, in the case of a cardiac surgery patient, establishing that a low cardiac output is related to volume depletion rather than pump failure shapes interventions and expected responses.

The expert clinician is always engaged in interpreting the present clinical situation in terms of the immediate past condition of the patient. Questions have to do with the direction of changes in the patient's condition: Is the patient's consciousness lighter? Is there a trend toward an increased or decreased respiratory effort? How do we account for the baby's increasing irritability? Is the patient becoming septic? What is the patient's baseline? The answers to these questions come in the form of comparable judgments over time (Taylor, 1993, p. 230). In situations that are challenging or atypical, the expert clinician is also engaged in interpreting and reasoning through the specific patient's condition or atypical presentation to prior and similar patients' responses. Expert clinical reasoning-in-transition can be said to occur for a particular patient but also across patient populations. This kind of ongoing clinical problem solving is far more common and crucial to patient well being than can be depicted in formal case studies or assessments made at one point in time. Formal case studies usually take the position of an objective outside (disengaged) third person view, and thus cannot depict the nurse's engagement with the specific patient or the situation. The quality of the nurse's (or any other professional's) skill of involvement with the patient/family, and with the problems and concerns in the clinical situation, determine what can be disclosed by the family/patient and what can be noticed, and acted upon by the nurse, as mentioned earlier.

We support the advancement of evidence based practice, but recognize that the objective application of clinical trials and other research findings must be critically evaluated and selected for use in attuned and fitting ways for particular patients. Accurate evaluation and judgment for a specific patient requires the kind of engaged reasoning we are describing.

The trend to use large population statistical studies about patient outcomes does not easily translate into the implications for a particular patient (Frankford, 1994; Tannenbaum, 1994). Clinicians can use these large randomized outcome trials only as guidelines, not prescriptions, when considering applications for a particular patient. The reasoning of basic science that uncovers physiological mechanisms and pathways is easier for the physician or nurse to translate to the particular patient and comes prior to the use of generalized statistics about prognoses or outcome data for large groups. Formal criterion reasoning, as used in the scientific process, provides a "snapshot" form of reasoning, that is, a single sample at one point in time used to compare with another single point in time. While scientific evidence is essential to good practice, the clinician must develop skills of reasoning that are closer to a moving picture where sequence, development, change, and nuance can be considered. Narrative understanding over time is required so that clinicians can determine whether their understanding has increased or diminished as the patient's condition changed. That is why we believe that developing skills of narrative reflection on practice is particularly helpful in developing expert clinical judgment. Narrative captures concerns, context, sequencing and consequences of the disease progression and therapeutic interventions over time (Benner, 1984; Benner & Wrubel, 1989; Charron, 2001)

We present many examples of narrative reflection and ask the reader to become engaged in the narratives in order to imaginatively feel the ambiguities and tensions of the unfolding clinical situation. Our thick description is comprised of many acute and critical care nurses' stories. Our thinking-in-action approach to teaching this practice uses strong practical situations that expert nurses themselves use to order and guide their actions. For example, if the issue is one of highly unstable hemodynamics, then all other tasks tend to be ordered in relation to stabilizing the patient's hemodynamics. Understandings of strong situations order the clinician's world of practical engaged reasoning. This strategy can be contrasted with traditional case studies that present an array of information about the case at a particular point in time. The case study is a good approach to considering all the issues in the clinical situation, but it does not capture clinical reasoning as it unfolds over time. Nor does the typical case study include the intents and concerns of the clinician. Narrative reflection allows the clinician to keep means and ends in relation to one another and tied to understanding the situation including the temporal sequencing of the situation.

Trying to spell out the elements that should go into the interpretation is a voluminous task, even an endless task ("limits of formalism" or "infinite regress" in philosophical terms). One literally cannot name all the elements of an actual past paced clinical situation. Additionally, to be useful, this information must be related to other salient data. Artificial intelligence workers have also noted the temporal sequencing problem, which is the difficulty in capturing changes in the situation that yield inferences, because of the sequence of events and the reasoning that occurs about the sequence. This is still an outside-in account and does not give the sense of insight or disimpeded action that is acquired by the thinker when moving through a transition in the patient's condition. All the physiological data must make sense in terms of the patient's physical condition and human concerns. An outside-in description of a clinical situation or an artificial intelligence approach to analyzing the data/task demands is close to how beginning critical care practitioners experience their work. By contrast, expert critical care nurses are always dwelling in meaningful stories of the patient's and family's situation, managing to keep an up to the minute clinical and human grasp of the significance of the situation. Expert clinicians must be able to reason about the <u>particular</u> patient and family. For example, it is not enough to simply "know that" most burn patients experience massive fluid shifts. The expert clinician must "know how" and "when" to initiate appropriate interventions based on how the particular patient presents in the clinical situation. This kind of practical reasoning is ongoing and open-ended.

SKILLED KNOW-HOW

The performance of interventions sets up the possibility of thinking-in-action; that is, as the patient responds to interventions, the nurse gains a better sense of what is going on with the patient. In an immediate post-op cardiac surgical patient for instance, a skilled nurse assesses peripheral rewarming by feeling the temperature change from the thigh down to the foot. She can feel the difference in skin temperature and gain a sense of the degree and extent of rewarming. This embodied skill enables the nurse to think-in-action about the influence of the warming blanket or the vasoactive drug infusions on the patient's progressive vasodilation and rewarming.

The central role of the body in skillful performance—skilled know-how—is primarily evident in observation. But, even with observation, many aspects of skilled know-how are not visibly accessible, as in the above example of perceiving the degree of rewarming while assessing the temperature change in the patient's legs. To learn this kind of skill, the clinician must distinguish the degree of temperature change by assessing the patient him/herself, understand the degree of rewarming in terms of how experienced clinicians describe it, and/or compare and contrast similar or dissimilar patients' situations in relation to the warming blanket temperature and particular drug infusions. Some aspects of skilled know-how are observable and can be learned by mimicry. However, mimicking a skill is not the same as skillful performance. For example, when one is learning how to do sterile technique, the body is slow to gain the rhythms of the prohibited and sanctioned territories of "sterile" and "dirty." But with time, these territories are meaningfully oriented for the practitioner, and motions become fluid and sensible in relation to gowning, gloving, and performing dressing changes.

How nurses situate themselves for observing and monitoring the patient is another form of skilled know-how (Hooper, 1995). Expert nurses learn to locate themselves in regions around the patient's bed where they can best see, hear, or touch the patient while they are charting, preparing IV drips, and completing non-direct aspects of patient care. Where nurses situate themselves sets up, in part, how and whether they can become attuned to the patient's condition and recognize a changing condition through the five senses. For example, even though the nurse may not be focally aware of listening to the rhythmic beat of a patient's heart, a dysrhythmia is immediately noticed when the nurse hears an irregular sound pattern.

Skilled know-how is an embodied way of knowing that is pervasive in all of the domains, and will be illustrated in the following chapters. Attunement, sequencing activities, and intervening all require skilled know-how, an embodied understanding of the task at hand.

RESPONSE-BASED PRACTICE

Excellent clinicians engage in an ongoing dialogue with the situation. A hallmark of expert clinicians is the capacity to read the situation and engage in a response-based practice (flexibly respond to the patient's changing situation and needs). Nurse educators typically isolate interventions and skills for students to practice in a learning laboratory but, in reality, nursing interventions are generated from actual clinical situations in addition to the nurse's plans. Expert practice is response-based and proactive (Benner, Tanner & Chesla, 2009).

For example, when cardiac surgical patients begin to emerge from anesthesia in the early post-operative period, they are commonly anxious and often become very hypertensive. Although textbooks and treatment protocols instruct clinicians to begin anti-hypertensive medications, expert nurses typically intervene first by trying to orient and reassure the patient in response to the patient's anxiety or fear. Many clinicians have learned that this kind of caring practice can alleviate the hypertension associated with the patient's emotions. However, if the nurse is not able to "talk the patient down" in a relatively short time period or the hypertension is sustained and presents a threat (e.g., vein graft rupture, increased bleeding), then the expert nurse additionally responds with a pharmacologic intervention to rapidly control the hypertension (Hooper, 1995). Similarly, when a pregnant patient is in labor and has expressed a strong preference for natural birth, there is often a point during the delivery, when the exhausted, suffering patient declares she can no longer push. However, it is often too late of an epidural anesthetic. It is then that the skillful nurse, guided by the patient's expressed preferences, coaches the patient to "dig deep." The expert strongly and intensely coaches the patient about how to breathe, when to push, and how hard to push, moment by moment. Minutes later the newborn wails and joy bursts forth. These examples illustrate the level of attentiveness needed at the bedside to respond to the patient's particular needs and preferences. It reflects how skillful nurses read the situation and how their actions are oriented by the kinds and sequence of the patient's responses. It also reveals the ethos of "do no harm" that is embedded in excellent practice. In acute and critical care, where many interventions have the potential for harm, expert clinicians prefer to try the least harmful but potentially effective intervention first.

It is the relatedness of expert practitioners to particular patients, families, and situations that we seek to preserve in this work. To make this theater of learning effective requires that readers imaginatively enter into the clinicians' concerns. Expensive and potentially harmful technological or pharmacological interventions are rendered safe or unnecessary by having skillful clinicians engage in caring practices and reading changing patient situations.

AGENCY

Agency is a term that we have borrowed from the fields of moral psychology and ethics that refers to one's ability to act upon or influence a situation. We found that both the sense of agency and the capacity for different levels of agency or influence varied at different levels of expertise (Benner, Tanner & Chesla, 2009). For example, the expert nurse develops a response-based agency, directly responding to changes in the patient and family as they occur. Advanced beginners have an enriched sense of responsibility and agency as compared to when they were initially doing clinical rotations in nursing school, but their actual agency is limited by their current level of clinical understanding and embodied know-how in actual clinical situations. At the competent level of practice, agency is enacted through achieving goals and making plans and choices. Experiential learning is required before the practitioner's actions are guided by recognizing patterns in order to respond to the actual situation. With sufficient experiential learning, the clinician becomes attuned to the situation. In our study of critical care nursing practice, we found that proficient nurses frequently told stories of having their expectations "turned around" or changed in the situation (Benner, Tanner & Chesla, 2009). Engaged reasoning that responds to patient changes characterizes proficient and expert performance. We infer that, with a certain level of experience, reading the situation becomes possible, and a more response-based, attuned agency is developed. This skill and capacity oriented view of moral agency links agency to more than "moral intent," noting that even a perfect moral intent without the capacity to perceive and respond quickly and effectively will limit all practitioners' moral agency. Attunement and skill of involvement also determines what the agent is able to notice and discern, so that moral intent, again without adequate skills of engagement will not ensure a high degree of moral agency.

Rubin (2009) found that experienced nurses who were not considered to be expert practitioners did not see or experience their agency in the situation. They imagined that they were just weighing objective facts and coming to procedurally guided conclusions. Clarifying and imagining one's influence or agency in a situation is at the heart of developing good clinical judgment. Clinicians can never truly stand outside the situation and objectively calculate static facts of the matter, because they are always engaged in the situation by their action, reasoning, and relationship with the patient and family. Expert clinical practice requires taking a stand by identifying and responding to the demands of the situation (Benner, Tanner & Chesla, 2009) and the conditions of possibility for expert practice include skilled know-how, perceptual acuity and an attuned emotional involvement.

PERCEPTUAL ACUITY AND INTERPERSONAL ENGAGEMENT

We want to highlight problem identification as well as problem solving in the examples provided in this work. Being a good problem solver is not sufficient if the most crucial problem is overlooked or the problem is framed or defined in misguiding ways. Sometimes the definition of the problem makes it unsolvable and redefining or reframing the problem creates new options. Focusing on problem identification (which problem(s) does the clinician perceive and seek to solve) requires perceptual acuity. One may have the appropriate intellectual understanding of particular clinical entities and ethical issues, but not have the attendant experiential learning and comparison of actual patient care situation to develop the perceptual acuity to recognize when these issues are at stake in actual situations. Perceptual acuity is linked with emotional engagement with the problem and interpersonally with patients and families (Benner & Wrubel, 1982). Thus, we will highlight the emotional skills of openness and responsiveness, and point out emotional tones that signal lack of a good grasp of the situation.

Perception requires skillful engagement both with the problem and the person(s). Perceptual acuity is much less studied than judgment, yet one can only make judgments about what is perceived. Hence, good clinical judgment hinges on skillful engagement. The skills of problem engagement and interpersonal involvement require experiential learning. For example, clinicians talk about problems of over-identifying with the patient and becoming flooded with feelings. It is equally a problem to wall off feelings so that the possibilities of attunement are blunted or shut down. The beginning nurse can feel a generalized anxiety over the demands of learning or the fear of making errors. At this beginning stage, dampening emotional responses can lower anxiety and improve learning and performance. But with the gaining of competency, emotional responses become more differentiated and more attuned. The practitioner begins to feel comfortable and "at home" in familiar situations and uneasy when the situation is unfamiliar. This differentiated emotional response is the beginning of gaining a sense of salience and developing attunement to the situation. At the competent stage, clinical learners can safely pay attention to vague or global emotional responses as a sign that they do not fully understand in the situation. At this point, they have a developing sense of when they do or do not have a good clinical grasp of the situation. These emotional senses of the situation are crucial to early problem search and identification. They are the sources of discovery and early warnings of changes in patients. Emotional responses also play a key role in perceiving the other's plight and in reaching out to the other (Benner, 1984; Benner & Wrubel, 1989; Stannard, 1997).

Excellent clinical nurse educators in academia and organizations coach students or developing nurses for an appropriate sense of salience in complex under-determined clinical situations (Benner, Sutphen, Leonard & Day, 2009). The novice, first year nursing student, as well as beginning nurses have difficulty grasping the nature of the clinical situation, i.e. what must attended to first, and want is less important at the present. Nurse educators begin early, helping students and beginners frame the nature of the clinical situation and deliberately set priorities for what they should do first, and for what is most important in caring for the patient. Lisa Day, for example, asks her students "what is at stake" in this patient care situation, and "what are the nurse's most appropriate responses to those particular stakes?" (Benner, Sutphen, Leonard & Day, 2009, p.133-141).

Throughout nursing education and clinical precepting nurses require situated coaching. The focus of the coaching changes qualitatively over time, with the novice and beginner requiring questioning and framing to help them grasp the nature of the clinical situation. At a later stage of development, when things do not go as expected, expert coaching is often required to help the competent nurse re-frame the problem, or focus attention, or determine effective nursing interventions.

Traditionally, emotion has been seen as opposed to cognition and rationality. But increasingly, it is recognized that emotions play a key role in perception and even act as a moral compass in learning a practice (Damasio, 1994; Dreyfus, Dreyfus & Benner, 1996; Noe, 2009). For example, at the competent stage, clinical learners feel "good" when they perform well and when they take the risks inherent in making sound clinical judgments. Nurses at this level feel disappointed and regret when an error in judgment causes the patient to suffer negative outcomes (Dreyfus & Dreyfus, 1996). These are essential aesthetic and ethical responses that guide the development of perceptual acuity and problem identification. Larry Blum (1994) has noted this in studying moral development and moral psychology:

> Thus moral perception, I argue, cannot be identified with moral judgment. In a given situation, moral perception comes on the scene before moral judgment; moral perception can lead to moral action outside the operation of judgment entirely; and, more generally, perception can involve moral capacities not encompassed by moral judgment. I argue also that moral perception should not be conceived of as a unified capacity, but that it involves multifarious moral and psychological processes (p. 31).

In their narratives of practice, acute and critical care nurses disclose emotional responses. Emotionally imbued concerns and relationships with patients and families direct clinical understanding and actions. We can learn much about the practice of acute and critical care nursing and the moral arts of paying attention and responding compassionately by reading these nurses' accounts. The vivid, immediate narratives can increase the reader's own moral and clinical imagination through situating thinking and action and knowledge use. We can also learn much from the situations where patients are not treated compassionately. This book seeks to facilitate experiential learning by making the perceptual skills and processes associated with problem identification more visible and by the learning strategies described in this book.

Interpersonal engagement is not synonymous with problem engagement though it is linked. Bearing witness to another's distress can cause anxiety and nurses may distance themselves for protection. If nurses selectively attend to <u>some</u> problems more than others, for example, dysrhythmias or cardiac output, they may not be able to engage with the whole clinical situation. Anxiety can disrupt attentiveness and helping relationships. Extreme disengagement may prevent the nurse from experiencing personal responsibility and agency in a clinical situation and is linked to the inability to develop good clinical judgment (Rubin, 2009). Thus, we will attend to the problematic and effective aspects of the skill of involvement throughout this work. For reasoning-in-transition (or practical clinical reasoning) to be possible, the clinician must develop interpersonal skills of engaging with the clinical and human situation at hand. We have called this the <u>skill of involvement</u>, which requires developing the skills of getting an open and attentive engagement with the clinical situation or problem and developing the skill of getting the right kinds and amount of interpersonal engagement with the patient and family (Benner, Stannard & Hooper, 1996, p. 1).

Establishing safe, effective boundaries between the self and "other" can be disrupted by over- or under-identification with the other. As Levinas (1985) points out the "other" needs to be considered other and not same. But they must not be considered "wholly other," because all human beings share a common humanity of embodiedness, vulnerability, suffering, finitude, and the possibility of tragedy. It is considered an error in ethical comportment in nursing or medicine to violate the established appropriate boundaries between patient and nurse or physician. Idealizing, falling in love with, or demonizing and dehumanizing patients are all boundary problems. It is also a boundary problem and a breakdown in ethical comportment when nurses or physicians engage in aggrandizement of the self, or grandiose thinking. Sometimes excessive, aggressive, but futile attempts to save a patient's life may start out well intended, but become an exercise in poor judgment and grandiose thinking. We use term, "skill of involvement" to depict aspects of troubled "self-other" boundaries (as in "boundary" problems), but we prefer to use it as a broader term to include the necessary positive learning and development of attuned, effective skills of involvement. These situated skills of involvement are thought of as a form of skilled know-how because the nurse develops appropriate emotional attunement and responses over time through experiential learning. The nurse learns safe and helpful closeness and distance by getting their interpersonal connections, better or worse, in actual nurse-patient-family relationships.

INTEGRATING ETHICAL AND CLINICAL REASONING

It is not possible in practice to separate clinical and ethical reasoning, because good clinical judgments reflect good clinical practice. Good clinical judgments require understanding what are considered possible good outcomes for the patient and family in particular situations. As Dreyfus, Dreyfus, and Benner (2009) point out, this is a circular, but not a viciously circular project:

> To become an expert in any area of expertise, one has to be able to respond to the same types of situations as do those who are already expert. For example, to play master level chess, one has to see the same board positions as masters do. This basic ability is what one calls having talent in a given domain. In addition, the learner must experience what society considers the appropriate satisfaction or regret at the outcome of the response. To become an expert nurse one should feel concern, not indifference, about the patient's and family's plight. To acquire ethical expertise, then, one must have the talent to respond to those ethical situations to which ethical experts respond and one must have the sensibility to experience the socially appropriate sense of satisfaction or regret at the outcome of one's action (p. 259).

Learning to make good clinical judgments and be a good practitioner requires ongoing experiential learning, reflection, and dialogue with patients and their families. Biomedical ethics has traditionally focused on procedural issues such as ensuring autonomy of the patient, informed consent, justice, beneficence, non-maleficence and truth telling (Beauchamp & Childress, 1994). These bioethical principles are all essential ethical concerns that must be translated into concrete visions for excellent practice, but they do not, in themselves, create concrete visions for excellent practice. Notions of good guide the actions of nurses and help them notice clinical and ethical threats to patients' well being. In addition to the ethical discourses of dilemma, or practice breakdown ethics, nurses need to be formed or ethically shaped by their practices of everyday care and skills of involvement with their patients. Expert practitioners are motivated and guided by their ability to do excellent practice. Other motivations exist and there are many threats to excellent practice, but the ethical pull of excellent practice itself is self-motivating. To be a good practitioner requires at minimum, to do one's duty to uphold the standards of good practice. Another moral source is the direct human pull of alleviating another's suffering or meeting the other as a fellow embodied human being. Nursing, like teaching, medicine, social work, and other helping professions, depends on solidarity with one's fellow human beings and on the professional standards of beneficence and non-maleficence for helping people during periods of vulnerability and distress. That is what it means to be "good" at their work. These notions of good internal to the practice of nursing (MacIntyre, 1981) again require teaching and coaching in particular clinical situations and cases. In order to learn everyday ethical comportment, student and developing nurses need integrative teaching about ethical concerns and notions of good they encounter in their everyday practice (Benner, Sutphen, Leonard & Day, 2009).

THE LINKS BETWEEN EMOTION, JUDGMENT, AND NARRATIVE ACCOUNTS

Narratives reveal the emotional colorings in clinical situations. For example, when using a narrative pedagogy, a student may link two clinical situations that occurred years apart because they had similar moral emotions or sense of personal risk. For instance, a master's student recalls advocating for a patient's right to informed consent early in her career and links this story to an incident twenty years later when she helped a group of patients to politically organize to get back lost healthcare services. In the later situation, she took even greater risks in order to advocate for patients, threatening her possibility for promotion. She interpreted her actions as developing strength and agency as a patient advocate.

Emotions are social and moral. Some settings enhance moral-emotional capacities and others impede them. Vetleson (1994) draws attention to the social conditions of emotions:

> The performance of our emotional capacities is not indifferent to the social setting in which it takes place; rather, a faculty such as empathy—giving rise to care, compassion, sympathy—is highly susceptible to changes in the moral subject's social environment, which means that the social environment may help encourage or impede the faculty's actual exercise. In this sense one social setting may cultivate empathy, whereas another may undermine it (p.81).

We found some settings so destablized and pressed for time and resources that nurses could no longer hold the system together and patient safety was threatened. This was called "letting the system fail" (see Chapter 11). The patients' and families' suffering could and did become invisible to nurses who detached themselves as a means of self-protection. We agree with Vetleson (1994) that this kind of separation and isolation are not due to an inability to recognize the universal principles involved, but rather a consequence of having lost the ability to meet the other and to identify with the suffering of particular others. The lost ability of emotional engagement has been called "burnout." Some work environments foster burnout of employees through work overload, lack of infrastructures to support safe and sustainable responsibilities, or administrative failure to prioritize the patients' good over other competing goods.. Individuals both constitute and are constituted by social situations. We found inspiring examples of moral agency in nurses who creatively subverted the system against all odds on behalf of patients and families. But there are real limits to daily heroism in situations of extreme workload and in systems designed more for cost control and profit than patient and family well-being. The nurses' stories present a mandate for redesigning healthcare systems for humane care and basic social services, so as to prevent unnecessary suffering and render technical medical interventions safe (Weiss, Malone, Merighi, & Benner, 2002).

It is a mistake to imagine that persons can be completely in command of their emotions. Indeed, if emotions were purely and completely at the command of the person's internal intentions, they would lose their relational and perceptual qualities which allow persons to read moods, emotional climates and possibility or danger in its most subtle forms (Damasio, 1999). Human beings' "fuzzy' recognition of similarities and differences in situations depend on emotional intelligence and health (Damasio, 1994).

THE ROLE OF NARRATIVE IN EXPERIENTIAL LEARNING

We believe that clinical knowledge that enables the clinician to practice in particular situations is understood and captured best by narrative understanding (Benner, 1984; Benner, Tanner & Chesla, 2009; Diekelmann, 1989). Clinical learning is experienced as a story. Drawing on the work of Taylor (1989), MacIntyre (1981), and our own research, we conclude that experiential learning is structured narratively. Therefore understanding experiential learning requires narratives to capture the agency, temporality, and practical understanding inherent in it. Memory itself has a narrative structure. Therefore, a good teaching/learning strategy is to dwell in and with stories that capture clinical understandings of situations. Feeling the risks imaginatively and participating in the narrative enhances one's situated use of knowledge. Clinical and ethical concerns organize one's story (Rubin, 2009). Where to begin the story, what to tell, what to leave out, and where and how the story ends provide access to the storyteller's understanding of the situation. Stories or narratives as Robert Coles (1989) create moral, and we add clinical, imagination. A more detailed description of the educational implications of this work is provided in Chapter 13.

DEVELOPING CLINICAL AND MORAL IMAGINATION

All practitioners move into and take up a practice through developing their imagination for being an excellent practitioner (Dysktra, 1999; Foster, Dahill, Golemon & Tolentino, 2005). Clinical and moral imagination refers to one's ability to envision being in a patient situation, being confronted by the patient's physiologic and human needs, recognizing the challenge of competing goods, feeling the risks and uncertainty, and feeling the constraints or possibilities inherent in the context in an unfolding situation. Developing a rich clinical imagination through study, example, and experiential learning is what enables a clinician to anticipate and respond to a wide range of clinical situations and human concerns. Nurses learn directly from their patients some of the milestones and challenges in recovering from illness, and this experiential learning helps them develop imaginative responses to these challenges and milestones. If nursing practice could be reduced to a collection of unvaried techniques and strategies, then clinical and moral imagination would not be required. Teaching and learning for any under-determined practice requires imaginative problem solving...interventions that are particularly well-suited to the concerns and situated needs of patients. In compiling these first-person experience-near accounts of excellent nursing practice, our clinical and moral imagination for nursing was enriched because we imaginatively entered the nurses' stories. We encourage our readers to do the same.

THE LOGIC OF PRACTICE AND NARRATIVE PEDAGOGY

Nursing and medicine, like other practice disciplines such as law, social work, teaching, and psychiatry, involve a curious mix of science, technology, and praxis. Praxis is broader than the science guiding it and includes the working out of knowledge, inquiry, and relationships in practice. The logic of practice is different than the logic of science or structuralism as Bourdieu (1980/1990, pp. 11-12) has pointed out:

> [Structural diagrams] are logical models giving an account of the observed facts in the most coherent and economical way; and they become false and dangerous as soon as they are treated as the real principles of practices, which amounts to simultaneously overestimating the logic of practices and losing sight of what constitutes their real principle...Practices produced according to perfectly conscious generative rules would be stripped of everything that defines them distinctively as practices, that is, the uncertainty and 'fuzziness' resulting from the fact that they have as their principle not a set of conscious, constant rules, but practical schemes, opaque to their possessors, varying according to the logic of the situation... Thus, the procedures of practical logic are rarely entirely coherent and rarely entirely incoherent.

Bourdieu was describing cultural and social practices and admittedly nursing and medicine are complicated by the fact that they also draw on natural and human sciences. Both nursing and medicine require: 1) ethical and clinical reasoning (i.e., reasoning-in-transition about the particular (Benner, 1994a); 2) the use of scientific norms and data; 3) social negotiation of clinical understandings with patients, families, and other clinicians; and 4) helping relationships with patients and families. These broad socially organized practices provide an inherent sense and coherence to the practice. Practice is embodied and embodied understanding contributes to the logic of the practice. As Bourdieu (1980/1990, p. 10) points out, complex social practices often occur "without any organizing intention, that was revealed by analysis, one had to look to the incorporated dispositions, or more precisely the body schema, to find the ordering principle...capable of orienting practices in a way that is at once unconscious and systematic."

We agree with Bourdieu (1980/1990) and with Dreyfus and Dreyfus (Dreyfus, 1979; Dreyfus & Dreyfus, 1986) that we are in danger of losing sight of the logic of practice and over-simplifying practice education by mistaking menu-driven lists of possible actions and classificatory information with what <u>generates</u> good practice. While memory and analytical decision supports are useful to the practitioner, they are not alone sufficient to guide practice. Good clinical practice requires more than decisions. Only good practitioners will be in the best possible position to make good use of information systems and decision supports at specific points in time. Good practice requires aesthetic and ethical understandings as Bourdieu (1980/1990) points out:

> This practical sense is, on reflection, no more and no less mysterious than the one that confers stylistic unity on all the choices that the same person, that is, the same taste, may make in the most varied areas of practice, or the sense that enables a scheme of appreciation such as the opposition between bland and bold, dull and lively, insipid and piquant, to be applied to a dish, a colour, a person (more precisely, their eyes, their features, their beauty) and also to remarks, jokes, a style, a play or a painting. It is the basis of those realities, over-determined and at the same time under-determined, which, even when their principle has been understood, remain very difficult to master completely except in a kind of lyrical paraphrase that is as inadequate and sterile as ordinary discourse about works of art (p.14).

In many instances nurses describe ethical and aesthetic perceptions of artistry in practice. We have presented these accounts of practice in the nurses own spoken language with the usual light editing required to transform spoken into written language.

Another reason for importing the narratives into a nursing textbook, in addition to keeping the logic of practice, is that narratives include the ambiguity and temporal unfolding of clinical situations. Narratives, to be an effective learning strategy, must be read imaginatively by the reader. Conjuring up the sense of risks and opportunities in the narratives will allow the reader to rehearse their own agency or sense of risk and responsibility in the situation. Connecting the sense of risk, opportunity, and satisfaction creates a sentient compass to practice issues that will aid the reader in developing perceptual acuity and sensibilities. Narratives depict embodied quasi-emotional, fuzzy recognition of impending changes complete with felt uncertainties that are common in practice. Academic settings err on the side of making problems clearer than actual clinical situations. Yet the expert nurse must become adept at reading open ended under-determined clinical situations.

We recommend augmenting case studies, which include all the information required for analyzing a clinical situation, with narratives (such as the ones included in this book), in order to help students confront the inherent ambiguities in complex and under-determined clinical situations. Such imaginative rehearsal is good for developing a sense of moral imagination and agency. Knowing moral principles is not sufficient for recognizing when the moral principles are relevant (Benner & Wrubel, 1982; Blum, 1980; Vetleson, 1994). For example, one can be against racism in principle, but fail to recognize racist attitudes and behaviors in practice, such as preferential treatment given to clients closest to one's own ethnicity. Narratives reveal perception because the narrator gives a dramatic account of noticing or having issues come into awareness in actual clinical situations. The narrator may exaggerate to make a point or leave out aspects considered irrelevant, therefore narratives must be read not as comprehensive or propositional accounts, but rather as accounts of experiential learning. Rational-technical accounts are still more comprehensive and economical for mastering the scientific and clinical facts of practice, but narrative accounts bridge part of the gap between textbook descriptions and actual clinical manifestations.

This textbook cannot replace the necessary science and procedural knowledge that the clinician must master. We strongly warn the reader against a too literal reading of the narratives as concrete instructions for actions. Rather, the narratives provide practical accounts of the logic of practice. Narratives demonstrate the ways that ethical, clinical, and scientific reasoning are linked in actual practice. They allow the reader to prepare for actual temporalities and ambiguities of practice, complete with the inherent contingencies and imperfections. Feeling the risks and ambiguities, as well as the possibilities, in actual clinical situations allows readers to imagine better possibilities while preparing for current realities. Each reader can bring new interpretations and nuances and enrich the text by critical reading and thinking-in-action. The clinician's understanding of the situation guides what is in the foreground and background. This grasp of the situation is embodied so that it orients attentiveness and action in the situation. One can never be beyond experiential learning or error. Patient safety demands that we learn from all system and practice breakdowns so that we continually engage in a self-improving practice. Mistakes do not start out as mistakes…they become mistakes as time unfolds (Weick & Sutcliffe, 2001). Being a human expert is not to be beyond learning or mistakes, but it does require the courage to stay curious and open to learning from mistakes.

SUMMARY

Nurses' work, illustrated by the interviews and observation of their intensive caregiving, demonstrates the care of embodied, sentient persons is a fragile practice. This work is animated by many lifeworld traditions and moral sources in our diverse sample. We are encouraged by the "dispersed forms of goodness" (O'Neill, 1996; see Chapter 11) evident in our interviews with, and observations of, nurses. The many concrete reports of protecting vulnerabilities, of providing comfort and safety, and of attentiveness and beneficence are a source of encouragement and are a remarkable achievement in the midst of rapidly changing work environments. But we also found that this societally important work is being threatened. We are alarmed by the discouragement and demoralization of nurses who are asked to do more than is possible and who are not given the time to do their caregiving work. When nurses are not given the time to be attentive, the large scale health care systems we have created become dangerous places.

REFERENCES

Beauchamp, T. L., & Childress, J. F. (1994). *Principles of biomedical ethics* (4th ed.). New York, NY: Oxford University Press.

Bass, D. C., Dyskstra, C. (2008). *For life abundant: Practical theology, theological education and Christian ministry*. Grand Rapids, MI: Eerdmans.

Benner, P. (1984). *From novice to expert: Excellence and power in clinical nursing practice*. Menlo Park, CA: Addison-Wesley.

Benner, P. (1984/2000). *From novice to expert: Excellence and power in clinical nursing practice*. Menlo Park, CA: Addison-Wesley.

Benner, P. (Ed.). (1994a). *Interpretive phenomenology: Embodiment, caring, and ethics in health and illness*. Thousand Oaks, CA: Sage.

Benner, P. (1994b). The role of articulation in understanding practice and experience as sources of knowledge in clinical nursing. In J. Tully (Ed.), *Philosophy in an age of pluralism: The philosophy of Charles Taylor in question* (pp. 136-155). New York, NY: Cambridge University Press.

Benner, P. (1994c). The role of articulation in understanding practice and experience as sources of knowledge in clinical nursing. In J. Tully (Ed.), *Philosophy in an age of pluralism: The philosophy of Charles Taylor in question* (pp. 136-155). New York: Cambridge University.

Benner, P. (In Press). Formation in professional education: An examination of the relationship between theories of meaning and theories of the self. *Journal of Medicine and Philosophy*, (In Press).

Benner, P., Stannard, D., & Hooper, P. L. (1996). A "thinking-in-action" approach to teaching clinical judgment: A classroom innovation for acute care advanced practice nurses. *Advanced Practice Nursing Quarterly, 1*(4), 70-77.

Benner, P., Sutphen, M., Leonard, V., & Day, L. (2010) *Educating nurses: A call for radical transformation.* San Francisco, CA: Jossey-Bass and Carnegie Foundation for the Advancement of Teaching.

Benner, P., Tanner, C. A., & Chesla, C. A. (1996). *Expertise in nursing practice: Caring, clinical judgment, and ethics.* New York, NY: Springer Publishing Company.

Benner, P., Tanner, C. A., & Chesla, C. A. (2009). *Expertise in nursing practice: Caring, clinical judgment, and ethics.* New York, NY: Springer Publishing Company.

Benner, P., & Wrubel, J. (1982). Clinical knowledge development: The value of perceptual awareness. *Nurse Educator, 7,* 11-17.

Benner, P., & Wrubel, J. (1989). *The primacy of caring.* Menlo Park, CA: Addison-Wesley.

Benner, P. (2000). The roles of embodiment, emotion and lifeworld for rationality and agency in nursing practice. *Nursing Philosophy*, 1(1), 5-19.

Blum, L. (1980). *Compassion.* Berkeley, CA: University of California Press.

Blum, L. (1994). *Moral Perception and Particularity.* Cambridge, MA: Cambridge University Press.

Bourdieu, P. (1980/1990). *The logic of practice* (Richard Nice, Trans.). Stanford, CA: Stanford University Press.

Bowker, G. C., & Star, S. L.(2000). *Sorting things out: Classification and its consequences.* Cambridge, MA: MIT University Press.

Charron, R. (2001). Narrative medicine, a model for empathy, reflection, profession and trust. *Journal of American Medical Association*, 286(15), 1897-1902.

Day, L. (1999). *Nursing care of potential organ donors: An articulation of ethics, etiquette and practice.* (Doctoral dissertation, University of California San Francisco, School of Nursing).

Day. L., (2009). Evidence-based practice, rule-following, and nursing expertise. *American Journal of Critical Care*, Sep;18(5):479-82.

Damasio, A. R. (1994). *Descartes error: Emotion, reason and the human brain.* New York: Putnam.

Damasio, A. (1999). *The feeling of what happens: Body and emotion in the making of consciousness.* New York, NY: Harcourt.

Diekelmann, N. (1989). The nursing curriculum: Lived experiences of students. In *Curriculum revolution: Reconceptualizing nursing education* (pp. 25-41). New York, NY: National League for Nursing.

Dreyfus, H., & Dreyfus, S. (1996). The relationship of theory and practice in the acquisition of skill. In Benner, P., Tanner, C. & Chesla, C. (Eds.), *Expertise in nursing practice: Caring, clinical judgment, and ethics* (pp. 29-47). New York, NY: Springer Publishing Company.

Dreyfus, H., Dreyfus, S., & Benner, P. (1996). Implications of the phenomenology of expertise for teaching and learning everyday skillful ethical comportment. In Benner, P., Tanner, C. & Chesla, C. (Eds.), *Expertise in nursing practice: Caring, clinical judgment, and ethics* (pp. 258-279).

Dreyfus, H. L. (1979). *What computers can't do: The limits of artificial intelligence.* (Revised ed.). New York, NY: Harper & Row.

Dreyfus, H. L. (1992). *What computers still can't do: A critique of artificial reason.* Cambridge, MA: MIT University Press.

Dreyfus, H. L., & Dreyfus, S. E. (1986). *Mind over machine: The power of human intuition and expertise in the era of the computer.* New York, NY: Free Press.

Dykstra, C. (1999). *Growing in the life of faith: Education and Christian practices.* Louisville, KY: Geneva Press.

Eraut, M. (2004). *Developing professional knowledge and competence.* Philadelphia, PA: Falmer Press, Taylor and Francis Inc.

Foster, C. R., Dahill, L. E., Golemon, L. A., & Tolentino, B. W. (2005). *Educating clergy: Teaching practices and pastoral imagination.* San Francisco, CA: Jossey-Bass.

Frankford, D. M. (1994). Scientism and economism in the regulation of health care. *Journal of Politics, Policy and Law, 19*(4), 773-799.

Gadamer, H. (1975/1960). *Truth and method* (G. Barden J. Cumming, Trans.). New York, NY: Seabury.

Geertz, C. (1987). Deep play: Notes on the Balinese cockfight. In P. Rabinow & W. Sullivan (Eds.), *Interpretive social science: A second look.* Berkeley, CA: University of California Press.

Greenspan, M. (2007). *Running toward: Reframing possibility and finitude through physicians' stories at the end of life.* (Doctoral Dissertation, Department of Social and Behavioral Sciences, University of California San Francisco).

Hooper, P. L. (1995). *Expert titration of multiple vasoactive drugs in post-cardiac surgical patients: An interpretive study of clinical judgment and perceptual acuity.* (Doctoral dissertation, University of California at San Francisco, San Francisco, School of Nursing).

Kassirer, J., & Gory, G. A. (1970). Clinical problem solving: A behavioral analysis. *Annals of Internal Medicine, 89,* 245-255.

Lave, J., & Wenger, E. (1991). *Situated learning: Legitimate peripheral participation.* New York, NY. Cambridge University Press.

Logstrup, K. (1995). *Metaphysics.* (Vol. 1). Milwaukee, WI: Marquette University.

MacIntyre, A. (1981). *After virtue: A study in moral theory.* Notre Dame, IN: University of Notre Dame Press.

Mc Niesh, S. (2008). *The lived experience of students' formation in an accelerated nursing program: Taking up the existential skills of the practice.* (Doctoral Dissertation, University of California, San Francisco, School of Nursing).

Noe, A. (2009). *Out of our heads: Why you are not your brain, an other lesions from the biology of consciousness.* New York, NY: Hill and Wang.

O'Neill, O. (1996). *Towards justice and virtue, a constructive account of practical reasoning.* Cambridge, MA: Cambridge University Press.

Polanyi, M. (1958/1962). *Personal knowledge: Towards a post-critical philosophy.* Chicago, IL: University of Chicago Press.

Rodriguez, L. (2007). *Student and faculty experiences of practice breakdown and error in nursing school.* (Doctoral Dissertation, University of California, San Francisco, School of Nursing).

Rubin, J. (2009). Impediments to the development of clinical knowledge and ethical judgment in critical care nursing. In P. Benner, C. A. Tanner, & C. A. Chesla (Eds.), *Expertise in nursing practice: Caring, clinical judgment, and ethics* (pp. 171-198). New York, NY: Springer Publishing Company.

Schon, D. (1987). *The reflective practioner: How professional think in action.* New York, NY: Basic Books.

Schon, D. (1991). *Educating the reflective practitioner: Toward a new design for teaching and learning in the professions.* San Francisco, CA: Jossey-Bass.

Stannard, D. (1997). *Reclaiming the house: An interpretive study of nurse-family interactions and activities in critical care.* (Doctoral dissertation, University of California, San Francisco, San Francisco).

Sullivan, W. & Rosin, M. (2008). *A new agenda for higher education. Shaping the life of a mind for practice.* San Francisco, CA: Jossey-Bass.

Sunvisson, H., Haberman, B., Weiss, S.M., (2009). Augmenting the Cartesian medical discourse with an understanding of the person's lifeworld, lived body, life story and identity. *Nursing Philosophy.* Oct; 10(4): 241-52.

Tannenbaum, S. J. (1994). Knowing and acting in medical practice: The epistemological politics of outcomes research. *Journal of Health Politics, Policy and Law, 19*(1), 27-44.

Taylor, C. (1989). *Sources of the self: The making of the modern identity.* Cambridge, MA: Harvard University Press.

Taylor, C. (1993). Explanation and practical reason. In M. Nussbaum & A. Sen (Eds.), *The Quality of Life.* Oxford, UK: Clarendon.

Vetleson, A. J. (1994). *Perception, empathy, and judgment, an inquiry into the preconditions of moral performance.* University Park, PA: Pennsylvania State University Press.

Weick, K. E., & Sutcliffe, K. M. (2001). *Managing the unexpected: Assuring high performance in an age of complexity.* San Francisco, CA: Jossey-Bass.

Weiss, S. M., Malone, R. E., Merighi, J. R., & Benner, P., (2002). Economism, efficiency, and the moral ecology of good nursing practice. *Canadian Journal of Nursing Research, 34*(2), 95-119.

2

Clinical Grasp and Clinical Inquiry: Problem Identification and Clinical Problem Solving

*C*linical judgment is considered "judgment" because certainty is missing. Thinking and judgment are required to act in situations that are ambiguous, somewhat underdetermined, unexpected, or markedly different from one's assumptive set or preconceptions. Excellent clinical practice requires attunement and timing that are responsive to the unfolding and ever-changing clinical situation. Through experience, one learns to sense what it is like to have a good clinical understanding or grasp of a situation, and what it feels like to be puzzled or have a lack of grasp. This is a form of embodied tacit knowledge, available only to nurses who have learned from previous situations that were similar or markedly different from the current situation. For the expert, clinical inquiry, which is the search for understanding or puzzle solving, is initiated by a lack or even a temporary loss of grasp. This is illustrated in the following exemplar from Julie Chappo, a medical nurse, involving a "very demanding and difficult" patient:

Nurse: One morning, my patient was Nike whom I previously had assisted with his care. His assigned nurse clashed with him and she traded patients because she felt that he was too demanding and she couldn't please him. He was a complex patient requiring almost one on one care. I had three other patients who each had issues that day so I was prepared to be busy. I read over Nike's chart to give more information that would help me in his care. I planned to spend extra time with him.

Nike was a 38-year-old who was admitted with hypoxia and CHF. He had multiple complications from Juvenile Rheumatoid Arthritis and long-term prednisone therapy. He was wheelchair bound and he had suffered several compression fractures. His stature had decreased 6 inches. He had a history of bowel obstruction and previous bowel surgeries. It was suspected that he may have aspirated and had a partial small bowel obstruction this admission.

On morning rounds Nike was sleeping and I immediately noticed the great difficulty he was having breathing. He was on oxygen and, even in his sleep, he was using his accessory muscles to breathe. I thought to myself that something was not right. His frail body was bent over and his abdomen was protruding. He had severe kyphosis.

I woke Nike and he seemed glad to see me. He recognized me from the weekend. We talked about his breathing and he told me his shortness of breath was a recent problem in the last 10 days. He had not been on oxygen at home. He stated, "I can't get comfortable in this bed." We conferred and decided I would get Nike in a more upright position in his wheelchair. His biox was good despite his shortness of breath. When I assessed his bowels, Nike stated that his abdomen was always distended. He had gone through laxatives and enemas the day before. His physician came into the room and also noted his "huffing and puffing." She ordered a CXR, KUB, and made him strictly NPO.

Nike did do better in his wheelchair. His breathing was easier so I had Nike work on his incentive spirometry. We set goals. Nike was more relaxed and we talked about his RA [rheumatoid arthritis] and the different treatments he had tried. We talked about his family and the closeness he had with his brothers. He lives with one brother and two live close by. They each take shifts caring for Nike. Nike said, "I like to make jokes with my family and friends and be the life of the party when I feel well." I monitored his respiratory status closely, checking his biox frequently. His lung sounds were diminished. The physician kept in contact with me through the day about his condition.

Nike tired easily and I got him back in bed. With any movement he became short of breath and it took awhile for him to recover. He was difficult to turn or position in bed. Nike needed his neck supported at all times. He would say, "Move my pillow, I can't breathe." I would do this and touch his shoulder and ask if this was better. He would say "yes," but it only lasted a few minutes before he needed repositioned again. I was frustrated trying to get Nike comfortable and ease his struggle to breathe. I kept my charge nurse informed throughout the day because I needed help coordinating the care of my other patients. I still had the feeling Nike was going to take a turn for the worse.

Later in the day Nike's condition deteriorated. His phone rang and he was too short of breath to talk. His brother on the phone was concerned and said he was coming to the hospital. Nike's respirations were up to 36 a minute and talking was too much effort. His biox was stable, but I knew this was not always the best indicator. I called his physician to report the change in respirations. I also reported Nike's low urine output. He had been incontinent, but had not voided in 4 hours. It was difficult to assess his bladder because his abdomen was so protuberant. I did a bladder scan, which revealed over 1000cc. The physician ordered ABG's and a foley catheter. After the foley was inserted and his bladder was emptied, Nike's respiration eased slightly. His abdomen remained distended and tight.

The results of the ABG's were not good. I called the physician and reported the results and that Nike felt worse. Nike's brother and a close family friend were at his bedside. The physician came quickly. Nike's friend stated that it scared him to see Nike this way. I told him I was glad that they had come to support Nike.

The physician spoke to Nike and his brother about the possibility of the need for a respirator and the need for a NG to relieve the pressure in his abdomen. Nike was frightened at what he heard. His hands were shaking. I held his hand and explained that he be moving to an area that could watch him more closely. Nike asked questions about the respirator. I told him the respirator would be used if needed to make his breathing easier.

I moved Nike to the Progressive Care Unit that evening. The transfer went smoothly. I had planned ahead and didn't let things escalate into a crisis. I coordinated the care of my other patients so I could be with Nike as needed. I had a feeling all day that Nike's respiratory status was on the verge of failing. I saw his physician a few days after Nike's transfer and asked about his progress. He had improved. She explained what had happened to him and she thanked me for watching over him so closely.

In conclusion, where one nurse felt Nike was very demanding and difficult; in getting to know Nike as I did, he was a very sweet man who was acutely ill. His shortness of breath, requests for frequent repositioning, and anxiety could be misinterpreted as being needy, when he really was in a respiratory crisis.

Julie, Nike's nurse, had cared for this patient in the past, but did not initially know what was occurring with the patient during this admission, so her initial perception of his responses and demands were shaped by another clinician. Although Julie, at first, plans around another nurse's understanding, she immediately notices that the patient is unexpectedly struggling to breathe. Julie's grasp of Nike's respiratory distress situates her to more accurately understand his irritability, restlessness, and rudeness as discomfort rather than as a "difficult" patient who cannot be pleased. Her openness to to discovering or making better sense of Nike's responses and to having her preconceptions turned around characterizes an expert clinician. Her openness, her attunement to the patient's behavioral responses being linked to his physiological ones, and her sense of the puzzle (her uneasiness that "something was not right") generates the problem search. Central to clinical problem solving are the ethical issues of discerning whether to probe the possibility that the patient's frustrating behaviors stem from pain, discomfort, or a physiological problem or to accept the deleterious labeling of him as "demanding". This is a moral judgment not only for the patient but also for the nurses. Julie corrects the other nurse's perception of this patient as well as her own. In situations of <u>breakdown</u> (a situation that does not go well) such as this, a nurse's clinical and ethical understanding of the situation can easily be clouded by the adamant, judgmental or harsh comments of others. Her judgment is altered and her uneasiness is better understood as the patient's physiological status unquestionably deteriorated.

This nurse's account of experiential clinical learning also illustrates the timing and logistics (x-rays, blood gases, bladder scan, foley, et cetera) for responding to the clinical changes or transitions in an emergent situation. For example, even after Julie initially gets the patient more comfortable, her suspicions that he is on the edge of deterioration makes her take immediate action to warn the physician when Nike cannot take the phone call. The exemplar or narrative account illustrates how the nurse gains a clearer grasp of the situation by engaging in <u>modus operandi thinking</u>. Modus operandi thinking is detective-like thinking where the clinician recognizes a wrong hypothesis or diagnosis, figures out the source of the breakdown, and hones in on a corrective intervention.

Learning the expected time tables and signs of progress enables the expert clinician to recognize when these are missing. Gaining an understanding, or clinical grasp, of the patient's situation is a perceptual skill that enables the clinician to recognize when he or she does <u>not</u> have a good grasp of a clinical situation. Recognizing clinical transitions in the patient's physiological condition and gaining a good clinical grasp of its meaning direct the therapeutic interventions. Thus, gaining a good clinical grasp is a skill that requires experiential learning, the requisite theoretical background, and the development of perceptual acuity about subtle clinical changes. The sense of whether or not one has a good clinical grasp of situation directs her worry and concern with subsequent exploration, problem solving, and intervention. Gaining a good clinical grasp is the orienting activity (i.e. the way the nurse situates his or her actions and plans as a result of paying attention when the patient's condition is changing).

For developing clinicians and for experts in unfamiliar situations, a good clinical grasp is gained by thinking in the situation and reasoning through transitions in the patient's condition.

TABLE 2.1
Four Aspects of Clinical Grasp

▩ Making qualitative distinctions

▩ Engaging in detective work, modus operandi thinking, and clinical puzzle solving

▩ Recognizing changing clinical relevance

▩ Developing clinical knowledge in specific patient populations

Through this practice of thinking and reasoning, clinicians develop habits of thought and action. Nike's nurse details her thinking and reasoning in the midst of the patient's physiological deterioration. Her ability to gain an accurate grasp hinges on monitoring and making sense of Nike's responses over time as various interventions and tests are performed. The nurse's subsequent actions are based upon these. This exemplar demonstrates that, no matter how well developed "best practice" and evidence-based protocols or guidelines become, clinical puzzles that arise everyday cannot be solved without engaged thinking and clinical reasoning in and through the <u>specific</u> context of each individual situation. A better or poorer grasp in clinical situations guides thinking-in-action. This chapter focuses on articulating four distinct aspects of thinking and reasoning within this habit of thought–clinical grasp. Table 2.1 lists the four aspects of clinical grasp that are pervasive in expert nursing practice.

As clinicians experientially learn in practice, fewer clinical situations present as puzzles to them because some transitions in the patient's condition are predictable. For instance, a pattern of hemodynamic changes are expected in hypothermic cardiac surgical patients in the immediate post-operative period when they begin to re-warm. Another predictable transition is the sudden rise in intracranial pressure in a head injured patient during suctioning and turning. In the following example, a predictable time of vulnerability after angioplasty is anticipated by the nurse:

Nurse: I turned the heparin off at 6:00 which is pretty standard protocol, and if patients are going to re-occlude, they re-occlude within an hour or so of turning off the heparin. At 7:10, she developed chest pains...we did a 12 lead [EKG] and I put the heparin back on and we gave some morphine for the pain. The pain abated some but the morphine didn't take it all away. The cardiologist bumped the first open-heart case and she was in the OR at 8:00.

Recognizing and responding to this predictable transition requires recognition of the change and then a rapid response and mobilization of resources. The nurse's understanding of known risks guides preparation of the environment and vigilance. Setting up for therapies is also guided by predictable transitions and time frames, as pointed out by a pediatric critical care advanced practice nurse regarding a seven-year-old child in septic shock:

Advanced Practice Nurse: Well, my immediate concern is to make sure the nurses know how to <u>recognize</u> septic shock and how to respond to it, because it's not something that we see very often and he [child in septic shock] doesn't look critically ill... Kids can be in septic shock and be awake and alert... That kid [pointing to another child in the unit] is easy to recognize; he or any other post-op cardiac surgery patient looks like they're critically ill because they're intubated, they have chest tubes, they have their own pacemakers, they're on dopamine, dobutamine, epinephrine, or whatever. It's easy to see that that kid's critically ill. It's not so easy to recognize this kid [in septic shock] is as critically ill, to be perfectly honest with you. He comes in with a blood pressure of 100/35, and has gram negative rods growing out of his blood, and has a systemic rash, and if <u>we</u> don't get lines in him, get a blood gas on him, get these antibiotics, get fluid boluses, start the Dopamine... If we don't do those things, 'boom, boom, boom, boom' like we're used to doing with that [other] kid, then we'll lose him. The next thing you know, he'll be bradycardic and we'll be intubating him emergently, and we'll never get caught up. This is the kind of disease that you have to <u>catch</u> in this stage or it becomes irreversible; you get irreversible acidosis and multi-organ failure, so... It's just recognizing that for nurses. And just really being on top of it... (Observational Interview).

This advanced practice nurse emphasized the life-saving importance of recognitional (or grasp) skills in this septic child's condition and clinical trajectory. In this situation, as in many, the timing of the recognition is vital. Early recognition, when the child is still awake, alert and stable, is key in preventing the irreversible cascade of multiorgan damage and failure. Her vigilance in ensuring that other nurses do not miss the narrow window for rescue points out the practical difficulty of giving someone else your grasp. A good clinical grasp of the child's emergent situation, despite his seemingly stable presentation, was essential to initiating aggressive intervention in order to prevent imminent, irreversible and rapid deterioration.

In expert practice, predictable transitions in the patient's status and responses are readily perceived and the nurse continues to have a good clinical grasp without experiencing confusion. However, a clinical transition is often recognized when the clinician senses definite changes, or a cluster of subtle changes that tell the clinician that she/he no longer has a good grasp of the situation. The working definitions of the situation no longer hold and a problem search begins. If plausible alternative explanations of the problem are readily apparent, then deliberative rationality (stepping back and reflecting on the most plausible and probable alternatives) can lead to a clearer understanding of the problem and provide new directions for intervention (Dreyfus and Dreyfus, 1986). Incidence and prevalence data can assist in evaluating plausible competing explanations. However, if no plausible alternative explanation fits the clinical signs and symptoms, stepping outside of all current understandings of the situation is necessary. Redefining and reframing the situation and a more comprehensive problem analysis are required. Critical thinking and letting go of prior assumptions are required in order to gain a new grasp of the situation.

The nurse enters the clinical situation with the goal of gaining a good clinical grasp. Initial assessments are oriented toward gaining a clearer understanding of the patient's clinical situation, responses, and trends. Central to gaining a good clinical grasp is discerning between competing explanations of the patient's condition or needs. Clinical grasp is anchored by prior understandings gained and anticipated possible futures learned from caring for previous particular patients. At the very heart of clinical judgment is the discernment skill of making <u>qualitative distinctions</u> which are judgments about qualities and changes in the patient that can only be made in the context of the situation (Benner, Tanner & Chesla, 2009; Rubin, 2009).

MAKING QUALITATIVE DISTINCTIONS

Recognizing what is salient and making important qualitative distinctions requires experiential learning and situated judgment. By qualitative distinctions, we mean those distinctions that can only be made in a particular, contextual, or historical situation. One may misinterpret the situation if the immediate history, the understanding of the relationships involved, or the context are overlooked or removed. The distinction is qualitative because one cannot make it by objectifying the situation; that is, one cannot decontexualize the aspects and features of the situation, quantify all the relevant variables, and still understand the relevance of the "facts" of the situation. For example, is the patient actively withdrawing for self-protection or is the patient losing consciousness? The clinician's understanding of the patient's response would be strongly influenced if the patient had just sustained a significant head injury. Another example from clinical observation is provided by a flight nurse who was transporting a baby from a community hospital:

> **Nurse:** He just sped up. He's 127 [heart rate] now. His heart rate was only 90, now he's 122; cuff pressure's 107/62; his CO_2 is 37; his sat's still 100%; now he's come back down to 116 (Observational Interview).

In this example, the nurse notices the baby's heart rate has "sped up." Without knowing that the baby had received vecuronium (a paralytic agent) earlier at the time of intubation, one could easily misinterpret the increased heart rate as something other than a sign that the vecuronium was wearing off. For this expert nurse, making the clinical distinction guided her ongoing grasp of the baby's condition and transition as normal rather than as a symptom of instability or an ensuing complication.

Making qualitative distinctions not only informs the nurse about a patient's normal responses, but also commonly assists the nurse to rapidly hone in on a complication and initiate immediate treatment. In the following situation, a 60 year-old man had been in a car accident, lost his left arm below the elbow, had a tracheostomy inserted in the ICU, recovered, and was discharged. He had been in the clinic for follow-up just a few days before being seen back in the clinic by a trauma advanced practice nurse. The following occurred while observing the advanced practice nurse and the patient:

> **Advanced Practice Nurse:** [Enters patient's room] Hi. How are you doing? H., I'm not sure if you remember me, I'm Beth[1].
>
> **Patient:** You changed my bandage...
>
> **Advanced Practice Nurse:** Yeah, I changed your bandage. How's it going?
>
> **Patient:** Umm, actually, not real good.
>
> **Advanced Practice Nurse:** What's going on?
>
> **Patient:** I feel like there's a blockage or obstruction in my throat. And I feel like I'm wheezing and stuff.
>
> **Advanced Practice Nurse:** Come sit down right here (on the exam table).
>
> **Patient:** When I breathe in or get hot or do anything real strenuous or...
>
> **Advanced Practice Nurse:** Hang on just a second because I have a feeling I want to track down one of the attendings real quick. [Quickly leaves the room to find the physician who is getting ready to leave] (Observational Interview).

---

[1]The real names of people and places, or other identifying information, have been changed in all of the stories throughout this book in order to maintain confidentiality.

The advanced practice nurse was later asked what she recognized:

Interviewer: ...when you said, 'How are you doing?' and he said, 'Not so good', then your whole way of being with him just changed, I thought.

Advanced Practice Nurse: Oh, it probably did. Well, I think too that I knew before I walked in the room that the patient was coming in—<u>he</u> requested the appointment, because I went up and looked, and he requested the appointment. So I knew that something else was going on with him. The only issue that we [trauma service] really had with him is that we did the trachea. And, his other injuries were well taken care of by other services, and so there wasn't a lot that we were really following him for. Before he was discharged, I was always concerned about his trachea just because once we took out the tracheal tube he still had a lot of discharge through the stoma. But I knew something was wrong with him. As soon as he talked, you could hear there was something wrong with him. And he ended up having subglottic stenosis and he's having surgery today [the morning after the clinic visit] (Observational Interview).

Knowing the patient's history and his normal voice helped the advanced practice nurse immediately recognize or "hear" that a major complication was developing and identify the problem. She immediately got the physician involved because she knew "he [the patient] has something big going on" and needed a physician to confirm it and refer the patient for surgery. Qualitative distinctions of this nature are often accompanied by an emotional quality as the clinician recognizes the meaning of the patient's responses. The patient's high risk for completely occluding his airway prompted the advanced practice nurse's urgent actions, and led to immediately taking the patient to surgery.

Some qualitative distinctions can be made only by knowing the particular patient's responses over time. Here, "knowing" refers to skillful discernment that is perceived through the body—the senses—but may be difficult to clearly articulate. During a clinical observation, a burn nurse tries to convey a meaningful distinction in skin temperature that guides the patient's fluid management after the physician decreased the intravenous (IV) fluid replacement rate:

Nurse: I probably would not have backed down as far as she [physician] did because she backed down our urine goals. I would have kept his urine output according to protocol. But she backed those goals down. So with her backing those goals down, yes, I'm comfortable with backing his IV fluids down. <u>However</u>, I will be very careful and scrutinize the patient very closely, because in under an hour, we went from 1100 down to 750 (cc's of IV fluid per hour), and that's a <u>huge</u> jump. And he may be just fine with it. No problem. But we just have to keep an eye on him.

Interviewer: So what are you keeping an eye on?

Nurse: His heart rate. His urine output. His extremities are still going to be cool, but you'll still be able to tell how he's doing just by looking at him and the first eight hours after a burn, you have the biggest capillary loss. So you have to give the most fluid during that period of time. So, basically his urine output, his heart rate, and he's going to be cool to touch, but make sure he doesn't get any cooler. Make sure he doesn't just totally shut down and that type of thing. He's going to be cool. You don't have real decent capillary closure—you begin to have capillary closure at the end of the first

24 hours, then you have complete capillary closure at the end of 48. So you don't really expect them to be really <u>totally</u> warm until the next day, but you don't want them ice cold. If they're ice cold, they're not perfusing. They're too dry.

Interviewer: Where did you learn that distinction? ...it sounds like a gray area, ice cold versus cold...

Nurse: Over and over and over. Just putting your hands on them. But something I teach my orientees is don't just look at your numbers. Put your hands on them. Because that tells you almost more than the numbers do because you have pain problems [which alter the numbers], you have all these problems with burns, so feeling their extremities is a really, <u>really</u> good way to tell how dry they are (Observational Interview).

This expert nurse is describing a qualitative distinction between cold and ice cold that can be perceived only by touching the patient. She points out how good clinical judgment depends on gaining a "feel" for this patient in order to keep track of his skin temperature over time. Because the objective data from the monitors can be skewed by multiple physiological changes, the numbers alone are less reliable as an indication of fluid status than the numbers plus a good clinician's perceptual acuity. The nurse's understanding of the complex pathophysiological processes and her experience have taught her that cool skin is normal for burn patients in the first 24 hours. However, "ice cold" skin warns of intravascular volume depletion, which will compromise end-organ perfusion and prompts increased fluid replacement. The nurse then talks about why this distinction holds significance for the patient:

Nurse: ...if [the burn area] is full thickness, they'll have to go in and take it [eschar] off, excise it surgically to remove it and put some graft on. But you always have an area outside of that that is partial thickness. If you give good fluid resuscitation, and if you perfuse that area, you're not going to increase the depth of burn so it takes us a couple of days to actually see, especially burns that are marginal. He has several marginal burns. Some on his upper arms. He may just have a partial-thickness or second degree burn, but we really can't make strong determinations of that until after a couple of days (Observational Interview).

Not perfusing the partial-thickness burn areas can potentially increase the depth of the burn. The nurse recognizes that vigilance in continually monitoring the patient's skin temperature can make a difference in his outcome as well as the types and extent of interventions necessary. This example highlights the direct link among clinical grasp, judgment, and intervention.

Although many distinctions can only be made by knowing a specific patient, other distinctions can be made based on knowing a patient population; that is, knowing typical responses and patterns, trends and recovery trajectories, and the anticipated complications in patient populations with similar clinical conditions. Patients who suffer from the same illness or disease not only have similar responses but will also typically have similar qualities of responses. For instance, patients in acute congestive heart failure have a cough, but the quality of the cough differs from patients who are coughing from emphysema or pneumonia. A heart failure patient tends to have a dry, hacky cough while the patient with emphysema tends to have a long, productive, hollow, and sometimes wheezy cough. Expert nurses learn to make fine qualitative distinctions, as exemplified by a burn nurse during a clinical observation:

> **Nurse:** ...I would suspect he may need some surgery to his legs, but he may not. It just depends. We'll just have to see over the course of—But that's definitely his deepest area [calves and thighs].
>
> **Interviewer:** [looking at the wounds] I still, I looked and looked after you told me, but I can't...
>
> **Nurse:** You just have to do it a lot. It was a different kind of pink. It was a bad pink. It wasn't a good pink (laughs as she struggles to describe the difference).
>
> **Interviewer:** Talk about, as much as you can, describe what good pink looks like versus bad pink.
>
> **Nurse:** Bad pink is paler, dryer, dryer is a big thing.
>
> **Interviewer:** So, the lower part of his legs—what was it that made his legs worse than the upper part? That was shiny? Deeper reddish...
>
> **Nurse:** Because it was kind of a ruddy pale and it wasn't just a pink. See, it is just a lot of gray. And you just have to do it over and over and over (Observational Interview).

This nurse struggles to articulate what she knows, not for lack of scientific knowledge or intelligence, but because these subtle qualitative differences are commonly what Polanyi (1962) refers to as "ineffable" or incapable of being described in words. Although qualitative distinctions in clinical practice are commonly rooted in insight and intuition, gained individually from tacit (incidental; trial-and-error) learning, this kind of knowledge can be deliberatively taught and coached, as noted by the Interviewer above, by focusing one's attention on specific attributes (Polanyi, 1962; Sadler, 1980). When called upon to clarify the subtle distinctions, this nurse makes more visible the wisdom she has tacitly learned by developing the visual acuity to discriminate between a grayish, ruddy pale, and dry pink color versus a shinier, brighter pink. The distinction alerts the nurse to areas that are at high risk for becoming deeper burns.

In this situation, the qualitative distinctions in the burn wound focus on visually noticing differences in color, sheen, and texture that can be compared simultaneously. However, many distinctions require noticing pattern of responses that change over time. Expert physicians have been prominent and vital in teaching nurses to make these qualitative distinctions in particular patient populations and in teaching the implications for intervention. For instance, an advanced practice nurse talked about learning from a cardiac surgeon:

> **Advanced Practice Nurse:** When I was just starting to work with cardiac surgical patients, I had a lot to learn. I was called by the nurse to see a 68-year-old woman who had returned from surgery after a mitral valve replacement. The patient's pulmonary artery (PA) pressures were extremely high, 70/36, and her cardiac index was 1.9 [low]. The nurse was titrating nipride because of the patient's hypertension and dopamine because of her low cardiac output. I expected from this patient's history that her PA pressures would be high post-operatively. But, my concern was, 'How high is high?' At that time, I had no idea what was 'normal' for her. When I arrived, Jill [the nurse] was just barely keeping up with the care of the patient. I started to help Jill and she

explained that one minute, the patient would be severely hypertensive and need high levels of Nipride and the next minute, her arterial pressures would plummet and she'd have to rapidly titrate the Nipride off. I did realize that she was 'chasing' the patient's pressure but I didn't understand what was happening. At that moment, the surgeon happened by and Jill expressed her concerns. As he watched the patient's hemodynamic changes on the monitor, I mentioned that I noticed the cyclic fluctuations in the arterial pressures. He then told Jill to start infusing crystalloids until the fluctuations stopped. I was so surprised! I said, 'Fluids? What about her PA pressures? They are so high.' He taught us that the numbers themselves in these kinds of patients were meaningless because there was no normal. In patients with valvular disease, you monitor trends in the numbers and judge the patient's responses to treatment in the early post-op phase by the direction and stability of the numbers. Then he pointed out that almost any time you see significant arterial pressure fluctuations and find yourself chasing the pressure with Nipride, the patient is hypovolemic, despite the numbers. He left and I was so nervous, but after a half of a liter of fluid had infused, the patient's arterial pressure began to stabilize, the PA pressures increased, and the cardiac index came up. I really didn't understand what I had just seen, so I spent the latter part of the day and evening reading about the pathophysiology and hemodynamics of mitral valve disease. The next day, I talked to the surgeon to clarify my understanding and then used the previous day's situation to inform the staff about the pattern Jill and I could now recognize and understand. Since then, I've learned that that pattern of fluctuation almost always means hypovolemia in any cardiac surgery patient, not just mitral valve patients.

This story highlights the essential clinical knowledge that expert physicians contribute in assisting nurses to develop clinical judgment and skillful interventions. Teaching qualitative distinctions and patterns of responses at the bedside in an unfolding situation commonly enables expert clinicians to grasp and point out to others the big picture, as well as the implications for intervention. Because physicians have, over the decades, helped teach nurses what was traditionally thought of as "medical knowledge," nurses have learned to diagnose and manage sicker and more complex patients. In turn, nurses continue to extend this clinical wisdom by teaching other nurses, medical students, and other physicians to improve the quality of care, limit instability, and limit unnecessary interventions.

Both Taylor (1985a) and Rubin (2009) have written about making qualitative distinctions. Taylor (1995) also uses the term "strong evaluation" to refer to qualitative distinctions that call for an ethical understanding about the notions of goods at issue in a situation. For example, he contrasts, "simple weighing" with strong evaluation. Simple weighing entails only preferences or desires, such as "shall I bathe the patient first or change the IV dressings?" Strong evaluations have to do with taking a stand on what is a worthy or good thing to do. When families, patients, and healthcare providers make ethical judgments about worthy treatments for acutely and critically ill patients, they are potentially making a strong evaluation of whether they are engaging in futile treatments and therefore merely prolonging suffering before death, or whether the proposed treatment has a good chance of saving the patient's life at a level the patient would choose. A strong evaluation can also be about whether they are giving up on a given therapy because of expense or fatigue rather than in the interests of a reasonable chance to save the patient's life. The earlier example of Julie, the nurse, calling the physician that Nick's respiratory condition was deteriorating when she recognized that he was too short of breath to talk on the phone is a strong evaluation of weighing the patient's distress against the probable need for intubation.

Prognostic scoring systems, such as the APACHE III, WPSS or IPSS may guide clinical judgment by assisting clinicians in making the best predictions of survival. However, these systems are reliable only at the very low and very high end of the scales, where it is relatively easy to predict survival or recovery. In the mid-range of the scales, expert human discernment and judgment are required (Knaus et al., 1991; LeGall, Lemeshow & Saulnier, 1993; Lemeshow et al., 1993). Thus, in the mid-range of the scales, regardless of the prognostic score, it is the patient, family, and clinicians who must make the strong evaluation about whether the treatment is humane and heroic or futile and unwise. The import of the decision is both clinical and ethical and is never just a simple weighing of predictive scores.

One strategy for enhancing clinical judgment is to keep a record of the qualitative distinctions that one makes in practice. Because qualitative distinctions are often based on the immediate history, the understanding of the relationships, and the context of the situation, these aspects of the situation would need to be recorded for newer nurses to best understand the distinctions being pointed out. Individuals or groups of clinicians could share stories that exemplify qualitative distinctions. Because a patient's changing condition often requires recognition and intervention from clinicians across disciplines, these distinctions could be contributed by and shared among multidisciplinary groups from multiple disciplines to enhance a community of learning.

Because many qualitative distinctions escape articulation but are easily pointed out in an actual situation, bedside teaching can strongly and effectively enhance learning. Differences in color, temperature, smell, sound, texture, tone, shape, and size can be experienced firsthand by the learner, with an expert to assist in comparing and contrasting what is observed. This method teaches the individual while simultaneously setting up a culture and community of attentiveness, dialogue, and team learning.

For example, the qualitative distinction made in the following interview excerpt is a fairly common one, but little has been written about this common observation; namely, the quality and meanings of a patient's emotional withdrawal and engagement. The nurse describes a chronic critically ill patient who required mechanical ventilation (also cited in Benner, Tanner & Chesla, 2009, p. 221). The patient's will to live and his quality of life are being questioned by the healthcare team:

Interviewer: It sounded like you had a feeling, a strong feeling that he wanted to live. How did that come about and do you know when it came about?

Nurse: I think he always had it. I think he was an incredible fighter. I would see him angry or I would see him withdrawn. But even withdrawn, he was actively withdrawn. He wouldn't look at you. You would try to talk with him and he would follow you, track you in the room and everything, but then he wouldn't look at you... He really derived a lot of pleasure from living. Again, I think they looked at him and they saw, 'this is as good as it gets, and this is really depressing, and he was really depressed and so why continue? This is torture.' What I saw was that this guy is definitely borderline whether he is ever going to get out of here or not but still he was glad to see you. He wanted to watch the ball games—a really big A's (baseball) fan—to me that is not someone who has given up. Somebody who is that manipulative or that active in planning my day is not someone who doesn't want to have to deal with living or doesn't really have the strength to go on.

Reading the patient and understanding his patterns of emotional withdrawal helped this nurse to make a qualitative distinction between interpersonal engagement and withdrawal ("active withdrawal") and passive withdrawal related to depression or relinquishing connections to his life in preparation for death. Central to understanding this patient is coming to know him (Tanner, Benner, Chesla & Gordon, 1993). Identifying central concerns and issues in this particular situation provides the orienting base for making this qualitative distinction that requires <u>reasoning-in-transition</u>; that is, reasoning through a changing situation. It also illustrates <u>modus operandi thinking</u> which refers to keeping track of events, sequences, and patterns to allow the nurse to make qualitative distinctions crucial to the clinical and ethical judgment that the patient has not given up on treatment and hope for recovery.

The earliest distinctions made by nurses as they develop in practice tend to be physiological because the typical priorities of care are necessarily focused on knowing the patient physiologically and managing the patient's physical condition. To become expert, however, clinicians must also learn to make strong emotional, social, spiritual, and ethical evaluations with and about the patient and family because these are inextricably linked to their clinical judgments and interventions. At times, the patient's non-physiological needs must take priority and, in some instances, the nurse is confronted to make this type of judgment <u>without</u> knowing the patient. Based on extensive past similar and dissimilar instances, the expert nurse may instantaneously grasp what is salient about the emotional or spiritual response of the patient without knowing the specific patient, in order to make a weighty distinction in a fleeting moment. In the following exemplar, OR nurse Judy Rumensky reveals how the patient's primary need grabs her attention and compels her to first respond to the emotional and spiritual needs over the physiological needs:

Nurse: It was a night from hell in our OR. We are a Level I trauma center on a hot August night (trauma season). We had all 8 of our trauma rooms going with a wait list of urgent cases that every surgeon was clamoring to go next. The only people free were the anesthesiologist supervising the CRNAs (nurse anesthetists), the orderly, and me. I was in charge.

I got a call from an excited resident saying a patient was crashing in the ICU, and they were coming to the OR. The few details I found out were that it was a 42 year old woman who had been in a motorcycle accident and sustained multiple traumas. She's been in the ICU for a month with a trach and on the vent. That night she began bleeding profusely from around her trach and was getting a mediastinal shift.

I quickly pulled a tech out of the workroom. I moved to the biggest room. I transferred the phones and asked the orderly to man them. The surgeon was new in town (first night on call) so I opened every chest instrument pack I had.

I heard the thundering hooves and ran down the hall to meet the gang of residents and nurses running down the hall with the stretcher. As I reached out to grab the chart, the patient grabbed my hand in a death grip and mouthed the words "Help me!" As I looked at the terror in her eyes, I knew that she sensed the gravity of her situation. She was bleeding out her trach, and the blood was all over the place. I am sure she could see that. We got into the room, she continued to hang onto to my hand, and her eyes never left my face. I can't remember the exact words, but I tried to calm her by telling her what we were doing, that we were taking good care of her.

I heard orders being barked, "Get more blood! Where's the suction? Get more fluids! I need some more gowns! More sponges and tapes!" I knew they were talking to me, but I couldn't let this patient's hand go. She was awake and alert and could see the chaos around her. We moved her to the table. The surgeon and his team went out to scrub. The anesthesiologist pushed the [propofol]. I kept holding her hand, looking at her and telling her I would stay with her. She finally went to sleep. I was the last person she saw. She did not make it through the surgery. Her innominate artery ruptured. Every time her heart beat, her innominate artery pulsed against the cuff of the trach tube and eroded. We weren't quick enough to repair the damaged artery.

I hope she died knowing some nurse had nothing better to do than hold her hand. Because I didn't.

Here, the patient somehow understands how dire her situation has become. Judy immediately grasps that the patient's "death grip," plea for help, and terror in her eyes are qualitatively different from the responses of most frightened patients. In a moment, as the nurse "sees" how very close death is, the patient's response makes a moral claim on her to be fully engaged and present, without distraction. Expert nurses commonly tell us that they never want to be the last person the patient sees, but when it happens, being able to make the distinction about what is at stake (the distinction between what is most important versus what's urgent) determined the nurse's embodied response. Caring came first.. Despite the extreme clinical demands, it was the ethical judgment that the patient needed as she closed her eyes. In those few moments, others in the room responded to the clinical demands until the patient was sufficiently medicated to fall asleep.

The nature of the qualitative distinctions described thus far all relate to perceptual grasp of the "patient's" condition (physiological, emotional, spiritual, etc). In contrast, developing nurses are confronted by difficult, weighty, and sometimes adverse situations that challenge them to make moral distinctions about who they themselves are as nurses and in relation to their patients. These distinctions are born from the notion of what it is to be a good nurse and subsequently guide the care that the nurse is able to compassionately provide. The nurse's ability to make good and strong moral distinctions can be transformative, as told by Jan Vincent:

Nurse: Tom was a 25-year-old married male who skipped work to spend the day with his girlfriend. After a day of drinking, they were in a horrific motor vehicle accident that resulted in his girlfriend's death. He became a quad[raplegic]. He looked a bit like Frank Zappa—tall, lanky with long flowing hair and a large mustache. His two front teeth were missing. In contrast, his wife was tall, soft-spoken and "bookish-looking." Their daughter was a miniature image of her mom. His parents were always meticulously groomed and always very polite. Tom was their only child.

Tom's physical care was challenging—vent-dependent, halo traction, etc. But after meeting his wonderful wife, parents and 4-year-old daughter, the greater challenge for me was to overcome the anger I felt about him cheating on his wife… During his [prolonged ICU stay], Tom's infidelity was <u>never</u> an issue for his wife and parents. Why should it be for me? It did not help that as a sequel to his head injury, he was always "mouthing/whispering" words in crude terms…Despite my issues with Tom's infidelity, I assured that he received the very best nursing care I could provide. Tom was my patient—not an unfaithful husband.

Tom's first weeks were critical. There were several "life and death" situations that occurred, and we did not know whether he was going to survive. It was during that time I realized how utterly helpless Tom was. His life was literally in my hands. I saw and felt the devastation his condition had on his family. Their emotional state was very fragile. One minute they were focused on the immediate would he live or die? The next they were concerned about long-term issues, financial as well as long-term care. My bias moved to a box in the back of my brain and I focused on the priority— Tom and his family.

Jan goes on to detail the comprehensive and meticulous care that she and the team provided. She tells how she became close to Tom, knew all the "idiosyncrasies specific" to his care, including his favorite position, favorite music, lip gloss, etc. After his prolonged ICU stay, he was finally transferred to a Rehab center:

> **Nurse:** Tom left, his family checked in with me a couple of times, and I called the Rehab center. Two weeks after discharge, Tom died after aspirating Jello. I was devastated. His parents dropped by the ICU several times after his death, always acknowledging the wonderful care Tom received. I was so thankful that I cast aside my personal feelings regarding infidelity and vowed not to judge patients that I really do not know. I am a nurse, first, last, and always.

Jan's honesty and reflection about Tom's infidelity, her struggle to understand the wife's seeming acceptance, and the distinction she makes that enables her to care for Tom in the best way possible exemplifies how many nurses come to terms with "difficult" patients and families. Mentioned, but rarely explored, in a clinician's educational preparation are ways of coping with or working through the many sources of moral conflict that challenge a clinician. Unlike ethical dilemmas that require difficult and competing choices, and where ethicists are more readily available for dialogue and support, moral conflicts of this nature, the everyday ethics of care, continue to either be worked out in daily practice by committed individuals or covered over without resolution for the clinician or patient. Narratives can uncover moral struggles that confound excellent care, make visible the moral distinctions that nurses labor to make, disclose the triumphs in everyday practice, and create a dialogue among clinicians to help developing nurses learn to better cope with inevitable burdens and help newer nurses develop into strong moral agents.

ENGAGING IN DETECTIVE WORK, MODUS OPERANDI THINKING, AND CLINICAL PUZZLE SOLVING

Modus operandi thinking keeps track of the specific situation, the way the situation unfolds, the meanings of the patient's responses that have occurred at the time that they occurred, what has been tried, and what has or has not worked with this patient. It is a kind of reasoning-in-transition; that is, gains (and losses) in understanding that are error-reducing or producing (Benner, 1994a; Taylor, 1993). This is a form of practical clinical reasoning as opposed to formal decision making models. Who could predict? Who could imagine? For example, a nurse from a neonatal intensive care unit describes how some basic interventions need to be tried before withdrawal of therapies is considered:

> **Nurse:** After a lot of hemming and hawing and consulting, the only thing that [the physicians] could figure out was that she [the infant] had hypoplastic lungs, which are pretty difficult to diagnose except on autopsy. Her lungs looked a little bit small on X-ray, but that's really not a very good indicator and the only other thing that might give us any indication would be to do a lung biopsy and she wasn't in any condition to have that done. So we treated her with high frequency ventilation for several days, weaned her off the vent for about a day, and then she had to go back on, and it was back and forth, and this went on for a week and a half. So it got to the point where the ethics committee decided that they needed to meet regarding her because, if in fact she really had hypoplastic lungs, the chances of her surviving long term are at best minimal, and

it was time to decide whether it was appropriate or not to continue. So, another nurse and I were taking care of her consistently and we had had a discussion prior to the meeting. We both kind of had the gut feeling that there was something more going on. It wasn't really anything that we could put our finger on, but we just felt like it wasn't time to just stop. And we voiced that concern during the meeting. We felt that, first of all, in the process of all this intensive care, there were some really basic needs that had not been met. One of those was good nutrition. She had been on TPN [total parenteral nutrition] for awhile but we had to keep her so fluid restricted because she had this tendency towards pulmonary edema, that she really wasn't getting good calories. Not enough certainly to grow or heal on. So we brought that up and the doctors, well, they pooh-poohed nutrition. You can't get better if you're not well nourished. What came out of the meeting was that we would try to improve her nutrition, the best being interval feeds if we could accomplish that. So we were going to get rid of her central lines—she had umbilical lines and we don't like to feed babies that have them in. So we were going to get rid of those lines and try to start some nasogastric feedings, whatever she would tolerate, and see if we could increase her caloric intake.

Interviewer: Was her CO_2 still a problem?

Nurse: It wasn't as much of a problem but she still required the ventilator, although we had managed to get her off high frequency ventilation by this time. So [the physicians] gave us a week to perform a nutritional miracle on the child... But the deal was we would have a week to try and get her ventilator settings down, improve her nutrition, and then at the end of that week we would reevaluate and see if there had been any miraculous improvement. Well, there wasn't a miraculous improvement but there was a significant improvement. She was able to come down on some of her ventilator settings, but we also had to start her on steroids, just as a last ditch effort... And she got better with the steroids. We didn't really accomplish the feedings because she didn't tolerate them at that point in time. But since she had made some progress on her ventilator settings, they decided to keep going with it. I thought it was rather interesting that she improved after the steroids because, if her problem was hypoplastic lungs, steroids aren't really going to do a whole lot for that. So that made me think that she had just had some viral infection or something that really wiped out her lungs, and that she had a lot of inflammation and damage. The steroids might make some difference with that. Or maybe she had both; I mean, certainly her lungs looked small on X-ray, so it's hard to tell. But she did get a little bit better.

Early in this exemplar, the physicians and nurses are involved in the problem search and the commonly occurring clinical detective work that keeps track of likely precipitating events and multiple clinical risks. When the infant does not respond favorably to interventions, the nurses who are closest to the situation or more fully engaged with this baby's realistic possibilities are unwilling to stop or withdraw life support. Because of their modus operandi thinking, the nurses knew that "there were some really basic needs that had not been met" and that "you can't get better if you're not well nourished." By keeping track of what had been tried and what needed to be tried, these nurses prevent premature withdrawal of life-sustaining interventions in order to give the infant a fair chance. As in this situation, modus operandi thinking improves clinical judgment and can influence or alter the patient's course.

As in the above situation, clinicians commonly engage in modus operandi thinking when they disagree on the patient's condition or on the appropriate intervention. Clinicians also become engaged in modus operandi thinking when they experience confusion about the patient's responses or others' interpretation of the patient's responses. For attentive clinicians, a lack of understanding or confusion prompt detective-like thinking. In the following story, the advanced practice nurse describes her confusion:

Advanced Practice Nurse: A girl, who was 15, came into the emergency room, with a [hemato]crit of 14. Brought in by private vehicle with blood all over the back seat and the story was that she fell in glass. And it was a weekend, and I'm rounding with the team and the team is telling me the story and it's like, 'okay,' and I walked in and here's this very small pale child laying in bed, and it looks like the whole bed had just kind of swallowed her up, and the only injury she has are on her wrists. On the inside of her wrists. And I thought...

Interviewer: Wait a minute. Huh?

Advanced Practice Nurse: Nobody thinks of this. And so it was really educating the team. Nobody, nobody thought of this. Nobody on the entire team thought that maybe this story wasn't true. And I remember fighting and then finally they clicked and they said, 'Oh,' and I remember getting child psych in and I was keeping that girl [hospitalized] and coming up with reasons to keep her in the hospital when the intern said, 'Oh no, no, she can go.' I was like, 'Wait, this is a family from [a country where suicide is disgraceful]. There are some issues here, and we need to deal with this girl. We need to make sure that this girl is safe, and I don't care if medically she is safe, we need to do something.' So a lot of that was, not only looking after the patient, taking care of the patient and making sure that the resources were there, but dealing with the medical aspect. And taking care and making sure that the medical team is starting to look at other things, and starting to question things, 'Well, does that story really make sense?' And it was amazing how they all just thought, 'Yeah, that just made perfect sense. Not a problem. That makes perfect sense that this little girl has completely bled out from two cuts on her wrist, and the family didn't bring her in until she had almost bled out.' So, we deal with a lot of those, and there are those kind of things where you walk away saying, you made a big difference.

Interviewer: You were talking with the team? Can you tell us more about what you did?

Advanced Practice Nurse: I think I came out and said, 'Are you people crazy?' (Laughter)

Interviewer: And their response was?

Advanced Practice Nurse: No, I think I just came out and said, 'Has anybody looked at this girl?' And they all just look at you, and it's like, 'Does this make sense? Has anybody really looked at where her wounds are and does this make sense to you?' And they really going to try and defend it...

Interviewer: Do you remember the conversation?

Advanced Practice Nurse: It was almost two and one-half years ago, probably. I think their attempts to defend it were pretty feeble. But it was more like, 'Oh, yeah, but the father brought her in. The father's the one that told us this.' And I looked at him and I said, 'So this father's telling you these stories?' And this is a father who [is very ashamed] and believes that this isn't something that your children do, and it was just trying to get them to [recognize this].

This example illustrates the nurse thinking-in-action; that is, thinking in the midst of the situation and gaining a sense of the whole in relation to the specifics. Having noticed the girl's wrist injuries without other bodily lacerations, the history about falling in glass no longer makes sense and the nurse engages in detective-like thinking and questioning, "Has anybody really looked at where her wounds are and does this make sense to you?" The intern's responses were not reassuring. Hearing that the intern is ready to discharge the patient, the nurse immediately understands the danger for the girl and that the intern has missed the ethical aspect of his decision. By asking her questions out loud and to the physicians, they come to a clearer understanding of the situation.

In the above situation, the advanced practice nurse has an assumptive set or preconceived notions about the possible configurations of lacerations in someone who has fallen into glass:

Advanced Practice Nurse: ...she doesn't have a lot of cuts on her...the story in and of itself didn't make sense that this person was bleeding to death in the back of her father's car and the only way I could see that she is going to have that low of a hematocrit, be bleeding that much, is she's got to have some big major cuts...

Assumptive sets are developed over time with experience in similar situations so that expert clinicians come to embody habits of thinking or perceptual habits (Hooper, 1995). Two matching wrist wounds do not fit the nurse's preconceptions and initiated a problem search.

Nurses with good perceptual habits are then "set to see", to notice, to grasp, to attend to, and to anticipate (Hooper, 1995; Merleau-Ponty, 1964). These habits of thinking and noticing then make it possible to readily identify wrong hypotheses or unexpected responses. In another case, the nurse expressed concern about whether or not the two younger children's scald burns were accidental, as reported by the mother and a 14-year-old:

Nurse: Well, I think that the big deal was—because they arrested the 14-year-old—or didn't arrest him, because she [mother] blamed the 14-year-old at one point too. There was another kid there and she said that the 14-year-old turned the faucet on. The key here is that the children had circumferential burns and there were no splash marks. So what that tells you is that the—especially the two- or three-year-old could've easily jumped up, jumped out, and these kids were burned from the waist down. And there's no signs of trying—even the little one—trying to get out. I mean she was 18 months; that meant she was walking. So these kids—when you see something that's abusive— something like that is pretty straight forward.

Interviewer: How would this look different from a non-abusive situation?

Nurse: You wouldn't see circumferential [burns] first of all. You would see tons of splash marks, you would see struggle like the kid tried to [get out] and usually it would only be like a little area or...

Interviewer: The splash marks would be in a sort of random pattern over other parts of...

Nurse: Mm hum. Depending on where the child was burned. You have to listen to the story and then you have to look at the child's burns, and you have to see it—and you learn to do this. You actually think about it mechanically in your head, 'Okay if this child was in this bath tub...' First of all if they're circumferential, usually that means the kids have somehow been forced down into a situation that they haven't been able to get out of. Because, even an 18-month-old is going to—if they get into too hot of water, they're going to struggle to get the heck out of there. And so, it was pretty obvious, pretty awful.

Upon seeing the pattern of the children's burns and the inconsistency based on her assumptive set, the nurse immediately begins to question the accidental nature of the situations. She perceives that the children were forcefully immersed in hot water due to the lack of splash marks. Without preconceived notions, one may accept the situation as accidental and return the children to a dangerous home environment without involving Child Protective Services. At the same time, the clinician must stay open to other feasible explanations for the burn pattern to avoid inappropriate family disruption.

In a complex clinical situation, clinicians can lose track of where they stand in relation to what they have learned about this particular patient's responses and condition. Keeping track of what has been learned is an active guardianship of an ongoing understanding of the clinical situation. It is an account of what makes sense in the situation and what does not make sense. Modus operandi thinking is situated thinking, an engaged reasoning that takes account of the patient's context, temporal sequence of changes, responses, progress, and failures.

Clinicians can also lose track of the complex and evolving situation when other team members are rapidly and simultaneously intervening or when the nurse must implement multiple simultaneous interventions, each of which alter the patient's responses. Under these circumstances, it may not be possible to understand which interventions improved, failed to affect, or hindered the patient's condition. Even though the clinician can see that the patient's situation is more or less stable, the clinician may not know <u>which intervention</u> made the difference and, consequently, have little understanding about what to do next. To prevent this kind of confusion, skillful clinicians try to implement one therapy at a time if the particular therapies affect the same kinds of patient responses (Hooper, 1995). For instance, in cardiac surgical patients, numerous vasoactive drugs commonly alter the same hemodynamic parameters. To avoid losing one's grasp, one nurse conveyed:

Nurse: When you start moving too many things at one time, you don't know what is happening, what's having the most effect. So, change one and get a feel for what the one thing does before you start manipulating the others.

The maxim "change one thing at a time," although not always possible or prudent, can assist less experienced clinicians in developing modus operandi thinking. It is also helpful for more experienced clinicians to point out, in context, the specific effects and patient responses to particular interventions.

Engaging in detective work to solve a clinical puzzle requires an openness, not only to the physiological issues, but also to any aspect of the patient's well being that can affect his or her condition. Openness is continually needed because very experienced clinicians can still be surprised and learn from situations when something unexpected affects the patient's illness or suffering. Liz Ciyou Allee, a hospice nurse, shares a narrative that invites us to imaginatively engage and think with her through her problem search in a gentleman dying of cancer:

Nurse: One night when I was in charge, a particular patient had been difficult to handle due to his symptoms being out of control regarding pain. I took six patients and included him in my assignment. After report, Larry was my first stop. I could hear him moaning way down that hall. As I entered, his very anxious wife was standing faithfully at her husband's side. She was stroking his hand whispering quietly to him. "It's ok, I'm here sweetheart. I love you...It's okay." His daughter was sitting in a chair in the corner crying quietly, hoping that no one would notice. They both looked up at me with a look of "can you please fix this?" I introduced myself as I laid my hand on Larry's shoulder. He opened his eyes and continued to moan. The questions started immediately, "Is it normal to have this much pain? Is there anything we should be doing that we are not? What questions do other family members ask that we have not asked?" I told them, "pain is different for every patient. Some of our patients never have pain and some have lots of pain. Keeping the room quiet and the lights down low with as little stimulation as possible would help some." I then turned to Larry and started talking with him. He rated his pain at a 10 on a 1-10 scale. When I asked him to locate his pain, he stated that he hurt all over. I was initially stumped because Larry was diagnosed with a glioblastoma—four of them total and there is usually little pain with this type of cancer, especially generalized pain. I checked his bedside record and saw that his morphine drip was going at 28mg/hr and it had been increased from 20 mg. since this morning. I titrated his morphine up to 30 mg. He also had 2 mg of ativan every 4 hours IVP, but with little effect. I asked my colleague to help me reposition Larry.

After assessing Larry I stepped out of the room to talk with my coworker. We were both a little stumped as to why he was having all of this pain. I reviewed his history and could not find any notes that would indicate other co-morbidities or any mets to the bone or other organs. I placed a call to the patient's physician and awaited a return call. When the physician returned my call, I discussed the patient's current condition and asked for a breakthrough pain med. The physician ordered dilaudid for breakthrough pain, hoping that the synergistic effect of the drugs would help. I re-entered the room with the dilaudid and talked again with Larry. He continued to moan in the bed. I spoke with the mother and daughter and again spoke with Larry. He stated that he had not had pain like this before and he just seemed to hurt all the way to the "core of his body." After giving the dilaudid IVP, Larry became a little drowsy, but continued to moan. His wife continued to sit at his bedside and rub his hand. Larry's daughter followed me out into the hall and asked if I thought it would be okay if they went downstairs for a bite to eat. I encouraged her to take a break, but to be aware that often times when family members leave, that is when the patient will take a turn for the worse or will have a change in their status. I also explained that they should not feel any guilt if this were to occur.

I re-entered the room with some scented lotion. Larry was lying on his left side so I warmed some lotion and began talking with him. I gently rubbed his back and talked about his family. I asked him about his pain and he said, "I still hurt all over." He suddenly began sobbing uncontrollably. I came around the bed and sat down next to Larry. He held out his hand and I held it as he cried. He then began to talk to me. "I don't deserve to be without pain. I was unfaithful to my wife last year. She has stood by my side through all of this and I don't deserve it." I asked Larry if he had talked with anyone else about this and he stated that "no," he had not. I offered to call the chaplain and Larry agreed. When the chaplain arrived, I talked with him about Larry. I checked on my other patients as the chaplain met with Larry. The chaplain returned 45 minutes later and told me that Larry had decided to tell his wife and ask for forgiveness from her. He stated, "Larry seemed much calmer."

I re-entered Larry's room to find him relaxed and appeared to be comfortable. I asked Larry about his pain. He looked at me and said, "I don't feel any pain now. I do feel a little anxious though." I gave him some ativan IVP. I sat at Larry's bedside awhile longer and assessed his vital signs and pain response. He did seem to be more comfortable. I left Larry and continued to care for my other patients. When his family returned they came and asked me to come to Larry's room. When I entered Larry appeared to be sleeping comfortably; however, his LOC had diminished and he was no longer arousable. I explained that this was a sign that Larry was taking a turn for the worse and once again called the chaplain. Larry passed away just before the end of my shift. He was not in pain and had a peaceful death. I came to realize that day that, in hospice patients, it is important to assess their spiritual well being as well as their physical health. I now include a spiritual assessment for each of my patients and take that into account when I am addressing a pain issue.

A patient with glioblastoma does not typically present such a perplexing pain management problem. Parts of the puzzle include the two salient differences in this patient's pain (the atypical generalized pain, but also its severity and character), the missed timeline of responding to fairly large doses of morphine, and the lack of response to multidrug therapy. Hence, Liz finds herself thrown out of familiar everyday practice, in a kind of breakdown situation, and proceeds, as excellent nurses do, to collaborate with trusted colleagues. Simultaneously, Liz is reasoning, not just through this particular patient's responses, but also through former patient's responses with this kind of glioblastoma and their transitions over time to figure out what is similar to or different from prior situations. With each intervention, Liz tracks the patient's response or lack of and the timing of each, which informs her that nothing has really helped. Despite the pervasive implementation of best practice guidelines on pain management across hospitals, no clinical guideline would point her to the nature of this patient's problem. Nurses do and will need to continue to engage in detective work and modus operandi thinking to solve the complex, and sometimes, hidden problems that create suffering.

This narrative account is a good example of engaged thinking-in-action, reasoning-in-transition, and learning about a gap in the educational preparation of most clinicians. But, it's also a good illustration of how the best of detective work does not always uncover a solution by itself. Here we notice that Liz's strong engagement with the patient as a person and her skillful, caring involvement are central to the eventual disclosure of the secret, the source and nature of his intractable pain and existential suffering. The practical knowledge around good detective work is typically learned "in" practice and is hard won through trial and error learning. However, teaching students and newer nurses to develop this particular type of thinking and reasoning is possible by instructing them to: engage and imaginatively enter similar situations via narratives; probe patient cues; explore their hunches with curiosity and persistence; stay open by carefully listening, hearing, and responding to the patient's concerns; dialoguing in a community of learners about possible understanding and interventions; and reflecting on what was learned and how their perceptions, perspectives, and/or practice may be altered (Hooper, 1995; Kyriakidis & Vitello, in progress).

RECOGNIZING CHANGING CLINICAL RELEVANCE

Recognizing changing clinical relevance is an experientially learned skill that enables clinicians to distinguish what is relevant or not in situations as they unfold and how the context and alterations in the patient's clinical possibilities alter the meaning as the relevance of the signs and symptoms and patients' responses to therapies change (Dreyfus & Dreyfus, 1986). Recognizing changing relevance for different signs or symptoms, or recognizing turning points or transitions in the clinical situation, are subtle aspects of clinical judgment. Changes in the point of scrutiny that cause the clinician to interpret clinical data differently (i.e. with changing weights and emphases) are hallmarks of proficient and expert clinical practice. In the following example, a cardiac surgical patient is being fluid resuscitated and the nurse is concerned about pain management when she notices that the patient's restlessness is greater than expected:

Nurse: And then, I thought about it, and I said, 'Wait a minute. This guy is a drinker, OK.' He needed something to calm him down. So I knew he needed something besides the morphine. So I suggested that to them [physicians]. Finally the ICU doc came in and I said, 'I think this guy needs something else'; so I told him I think he needs [ativan]. And he said, 'Yeah. I think that's really right.' And so, after giving that, it really calmed him down...The concern with the fluid resuscitation was to make sure that he is really getting the amount that he needs since he is also diuresing. The formula for fluid replacement is not really strictly followed, but it's just like a guide-line. So at the time, my concern was the fluid resuscitation and the pain management. ...at about 2:00 p.m....he was really diuresing a lot, so we slowed the IV fluid rate down to 250 cc. But then in the afternoon, they were making rounds and the trauma team said, 'Oh, I think he can be taken care of on the floor.' And I said, 'Wait a minute. I don't think so, because he's still being fluid resuscitated, and also the pain manage-ment is a problem'... But the ICU [resident] was sympathetic with me and I think that he believed that pain management was the main problem. And I don't think the floor can handle that.

Interviewer: The ICU resident was in agreement?

Nurse: Yes. So I said, 'The problem is pain management, and with him being an alcoholic.' Because he tended to be really restless and toward the end of the day, I noticed that after I gave him some [ativan] he would wake up in about 3 hours and start getting up and saying, 'Can I go out and walk outside?' And I would say, 'Why?' 'I want to smoke.' And I said, 'No. No. You can't.' And he would listen, but he is really restless... So I wrote in the nursing care plan, #1 problem—Potential for DT's [delirium tremors].

The nurse's account demonstrates her shifting understanding of the patient's needs as, first, fluid resuscitation, then pain management, and then managing alcohol withdrawal. Getting stuck on one of the problems would have clouded the nurse's judgment and per-haps precluded or delayed needed treatment for the evolving complication of DT's.

Recognizing changing relevance sometimes occurs as a result of a sense of lost under-standing of, or attunement with, the situation. The preconceptions about the clinical issues and what is clinically relevant are no longer appropriate. Therefore, the account takes the form of noticing relevant evidence that does not match the clinical expectations. The ability to recognize changing relevance marks the beginning of proficiency. It signals a beginning ability to read the situation in its own terms and particularity, rather than matching the situ-ation with expected clinical goals, processes, or outcomes.

Because the skill of recognizing changing clinical relevance is essential for developing expertise, there is a tremendous need to focus educational efforts on acquiring this skill. However, recognizing changing clinical relevance is a perceptual or embodied skill (skill of perception or of the body) and, therefore, requires more than a simple transfer of knowledge or facts. It requires practice with observing and thinking through changing situations. An emergency department nurse points out the importance of this skill:

> **Nurse 1:** Because I do a lot of triaging patients. John Q Public arrives at my door saying, 'I need to see a doctor.' And it's just amazing how it doesn't even take me a quarter of a second now to know as soon as I see someone and they sit down, if they're able to sit down, if I'm going to let them stay; or I'm going to send them to a clinic; or if I'm going to pick them up and put them on a gurney or something. It's like this nurse radar that you get after about five years I think; it certainly wasn't immediate. And it's things that you don't even really realize—that you can't articulate anymore...you just look and you just know. It's odd.
>
> **Nurse 2:** My eyes are so much smarter than they used to be.
>
> **Nurse 1:** Mine too.
>
> **Nurse 2:** They take in a lot more, because it's the fastest thing. Everything else is kind of slow. You've got to put a stethoscope on to listen for breath sounds and take your 15 seconds to get vital signs but your eyes can take in stuff really fast.

Acquiring perceptual acuity or any embodied skill involves learning through the body, through the senses. It entails learning new embodied habits of attentiveness, thinking, and acting. Although many clinicians have acquired embodied skills such as recognizing changing clinical relevance by themselves, over an extended period of time, and through "trial and error" (getting it wrong and getting it better), innovative and practical teaching strategies can improve the readiness and attentiveness to this type of learning and reasoning.

Developing a skilled or adept body and the ability to "see" (grasp) necessarily occurs in an evolving patient situation. Thus, the best learning occurs at the patient's bedside with a skilled clinician who is precepting or through interactive audiovisual learning modules. Benner, Tanner & Chesla, (1992; 2009) point out that learners may best learn this kind of skill once they have mastered the "task world" so that their concerns can be refocused on other aspects of caring for the patient. In order to "see" a change, the clinician must notice or have pointed out to them what the patient looked like prior to the change. Then, the skilled clinician/teacher can point to and describe (as much as possible) the changes they are noticing as they occur. Another example of teaching this skill is that, as a more advanced clinician (e.g., colleague, clinical specialist, physician, educator) rounds on a particular patient and anticipates a particular change, the experienced clinician can describe the specific changes that they anticipate which therefore shapes the learner's attentiveness in a contextual way. Good clinical practice always requires situated cognition (Lave and Wenger, 1991). Learning this discernment requires attentiveness to general and specific patient responses and, over time, comparing and contrasting a specific patient's responses to those observed in other similar and dissimilar patients.

DEVELOPING CLINICAL KNOWLEDGE IN SPECIFIC PATIENT POPULATIONS

Clinical knowledge is typically developed in relation to specific patient populations (e.g., cardiac surgical patients) and, often, sub-populations (e.g., patients with cardiac valve replacements). By clinical knowledge we mean the flexible integration of the best of scientific knowledge with the practical knowledge born from experiential learning. The experience of frequently caring for patients who have the same or similar conditions affords the clinician the conditions for comparing and contrasting different patients' responses to the same conditions, therapies, and complications over time. It requires attentiveness and remembering past trial and error learning in particular instances. Focus on fewer specific populations enables the clinician to become more attuned and develop better skills of recognition, thinking and reasoning, puzzle solving, anticipation, managing, and advocating for what patients need (Kyriakidis, research field notes, September 2, 2007). In fact, Kyriakidis and Vitello (in progress), who studied the clinical development of beginning (newly licensed) nurses over their first two years, found that clinical knowledge and skillful performance were improved when beginners started their practice in a specialty or focused their learning and care of fewer specific patient populations. Many past judgments allow the clinician to learn typical responses and trajectories with particular patient populations. These understandings compel us to rethink the advice commonly given to new nurses about starting their careers on a general medical-surgical unit where there are rarely specific patient populations. Although there are different challenges, specialty or subspecialty units, which narrow the scope of clinical conditions that must be learned before safe care is possible, may provide a better developmental path. Nurses who are on general units may benefit from focusing on the care of particular types of patients (eg., heart failure, confused elderly, abdominal surgery) over time before being assigned to care for patients with diverse conditions. Similarly, consistent patient assignments that allow the new clinician to come to "know the patient" and know the condition have substantial benefits for the patients and clinician over the too often fragmented assignments of a different group of patients daily.

Many of these issues are illustrated in the following excerpt from the ongoing research study of clinicians who care for our wounded soldiers injured in Operation Iraqi Freedom and Operation Enduring Freedom in Afghanistan (Benner, in progress). Lucille Raia, a rehab nurse, gives us a glimpse of the new clinical knowledge development in this specific patient group as she encounters an atypical presentation of an infection:

> **Nurse:** I was an experienced, yet new nurse on a general rehab floor that was fast changing into a polytrauma unit to care for the servicepersons returning from [Iraq and Afghanistan]. It was early in our experiences with returning active duty. The staff, team, and organization were unfamiliar with the breadth and depth of their physical and emotional injuries as well as their presentations. Compounding the individual's care were the dynamics, involvement, entitlement, [expectations] and sometimes anger toward the healthcare team, especially nurses, that the families and significant others displayed.
>
> A young 21 year old soldier had sustained multiple injuries involving abdominal, orthopedic, and traumatic brain injuries (TBI). His rehab course was uneventful except for a persistent low grade fever of unknown etiology. Mr. G was ambulatory with a cane and was preparing to be discharged to home with his mother….[one evening], Mr. G appeared tired and slowed. His mom said he had been awake complaining of [abdominal] pain. I found Mr. G to be weaker, still with a fever, and a noticeable gait change.
>
> The doctor was call and ordered Infectious Disease and surgery consults, labs and xrays to rule out bowel infarct and infections; however, Mr. G worsened and became more somnolent. Mr. G was in bed and his nurse tried to arouse him. I went into his room, and Mr. G began seizing. He was unresponsive and we called a code…. Mr. G was intubated and stabilized. He was transferred to the ICU. After two days,

> Mr. G died [from] bacterial meningitis. The organism was indigenous to Iraq where the young man had been injured. Also, when first injured he had been treated for meningitis but this was unknown to [our] staff....Staff re-questioned their assessments and interventions...Our learning curve unfortunately for these seriously injured patients needed to be less prolonged...these patients are not our traditional Veteran's Administration rehab hips, knees, and the like, but traumatic seriously recently injured individuals who were not presenting in the same way as our other patients had.

The nurse points out the limitation of recognizing, and therefore making accurate judgments, when working with new and unfamiliar conditions, organisms, or patient groups. For the nurses on this polytrauma unit and among the many clinicians who care for our wounded soldiers injured in Operation Iraqi Freedom and Operation Enduring Freedom in Afghanistan and cared for in the field, in transport, and in the U.S., the breadth and depth of knowledge is expanding daily (Benner, in progress). Although much of the care is similar to the care of soldiers in recent, past wars, we currently have the ability to save many, many more soldiers who suffer polytrauma than in wars past. This, coupled with infections from novel organisms and the pervasive multidrug-resistant organisms created by the public's misuse of antibiotics, has compelled urgent and rapid advancement of new clinical knowledge and has altered the type, amount, and specificity of prior interventions and rehabilitation. For instance, the recognition that over-resuscitation was causing abdominal compartment syndrome, which is almost always fatal, was recognized by nurses and resulted in significant changes in fluid resuscitation of seriously injured soldiers (Colonel N. Molter, personal communications, March 23, 2010). Another example is the very careful and limited use of specific antibiotics for the multidrug-resistant organisms infecting many soldiers.

As noted above, the novel challenges described above are compounded by the unprecedented incidence of traumatic brain injuries (TBI) incurred by our soldiers from multiple exposures to blasts or improvised explosive devices without any apparent external injuries as well as the multiple and frequent amputations (Benner, in progress). Thus, the call for new knowledge development far exceeds physical rehabilitation of the body. The sheer numbers have provided the needed experience and demand for rapid knowledge development, quick identification of patterns, of frequent avoidable complications, and for assessment of recurring complications from particular injuries, such as direction of the blast for the soldier, recurring infections from "dirty" bombs and so on. Only with reflection about and articulation of this frontline learning can nurses and physicians develop more astute clinical observation and clinical judgment. Narratives of significant cases and learning, such as the one above, can help improve nurses' clinical care, problem solving, anticipate complications, and recognize early warning signals. In order to make this knowledge cumulative and available for clinical inquiry, research and improved patient care, this experientially gained knowledge has to be made visible and public. It has to become shared knowledge.

As with our wounded soldiers, there is a steep clinical learning curve when a clinical group begins treating a new population of patients (eg., face and organ transplants, the early period in the AIDS pandemic) or a known population with new conditions (eg., new multidrug-resistant organisms). To develop expertise, clinicians must constantly learn and refine their practices based on new patient responses, populations, other clinicians' practices, and in response to larger system changes. In turn, this knowledge, made public, can be examined for developing new clinical research to further test and expand this clinical knowledge. For example, the clinical learning associated with babies born to substance- and poly-substance addicted mothers increased as the birth rates of such infants increased. The following nurse charts some of the active clinical learning of peers on her unit as they began to treat more substance-addicted babies experiencing neonatal abstinence syndrome:

Nurse 1: Babies who are born to substance addicted mothers are very jittery, moving the arms.

Nurse 2: Right. What they call hyperactive moros. I mean when we started scoring him, which is another thing that the task force has instituted, that babies in whom we suspect there may be a problem, we've now got the scoring sheet that we adapted from the one at a different hospital...and also we've been using their video where it's clearly explained how you score infants. So it's not a subjective thing. It's not, well this baby is jittery because it cries a lot. We have a lot of babies in the Well Baby unit that cry a lot, and there's nothing wrong with them, that's just the way they are. But there are babies that cry a lot and have loose stools, and have hyperactive moros, and poor feeding and regurgitation, and you go down the list and pretty soon you find you've got yourself a score of 15 or better and you know that something is going on.

This interview excerpt is instructive because it demonstrates the clinical learning about making distinctions between the patterns of crying in healthy newborns and neurological responses of babies who are withdrawing from any number of the various addictive substances. In addition to reading the growing scientific literature on the manifestations of addiction in infants, clinicians had to learn what these manifestations <u>actually</u> looked like in practice and how they were distinguished from variations with other conditions. The variations in clinical practice are many, both on the side of the "normal," non-addicted baby who cries a lot and the addicted baby who has a high-pitched cry, cries inconsolably and has other manifestations of neurological irritability.

Similarly, new clinical knowledge is developed when clinicians begin caring for patients with increasingly complex or multisystem problems. For instance, although a particular type of surgical patient may be familiar to a unit or nurse, the increasing complexity of patients' comorbid conditions confuses, complicates, or produces different patient responses to interventions. Another area of continued clinical knowledge development is accompanying the escalating mandates to perform increasingly invasive surgeries on an outpatient basis and discharge patients from acute care settings earlier and earlier. The "push" toward decreasing patients' in hospital stays motivates changes in medical practices and therapies which, in turn, changes patient trajectories, expected responses and outpatient and home care.

The clinician's understanding of specific clinical situations and expected trajectories of particular clinical populations locates and guides clinical judgment. This is illustrated in the following neonatal ICU nurse's discussion of distinctions she makes between normal and premature infants:

Nurse: I know I approach a full term baby differently than a preemie. With a preemie, you are just much more gentle because they get over stimulated so much more quickly. A full term baby can handle pretty much anything, even if he's really sick. Just being very careful about noise and being very careful about handling, turning, drawing blood, starting IVs, and all those interventions.

Interviewer: So it sounds like touch is a really important nursing intervention [with preemies].

Nurse: Yes, it is. It makes the difference whether or not you'll have a good shift with the baby, depending on how you handle him. Because if you let Ricky [the baby] cry too long, there was just no calming him down afterwards. And he had a cry that everybody knew, so as soon as you heard the first wail, it was like, 'Okay, somebody take this kid, I have to go see Ricky.' It made for some interesting days and nights. But he's going home tomorrow.

The nurse's understanding of Baby Ricky is situated in her understanding of the common differences in the patterns and responses of premature and normal infants. Premature infants require more skillful use of touch and stimulation. At the heart of this discussion is that the nurses have come to know this infant extremely well and their knowing and responding to Baby Ricky's particular patterns are essential to his recovery.

Because clinical knowledge is ambiguous and views on optimal treatments vary, clinical knowledge must be interpreted, negotiated and may be contested so that definitive research is needed. The judgment, skill, and art of communicating and negotiating clinical understandings is taken up in Chapter 10. The following exemplar by Emily Dever, an ED nurse, points to an instance where the nurse's embodied knowledge, her ability to make a fine qualitative distinction about a population-specific problem, and her immediate but non-reflective interventions are described. It shows how the nuances or distinctions in the nurse's clinical knowledge development alter the need to interpret and negotiate what is ambiguous, end the problem search, and prevent extensive interventions that, in this instance, accompany a code:

Nurse: "Joy" was a 3 month old with a congenital heart defect. Mira [new nurse giving report] thought "the defect was a hypoplastic right heart". I vaguely recalled Joy being here within the past month and that she had pulmonary stenosis as well, but I had never cared for her. "I'll read the doc's H & P when report is over" I thought to myself and let Mira continue. Joy had come in last night in respiratory distress, had been intubated and a central line placed. No drips and except for some sedation PRN. Nursing didn't seem to know what had started her spiral leading to the intubation. I glanced over at the central monitor; it wasn't alarming but Joy's heart rate was 215. I asked where she had been running as I got up to go to her room. "A little tachy on and off but she's been fine" was the reply. Mira didn't seem alarmed at the HR. I wondered why her alarm limits were set so out of range. As I was headed to the room, my attending pediatrician was about 5 feet away. I looked at him and asked if Joy had been echoed and that she was very tachy. He replied that "cardiology didn't want an echo last night but perhaps when they came in this morning they might change their mind and order one".

All the lights were out and even in the dark I could see that Joy was dusky blue. Her biox wasn't picking up. I put one hand on her and I knew why—she was ice cold peripherally. She was intubated, eyes closed, nasal flaring, retracting and I could hear her wheezing from the side of the bed. Centrally she felt hot and that jogged my memory that she had a brain injury that caused her to have temp instability as well. I couldn't palpate a radial pulse but found her brachials easily. I thought to myself, "at least she shouldn't be too hypotensive as well but her cardiac output is definitely down". I quickly flipped the vent 100% breaths button and decided not to bag her. Sometimes children, particularly heart babies and BPD [bronchopulmonary dysplasia] children, do worse when you interrupt the circuit and attempt to bag. They're sensitive to the volumes and get out of sync and start to clamp down harder. I'm sure Joy had a little combination of both... [she tells her peers] "She's about to code". I asked the secretary to tell RT [respiratory] I needed her right away then turned to Dr. B. who was on the phone with cardiology. I looked right at him and said, "I need you NOW, she looks like—!" Everyone responded.

I flipped on the overhead lights. Something in Joy's color made my gut go off and I asked the night EMT to get a DEX (glucometer DEX) for me from a heel stick. I asked the [others] to hang some normal saline and to get some meds while I completed a little more assessment to determine what was going on. Dr. B. came in. I'd already made up my mind that while I started getting labs and assessing the situation that he had about 3 minutes to start giving me orders before I called the ICU attending to come down. Dr. B is wonderful but all the ER doc's are pediatricians, not extensively trained in intensive care. Dr. B agreed she looked pretty bad and added "she looked fine when I was in here at 0630."

As I found my central line and was drawing labs, I looked up and sighed relief to see Dr. M., one of the ICU attendings, strolling in. The EMT informed me that he couldn't get any blood for a DEX by heelstick which I thought would be quicker and worth a try, but she was too clamped down. "It's okay. The central line drew pretty easily and I'm running the whole iSTAT." I was still debating whether this was cardiogenic, septic or something else. Dr. M had followed her all night and didn't feel it was cardiogenic, so no Lasix. RT was here and back-to-back treatments were started. Joy's blood pressure was in the mid 80's by Doppler. I started the NS bolus, tried some Ativan for sedation and some Tylenol that I was doubtful she'd absorb. Her axillary temp was 39.5! I knew it was higher since her perfusion was poor. I placed some cool packs under the blanket behind her scapulas and prayed she wouldn't seize. Her DEX came back less than 20 and I started a D10 bolus. It clicked!! I thought to myself "that's why my gut went off with her color". It wasn't quite the shade you see with hypoxia; it's what I had seen several times over the last year with profound hypoglycemia....sort of a grey-blue, hard to describe but just plain ugly.

The treatments and sedation were helping. Her flaring and retractions diminished and the wheezing ceased. She was moving good air. Guess that validates the non-cardiogenic part. I was on my second NS bolus and was again questioning the fluid with her cardiac status. Dr. M had been in touch several times over the night and was looking back through the I/O sheets. I hadn't even had time to look at her chart. Looked like Joy had responded a little too well to her earlier Lasix. It was shortly after that her HR began to climb and she was dry.....

Joy was responding nicely to the treatment plan. It's amazing what a little sugar and fluid (among other things) can do for you. Joy was responding and looked 200% better. Her perfusion was better, her labs were better and her HR was calming down to the 170-180 range. Her B/P dropped into the 70's as her perfusion improved, we knew it would improve once her fluid status and temp were better under control. We were having trouble synchronizing the vent for her, even with sedation. Dr. M tried different vent modes and bagging rates/volumes. In the end he decided we needed to paralyze her and take control so she could rest and we could ventilate better. I gave more sedation and started the sedative drip before the first dose of paralytic. I talked with Dr. M and we decided to leave any remaining paralytic doses PRN for now to see if we could overcome this. She did much better after the paralytic. Joy is fragile. She doesn't have any reserve and the slightest stressors can set her into a spiral....hence, her repeated admissions with distress and respiratory failures. I still couldn't get a feel for what had led to her initial distress this time. Dr. M and I conferred on various theories.

Things were under control within the hour or so. I made a mental note to check on Mira next time I worked with her. I wanted to make sure that she was ok and if there was anything I could help her learn as the "red flags" of pediatrics. It's a horrible feeling to give someone report and then find out the patient isn't quite as you thought they were. I also wanted to send Dr. M. an e-mail thanks for his uncanny sense of timing and for making rounds in the ER.

Joy was a complex patient. Even though I can't explain it to anyone, I still believe there is a different color of "blue" that accompanies profound hypoglycemia versus other "blue" states like hypoxia. I guess I'd say it's more of a grey-purple than blue. Joy's certainly not the first hypoglycemic or complex patient that I've cared for. I've just never really thought of hypoglycemia as having a particular color change associated with it, and I'm sure not every patient is the same. It's one of those things you always think about but sometimes is further down your list of troubleshooting. It moved up my list. It's fun to see the facial expressions of my seasoned colleagues when I mention it. They all stop and think about it for a moment, some laugh and others slowly nod their head and agree followed by a story like "You know, I remember this patient…." It's nice when we can share stories and learn from each other.

Included in this account are the realization and articulation of past experiential learning; that is, how the nurse qualitatively and immediately recognizes profound hypoglycemia. Additional physicians and nurses have confirmed the diagnosis associated with this qualitative distinction, adding that the grayish blue color appears as a faint, undertone and is a distinctly different blue than hypoxia and a different grey than sepsis. What is stunning about Emily's perceptual grasp is, not only has she learned to make the distinction tacitly from astute observation in past situations, but here she actually differentiates the subtle color difference in Joy when one would typically be "set to see" the "blue" from hypoxia due to the multiple cardiac anomalies and bronchopulmonary dysplasia.

In addition to Emily's expert clinical knowledge, judgment and management of Joy's individual medical conditions, this narrative reveals how nurses find themselves in the midst of the ambiguous, complex puzzles of multiple coexisting conditions, where any one or all of the medical conditions could be producing the crisis. Despite the complexity, her embodied response is to get a DEX when she recognized the grayish blue color. As importantly, because of the complexity and urgency of this situation, there was absolutely no time and no margin for error, particularly about a diagnosis that was based on findings that escape clear articulation, so she was compelled to initiate multiple instantaneous interventions until her strong suspicion is confirmed. For developing clinicians, gaining an accurate grasp can be the hardest skill to learn because it requires attentiveness, sustained curiosity, reflection, articulation and public comparisons made with expert clinicians who already know how to make the qualitative distinction. Emily helps us understand how the most probable causes of Joy's crisis stood out as secondary. She details her reasoning and her modus operandi thinking that includes "if…, then…" thinking. This kind of contingency thinking and action is based on and refined through clinical experience. Engaging in detective-like modus operandi thinking also allows the nurse to engage in clinical forethought, to anticipate what is likely to occur in the next clinical situation that seems similar to prior experiences (see Chapter 3). Working in this pressured situation and in the midst of the ambiguity, the multiple, immediate interventions for each of the probable problems supported Joy until the glucose came back at less than 20. The quantitative measure, understood by many as the "legitimate" data, came later but validated Emily's intuition about hypoglycemia, her tacit grasp of the situation and confirmed the nature of the problem and guided her ongoing interpretation of the baby's responses and needs.

In this situation, it is remarkable that no one noticed or expressed curiosity about why Emily acts upon her perceptual grasp of the skin tone without hesitation or how she expediently diagnosed the problem. Nurses often experience the challenge of acting upon tacitly learned but ineffable (inexpressible) knowledge in confident and strong ways when the stakes are so high. It's even harder in environments where formal or scientifically derived knowledge routinely trumps or is valued to the exclusion of hard-earned practical wisdom. It is not uncommon for qualitative distinctions like this one, when shared, to be disregarded as "unscientific" (unable to be measured or quantified) and cause experts to abandon the effort of articulation and subsequently of extending this knowledge in practice, or to even confirm or disconfirm scientific evidence. Emily briefly acknowledges her triumph as ordinary, saying "it's amazing what a little sugar and fluid can do for you."

Knowing how to manage the physiological conditions in a particular patient population is only part of their care. Recovering from an illness requires emotional determination to bear the work, sometimes the pain, and the exhaustion to build the endurance needed to transition toward self care. Expert nurses learn to "read" the patient's ability and pace, as s/he participates in recovery, to know when to push, when to support and when to step back and relax. For example, nurses learn to judge how patients in this specific population are coping with the weaning process by making astute judgments and qualitative distinctions about different patient responses, as illustrated in the following example:

Nurse 1: You can tell when you're weaning someone that they aren't doing well. They get diaphoretic, cool, clammy. Their pressure goes up, their heart rate goes up, their respiration goes up. They just look terrible. And you don't need to have a number. You know their CO_2's climbing and their O_2's dropping, they're getting acidotic.

Nurse 2: And this lady, you saw those things or did you see them and you finally knew?

Nurse 1: You see them on every COPD patient. You only need to see it a few times to know what they're doing.

Interviewer: And you have a degree of comfort with interpreting those symptoms?

Nurse 1: Yes. Oh, yes. I mean, it's obvious that they're air hungry. They either need their respiratory rate pushed up or they need to be put back on the vent, or they need to rest. And different people present in different ways. You just have to find out what those people present with. Some people don't get diaphoretic and cold and clammy. Some people's heart rate and blood pressure just go up and their respiratory rate goes up and they look uncomfortable. Other people want the table and the pillow and they lean over.

Interviewer: And that's a bad sign, the table and the pillow?

Nurse 1: And purse-lip breathing when they have a trach in, yeah.

These interview excerpts illustrate the common distinctions that expert nurses learn to make when working with specific patient populations. The language reflects a deep familiarity with common patterns, signs, symptoms, and clinical distinctions. Talking with colleagues about the distinctions they are making in particular patients is crucial for learning to make more refined clinical judgments about specific patient populations. The verbal accounts of the distinctions can alert one to look for certain things, but to learn <u>how</u> to make these distinctions, one must observe them in particular patients and contexts. Asking one's colleagues to describe what seems "obvious" to them can uncover distinctions that the clinician may not have articulated in the past. Learning to be a good clinical detective requires success with past detective work. The process is circular, as is all interpretation; questions foretell possible answers but, as the above examples illustrate, the beginner can move from being a map reader to one who knows the terrain well and is at home in making qualitative distinctions about the terrain or body of water for navigation (Bourdieu, 1980/1990). As one neonatal ICU nurse who was describing stimulation and comfort care for growing premature infants noted, "You're a better monitor than anything that Hewlett-Packard ever made." This is confidence born of many years of direct observation and handling of premature infants on monitors. The nurse has confidence in her ability to make qualitative distinctions and to notice subtle changes in the infant.

CLINICAL GRASP AND RESPONSE-BASED PRACTICE

As previously discussed, an expert clinician's interventions are response-based, that is, in response to the patient's situation. A good clinical grasp is essential to developing the capacity to respond rapidly to changing situations (Benner, Stannard & Hooper, 1996); that is, the expert nurse's immediate understanding of the situation directs what intervention is initiated, when it is initiated, and the way in which it is used. Included earlier, Emily Dever's exemplar about Baby Joy, who had severe hypoglycemia, points out how the baby's greyish-blue color guided thinking and intervention regarding her near-code. What was stunning when Emily only peripherally noticed Joy's skin tone was her immediate response to order the DEX, without stopping to think about the meaning of the skin tone. Her grasp was so closely linked to her response that we refer to this as an embodied response. The instantaneous and high priority therapies developed in acute and critical care units require ongoing clinical grasp in ever-changing, complex situations. This is learned by experience in making qualitative distinctions, by modus operandi thinking, by recognizing changing relevance in patients' clinical signs and symptoms, by coming to know the clinical trajectories in specific patient populations, and by knowing particular patients within those populations.

Since inexperienced clinicians can never be prepared to recognize every problem and appropriately intervene in every situation, learning will inevitably occur in situations of breakdown. Experiential learning is often gained through hard lessons, time-constrained situations, and emergencies, as illustrated in a flight nurses' interview:

> **Nurse 1:** Well, there is one call that will always stay with me. This was very early [in my career]. It was a 60-year-old male trapped in a vehicle on [the highway] and when we arrived, we landed [helicopter] and there was still extrication to go on, so basically, at that point, your job is first to do what you can with the patient, staying out of the firefighters' way, and there was really nothing we could do at this point because there were so many firefighters working on getting him out of the vehicle. But I could see his leg, how entrapped his leg was, and he was bleeding a lot from the femur, but the man was awake and alert and being calm. <u>Someone</u> was in the—it was you and I (speaking to Nurse 2), someone was in the car with him keeping him calm.

> **Nurse 2:** Yeah, there was a firefighter in the car.

Nurse 1: Keeping him calm, talking with him the whole time. And, once we got him out, it looked like he had a femur fracture and really his respirations were fine. So...

Nurse 2: You couldn't move him because they were extracting his lower legs...

Nurse 1: That's right, that's right he <u>wasn't</u> moving his lower extremities. Yeah. But that doesn't remain in my memory as significantly as a lot of things on the call. So [later] we get him in the helicopter, and I believe he has an IV...but he was talking, and that's unusual that we get to talk to them. And he thought it [the accident] was his fault. He was upset that he thought it was his fault. So basically, at that point, my inner nature is always, 'It doesn't matter right now. What matters is that we get you to the hospital. That's all that matters right now. You can deal with all that later.' And then he started having some significant back pain, some increasing back pain. And at this point, I had his IV—thinking trauma patient—I had his IV opened up wide, and he was normotensive, if not a little hypertensive. Maybe 140/90 or something like that. So, regardless of the blood pressure, I kept the IV open wide. And his back pain kept getting worse. And I just really didn't associate it with anything except for trauma, maybe belly, maybe broken back, wasn't moving lower extremities. And then he started getting a little scared. I mean he was holding onto my hand the whole way. And I said, 'You're going to be just fine. Your vital signs are very stable. You're going to be just fine.' But I'm telling him, 'You're doing very well.' I explained to him in very laymen's terms the [oxygen] saturation and his breathing well, et cetera. Well, to make it a hard story, he does die in the OR. He had a traumatic triple-A [abdominal aortic aneursym]. [The nurse becomes very tearful]. So, from that story, and a subsequent article on [Nurse 2]'s part, I have since learned the signs and symptoms of a dissecting aortic aneurysm. And I'll <u>never</u> forget them. And <u>only</u> open fluids wide open if they've got a low blood pressure. You know? Don't just think trauma patients need fluids. That was hard. I'll carry that with me [tearful].

Interviewer: That kind of knowledge is hard won, very hard won.

Nurse 1: I won't forget it.

Contained within the experience is the remorse over not understanding the meaning of the worsening back pain, increasing the IV fluids, and telling the patient that he would be fine. These are passages on the way to gaining a sense of the veracity of one's clinical grasp. The nurse details early reasoning but has not yet gained the ability to see the unexpected in the deteriorating situation. The nurse's grasp of the kinds and depth of possible and likely complications are simply limited by inexperience. Clinicians cannot be beyond experiential learning. They can only be responsible for incorporating what was learned into their clinical grasp of future situations. The above story becomes a paradigm case for this nurse because she learns to recognize the clinical picture of a patient with a dissecting aortic aneurysm and will forever remember it.

In everyday practice, one's clinical grasp not only guides one's own responses to the patient, the nurse is positioned to pass that clinical understanding on to physicians who may or may not be physically present or may not have ever seen the patient. More often than not, the intended shared understanding between the two clinicians begs a response or intervention. Therein lies a major source of breakdown in the care of patients, when one's clinical perspective is not or should not be accepted and therefore a needed intervention is not initiated. Failure to rescue is among the potential consequences. As one might suspect, breakdown is far more prevalent when clinicians do not know each other or work well together.

In contrast, intricate and delicate interventions, procedures, and surgeries are currently evolving in which the safety and success depend on the accurate clinical grasp of one clinician directing the skillful performance of another. Expertise and hard won trust are essential to enable the nurse anesthetist-physician team to work together as if they were one person. This is best exemplified in an excerpt from Tammy Freehling, a nurse anesthetist (CRNA), while working with a neurosurgeon who is performing an awake craniotomy. The CRNA must carefully balance sedation to keep a sleepy patient awake, calm, still, and responsive during the microscopic excision of the brain tumor that is impinging on her speech and motor centers. Not every patient with this brain tumor is a candidate for staying awake while having the skull opened, so Tammy takes a few brief moments to assure that Debra, the patient, is a good candidate. She also needs to establish a good rapport, knowing that her constant "read" of Debra's functional abilities and subsequent guidance to the surgeon will depend on Debra's every response to Tammy's requests:

CRNA: When Dr. Ray seeks me out weeks prior to a surgery, it's serious. For awake craniotomy, I know that either motor function or speech is on the line and the stakes are particularly high for this patient Debra is only 26 years old, mother of two youngsters, devoted wife and part time cashier at the local grocery store. Her difficulty with expression started six weeks ago, just a stammer here or there which progressively grew into longer pauses, effort getting words out, and then, unintended words. When he tells me that he needs my help, there's little to do with my providing anesthesia. It has everything to do with my nursing assessments. Across the drapes, the vigilance of a Rottweiler guard dog for any speech or motor deficits is needed. Dr. Ray knows that I'm loud and persistent if there's any detectable change.

[Pre-op, before approaching Debra,] I took a minute to watch her from a distance to get a general idea of her emotional state. She was calm and holding hands with her significant other. Her IV was already in place which can be a source of anxiety. No worry lines on her forehead. No extraneous body movements indicating tension. Once again, I've trusted her surgeon to select an appropriate candidate who can withstand the emotional strain of the next few hours. He typically selects patients for awake crani who possess a special combination; someone able to understand how much the outcome depends on their feedback during the surgery and someone who can maintain composure in face of so many unknowns.

For now, my biggest challenge lies in this next few moments...establishing a trusting relationship. [We exchange greetings, introductions, and procedure timeframe.]

I began our discussion, "So Debra, I'd like to spend some time taking you through what to expect. You might wonder how in the world we're gonna get you through having your head opened without hurting you and without it being scary. Our medicines are pretty amazing. We've had over a decade of working on getting just the right amount of "comfort medicines" while still being able to check your neuro exam. Without getting too specific, these meds in your IV will give you a really nice balance of relaxation and relief from anxiety... It is likely however that you will remember what goes on in the OR. This is why you'll have us right there to let us know if you're hurting or uncomfortable. The patient asks, "So, you'll be right there with me?" I tell her, "Yes, either Dr. M [an anesthesiologist], or I, the whole time. And throughout, you'll be able to talk directly to us." Debra asks: "So I'll remember....?" I respond, "Yes, you'll likely remember quite a bit. During the surgery, Dr. Ray actually needs your help and your involvement. We are VERY interested in your ability to move and to speak. So, we'll be putting you through a little workout at times. When Dr. Ray is close to the motor strip in your brain, I'll be asking you to smile, stick out your tongue, squeeze my fingers and wiggle your toes. During the period while he's working to remove tumor, I may be asking you to do this over and over again. And because he's working on the left side of your brain, I'll be watching real close as to how your right sided movements compare to your left side. Similarly, when Dr. Ray is very close to the speech center, I'll be very interested to watch and hear you speak… The whole time that he is working close to your speech center, it is all important that he can tell if your speech is at all affected. So I will be visiting with you about anything that you'd like to talk about… You'll be sleepy. You'll want to be left alone to take a nap and you'll wonder, "why won't these people let me take a break?" I promise you that as soon as Dr. Ray is at a stopping point, I will give you a rest every chance we get. It's common for people to be sleepy when their brain is being worked on AND some of the medicines that I've used to make you comfortable add to the sleepiness. We will find a nice balance of comfort and wakefulness."

Debra asks, "Will I hurt very much?" "Honestly, you'll have some headache as the surgery proceeds. What's important is that Dr. Ray knows that it can get a bit uncomfortable so he's very good about letting us know when you can sleep. Toward the end, we let you get a nice rest and work in more pain medicines to get rid of that headache." Debra is a bit teary, but ready to get started.

Tammy begins building a very focused but good relationship with the intent of providing a source of comfort and security during this frightening time. Going to sleep calmly improves the chances of waking calmly, particularly if the patient knows and trusts the anesthetist. An anxious and thrashing patient with an open skull is to be avoided if at all possible. Second, the brief discussion sets up the patient's role in the functional mapping of her brain. Third, Tammy conveys the importance of being able to constantly and closely monitor and safeguard viable brain tissue and how that is linked to the barrage of questions/commands that will ensue.

During the first one and a half hours, the "surgeon works diligently to expose the left frontal lobe down to the Sylvian fissure with the temporal lobe in view. As Dr. Ray peels gray tumorous slime off healthy pink convulutions of brain," he is ready for Debra to emerge from heavier anesthesia. One of the most stressful times of the procedure begins:

CRNA: "Debra, wake up" I say shaking her shoulder. No response. Again, I repeat myself. No response. "Thomas, hold up!" Dr. Ray knows when I call him by his first name that I'm <u>real</u> concerned, but it avoids the patient sensing my concern. Dr. Ray stops. He waits to hear a response. I shake my head, side to side indicating "no good" to let him know that I'm not sure where we are. So often patients get sleepy during the procedure even though all the anesthetics have been off for hours, but I can't see facial symmetry, mouth or tongue movements, or hear her enunciate. Dr. Ray's progress on the tumor can only proceed if speech remains intact. My worry is that the speech center has been inadvertently sacrificed. This time louder and with a more aggressive shake I persist, "Debra, if you hear me, squeeze my hand." Finally she gives a strong squeeze. A concerned Dr. Ray looks to me for a nod that she followed my command. Still reluctant to proceed, he intervenes, loud and upbeat, "Deeeebra, are you doing okay?" Groggily, she returns, "Yeeess, I'm okay," as I intently observe to see if she's struggling or just slow. Then, I'm elated when she loudly, brusquely, and very irritatedly yells, "I just wanna sleep!" Clear as a bell, deliberate and without hesitation….she conveys her thoughts. No facial droop, slur, or difficulty word finding. Dr. Ray replies, "Good job Tammy-O, keeping her talking." Energetically, he adds, "Hey Debra, things are going really well but now is the time that we need you to talk. Can you speak loud for us?" Now with eyes brighter she offers, "I'll try."

After tumor removal around the speech center, Dr. Ray is ready to move on:

CRNA: Okay, Tammy-O, we're going to move on to motor function." Dr. Ray gives me the settings for the stimulator that is connected to a probe he uses to evoke motor responses in her right brain so we can visually "map" the motor strip. As he touches the stimulator to the brain, I respond by naming the region that I see: Okay, HAND. Please repeat." He stimulates the same spot. "Yes, definitely HAND." Now that he's located the motor strip, things can go faster. The loudness or acceleration of my responses correlate with the strength of Debra's response. "FACE – grimace." He repeats each time, listening to me to hear consistency. "FACE again…now tongue jutting forward." With each location , he actually tags the spot with "A, B, C, etc" on the brain's surface. Finally we have the motor strip mapped all the way down to the feet.

He positions and refocuses the microscope, ready to resect the tumor again. "Ready, Tammy?" I must situate myself with a flashlight under the drape when the lights are dimmed during microscope use. "Yep, we're ready." Having explained to Debra that she's to follow the next motor commands in a series, I take her through the first 'run': "Eyes wide open, smile, stick your tongue out, squeeze my hands, raise your right arm, bend you knee, wiggle your toes. Debra, you're doing just great. Now we're going to repeat this over and over again. Okay?" She nods. Dr. Ray looks over at me and I say, "We're good!" He begins resecting again. "Now Debra, let's start at the top again. Eyes wide open…Good. Big, big smile….Nice. Stick your tongue out….Midline good. Debra, I'm going to reach across your belly so I can feel both sides. Another big hand squeeze…Excellent!" And so on. I follow each request of Debra with a response to Dr. Ray that he can continue. We proceed with each run of motor exams in a steady cadence, ALWAYS in the same sequence. The cadence and sequence assures Dr. Ray we are examining the whole motor strip, enabling him to continue confidently.

In the midst of Debra's "workout," Dr. Ray tells Debra that he almost has the tumor all out when I notice her shaking. Her jaw is cocked off to one side and eyes are rolled up in her head, "Thomas, she's seizing." I crank up the O2 in her nasal cannula, and do a modified jaw thrust, which I confirmed prior to surgery, to keep her airway open. Breathing remains spontaneous during and after the seizure. Dr. Ray douses the surgical field with cold saline and the seizure ceases.

Debra's post-ictal period is brief and within 5 minutes she responds verbally. I breathe a sigh of relief to find that she's easily reoriented. On occasion following a seizure, some patients arouse in a panic, trying frantically to move their head. With good fortune, Debra tells me that she is doing fine and Dr. Ray completes the resection. It's a relief for us all when the house lights come up and he proceeds with closure. I give Debra much-deserved analgesia. Moments later, I hear a snore. This time, her sleep goes undisturbed.

Here, the CRNA gives a glimpse of how exact, concise and negotiated communication about every assessment of the patient's responses literally determines where, how much, how fast, and whether the surgeon proceeds. During these 5-6 hour surgeries where the surgeon is working as fast as is safe, there is no time to lose on thoroughly articulated descriptions of every expected patient response while there is plenty of time to invest on any undesirable ones. Haste, lack of clarity, stuttered pauses or any breakdown in the team's well-developed communications and collaboration can cost Debra her speech or motor function. These communication patterns are developed experientially among specific clinicians working closely and consistently over time. Expert clinicians have taught us that they are unlikely to accomplish this level of success when they have not worked together, do not "know" each other and lack communication patterns that are mutually understood. Although this team's style of communications can appear social, their style, mood, and tone embodies what is at stake for Debra. Revealing their ethic of responsibility, they comport themselves in a way that enhances everyone else's ability to perform smoothly, including the patient, who hears every conversation and constantly participates in it. Recognizing the significance of this level of communication and the essential logistics for creating a cohesive team in which each "knows" the other carries important implications for managers who plan and schedule the clinicians for procedures and surgeries of this nature.

Another striking difference about the CRNA's practice with these specific patients is the shift in the kind of clinical judgments and interventions that dominate care. Here, skillful use of anesthetic medications to alleviate pain and provide comfort is required, but as importantly, the key interventions center on engaged and skillful involvement with the patient for a prolonged time period as a major source of anxiety relief and comfort. This unusual comfort measure in the unlikely setting of the OR can be instructive to those who are developing meaningful ways of comforting.

TEACHING AND LEARNING CLINICAL GRASP, REASONING-IN-TRANSITIONS, AND MODUS OPERANDI THINKING

Nurse 2 in the above interview about the patient with the dissecting aortic aneurysm points out one of the strategies for teaching clinical grasp. After the incident, he learned and then discussed with Nurse 1 that postmortem findings following severe trauma typically show that aortic shearing or tearing commonly lead to death at the scene. He studied the topic and then wrote an article that was published in a newsletter:

Nurse 2: So for patients who die at the scene, it wouldn't be uncommon for them to have a triple-A [repair of a dissecting aortic abdominal aneurysm]. It wasn't in my mind that this guy had a triple-A. As far as we knew, that I knew, he was paralyzed and he was normotensive, and I didn't think it was a triple-A. It wasn't until I went back and did some investigating and ended up writing this article for the newsletter, that I realized that patients who have triple-A's, traumatic triple-A's, can actually exhibit paralysis. So next time I have somebody who's paralyzed, whether it is from a broken back or whether it is from a triple-A, I'll always be thinking that in the back of my mind.

Nurse 1: Having <u>extreme</u> back pain... Because by the time we got there, he was having agonizing back pain.

The nurses from this particular group interview had established an active tradition of community learning by sharing their experiences, good or bad, with the rest of the group. They also routinely review difficult situations in a multidisciplinary team conference and can ask for review of any case they deem important or where additional learning is needed. In this way, these clinicians as a collaborative team are continually learning from their own as well as their colleagues' practices.

Collaboration plays an important role in the development of clinical grasp and expert judgment (see Chapter 12). However, when a collaborative team is not available, clinicians can develop their perceptual skills by reflecting on their own judgments over time, in unfolding situations, to either confirm or disconfirm their initial clinical understandings. Like confirmation of one's clinical grasp, disconfirmation helps learners acquire valuable knowledge. Discovering what was overlooked from a incorrect understanding can not only assist in sensitizing and attuning the learner to context-sensitive patient responses, but can also teach the significance and meaning of specific responses.

A preceptorship is a strategy for developing clinical judgment. This involves having a more experienced clinician (including other disciplines, nurse, physician, etc.) point out patient responses, patterns, trends, and distinctions to less experienced clinicians. Preceptorships are common for orienting new nurses but uncommon beyond six months after the beginning of employment. As Benner, Tanner and Chesla (2009) have described, clinical learning is qualitatively different at the proficient stage of development, after new clinicians master the task world. It is at the proficient stage that learners rapidly develop their perceptual skills in reading situations as they unfold. Hence, nurses at the proficient stage would greatly benefit from a preceptor, coach, or mentor-type relationship in which the expert points out fine qualitative distinctions and early transitions in patient responses in similar and contrasting situations. This type of teaching\learning promotes open dialogue so that the learner can also explore appropriate interventions in particular instances.

It may seem obvious that "knowing the patient" is central to developing good clinical grasp, reasoning-in-transition, and modus operandi thinking. However, an advanced practice nurse describes a situation that highlights the ongoing importance of teaching and reinforcing this as a basis for clinical understanding:

Advanced Practice Nurse: A woman was in a very simple motor vehicle accident. She was <u>reported</u> as having possible intra-abdominal injuries, and an ultrasound showed something questionable on her liver. She had had this history of breast cancer and had a mastectomy. The attending physician in rounds wasn't one of our usual attendings, so this particular attending went off into a big long teaching session on this woman and her risks and how she'd had met[astasi]s and all of a sudden, we had this very sick dying woman on our hands that was in a simple motor vehicle accident. And the person, you'd ask him, 'Well, when was the mastectomy?' and 'What kind of cancer and how many nodes?' And none of the answers to these questions were known. I remember getting up—we were sitting in a conference room—I got up and walked across the hall into the patient's room and said, 'Excuse me, ma'am, can you tell me about your breast cancer?' She said, 'I've never had breast cancer.' I said, 'Really? And why did you have a mastectomy?' and she said, 'The doctor made a mistake. And I have never had—' she said, 'The biopsy came back and I never had breast cancer.' And I said, 'Okay, thank you very much,' I walked back and said, 'She's never had breast cancer, folks.' And one of the attendings, not one of our usuals, turned around and said, 'How did you know that?' I said, 'I asked the patient.' 'Well, how did you know to ask the patient?' 'Well, it was that or to condemn this woman to liver metastases from her breast cancer, and we should get some [facts]'... 'This doesn't make any sense and nobody here knows the story.' And the attending was getting sucked into this, and 'nobody knows the story.'... And every one was very surprised, and I just remember him turning around and going, 'God, <u>how</u> did you know that? And how did you know to ask that question?' And that was the question I think I couldn't believe that he asked the most, 'How did I know to ask that question?'

As the nurse became puzzled during rounds about how a patient in a simple accident suddenly became very sick and dying, she raised some basic questions about the patient's history, questions that would have presumably been addressed in the admission history and physical exam. Although it is disturbing that no one knew the answers, it is more disturbing that the attending would ask, "<u>How did you know that</u>?" and "How did you know to ask the patient?" For this nurse, talking with the patient as the most important and primary source of information were taken-for-granted; yet, many clinicians need to learn this critical aspect of practice. A group of advanced practice nurse conveyed numerous, similar instances where the interns and residents would ask, "How do you guys know all the things that we don't know? Who tells you all this?" One nurse's strategy was to:

Advanced Practice Nurse: ...talk to the nurses taking care of the patient because they will confide in you a lot and then you follow-up... And you just have to know the nurses and know their skill levels and know who's really reliable and know who doesn't give a really reliable assessment. But I think the important part is just listening.

The advanced practice nurses go on to say that the good clinicians are the ones that "<u>will</u> listen to their patients." The more expert clinicians discussed the need to role model how to ask questions and listen to patients. The nurse practitioners talked commonly about "leading by example" or role modeling (see Chapter 12). Leading by example includes interacting with the patient themselves and showing others how to probe based on what the patient did or did not talk about. This interactive clinical learning strategy involves coaching the learner to probe and listen more attentively. In addition, follow-up dialogue helps push the learner to think, particularly when the teacher asks, "if (this)..., then (what)..." types of questions. The "if..., then..." questions assist in teaching\learning modus operandi thinking. These experts also find that when opinions about interventions differ, it is fruitful to share anticipated outcomes or complications with the newer clinicians, as they become more open to learning when the predictions came to fruition.

Teaching some aspects of clinical grasp would be extremely difficult outside a patient setting because the distinctions that must be learned are relative to each particular patient's "baseline" because many of these distinctions can only be compared and differentiated through the bodily senses. Differences are recognized by constant comparison. The development of clinical scenarios on CD-ROM may be the one of the best educational tools to assist learners, outside the clinical setting. However, of the senses needed in developing perceptual acuity, CD-ROM can only provide visual and audio information. To assist in learning through smell, "scratch and sniff" tools could provide information that escapes articulation; the odor in particular situations can point to, and sometimes even make, the diagnosis. For instance, the smells of melena, pseudomonas, renal failure, and diabetic ketoacidosis, to name a few, combined in an educational package with a CD-ROM program could enhance embodied learning. Each of the above strategies teaches the learner to become more attentive and to reason-in-transition.

SUMMARY

A good clinical grasp of the patient's situation is central to expert clinical and ethical judgment. Learning to make qualitative distinctions, keep track of what has been done and what worked, recognize changing clinical relevance, and develop population-specific clinical knowledge are essential aspects in developing a good clinical understanding of patient situations. Although reading about these aspects of practice can be helpful to learners, gaining this practical knowledge requires an embodied way of knowing that <u>cannot</u> be fully learned except through experience. In a human practice where individuals will always have unique responses to therapeutic interventions, expert practice will always call for clinicians who are able to clinically grasp the situation and alter interventions to best respond to a particular patient's needs. This, in turn, calls for excellent clinicians who can and are available to teach others these skills.

REFERENCES

Benner, P. (Ed.). (1994). *Interpretive phenomenology: Embodiment, caring, and ethics in health and illness.* Thousand Oaks, CA: Sage.

Benner, P., Stannard, D., & Hooper, P. L. (1996). A "thinking-in-action" approach to teaching clinical judgment: A classroom innovation for acute care advanced practice nurses. *Advanced Practice Nursing Quarterly, 1*(4), 70-77.

Benner, P., Tanner, C., & Chesla, C. (1992). From beginner to expert: Gaining a differentiated clinical world in critical care nursing. *Advances in Nursing Science, 14*(3), 13-28.

Benner, P., Tanner, C. A., & Chesla, C. A. (2009). *Expertise in nursing practice: Caring, clinical judgment, and ethics.* New York, NY: Springer Publishing Company.

Bourdieu, P. (1980/1990). *The logic of practice* (Richard Nice, Trans.). Stanford, CA: Stanford University.Dreyfus, H. L., & Dreyfus, S. E. (1986). *Mind over machine: The power of human intuition and expertise in the era of the computer.* New York, NY: Free Press.

Hooper, P. L. (1995). *Expert titration of multiple vasoactive drugs in post-cardiac surgical patients: An interpretive study of clinical judgment and perceptual acuity.* Doctoral dissertation, University of California at San Francisco, San Francisco School of Nursing.

Kelley, P. & Benner, P. (in progress). *Caring for wounded warriors from Iraq and Afghanistan with antibiotic-resistant organisms.*

Knaus, W. A., Wagner, D., Draper, E., Zimmerman, J., Bergner, M., Bastos, P., Sirio, C., Murphy, D., Lotring, T., ... A. Damiano. (1991). The APACHE III prognostic system: Risk prediction of hospital mortality for critically ill hospitalized adults. *Chest,100*(6), 1619-1636.

Kyriakidis, P.H. (Research field notes, Social and Environmental Conditions that Support or Impede the Development of Expertise, September 2, 2007)

Kyriakidis, P.H., & Vitello, J. (in progress). *Applying Benner's research to entry level registered nurses: An investigation of development and retention.*

Lave, J. & Wenger, E. (1991). *Situated learning: Legitimate peripheral participation.* New York, NY: Cambridge University Press.

LeGall, J., Lemeshow, S., & Saulnier, F. (1993). A new simplified acute physiology score (SAPS II) based on a European/North American multicenter study. *JAMA, 270*(24), 2957-2963.

Lemeshow, S., Teres, D., Klar, J., Avrunin, J. S., Gehlbach, S., & Rapoport, J. (1993). Mortality probability models (MPM II) based on an international cohort of intensive care unit patients. *JAMA, 270*(20), 2478-2486.

Merleau-Ponty, M. (1964). *Sense and non-sense* (H. Dreyfus & P. Dreyfus, Trans.). Evanston, IL: Northwestern University Press.

Molter, Colonel N. (personal communications, March 23, 2010).

Polanyi, M. (1962). *Personal knowledge: Towards a post-critical philosophy*. Chicago, IL: University of Chicago Press.

Rubin, J. (2009). Impediments to the development of clinical knowledge and ethical judgment in critical care nursing. In P. Benner, C. A. Tanner, & C. A. Chesla (Eds.), *Expertise in nursing practice: Caring, clinical judgment, and ethics* (pp. 171-198). New York, NY: Springer Publishing Company.

Sadler, R. (1980). Conveying the findings of evaluative inquiry. *Educational Evaluation & Policy Analysis, 2*(2), 53-57.

Tanner, C. A., Benner, P., Chesla, C., & Gordon, D. R. (1993). The phenomenology of knowing a patient. *Image, 25*(4), 273-280.

Taylor, C. (1985). *Human agency and language: Philosophical papers 1. (Vol. I)*. Cambridge, England: Cambridge University Press.

Taylor, C. (1993). *The quality of life*. Oxford, England: Clarendon.

Taylor, C. (1995). *Philosophical Arguments*. Cambridge, MA: Harvard University Press.

3

Clinical Imagination and Clinical Forethought: Anticipating and Preventing Potential Problems

*C*linical forethought refers to the habits of thought that allow clinicians to anticipate likely clinical eventualities and to take the actions warranted. Clinical forethought requires prior experiential learning with similar patient care situations. It also requires clinical imagination. Making interventions as a result of the patient's clinical manifestations in the moment require thinking-in-action that is aided by anticipation. We have placed this chapter early in the book so that the reader will notice this pervasive habit of thought in subsequent chapters. We have placed it early because an underlying premise of this work is that, like clinical grasp (see Chapter 2), clinical forethought entails aspects of clinical judgment and wisdom that are seldom articulated, despite the fact that clinical forethought is pervasive in the everyday logic of practice.

Clinical forethought both shapes and is shaped by the practitioner's clinical grasp, which can be thought of as an immediate understanding of the clinical situation. When clinicians engage in clinical forethought, they commonly project possible clinical eventualities that may occur with a particular patient and family and that may influence planning and orchestrating care. Clinicians prepare the environment by anticipating possible clinical eventualities. These habits of practice guide thinking-in-action. Because clinical forethought is always embedded in particular situations, over time, it becomes such a habit of thought and a patterned way of approaching clinical situations, that it becomes intuitive. By intuitive, we do not mean wild guesses or extrasensory perception. Rather, we use the term *intuitive* to refer to pattern recognition, a sense of salience, and a sense of concern or heightened attentiveness based upon experiential learning in whole past concrete situations (Benner & Tanner, 1987; Benner, Tanner & Chesla, 2009). This experience-based wisdom creates perceptual awareness, which refers to a knowing without necessarily having a specific rationale or making explicit all that goes into one's sense of the situation (Benner, 1984; Benner & Tanner, 1987; Benner, Tanner & Chesla, 2009; Benner & Wrubel, 1982; Dreyfus & Dreyfus, 1986). Although expert nurses can probably give the best account of their clinical interpretation, the aspects of their understanding, based on past whole concrete situations or on the recognition of global changes in the patient, may be vague or not easily articulated. It is an example of the clinician knowing more than he or she can say (Polanyi, 1958/1962). This should be distinguished from a confused, ignorant understanding of the situation because the clinician accounts for the relevant evidence, gives the most probable rationale, and points to the vague, more global observations. Sometimes nurses refer to intuitive thinking as "common sense," because what they "see" and understand is so familiar that it simply appears to be good sense, as illustrated in the following interview excerpt:

> **Nurse:** I think the good OR nurses, first of all, all have common sense. And the other thing that I've found over the 26 years that I've been in it is 'always go with your intuition.' Every time I don't go with my intuition, when I think there's going to be a problem and I'm thinking, 'I really should get out those surgical sponges, you know, I have a feeling this patient's aorta is going to fall apart.' Every time I don't do it, it always happens. And I'm always going, 'You thought about this, why didn't you act on what you were thinking about,' you know? And I'm going, 'Oh well, maybe it'll be okay.' But it always seems to happen. So, every time I get those feelings and I don't always act on them—but I should always act on them because 95% of the time I'm correct.

"Common sense" or intuition based upon 26 years of experience is frequently correct, but even if it is not correct, the anticipation itself allows for disconfirmation and correction. Clinical forethought is crucial to recognition of early changes in the patient, because it prepares the nurse to "see" or recognize what is likely to transpire, and to act based on these early changes. Paula Reiss, an ER nurse, shared a clinical incident that demonstrates the kinds of habits of thinking and action we are describing. This particular exemplar is stunning because one can see Paula's constant, complex grasp and thinking ahead in order to prepare for the likely eventualities for the patient, the mother, the physicians, and the student nurse. Without having to stop, analytically think or plan, this expert continuously coaches others to prepare them for what shows up as "common sense" in managing this crisis:

> **Nurse:** In through the ER doors came a young mom carrying her baby. One glance at that infant brought Tina and I to our feet. Something about the one little arm I could see from across the room. Pale. Mottled? Too limp. The mother started to speak, "His apnea monitor just keeps going off and now he's hard to wake up!" "Hey Dr. Z, care to join us? Hey Andie, could you call RT for us?" *"STAT!!!"* I whisper to her as I walks by. I quickly but gently lead our [mother and child] into one of our bigger resuscitation rooms. One of the student nurses joins us as well.
>
> Mom lays her most prized possession on the cold crisp white sheet for our inspection. Indeed a limp, mottled-appearing baby: shallow respirations, a reassuring tachycardia (at least he has some fight in him) and a vacant look to those little eyes I've seen too many times before—and I don't much like. "He sure is a cute one!" I say to mom. "We're going to do some things here kind of quickly to see if we can't get him to feel better. Do you want to stay?" (Under my breath I said, "Tina do you want to do airway?") Continuing to talk to mom, "You can—and it's fine if you don't want to stay right now too. No wrong answers here."
>
> "Oh I have to stay," she said. "I just can't leave him. I promised him I'd never leave him!" Tina is adeptly setting up the Ambu and securing it to his little face as I am looking for [IV] access. I invite Dr. Z. to join Tina at the head of the bed. Dr. Z is someone who

functions well in a code if the environment is a controlled one: [a stressful climate] in the resuscitation room just throws her over the edge.

I calmly ask the student to go out to the desk, ask for the resident and another nurse to join us. I continue to smile and comment on the cuteness of this baby. Calm is good. The student returns to the room and I direct her to get mom a seat and point to the perimeter of the room, (but where she can still see) and to pull up a chair next to her. "I'll keep you posted about what we are doing over here, and please feel free to ask any questions" I say to mom. To the student: "And get two warm blankets, please." One for Jacob. One for mom," who is shivering on this hot July day.

I figured out a long time ago that you can keep a resuscitation under control by kind of chatting with the parents about what is going on throughout in a calm and reassuring fashion. It's a discreet way of spreading reassurance throughout the room and reminding the other health care providers what the order of things should be.

RT is here too, as is our third nurse, Ellie. I explain to mom that we will be putting a special tube in his air pipe to help him breathe better. The resident comes in and I tell mom that this doctor and I are going to spend a little more time looking for a place to put an I.V. I've already laid the IO [intraosseous access] on the bed: I 'm thinking the resident will need to move mentally in that direction pretty quickly and might need a minute to rehearse the procedure in her head. Eyeing it, she whispers, "I've never done an IO." "I'll help you" I whisper back. Ellie is laying out the "holy water" (code drugs). "Can you scribe (do documentation)? I say, ripping the piece of 3 inch adhesive tape from my pant leg where I'd written initial vital signs.

Help as I might, the resident just could not get that IO to pop in. I look up at Dr. Z who is holding the ETT while RT tapes it and ask, "What do you think about a central line?" "Okay," she says. Ellie steps out for a second to call for a surgeon. Surgery staff come pretty quickly. I address them with a cheery hello so as to keep the same level of calm and control in the room. No need for tense surgeons. "These doctors are going to put the tube in we need to give baby Jacob some fluids" I say to mom. Dr. S smiled and said hi to mom while I set out the central line equipment, then set up some warmed normal saline in anticipation of a fluid bolus.

A controlled airway, assisted ventilations, glucose stores replenished, a bolus of fluids does baby Jacob a lot of good. His color is already a little better. Cap[illary] refill is almost down to 2 seconds. We are moving in the right direction. "What questions do you have?" I say to Jacob's mom. I note that the student is doing a great job—our baby's mom is kind of tucked in over there, with the young student's arm securely around her shoulders. I note that the student and the mom look to be about the same age.

"Will he have to stay over night in the hospital?" "Building blocks," I think. "One step at a time about how sick her sweet baby is." "Yes, he'll need to stay." I'll tell her as much as she's able to hear right now. That's all she wants to know for now, and I respect that. She'll ask more questions when she is ready.

[By now], the portable chest X-ray is clear. We know the results of the labs we need to know emergently, and the rest are pending. An ICU bed is ready—so we transport Jacob and his mom to the ICU.

It turns out that baby Jacob had an undiagnosed metabolic problem. Three days later Jacob was found to be a pink, happy, active baby boy. ETT tube and central line gone, cooing and playing happily with his toes. Truly now, a cute one.

Paula's experiential wisdom enables her to flexibly notice and keep track of the multiple emergent interventions that Jacob needs while she simultaneously anticipates and prepares for what each person in the resuscitation room needs to do and when. Her skillful foresight ensures that each person has a valuable role, is focused on Jacob and his mom, and remains calm to enhance the ability of each to capably cope and perform. She can imagine what is coming next while concurrently imagining what contingency plan may be needed if the inexperienced resident has procedural difficulties.

Clinical forethought requires imaginative use of past clinical experience and scientific knowledge. It is always situated, and anchored by clinical imagination. The most effective clinical forethought is based on both scientific understanding and experiential learning of clinical trajectories, however, clinical forethought does not have to be precisely correct in order to be a useful basis for thinking-in-action. To be useful, it only needs to be in the right direction or region of the problem and to be capable of being confirmed or disconfirmed by tests and assessments in the actual evolving situation. Clinical forethought works best when it is held tentatively and when it flexibly changes if the patient's condition unfolds in an unexpected direction. Rigid adherence to what one has anticipated and planned for, can be a source of error in this habit of thought because it prevents seeing the unexpected. The OR nurse, above, with so many years of experience, has a large repertoire of background experiences that enable her to see situations with a prepared mind. Such a prepared mind is based upon habits of thought—cultivated habits of thinking-in-action about expectations and articulating them and paying attention to when they are confirmed or disconfirmed.

Good clinicians draw on the best scientific evidence available to make sound clinical judgments and, as clinicians, they can contribute to the development of scientific knowledge through discoveries made directly in practice. Their discoveries can help prioritize research agendas. Many good questions and puzzles for scientific studies come from clinical practice. Communicating these puzzles and questions or directly engaging in scientific studies to solve these puzzles advances clinical knowledge and practice. Science is <u>necessary</u> for making good clinical judgments and for thinking-in-action in particular clinical situations; however, science alone is not <u>sufficient</u>. Effective clinical forethought requires the best scientific understandings of a particular patient problem and clinical wisdom gained through experience. In addition to scientific knowledge, the clinician must seek to interpret a particular patient's clinical situation and respond to demands and possibilities in a timely manner. The clinician must sense what is at stake for a particular patient and family, and be committed to working towards the patient's best interests. We need a greater emphasis on developing these habits of thinking in basic and graduate nursing education programs, staff development, and continuing education programs.

Categorizing and cataloging nursing diagnoses, interventions, and outcomes overlook the ways that these are generated and interrelated in actual practice. Expert nurses do not follow the mentalistic assumption that the thinking nurse goes to a catalogue of diagnoses and matches the diagnoses with corresponding interventions to achieve pre-determined, generalized outcomes. As Logstrup (1995) points out, subsuming or classifying things under categories is not the same as productive thinking. Classification systems may work for information management and record retrieval, but they do not present an accurate account of the habits of thought, thinking-in-action, or reasoning-in-transition involved in actual clinical practice.

Learning to think-in-action in any practice—medicine, law, nursing, teaching, or social work—is based on learning prototypical situations and then filling out these prototypes with actual clinical experience so that the prototypical cases become more nuanced

TABLE 3.1

Clinical Forethought

Anticipating and Preventing Potential Problems

▨ Future think

▨ Clinical forethought about specific diagnoses and injuries

▨ Anticipation of crises, risks, and vulnerabilities for particular patients

▨ Seeing the unexpected

and particularized in specific patient encounters. To this end we describe how thinking-in-action and reasoning-in-transition are aided by anticipation.

Though clinical forethought is integrally related to ongoing clinical grasp, it is a distinct habit of thought and action that deserves its own description. The goals of Chapter 2 and 3 are to bring clinical grasp and clinical forethought in from the margins of informal learning and into mainstream educational curricula. Both are hallmarks of practical reasoning across transitions in the patient's condition, or the clinician's understanding. We believe that the general characteristics of clinical forethought and clinical grasp are applicable to areas of nursing beyond acute and critical care even though the clinical content and contexts might be quite different. Four common aspects of clinical forethought are described in Table 3.1.

Future think is the broadest category of this logic of practice (Benner, 1984). Gaining increasing amounts and quality of information about specific diagnoses and injuries and acquiring knowledge information about particular patient responses shape clinical forethought in increasingly detailed ways.

FUTURE THINK

Future think is the overarching aspect in this habit of thinking. It was first described in *From Novice to Expert* as the habit of thought common to nurses that enables them to respond quickly to likely clinical eventualities (Benner, 1984). Clinical forethought also sets up a problem-solving context for evaluating a particular patient's responses, for instance, knowing what to expect after a surgery and how to prepare the environment (e.g., marshal needed supplies, fluids, and medications) which potentiates a quick response. Clinical forethought thus enables nurses to organize the complex environments of critical care, operating room, and post anesthesia areas and to make sure that needed tests are ordered and supplies are available. The following excerpt illustrates the kind of clinical forethought common in surgery:

Interviewer: How would you expect things to proceed with this patient? What are things that you are looking...?

Nurse: Well, one thing that I already talked to my tech about was I wanted to have a vascular pack ready. Now that's only for an emergency. This surgery is on the side of his neck, it's near his carotid and near his jugulars. This is strictly a soft tissue biopsy. We expect a minimal amount of instrumentation and not a very complicated procedure. But what I'm thinking about, and what the tech doesn't have the background to think about, is that because of all the vessels, we could get into some bleeding problems and I want her to have the items ready—I don't want to <u>leave</u> the room at a critical time and go get them. So I already asked her to take care of getting a couple of other items. The other thing that I consider is that because we are around the carotids and we can get vagal stimulation, they like to have certain medications on hand. I know those are there already, but if—these are just things that I'm thinking about...

Interviewer: Specifically what medications were you thinking...

Nurse: Xylocaine and atropine (Observational Interview).

Knowing the anatomy and nature of the surgery are required for this kind of clinical forethought, but nurses also learn to prepare for the specific practices of particular physicians, and even for staffing levels. For example, the nurse may prepare the environment more fully if she knows there is no one available to get supplies. The nurse may also prepare slightly different sutures or instruments depending on the surgeon's typical preferences (Hooper, 1995).

Clinical forethought not only enables nurses to prepare environments for potential eventualities, it also propels nurses to prepare the patient for a possible crisis. This aspect of future think is illustrated by the common example of having the needed IV access available, in this instance in the neonatal ICU as cited in Benner, Tanner, and Chesla (2009, p. 150):

Nurse: Actually he did this little tiny code where we did chest compressions for a few minutes, and then right after he did that—this is where my expert clinical judgment came into practice—I said, 'I need to get an IV in him just in case he does this again.' And two people said, 'No, you don't need to do that, he's okay.' So I slipped an IV in anyway, which is no small feat on a kid from our unit that's four months old. Their veins are usually so trashed [from prior multiple IVs]. Anyway, I got an IV into him and within twenty minutes, I needed that IV because he then really went into a full code and needed IV drugs.

Learning that a "tiny little code" is often an ominous forewarning of a crisis helps nurses develop predispositions to intervene early in order to prevent or mitigate an ensuing crisis. Similarly, sets or predispositions to act quickly during emergencies come from clinical forethought and reflection on and learning from practice after emergency procedures. Since the focus is on achieving the best ends possible in a resuscitation, the teamwork required for this work is invisible except when it is not there:

Nurse 1: I think you're right about saying that <u>which</u> doctor it is isn't as important as the team, because they're asking for atropine and get me this and get me that, and it magically appears in their hand. And they have no concept of what five different nurses are doing and how we're anticipating them. They just want it there 5 minutes ago. It appears and they're not aware really of where things are coming from or who's keeping track of anything.

Nurse 2: Doing things even before they ask. You have it in your hand and they say 'Give it' and you say 'Okay' and it's right there.

Nurse 1: Let's set up for a chest tube and you're standing there already set up.

For emergencies, mock codes help prepare the nurse to prepare for the next most likely patient intervention. However, what Bourdieu (1980/1990) points out for team sports also applies to clinical practice. Practice in the actual situation, complete with time demands and variation in the patient's responses, is required to learn to respond quickly and reliably. The practical details of anticipating what will be needed to respond rapidly to a crisis is illustrated in the following excerpt from the operating room where the anticipations are life-saving:

> **Nurse:** We possess the ability to make very critical judgments in the situation... For instance, today, I was scrubbed in an operating room. My circulating nurse is a very good nurse but she's not as experienced as some of our [OR] nurses are. We were doing a bilateral lung transplant and they put a clamp on the patient's left atrium, which is normal for that procedure, and the patient became bradycardic. And you could hear it on the monitors. His heart just got slower and slower and slower. And I know from experience, from having gone to ACLS and just from having assisted with heart surgery for a long time, that when a patient does that there's a chance they can go into brady-cardic arrest. One of the things that you can do—that you're lucky enough to be able to when the chest is open—is to put in epicardial pacing wires and hook him up to a pacemaker. And that can be done relatively quickly if there's a problem. Now, the doctor could look up, or somebody could look up and say 'We're getting bradycardic,' and then they could tell an unskilled person, 'Okay, get some pacing wires,' and the person would get the pacing wires. But they wouldn't realize that they would have to go through the cascade of getting the pacemaker and getting the pacing cable. And yet things can be abbreviated when there are people in the room like us who can make critical choices.
>
> When I heard that man's heart slowing down and it was getting slower and slower, I turned to my circulating nurse, and said, 'Get two pacing wires, get a pace-maker, I want a pacing cable, set them all right here and give the anesthesiologist the pacemaker'—and none of them had even thought of that yet. And it's not because I'm brilliant or a genius, it's just that I have the ability to make <u>critical</u> decisions. I've seen it before, you know? I know what the actions are. And it just abbreviated the whole situation—everybody was very comfortable and nobody got upset. If that had gone for two or three more minutes everybody would have been flapping their arms.
>
> Something very similar happened last week. There was a child who became bradycardic on induction and they didn't have an IV, and they were just barely getting things started, and the resident was new and flapping around and the attending was a little perturbed too. And when this child was becoming bradycardic I knew one thing that you do when a child becomes bradycardic is you give them atropine. And they had just gotten an IV started and instead of waiting for them to tell me what to do, I walked back to their cart and found the atropine syringe and just handed it to them and they immediately gave it like, 'Oh yeah!' and it's only because I've been doing it for a long time, and I think those of us who are very experienced just have the ability to make critical decisions in that way, to smooth things out and recognize situations.

This is a good example of what we mean by thinking-in-action and clinical fore-thought. Once the possible clinical eventualities become clear, the nurse anticipates the needed interventions for these eventualities. The nurse skillfully grasps the significance of the slowing heart rate and prepares, both mentally and physically, for the possibility that the patient may experience cardiac arrest. Realizing that she is more experienced than the circulating nurse (who, therefore, may not have anticipated and prepared for this contin-gency), the scrub nurse orders the pacing wires, cable, and pacemaker and has them ready to hand over to the surgeon. Although she claims "she's not brilliant," she has effectively learned from experience. Grasping the pattern enables the nurse to instantly "think ahead" to prepare for and prevent cardiac arrest.

In the child's situation, the nurse's anticipation and prompt intervention were life-saving. In addition to anticipating the patient's clinical needs, the nurse also anticipated what was needed by other team members and intervened to keep them calm and subsequently performing smoothly.

This kind of clinical wisdom developed by nurses over time is life-saving, local, and specific knowledge. It is an example of clinical imagination. The nurse's quick responses are part of the essential attentiveness required to maintain safe systems for highly technical medical interventions, such as ordering routine lab tests, anticipating what supplies will be needed, et cetera, as illustrated in the next interview excerpt:

> **Nurse:** Well, I take an inventory. I find out what's on hand in the room, where everything is, do I have enough of everything in order to take care of this patient? Like I'll make sure I have enough meds, enough equipment—if they're on a low-flow air bed, do I have enough chux if I want to change this patient? It's organized. It's knowing that you have everything to take care of that patient, and how to go about ordering it. If it's not there, you just have to do it. You don't wait for someone else to do it. And when you get report you ask these little questions like, 'Did you send the Pro time? Because I have to give a coumadin dose tonight.' Just the little things that...

> **Interviewer:** This is another discourse the experts always bring up: Does the lab work that has been ordered make sense? Are you still doing things that no longer make sense? Do you want to talk about that a little bit? I mean, it's catching the forgetfulness, or if someone has to have blood drawn, did they think to order everything? Do we need another order, that sort of thing?

> **Nurse:** Oh, you have to think of every system and the doctors even forget things. I'll sometimes make a list for the doctors. After I've done all my inventory and my assessment and everything, I'll have a list of questions for the doctors to clarify things that would help me take better care of that patient: if they're on the balloon, do they check their platelets twice a day, or, if they've gotten platelets, do they do a one-hour post-platelet count? There's just little things that get forgotten.

Making sure that things are not forgotten requires thinking about demands, resources, and constraints in the immediate future. Nurses use informal surveillance systems to make sure that typical treatment protocols are not accidentally being altered. This kind of safety work is further discussed in Chapter 8, but it is the kind of future think that nurses use to make sure that best practices are carried out. The practical demands of orchestrating future interventions congruent with the patient's needs and responses require keeping track of the thinking-in-action as it is occurring in order to anticipate the next intervention.

Preparing environments by making equipment and supplies available is traditional women's work in the domestic sphere. In patient care settings , this hidden women's work is extended into a highly technical, fast-paced environment. Future think includes anticipating and arranging times of interventions that maximize the patient's rest and anticipates the patient's most likely schedules at home:

> **Nurse 1:** When I admit people after surgery, I try to time the meds so that they know that they're not going to have to be disturbed, and I think more people are thinking about that too...changing their med times so that patients can have that time [to rest].

Nurse 2: Dressing changes at 3:00 in the morning burn me up.

Nurse 3: I used to work rehab and our thing was let's put the medications on this patient's schedule. Are they going to wake up at 1:00 in the morning to take these meds? No. Are they going to wake up at 5:00 in the morning to take these meds? No. So let's put it on their schedule; not the nurses.

Nurse 1: Another thing I've tried to do is select the pigtails [a long tubing] on the IVs as long as possible so that if you have to hang an IV at 1:00 in the morning, you can hang it through the main line and you can hang a med in the semi-dark.

In the small group interview, the conversation moves into the usual habits of clinical forethought that allow for the patient's rest and a smoother transition to home.

Transporting the patient from one unit to another, to diagnostic, and interventional X-rays all require clinical forethought to arrange for the needed supplies and transport equipment. This is particularly true for air and ground emergency transports but as illustrated below, equally true for within hospital transfers. In the following example, a patient had to be prepared to go for a cardiac catheterization to remove a portion of IV tubing that bent and broke lose. The nurse in the interview describes her future think about setting up for the transport and for the procedure.

Nurse: I also knew he had to have his antiarrhythmic medication before he went down. I didn't want him to have it delayed any longer. I kept thinking of all these medications that I needed to give him. But the most important thing was, let me give him his antiarrhythmic before we go down. I wanted to do that. And it actually went really smoothly. I couldn't believe how smoothly it actually did go. We could have gotten into a lot of problems going down there too soon and making sure that he did have an O_2 setup and everything else on the bedside there. We went down and they fished it out with no problem.

Interviewer: So the patient arresting was your number one concern. What were some of your other concerns, in that immediate situation, that hour that you were waiting?

Nurse: That was my main concern and also looking ahead. You always have to look ahead, like what can I anticipate? I told the nurses that I needed a rack for the bed so that we could bring down the IV pole or whatever and different things hanging on there. I needed that. I needed the oxygen tank; please get the respiratory therapist. Get everything ready. I want to be ready to go down when they say we can go down. I don't want to waste any time with this because we can't afford to delay this intervention (Observational Interview).

This detailed planning requires engaged reasoning about the procedure and also illustrates the next two aspects of clinical forethought: clinical forethought about specific diagnoses and injuries and anticipation of crises, risks, and vulnerabilities for particular patients.

CLINICAL FORETHOUGHT ABOUT SPECIFIC DIAGNOSES AND INJURIES

Thinking ahead about the clinical eventualities anticipated for patients with particular diagnoses or injuries enables the nurse to arrange possible equipment and prepare the immediate environment more specifically for likely eventualities. For example, in the specialty practice of emergency transport, nurses talk about getting an early sense of the seriousness of an injury in order to determine whether an airway will be needed before the accident victim is extricated from the vehicle or can wait until access is more controlled. The basic resuscitation guidelines shape their mental preparedness:

Nurse 1: Everything we do, whether it's medicine or trauma, everything comes down to A-B-C [Airway-Breathing-Circulation]. But yet you have to have all this information to be able to get to that point. We are giving people the best level of care that's possible for them and we're doing the simplest thing.

Nurse 2: The very basics.

Nurse 1: The very basics. The information that gets taught in BLS and CPR (Basic Life Support, Cardiopulmonary Resuscitation). Though we have a few extra tools to make sure that we get an airway [intubation and cricothyrotomy equipment], we're doing a few extra things to make sure that they're breathing, and we're simply putting in IVs or doing CPR to make sure they have some strong circulation. But you have to go through such a big process and such a large amount of knowledge to be able to come to that point, that I don't think people really realize that.

Interviewer: No, I do.

Nurse 2: (Laughs). Yes. And we need a really big knowledge base, but a lot of this job is very intuitive...for us. Because you don't always have a lot of information. And you gather it as you go or sometimes you don't get a lot of information, period. So, I think that people who don't do well in this job are people who can't be intuitive.

Nurse 3: That's true.

Nurse 2: You have to be able to look and say, 'This person's bad.' And then you know that the only thing you're going to do is A-B-C. You have to be able to do it. Now, that may be a little different for some of our inter-facility patients where you have to get the ICU gears going. You can say, 'This guy's really bad.' And then you have to think about all of his drips and potential for all of his drips. The potential complications from his pulmonary system, his renal system, his hepatic system. You think about all those things but you have to apply them to that hour that you have with him. 'What am I going to do to keep this guy alive or make him better before he gets to our hospital?' And it all comes back down to A-B-C. What's going to work?

The "simplest things" that the flight nurses are doing are based upon both clinical grasp and clinical forethought. However, as discussed in Chapter 2, constant on-the-ground learning with specific patients and patient populations informs thinking, can hone judgment and literally alter one's habitual interventions,. For instance, we have new clinical knowledge developed by health care providers in the Afghanistan and Iraq wars. The injuries are often traumatic amputations and massive injuries as a result of explosive devices. Health care workers embedded in the troops have quickly learned to consider C, circulation prior to airway and breathing if the patient is rapidly hemorrhaging massive amounts of blood. Providing oxygen if there is not enough blood to circulate will not help. The results of this situated learning and altered habit have, in turn, dramatically changed thinking to the point that pre-emptive measures around circulation have been implemented; that is, soldiers now loosely apply tourniquets to all four limbs prior to going into the field so bleeding from injuries can be immediately stopped with one hand (Colonel N. Molter, March 23, 2010), Also health care providers have learned not to give too much fluid in the field that will further dilute the patient's blood supply and likely cause delayed clotting.

In the above interview, recognizing that the patient is really "bad" depends upon knowing much about the plausible physiological injuries, but it also depends on having seen many critically and not so critically injured patients before, so that early recognition and discriminations can be made. This recognition skill is what we mean by clinical grasp. Clinical forethought prepares the nurse to act by having the appropriate equipment and medications ready, figuring out the situational limits to actions in the field, or in the hour or minutes before hospitalization, and taking those actions efficiently and reliably.

Simplification of the situation depends upon having a deep background understanding of many similar situations and the practical implications of those situations. It is misleading to think that since all the "background" knowledge is not brought to bear on each problem, that this fund of theoretical and experiential clinical wisdom is not necessary, and therefore less educated workers trained in the life-saving techniques could achieve the same results. A less prepared worker would literally not see or perceive the same things, since the foreground one sees is dependent on their background understandings. The person prepared to learn directly from each clinical situation develops a deep background understanding that enables them to zero in on the most relevant issues and distinctions in the situation (Benner, 1984; Benner, Tanner & Chesla, 2009; Dreyfus, 1992). As pointed out in Chapter 2, this ability to make qualitative distinctions cannot be simply trained by using pre-set protocols. Using protocols or following algorithms requires knowing when to use them and when to adjust them to the demands of the situation. Good thinking-in-action and clinical wisdom gained from clinical inquiry are required. What these experienced specialty nurses perceive as a simple reading of the situation and an instance of "common" sense is not at all simple or common for the under-prepared and inexperienced person. The inexperienced person or the expert person who does not know the patient population or the patient are more effective if they follow protocols precisely since they do not yet have the experiential bases for making situated adjustments based upon the patient's particular situation.

Good nurses use clinical forethought about the needs of patients with particular diagnoses every time a patient is admitted to their care. They first prepare the room based on whatever ambulance, emergency department or operating room report they can get. They actively start rehearsing the most likely scenarios so that they can be prepared and ready with equipment, fluids, physicians' orders, and medications at hand to respond instantaneously.

Nurse: This is about a 30-year-old man who was on a mountain bike and was hit by a car. He was thrown and fell on his right side. He had a right flail segment, a right hemo and pneumothorax, and a chest tube on that side. He also sustained a liver laceration. His liver was displaced into his thorax. His diaphragm, and possibly his phrenic nerve, was severed. He was not wearing a helmet and sustained a bleed into the left lateral ventricle in his brain. He also had a parietal hematoma. He was intubated... He had received six units of blood in the OR and five liters of crystalloids. But, he came back with two peripheral IVs. And no, they weren't thinking about how this patient needs nutrition, needs IVs, needs a central line. He's received a lot of fluids and we're monitoring him. Plus he has a liver laceration. So, he needs good IV access.

Interviewer: Why?

Nurse: In case he bled out really quick. If they bleed out, they bleed out quickly and they need to be taken to OR and you need to pump blood products in them stat (Observational Interview).

This kind of clinical forethought is crucial for preparing the environment and the patient for likely clinical eventualities. Upon admission, the nurse in neurosurgical ICU does not know very much about specific patient responses, and she goes on to mention that she hopes to get more information from the anesthesiologist about the patient's blood pressure patterns and responses to medications. Needing to know about specific patient responses sets up patient specific forethought and until the nurse gains that grasp, the nurse is less adept at anticipating and "staying on top" of potential complications or issues.

Clinical forethought about a patient with a specific diagnosis influences a nurse's interpretation of the patient's responses. In the above story concerning the mountain bike accident, the nurse goes on to coach a new graduate nurse about recognizing physiological transitions in patients with head trauma, explaining that seeing someone "resting comfortably" could mean that they are worse, not better. Her warnings are based upon first-hand experiential wisdom gained from having mistaken a patient's lower level of consciousness for "resting more comfortably." Such tragic instances of caring for a patient with a particular diagnosis shapes attentiveness and clinical forethought in future situations. Passing along such warnings makes cumulative wisdom possible, preventing needless repetition of errors. The following interview excerpt is a good example of the way that a prior experience where an infant died with staphylococcus sepsis makes this nurse vigilant for early signs of a trend:

Nurse: Well, after that whenever I took care of an infant with a diagnosis of potential staphylococcus sepsis, even though the child might have been awake, alert, and looked wonderful, I worried every minute and I followed his chemistries carefully and if they changed [to] what I thought was adverse, I'd have the doctors do whatever I thought. If I thought coags needed to be done, a DIC panel, or if I thought renal function studies needed to be done, whatever I thought needed to be done to follow the trend. Once the trend starts, there's not too much you can do, I guess, once it's started, other than give appropriate antibiotics. So then it becomes imperative to identify the organism. So then you have to become real assertive, 'Have you got the gram stain back?' 'What are the cerebral spinal fluid results? Did you do a urine culture?' You get real pushy about what's causing this condition, because if it's a staph sepsis, you know your baby is going to get very sick very quickly, and you're not going to be able to change the outcome. Early diagnosis and treatment, like in so many things, is the only thing that will save the infant.

Interviewer: In this case, just for my own peace of mind, did they do all of the blood work and then treat experimentally? Start on antibiotics?

Nurse: They put him on broad spectrum antibiotics.

Interviewer: But in this baby's case they had done all of the blood work...

Nurse: Yes, but the baby became so sick so quickly before the cultures had come back. By the time they identified what the organism was, the cascade had already begun, and once that cascade begins, they develop capillary permeability and they're in a continuous state of shock. Some children can be in shock for days, but if you can get them and treat them effectively, efficiently, as soon as possible before it becomes a septicemia, then the child has like a 50% chance of surviving, which is not terribly good odds, but you can save some of the children. Children do not have to die from septic shock if you can prevent them from developing it.

An actual experience such as this fills in the sense of timing in a way that no textbook description of symptoms can. It is also a good example of the use of <u>one</u> prior experience. The nurse has no other cases on a continuum, though she knows that it is possible to save lives by early detection and treatment. Single case experience needs to be tempered by comparisons with aggregate data and with subsequent variations added by a range of experiences with similar diagnoses. Though one's experience is sufficient to give the nurse a sense of how quickly staphylococcus sepsis can deteriorate into a grave condition is a life-saving kind of experiential wisdom that generates her vigilance and forethought. She now knows the terrain and the timing issues from first-hand experience. With additional experience, she will understand more directly about how to read and anticipate particular patients' responses.

Learning the typical clinical course of a diagnosis or injury provides nurses with an understanding of clinical trajectories and thus with essential knowledge for clinical forethought. Recovery from cardiac surgery becomes a known clinical trajectory with a background set of expectations and forecasts, as illustrated in the following observational interview excerpt:

Interviewer: Any expectations as to how his postoperative course will go and what his ultimate outcome will be?

Nurse: I think he should do reasonably well. Probably nothing spectacular in view of the fact he has vascular disease. He is 70 years old... In terms of the next couple of days, he will be slower to extubate, slower to mobilize fluids, just a slower course.

Interviewer: What guides those generalizations or hunches?

Nurse: The fact that he has COPD [Chronic Obstructive Pulmonary Disease], might make getting him off the ventilator hard. The goal is usually to extubate by tomorrow morning. By the way it looks now, we will not with him. Usually with a 'normal' heart, we extubate at 8:00 a.m. But with him, the earliest we would extubate him is the following day.

Interviewer: So just the whole weaning process?

Nurse: The whole weaning process will be slower. Speaking of which, I had better check a blood gas since we reintubated him (Observational Interview).

Expected timetables provide an informal set of expectations that project clinical forethought. In this case, the nurse recognizes this patient as a member of a subgroup of cardiac surgical patients—those with chronic lung disease. With experiential wisdom, the nurse finds that her expected timetable is extended in this subgroup of harder to wean patients. We have many such examples where recovery trajectories become routinized expectations, and deviations from these timetables become sources of problem-solving.

ANTICIPATION OF CRISES, RISKS, AND VULNERABILITIES
FOR PARTICULAR PATIENTS

Clinical forethought based upon understanding a particular patient's illness and responses to therapies reflects a historical and narrative understanding of a particular patient's clinical condition and patterns of responses to therapies. Experiential wisdom based on prior experience can be refined by understanding a specific patient's patterns. The common thread to anticipating a possible crisis is that of pattern recognition based on the particular patient's history. Recognizing specific patient vulnerabilities and risks allows the nurse to anticipate possible future complications or crises and prepare for or prevent them. This kind of clinical forethought enables the nurse to identify a region within a risk field and monitor clinical trends. Understanding a patient's fragile condition and anticipating the complications are inextricably bound with the skill of knowing the patient (Benner, Tanner & Chesla, 2009). The nurse with a good map of the patient's vulnerabilities, such as co-morbid conditions like diabetes, is in a better position to locate the risks and thereby anticipate and prevent problems for particular patients. For example, a nurse anticipates changes likely to occur after cardiac surgery:

> **Nurse:** Because I knew if he was warming, he would dilate and third space much of his intravascular volume. With the nipride going, his blood pressure would drop very quickly. So I didn't want to wait until his systolic blood pressure hit 90 to start fluid. I wanted to know when it hit 95 so I could turn off the nipride (Observational Interview).

Patient responses to particular therapies are predictable within regions and therefore anticipated along with therapies to respond to those transitions. In this case, weaning the nipride off before the patient became hypotensive allows the nurse to better manage a rapidly developing and potentially dangerous transition.

Knowing a particular patient's critical illness sets up a sense of potential crises, specific risks, and vulnerabilities. Nurses situate the patient's problems almost like a topography of possibilities. In this way, nurses' clinical forethought based on knowing a <u>particular</u> patient guides their anticipations and expectations. This is illustrated in the following patient who had pancreatitis and developed respiratory problems, septic shock, and adult respiratory disease syndrome (ARDS). The patient's blood gases and blood pressure began deteriorating despite therapy:

> **Nurse:** It was evident that she was really deteriorating and it looked like her sepsis was, I'm not sure if it was the ARDS? Or was it the sepsis? Was it a combination of both things hitting her at the same time? Because she started getting hypotensive and we're having to give more fluid and then we're having to add vasopressors—and it was the type of situation where I knew things were going down the tubes and they were going down fast. And I knew she was going to arrest that night. I just knew it... It's like you're trying to climb up the side of a cliff and you just keep sliding down. You just don't get anywhere with them. They're not responding the way you want them to or the way they should. You're supporting them maximally and they just keep deteriorating—we kept going up on her FiO_2, her $P[a]O_2$ kept falling. We're giving her fluid. We're giving vasopressors, her blood pressure's not going anywhere—next thing you know, she's on her head [placed in a Trendelenburg position as a desperate attempt to elevate blood pressure to perfuse vital organs]. And I said to the doctor, 'The family's here. I talked to them. I told them things aren't going well, but somebody better get

out there and just medically let them know exactly what's going on.' A new nurse came on and I stayed around, got her settled, and had a couple of senior nurses who had easy assignments come in and help her, so I could work myself out of the room. Sure enough, 5 hours later [the patient] arrested.

The patient's responses to the therapies are evaluated and the patient's deterioration is recognized as each measure fails to bring about the desired response. This has practical implications for setting up the next therapy. Eventually the nurse forecasts a cardiac arrest. Both clinical forethought and grasp of the patient's condition go hand in hand. The metaphors used are apt descriptors of the patient's transitions—climbing up a cliff and then sliding back down. The transition is characterized, not just as decision points along the way, but as a growing understanding of the patient's particular responses. In rapidly changing situations such as this one, the nurse's forethought includes informing the family as the situation unfolds.

Knowing a particular patient's responses is both life-saving and comforting for a patient, family, and other clinicians (Benner, Tanner & Chesla, 2009). For instance, when continuity of care is disrupted, nurse's descriptions of patient responses provide the possibility of passing along clinical forethought to other nurses. The following example describes the responses to renal dialysis in a complex post-cardiac surgery patient who had suffered a major stroke and multiple complications:

Interviewer: I'm curious. In report for nurses coming on who didn't know him as well, were you able to tell them about some of your perceptions from that day? Did you feel like you could convey some of that?

Nurse: Oh, we all did. We talked about him all the time...Yeah. Or people would say, 'Oh good, you're here today, Bob will be glad.' Or Linda would come in, or one of those co-primaries that took care of him a lot. We talked about him all the time.

Interviewer: So you would be able to at least transmit somewhat in report that: 'Today is a bad day and he is not able to walk or all of that'...

Nurse: Oh yeah, and especially related to dialysis...that really was over the line for him. And it got back down to the point where he was interactive all days except Monday, Wednesday and Friday when he was dialyzed... He would close his eyes during dialysis and anywhere from an hour to the rest of the afternoon after dialysis till he would start looking around and he did or didn't want to do something.

If the patient's predictable response to the dialysis had not been communicated, other nurses would have perhaps engaged in erroneous hypotheses and/or interventions, not anticipating the patient's vulnerabilities related to dialysis. This points to an important clinical implication: Nurses need to have interactive shift reports, because many crucial pieces of patient and family information are conveyed from shift to shift that cannot be expressed in written form. Interactions support questions and answers or probing which brings out essential details that aid grasp and forethought. With the current emphasis on cost control, many units have experimented with alternative and less costly approaches to "between shift reporting" (including unidirectional taped reports). Preventing patient complications based on reports that include dialogue and visual confirmations about patient changes however, is often far less costly, both to the patient and to the healthcare institution.

Anticipating particular patients' likely responses is a form of informal hypotheses generation and is crucial to confirm or disconfirm the clinician's judgment about the patient's condition. In the following example, a nurse being observed and interviewed at the bedside describes her thinking-in-action with a heart transplant patient:

Nurse: Now, I've slowed his vasopressors down and his pressure's hanging right about 90, so I'm happy and hoping that maybe with his improved oxygenation he'll do better. I'm also going to check another cardiac output and check his SVR [Systemic Vascular Resistance] since we started that levophed again. Because if his SVR is too high again with all that levophed and milrinone on board, then blood is going to back up into his lungs anyway because his heart won't be able to generate pressures against that SVR. So, I have to keep an eye on that, too. I'm surprised, actually, that his SVR isn't higher, it's within the normal range. He's not real, real clamped down. But like I said, if he starts generating SVRs higher than that, then it's not good. He's a real interesting patient, trying to figure out what all is going on. Everything leads to everything, like at first I was trying to figure out—I kept thinking to myself—well, why does his pressure keep going down when I keep turning that bolus off? But then I was thinking because it's right there, it's dumping into that right atrium and that's just what his heart wants is that filling pressure. So. I've slowed his fluids down and he's actually maintaining his pressures, so I hope he does that. As I said, I hope his improved oxygenation might help, too. You never know. Sometimes you don't know unless you try and you have to keep trying things every 15 or 20 minutes. Well, I know it didn't work last time, but we'll give it another shot. Maybe, maybe something has changed in the meantime. And I'm hoping against hope he's not infected because once transplants get infected it's real hard to get over it. There are so many opportunistic infections that can get to them. They're just like an AIDS patient in a lot of ways (Observational Interview).

The development of an empirical, response-based practice is evident in this interview excerpt. Because the patient is unstable, everything shows up as a puzzle. And the puzzle is particularly complex for this inexperienced clinician because everything leads to other things. The nurse predicts the responses she expects and this aids in her clinical grasp. For example, she is concerned that the levophed and milrinone have caused the SVR to increase. If the SVR is too high, she predicts that the patient's cardiac output will drop and subsequently lead to pulmonary edema. In addition, the nurse slowed the fluid infusion since unnecessary volume can easily result in edema throughout the body. But, she simultaneously knows that the patient's cardiac function is somewhat dependent upon maintaining higher filling pressures, as reflected in the blood pressure drop whenever his fluids are slowed. This kind of forecasting for a particular patient helps the nurse understand the patient's condition and enables her to prepare for untoward clinical responses.

Clinical forethought based upon a good clinical grasp of the patient's particular strengths and vulnerabilities is made possible by continuity in caring for patients. In very fragile patients, this experiential understanding of the particular patient is superior over any care plan or clinical pathway in guiding patient care because it attends to transitions in the patient over time, and makes adjustments to therapies quickly. This is illustrated in the fine grained understanding of the clinical implications of suctioning a very fragile premature infant. The nurse prepares and uses a second nurse to assist in order to prevent the kind of deterioration that would take hours to correct:

Interviewer: What are you expecting? I mean do you have in mind what sort of a course you're expecting over your shift today?

Nurse 1: Well, he probably—I mean hopefully—I'm not hoping that this baby is going to turn around and suddenly get dramatically better. It's probably going to be a little slower than that. What I really want to do—what we want to <u>avoid</u> is having the baby drop his PaO$_2$ significantly lower and have more problems with his blood pressure, and then progress to the point where he needs ECMO in order to live. And so really my goal is just to maintain at this point and not to make his condition any worse than it already is because he may get to the point where we can't fix him except by ECMO. So we're just trying to maintain the status quo and not get worse.

Interviewer: Have you done that yet today?

Nurse 1: ...I haven't done it yet today. I actually—a nurse practitioner and I have a date to suction him shortly. The other thing that we need to do is—we normally turn the babies at the time that we suction them. So I'm going to suction out his airway, which also may cause him to decompensate because he's going to lose his oxygenation for ten or fifteen seconds. So that's the first thing you worry about is his respiratory decomposition, and also...

Interviewer: I know you turn babies and disconnect them routinely. Why would it be such a problem for this baby...?

Nurse 1: Well.

Interviewer: ...or would it be such a problem?

Nurse 1: It would be a big problem; it probably will be a big problem, although the night nurse said he did pretty well with suctioning. But it's a problem—these babies are much more fragile. Normally babies who are sick but not terribly critically sick, you detach them for a few seconds and they decompensate briefly but they generally recover. Sometimes babies with pulmonary hypertension are extremely slow to recover—they lose a lot of ground. Once they decompensate and their PaO$_2$ falls, their pulmonary hypertension can worsen instantly. They can vasoconstrict down a lot, and just putting them back on the ventilator doesn't make it automatically get better immediately. Sometimes it can sort of set off a chain of events; it can take a couple of hours. I don't know that that will be the case with him, but you're always as quick and efficient as you can be turning them and you assume that they're going to decompensate and so, be prepared to hand ventilate, possibly also increase the drug infusions, whatever he needs.

Interviewer: Perhaps we can watch you do that?

Nurse 1: Yes. Can I go ahead and suction [speaker asks second nurse who will assist with suctioning]?

Nurse 2: Yes.
[A time lapse occurs, after a successful two person suctioning of the infant with no decompensation of the patient. The medical resident explains that he will tinker with the ventilator settings.]

Interviewer: How do you feel about that [tinkering]?

Nurse 1: I wish they wouldn't.

Interviewer: Why?

Nurse 1: I want to go to lunch. No, I mean it could make the baby get better or it could start a downward spiral, and then we'd spend the rest of the day trying to get the baby back to his baseline. You do have to try things at some point, but preferably you try [when the baby is ready].

Interviewer: What are going to be your responsibilities if they start tinkering?

Nurse 1: Well, I'll watch his monitors a little more closely than I have and then watch his blood pressure very closely. Usually the standard is to get a blood gas about 10 minutes after a ventilator change is made to see which direction we're going. Sometimes babies will change dramatically. As soon as a change is made, sometimes they can take an hour or so before the lungs open up more, or if the lungs are going to collapse down, get atelectatic. It might be awhile before you see it. So I'll really have to watch him closely for the next hour or so (Observational Interview).

The nurse recognizes that this particular infant is more fragile than most with this clinical illness. Here she details her reasoning about the physiological sequence of possible deterioration. Given the specific pulmonary and hemodynamic changes that are possible, she anticipates and is prepared for rapid and instantaneous interventions (such as hand ventilation and drug titration) that might mitigate decompensation. This example highlights how a strong understanding of the sciences is intricately integrated in everyday practice with clinical wisdom gained from experience with similar kinds of babies. Best practice requires both scientific and practical knowledge.

The nurse's statement, that she wants to go to lunch, is not a flippant response; it is a practical response to planning the close observation that will be required after the "tinkering." She knows she will not leave the baby immediately after the "tinkering" because she knows the baby's baseline and is in the best position to detect and correct early problems. She moves easily back and forth between the general case of premature infants with pulmonary hypertension and this particular premature infant. Her clinical forethought is fine-grained and immediate, forecasting the next hour, and the next few days if the baby's condition deteriorates.

Given the erosion of primary nursing as a form of nursing care delivery in favor of teams with assistive personnel, continuity of care is more difficult than ever for nurses to achieve. Yet, this finely trained forecasting would not have been possible had she not worked extensively with the same patient. An implication of this work is that hospital and unit administrators need to re-evaluate nursing care delivery as it relates to the prevention of both actual and potential patient complications. The skill of thinking and planning ahead will gain even greater importance in everyday practice as cost constraints cause reductions in the number of excellent clinicians at the bedside. Nurses will need to anticipate the potential eventualities of each patient and determine which patients will need the closest observation; yet, this is jeopardized by the limited access nurses have directly with patients. There is a limit, however, to any nurse's ability to detect and correct problems early when fewer expert nurses are available to attentively monitor a fragile patient's condition as it unfolds. Because both scientific and practical knowledge are required to develop clinical forethought and grasp, under-skilled assistants can never be expected to replace highly skilled clinical thinking-in-action.

SEEING THE UNEXPECTED

One of the hallmarks of expert nursing practice is the ability to notice the unexpected (Benner, Tanner & Chesla, 2009). Clinicians come to expect certain recovery trajectories and responses to therapies. When these expectations do not occur, the experienced clinician begins to pay more attention to the patient's responses. The fund of clinical expectations gained over time allows the experienced clinician to notice what is absent, and this search process is based on an implicit form of clinical forethought, namely clinical expectations. This is illustrated in an excerpt from a clinical observation where a burn nurse notices that the newly admitted patient's urine output is much lower than expected or hoped, given his fluid infusions:

> **Nurse:** [Looking at the patient's urine output.] So, okay, he needs to make an awful lot of urine that he's not making. He was—let's see, what was he last hour? He made 60 cc. Last hour, right? [Orientee nods yes] Okay, so we're 15 minutes into this hour and right now all we have is a little 'sweat' in here [checking the urine drainage tubing]. I don't know, we've got a little bit more (Observational Interview).

As the nurse looks at the urine drainage, she is disappointed to find only "a little sweat," meaning a very small amount of urine. Because urine output is a key indicator of the patient's fluid status, the nurse grows increasingly concerned that the patient was inadequately fluid resuscitated in the emergency department and that his fluid infusions need to be increased. Over the next hour, her multiple interventions, which include monitoring the urine output every 10 minutes, calling the physician to increase the fluid infusions, and watching his blood pressure, were prompted by noticing the unexpectedly low urine output in relation to fluid infusions. Within an hour of increasing the fluid infusion, the patient's urine output improved and the nurse gradually become less intensively vigilant in monitoring the patient's output.

Seeing the unexpected based on implicit or tacit clinical expectations requires engagement with the patient and openness so that missed expectations and counter examples are noticed. This habit of thought prevents overly routinized habitual responses based on conscious, deliberative clinical forethought. Over-reliance on explicit clinical forethought can hinder reading the situation for its particularity. Checklists are useful for standardized and routinized practice; however, keeping imaginative clinical forethought at the forefront of everyday nursing practice ensures that the nurse think about and pay attention to those aspects of the situation that require assessment, planning and timely interventions.

SUMMARY AND IMPLICATIONS

Clinical forethought improves by effectively learning from experience. It is based upon developing imaginative practice based upon effective situated knowledge use from experience and from theory and science. Developing and enriching clinical forethought requires attentiveness and reflection on practice. If clinical learning is effectively shared with co-workers, clinical forethought can also improve on the unit level so that earlier detection and treatment of hemodynamic instability, pulmonary edema, cardiac arrhythmias, et cetera reduce the need for emergency resuscitation. Cumulative wisdom develops at the unit level when experiential clinical learning is made public and everyone gains insight about particular patient transitions.

Developing cumulative wisdom can be a unit objective. Preceptors can be reflective about and verbalize their clinical forethought for orientees. Often expectations, habits of thought, and routines become taken-for-granted. By reflecting on them in order to teach new nurses, the preceptor can discover and articulate areas of experientially gained clinical wisdom that can then become a part of the pooled wisdom of the unit (Benner et al., 1996, pp. 193-231). Similarly, preceptors can coach orientees to actively develop clinical fore-thought by asking them what they expect, how they think the situation may unfold, and what preparation is needed for each eventuality. This teaches thinking-in-action and contingency planning. Questions compel the orientee to develop the habits of thought that are necessary to become an expert. Further, preceptors can teach and role model by asking physicians and other colleagues what they are anticipating in particular patient situations. Multiple perspectives contribute to collective wisdom so that the orientee can learn to better anticipate the course of treatment holistically. Reflecting on how others think-in-action can assist the orientee in developing habits of clinical forethought.

Becoming aware of times when clinical forethought was held too rigidly and blunted recognition of patient transitions requires reflection. Comparing one's perceptions and expectations with other clinicians can broaden one's own forethought and action. Verbalizing one's clinical forethought as tentative hypotheses to be confirmed or discomfirmed enhances experiential learning and improves clinical inquiry skills.

REFERENCES

Benner, P. (1984). *From novice to expert: Excellence and power in clinical nursing practice.* Menlo Park, CA: Addison-Wesley.

Benner, P., & Tanner, C. (1987). Clinical judgment: How expert nurses use intuition. *American Journal of Nursing, 87*(1), 23–31.

Benner, P., Tanner, C. A., & Chesla, C. A. (2009). *Expertise in nursing practice: Caring, clinical judgment, and ethics.* New York: Springer.

Benner, P., & Wrubel, J. (1982). Clinical knowledge development: The value of perceptual awareness. *Nurse Educator, 7,* 11–17.

Bourdieu, P. (1980/1990). *The logic of practice* (Richard Nice, Trans.). Stanford, CA: Stanford University.

Dreyfus, H. L. (1992). *What computers still can't do: A critique of artificial reason.* Cambridge, MA: MIT.

Dreyfus, H. L., & Dreyfus, S. E. (1986). *Mind over machine: The power of human intuition and expertise in the era of the computer.* New York: Free Press.

Hooper, P. L. (1995). *Expert titration of multiple vasoactive drugs in post-cardiac surgical patients: An interpretive study of clinical judgment and perceptual acuity.* Doctoral dissertation, University of California at San Francisco, San Francisco, School of Nursing.

Logstrup, K. (1995). *Metaphysics. (Vol. 1).* Milwaukee, WI: Marquette University.

Molter, Colonel N. (personal communications, March 23, 2010).

Polanyi, M. (1958/1962). *Personal knowledge: Towards a post-critical philosophy.* Chicago, IL: University of Chicago Press.

4

Diagnosing and Managing Life-Sustaining Physiologic Functions in Acutely Ill and Unstable Patients

*P*atients who become acute or critically ill or injured are either no longer able to independently maintain physiological stability or are at high risk for rapidly developing physiological instability. Their critical conditions define and orient the interventions and practices of acute and critical care nurses. Instantaneous interventions and the constant readiness to provide them are central to critical care nursing practice and are the principle reason that patients are admitted to critical care areas, particularly since these patients are typically life-dependent on continuous intensive care and the supporting technology (which includes pharmacologic agents, and/or blood and fluid products in addition to equipment). Although the primary focus and data are on critical care, nurses in all acute care areas find themselves diagnosing and managing unstable patients with some frequency. Thus, a major domain of clinical knowledge, basic in the care of all unstable and critically ill patients, is the continuous diagnosis and management of unstable, and often life-threatening, physiologic conditions and/or situations.

Based on extensive study of critical care nursing practice, there are at least five aspects of diagnosing and managing life-sustaining physiologic functions in unstable patients. The purpose of this chapter is to: 1) describe the link between and often simultaneous occurrence of diagnosing and managing an urgent clinical problem and 2) articulate the key aspects of this domain. The articulation of these five aspects will show how the context in specific situations alters the kinds of demands for intervention. Clinical judgment and practice can differ significantly when the nurses' responses are dictated by a standardized guideline or protocol rather than by demands of specific patient situation. Because of the trend in current thinking and practice to try and standardize the physiological care of patients with similar conditions, an additional purpose of this chapter is to: 3) emphasize the place that protocols and guidelines should and should not have in expert clinical judgment and practice.

The five aspects that characterize this domain are listed in Table 4.1. The key feature that distinguishes the first three above physiological aspects of caring for critically ill patients is the urgency of the situation which, in turn, is determined by the instability of the patient's condition. How critical the patient's condition is does not always determine how unstable the patient may be. For instance, a patient with multisystem organ failure (MSOF) may be much more critical than a hemodynamically stable patient with an acute myocardial

TABLE 4.1

Diagnosing and Managing Life-Sustaining Physiologic Functions in Acutely Ill and Unstable Patients

▨ Diagnosing and managing emergent and/or life-threatening situations (crisis,resuscitations)

▨ Diagnosing, monitoring, titrating, and providing instantaneous interventions in unstable patients to avert a crisis and to maintain vital functions and physiological stability

▨ Diagnosing, monitoring, preventing, and managing vital, but non-emergent fluctuations in physiological functions

▨ Coordinating and managing multiple instantaneous interventions

▨ Coaching and assisting patients in weaning from life-support technologies

Note: In each case, these interventions must be tailored to the particular patient's response, pathophysiology, clinical history, and expected clinical trajectory

infarction (AMI). However, if the AMI patient suddenly develops ventricular fibrillation, that patient's immediate condition becomes more unstable and more urgent (a crisis) than that of the patient with MSOF. Hence, the above categories are not necessarily indicative of the patient's severity of illness, but instead focus on how the patient's physiological condition orients the nurse's thinking, judgments, and practice.

The first aspect, "diagnosing and managing emergent and/or life-threatening situations," directs attention to how nurses instantaneously respond to or intervene in crisis situations and to how the context of the crisis influences the nurse's clinical judgment. The second aspect, "diagnosing, monitoring, titrating, and providing instantaneous interventions to maintain vital functions and physiological stability in an unstable patient," focuses on the clinical judgment and skillful actions required to instantaneously intervene in order to prevent an unstable situation from deteriorating into a crisis. Although there is no definitive boundary between an unstable situation and a crisis, there are many situations that are clearly in one realm or the other and the types of patient needs orient the nurse's practice differently. The third aspect highlights how nurses monitor and manage non-urgent, non-life-threatening fluctuations in physiological conditions in order to maintain optimal function and/or to prevent undesirable changes that may result in instability or lead to a crisis. Typically, immediate interventions to manage critical situations (included in the first three aspects) are taught in isolation of each other. In actual practice, however, an unstable patient's condition often demands numerous, simultaneous therapies. Therefore, the fourth aspect articulates the clinical judgment and skilled actions needed for coordinating and managing multiple instantaneous therapies. While the first four aspects of this chapter describe the incorporation of technology, particularly pharmacologic agents, in the care of the critically ill, the last aspect addresses how nurses coach and assist patients in becoming free of life-support technologies. In each aspect, the interventions must be tailored to the particular patient's responses, pathophysiology, clinical history, and expected clinical trajectory.

THE INSEPARABLE LINK BETWEEN DIAGNOSIS AND INTERVENTION

Most every nurse has been educated to believe that thinking, reasoning, and judgment in clinical practice are based on the nursing process. We learned that the components of the nursing process occur logically and sequentially in practice: assessment, diagnosis, intervention, and evaluation. For beginning and less experienced nurses, this process provides a sound method for developing one's thinking patterns. It may also be used by expert nurses when they are faced with reasoning through a new, complex, or puzzling situation. However, numerous and concurring studies of expert critical care nurses (Benner, 1984; Benner, Tanner & Chesla, 2009; Corcoran, 1986a; Corcoran & Tanner, 1988; Hooper, 1995; Stannard et al., 1996) have informed us that expert nurses do not continue to think or make clinical judgments in an linear fashion when they are in familiar, everyday practice. In familiar situations, expert nurses have already diagnosed and begin initiating treatment at the moment they recognize the clinical problem. For instance, in dysrhythmia monitoring and detection, at the moment an expert nurse sees a patient have a run of ventricular tachycardia or ventricular fibrillation, without thinking, her or his body is already in motion to respond to the life-threatening event. Delivering a precordial thump, reaching for amiodarone, or turning to the defibrillator are automatic responses based on the demands of the situation. It is this kind of skillful body or embodied intelligence that expert nurses develop which makes them best able to manage life-threatening physiologic conditions or events in unstable patients. In the care of the unstable and critically ill, this skill is often life-saving.

Excellent care of critically ill and injured patients requires ever-advancing skilled clinical knowledge as the acuity levels and complexity in patient care increases, particularly in the very old and very young who are admitted to acute and critical care units and discharged to home. To provide complex, multiple, and instantaneous therapies, the nurse must be able to take appropriate action almost simultaneously with identification of the problem. Tom Lowndes, a Florida Nurses' Association Awardee, shared the following exemplar, highlights the inseparable link between diagnosis and treatment. Further, it captures various aspects within this domain of practice:

Nurse: Rita was just an unsuspecting patron at a local restaurant one evening. As she was leaving the restaurant, and walking toward her car, a stranger ran after her, spun her around and stabbed her in the chest with a knife. The blade passed through the left ventricle of her heart, front to back. The man who had stabbed her was gone just as quickly as he had appeared, leaving Rita dying in the parking lot.

The restaurant was about 4 blocks from the hospital where I worked. But with a wound like that, 4 blocks is not close. Rita made it to our hospital because that restaurant was a gathering place for paramedics, fire fighters, and police officers, and there were plenty gathered there that evening. Rita got to our trauma center Emergency Department within about 2 minutes. As the ambulance drove up, one of our thoracic surgeons was leaving the hospital through the main Emergency Department doors. A few minutes later Rita was wheeling down the hall towards the operating room with 3 units of blood running, her chest already open, and Dr. R. doing open heart massage. Believe it or not, Rita survived the surgery and was in the Intensive Care Unit the next afternoon when I arrived at work.

My orientee (Anna) and I were assigned to care for Rita. As we walked into the Rita's room, Anna just stopped at the doorway and stared. She was stunned by the complexity of what we saw. Machines and monitors and tubes virtually filled the room. I stopped to look around the room too, but I was up near the bed, close enough to reach out and take hold of Rita's foot. It was warm. Her heart rate, rhythm, and blood pressure looked good. The ventilator gave her each breath with ease. A few drops of light red fluid trickled through the tube that drained her chest. There was clear light yellow urine in the drainage bag. 'Well Anna', I said, 'things are looking pretty good here.' Anna's expression told me that she thought I was crazy.

Anna and I spent the first couple of hours tracking down each line and tube from end to end. We untangled and labeled each one, taking note of what was running in and what was coming out. We checked each IV bag, and I explained what effects the different drugs were supposed to have, and how to calculate the doses and IV rates. We zeroed and calibrated the pressure transducers, and I explained how to recognize the waveforms on the monitor, and how to make sure that the measurements we took were accurate. We evaluated the physical findings—lung sounds, heart sounds, pulses, skin color and temperature, etc.—and discussed what we did find and what we might find in a trauma case like this.

Rita had not been conscious yet. There was no way to predict how things would turn out. Would she have brain damage? Would she ever wake up, and if she did, would she want to? Would she have renal failure? Would other major organs fail? Would infections develop? There was so much information that it's just impossible for a new nurse to have a sense of what is important. To me, every detail was a clue to what was going on. Urine output wasn't merely a product of the kidneys; it was a product of adequate cardiac output, a proper balance of preload and afterload. It was a sign of good prognosis. If the kidneys were working, they had not been ischemic too long, and that meant brain function might have been preserved. When I looked at a bag of urine I was looking at the promise of recovery for this woman. When I looked at the monitor tracings and the chest tube drainage I could see that her heart was okay. The pericardium was not filling with blood and there were no signs of tamponade. When I had walked in and almost subconsciously reached over to feel the warmth of Rita's toes, I was gathering information about her survival. I could see it was going to be one of those days when I would go home with a scratchy throat from having explained why ICU nurses consider decent urine output one of the most important vital signs.

A short time later, while I was out of the room at the nurses' desk, the ventilator alarm began to sound. I reached her bedside immediately, and could see that all that was calm moments ago was in chaos now. 'What's going on?' I thought. 'Is she seizing?' Her head was lifted off the pillow with convulsive coughing. The needle on the pressure gauge was hitting the red zone and the high pressure valve was venting with a loud hiss with each breath the ventilator tried to give. But the motions were not really seizure-like. My mind was racing while I methodically raised hypotheses and tested each for validity. 'Is the ET tube blocked? No. Has the ET tube moved? Can't tell. What do the lungs sound like? Right side OK, left side nothing. LEFT SIDE NOTHING!! What's going on here?' Anna was asking me if she should go get some morphine because that worked yesterday on a patient that had been coughing and bucking the vent. 'Yeah go get some morphine' I said, thinking 'lack of morphine is not the problem here.' As I was taking her off the vent and connecting the ambu bag I'm thinking, 'No breath sounds on the left, no breath sounds on the left, could be the ET tube is in the right mainstem' and I looked at the O_2 flow meter to make sure it was turned on. It took both hands on the ambu bag to force a breath through the ET tube. Rita was dusky and tachycardic, and her neck looked funny. I reached over and palpated, her trachea was shifted way over to the right. I'm thinking, 'she's got chest tubes already; she can't have a pneumothorax...' I gave the ambu bag to a respiratory therapist that had come in and said, 'Anna give that morphine, then go get a chest drainage system, a couple of sizes of chest tubes, and a bottle of sterile water.' I beeped Dr. T., the resident on call, 'come to ICU STAT.' The supplies arrived, I said, 'Open the package. You're going to learn how to set up for a chest tube.' Dr. T. called me back. He said, 'what's going on, I almost fell off my chair when your page came through, I've never had a stat call from you.' I said, 'Get down here now. This lady with the stab wound through her heart has no breath sounds on the left, we can hardly bag her, her trachea is deviated to the right, she's turning blue...' Dr. T. broke in, 'get a 14 gauge needle and stick it in her chest on the left side, I'm just upstairs, I'll be there in less than a minute,' then the phone went 'click.' I looked over at Anna, so far she had the wrapper off the package. I said, 'Dr. T. will be here in a minute, we have to have this ready,' then I went to the med cart and found the biggest needle we had, it was an 18 gauge. I went back in the room and nothing had happened with the chest drainage system. I said, 'Anna, go get some betadine, some xylocaine, and some 8 ½ gloves.' I looked at Rita's chest wall and at the 18 gauge needle and I decided to set up the chest drainage system. Dr. T. arrived and tossed his lab coat on an IV pump, put his stethoscope on, and checked for breath sounds. Anna came back with the gloves and the betadine. Dr. T. took the 18 gauge needle and stuck it in Rita's chest wall, then poured some betadine over it. Brown bubbles sputtered on the hub of the needle. Almost immediately it was easier to ambu. The chest drainage system was ready, Dr. T. put the chest tube in without a local (Anna had forgotten to bring the xylocaine). I listened to her lungs, 'breath sounds both sides now.' Rita's breathing was calmer, and we could put her back on the vent. Then I noticed her eyes were open, she was kind of looking around dazed-like. I put two of my fingers in the palm of her hand and said, 'squeeze my hand.' She moved her hand a little. 'Good sign' I thought! 'Now Anna, is there more morphine in that syringe? Let's give her the rest and get a chest X-ray.'

Things went smoothly for the rest of the evening. Anna looked a little shell-shocked for a while, and I have to admit, I could empathize. I would have stuck that needle in Rita's chest if I really had to, but it made me remember what it's like to have a patient's life depending on you to do the right thing the right way, even if it's something you've never had to do before.

Later on Anna said, 'How did you know what was happening? How did you know that morphine was not going to help?'

I didn't have a good concise answer, but I tried to explain by this example: 'Suppose you had a scissors and a hemostat in your lab jacket pocket. If I asked you to hand me a scissors, would you be able to reach into your pocket and pull out the scissors?' Anna said, 'Yes.'

I said, 'So, based on your past experiences you would be able to feel the difference between the two instruments without having to see them side-by-side, right?' Again, Anna said, 'Yes.'

I said, 'In a way that is similar to how I knew that Rita was not just bucking the ventilator. I know how things are supposed to look, and when something unusual happens, it gets my attention. Both of us see the same distracting bits of information, thousands and thousands of them. I have the benefit of experience, so I can recognize the patterns in the chaos, or see something out of place in the pattern and I have a sense of when it is trivial and when it is of great consequence.

You won't learn it from a textbook or from an algorithm. It's the result of paying attention at the bedside every day, all the time. One day you will find yourself visualizing and conceptualizing what is going on inside your patient when the blood pressure drops, or the breath sounds are absent. When that begins to happen, then you will understand what I have been talking about. It is something that can be learned, and it is something that needs to be nurtured, but it is not something that is easily taught.'

Within seconds of recognizing an urgent and unpredictable complication, this nurse diagnosed and confirmed the diagnosis of pneumothorax. At the moment he grasped the meaning of the patient's shifted trachea, dusky appearance, tachycardia, and the force needed for ambu bag ventilation, the nurse was already instructing the orientee to gather a chest drainage system and several sizes of chest tubes to prepare for the life-saving intervention—insertion of a chest tube. Diagnosing is not within the physician's realm of practice alone. It is critical that nurses also legitimately diagnose in order for instantaneous life-saving interventions to be possible and timely and to prevent the patient's condition from progressing into a respiratory and/or cardiac arrest. In this situation, the nurse's astute and early detection of the patient's pneumothorax enabled the resident to promptly hone in on the problem to verify the diagnosis and provide treatment within minutes.

A clinician's recognitional skills, immediate skillful bodily responses, and the synchrony of skills and responses cannot be developed based on factual knowledge alone, even though it is requisite for good practice. In contrast to Tom Lowndes' exemplar, a beginning nurse demonstrates how experience is central to the development of a skillful body in response to a crisis:

> **Nurse:** ...the patient was in atrial fib[rillation] for most of the night and she had been in for a Femoral-popliteal bypass and had a host of other problems, too... I remember I had the curtains part way closed because she wanted to sleep and so I couldn't see the monitor... But she started to brady down and they caught it on the monitors out at the desk, and everyone rushed in and I looked up to see all these people rushing in and they were rushing to my patient (laughs). And I was just like, 'Oh, my God.' So I jumped up and her rate had decreased and they were trying to rouse her. And it was like, 'Get the atropine.' And I said, my first thought was to run out to the stock and get it even though each bedside has its own basket with epinephrine and atropine and the tongue blade and an oral airway, and a nasal airway and everything. And just for that moment, I just completely blocked out that it was right at the bedside, easily available. And as it turned out, what she did, she bradyed down and then she converted subsequently back to a normal sinus rhythm and that was just her heart going through the conversion. So it turned out fine...her heart rate sped up and she was easily rousable and she was a little irritated that we woke her up (laughter), and she was fine...

> **Interviewer:** Atropine in the basket has become salient to you and will the rest of your career. (laughter) Just as heart rate, I mean that's the interesting thing about this. It's...

> **Nurse:** You learn from your mistakes.

Unlike the experienced nurses in this situation, the new nurse learned about the patient's dysrhythmia and potential crisis from those who were rushing to care for the patient. Not yet able to immediately grasp what actions were needed, the new nurse responded upon hearing someone else call for atropine. Although this nurse intellectually knew that there was atropine stored at the bedside, her habitual response was to go the stock area where she was accustomed to getting medications on a daily basis. Bodily responses in crises arise from the development of habits—habits of thinking and habits of doing—which are commonly learned from breakdown situations such as this. As the nurse points out, "You learn from your mistakes."

Although most habits of thinking and responding are learned in practice rather than in a classroom or book, courses and training programs that include the practice of skills or that demand proficiency in particular skills can be very helpful for beginners. For instance, the Advanced Cardiac Life Support courses [ACLS for adults and PALS for pediatrics] focus on common types of crisis situations in which proficiency in knowledge and skills are required for certification. Clinicians repeatedly rehearse emergency interventions to various types of crises as a way of developing bodily habits (embodied responses) and patterns of thinking. Courses such as these are invaluable when seconds count in an actual situation.

DIAGNOSING AND MANAGING EMERGENT AND/OR LIFE-THREATENING SITUATIONS

This aspect of managing unstable, critically ill patients may seem to be the most familiar type of care in critical care settings. It is characterized by the recognition and treatment of numerous types of crises, including respiratory and cardiac resuscitations. A crisis may be momentary or last for hours, depending on the cause, the interventions, and the patient's responses. Despite the concentration of life-threatening situations in critical care areas, patients experience emergent conditions in every patient care area. What is common is that all life-threatening situations require instantaneous interventions.

This specific category in this domain differs from the domain of judgment and skill articulated in Chapter 5, "The Skilled Know-How of Managing a Crisis." Here, we will highlight the physiological aspects of managing a crisis, where the clinician is the direct care provider. That role and the accompanying skills are distinctly different from the role and skills of organizer, coordinator, and facilitator when assisting in managing a crisis, which is the focus of Chapter 5. It is not uncommon for the nurse providing direct care to also take on the other roles simultaneously during a crisis. Our intention is to bring both roles to light so that the development of expertise in each may be improved. The multiple roles that nurses serve are exemplified in a clinical situation in which Lisa Salines, a labor and delivery (L&D) nurse, manages the emergent situation, helps orchestrate the team's efforts, and simultaneously coaches a float nurse as she learns how to manage the emergent delivery. Here, Lisa assists a float nurse, Mary, with a patient arriving via ambulance and who is bleeding:

Nurse: Amy was a 33 week gestation pregnant woman, whom was bleeding vaginally. I knew this could be very serious and require an emergency Caesarian Section (C/S). Amy was very anxious, breathing with her contractions and obviously in pain. My Clinical Leader asked me if I could help Mary and I said, "No problem." I just had a feeling that we were going to have to move quickly, Amy was breathing hard through her contractions and was unsettled. Amy was holding her firm abdomen and she was grimacing in pain, as if her pain was from a placental abruption. Her actions and vaginal bleeding as we helped the ambulance drivers transfer Amy to the L&D bed clued me in. I knew Mary and I had to assess Amy and act fast. I immediately applied the Fetal Heart Monitor and explained to Amy that her baby's heart beat was healthy and strong. Amy was also contracting. By that time we changed her into a hospital gown, Dr. Cook was here and did a sterile vaginal exam.

Dr. Cook, Mary and I were all looking down when Dr. Cook took her hand out. There were two softball size blood clots that came out with the glove. Instantly, I knew by Dr. Cook's surprised expression that Amy definitely needed to have this baby. Dr. Cook informed Amy that she needed to deliver her baby by C/S. In the meantime, I got equipment to prep Amy for surgery. Mary was very nervous; she grabbed my arm with both hands and asked me not to leave her. As she froze in her tracks, she looked terrified. Mary reminded me of me when I was new. Mary was really happy I was there. She gave me a look like: thank you, thank you, thank you for your help.

I anticipated what was needed, asking Dr. Cook for orders before she could even say them: like I.V., antibiotics, foley and skin prep. In the meantime, Mary and I were talking to Amy, reassuring her. I told her that "she was in the best place she could be. We were all there to help her and her baby." We were talking to Amy so she would not be so afraid while she was being attacked from all angles to get her ready for the O.R. Amy knew her baby was early and was terrified for the safety of her baby. I told her that our team of Neonatologist and Special Care nursery nurses would take great care of her baby.

Mary and I finished getting Amy ready: giving her an I.V. bolus and antibiotics, electric razor shave prep and inserting her foley catheter. I also reminded Mary to just quickly write anything we did on the fetal heart monitor strip or on her scrub pants so that we could go back later to document. As we moved Amy to the O.R., I tried to comfort Amy, by telling her that "once her husband arrived we let him come in to the O.R. to be by her side…."

After anesthesia was finished, I grabbed a warm blanket to cover Amy. I coached Mary, by reminding her to apply the bovie pad to Amy's right thigh and ask if Amy has metal plates or screws in her right leg, check the Fetal Heart Rate and apply the safety strap across Amy's thighs. I then went to the head of the bed to hold Amy's hand. She looked as if she was about to cry. I sat and talked to her and tried to take her mind off what was happening: "Is your baby a girl or a boy? What is the baby's name going to be?" I talked with her and told her that "her husband will be here soon" and shortly Mary brought her husband in to take over my job. Amy was relieved to see her husband's face.

Just seconds later we heard a vigorous cry and Dr. Cook said, "It's a boy". Amy cried tears of joy to hear the good news. The neonatologist explained that their baby needed to receive supplemental oxygen, but he was otherwise doing great. The nurse brought her baby over to see Amy and her husband before taking him to the Special Care Nursery. Amy couldn't thank us enough for all the support and help we gave her. Dr. Cook came in to let Amy and her husband know that Amy was very lucky she came to the hospital when she did, because her placenta had abrupted. Everyone was safe and sound. I left the room and Mary came out to thank me for my help. It's a great feeling when everything turns out fine in Emergencies like these. I heard later that week, that Amy and her baby were doing great.

Lisa has gained the experiential wisdom to grasp the salience of the early bleeding and pain. Hence, she already has a strong sense of the nature of the problem before even seeing the patient. All three clinicians immediately diagnose the placental abuption when the blood clots are extracted. Notice that, without pausing to think, Lisa is already moving to retrieve the equipment they will need to get Amy to the OR. This embodied intelligence enables expert nurses to rapidly manage emergent situations without having to focus specifically on what they are doing, allowing them to simultaneously orchestrate the team and coach others about what is needed <u>while</u> they are providing care.

In expert nursing practice like this, many of these crises are recognized before the patient deteriorates significantly or actually arrests. Because numerous and diverse conditions and complications can rapidly deteriorate into an arrest, the most appropriate and timely intervention is often determined by the context of the situation. In addition, depending on the urgency of the patient's condition, the nurse may have to initiate therapy without a physician's order in order to prevent the crisis from evolving into an arrest.

Anticipation and/or early diagnosis of a crisis requires that a clinician have similar experiences in past situations in order to notice and understand the meaning of early warning signals. In many situations, the clinical judgment needed to accurately diagnose a problem in its early stages is the life-saving skill. Below, a surgical ICU nurse articulates what she noticed and the actions taken that prevented the patient from fully arresting:

Nurse: Well, just a couple of weeks ago, it was the first time I had a patient who was having a cardiac tamponade. He'd had surgery. Pretty classic symptoms, but it's a very subtle thing...We had to open up his chest. And it was a very <u>calm</u>—I mean, it wasn't completely calm, but it went very well and it was very <u>organized</u> and the fellow came in. It was a cardiovascular fellow because he's the only one who can open the chest. So I was assisting. I was like, at the bedside, gowned, putting my finger on the bleeder and helping to take the staples out and do all that. And it just was—that situation just felt so much more in control. Although if someone looked at it, it would look so <u>out</u> of control because blood was pouring out of his chest. His chest was open. We were pumping in blood. I mean there was stuff all over the room. It looked out of control, but it really <u>wasn't</u>, and the guy did fine and went home... He was not doing a lot of bleeding out of his chest tube, like a moderate amount, but his cardiac output slowly went down and his blood pressure was going down, and it seemed like the only thing that he responded to was fluid. And then his CVP was going up and his PA pressures were going up and...I didn't notice a pulsus paradoxus. He could have had it. All I noticed is that he had also been diagnosed with an [aneurysm] <u>and</u> he had really bad vasculature. When they had sewed one of the grafts onto his aorta, it just sort of <u>split</u> where they—but they didn't know it at the time until after they closed his chest and they saw this big thing flapping around in his aorta and it was an aneurysm. And he had an aneurysm that spiraled all the way down to his <u>renals</u>. He had such a friable aorta. And so they had to go back in, put him on bypass, disconnect that graft, put an aortic graft in, and then reconnect the venous graft. So it was a big long surgery. But he was doing okay. That's the normal case of tamponade and you get an X-ray which pretty much confirms it. <u>If</u> you can get one before it actually gets too bad. And that's what you do, you notice these signs and...

Interviewer: What did you notice and what did you do about them?

Nurse: The low blood pressure, the falling cardiac output, the increased CVP... Those are all pretty classic signs of tamponade. But in order to make sure that it was tamponade and not some sort of <u>dissection</u> of his aorta, because he had such a bad aorta, we did an echo [echocardiogram]. We had the echo tech[nician] come in the middle of the night. And when he just <u>touched</u> the echo to the guy's chest, he would drop his blood pressure. That's how much of a tamponade he had. It's amazing...it would cause him to, to lose his blood pressure to the 60's and we'd have to stop. And we were giving him fluid....

Interviewer: And what did you see—what had the X-ray shown?

Nurse: A widened mediastinum which shows the silhouette of the heart as really, really big because there's a big clot around it. But before we even got the X-ray, just his clinical symptoms. And I called the fellow in because his blood pressure dropped <u>really</u> low, like to the 40s and then I had increased some of the vasopressor and hung some fluid, and it came back. I called the fellow while I was doing all that... He got here and then we just ended up opening his chest because he went into—he actually didn't go into V-fib, but he had no pulse, which is what he had on the monitor, or barely, like when it was in the 30's. So we had to open his chest and evacuate it the clots.

The patient's earliest symptoms of an evolving complication were his decreased cardiac output and low blood pressure. For many cardiac surgical patients, these are typically signs of worsening myocardial function or hypovolemia. However, this nurse's early diagnosis of the tamponade was possible, in part, because she knew the patient's past and immediate history (e.g., bad vasculature, friable aorta, intraoperative vascular complications). Her diagnosis was then confirmed when the patient's CVP and PA pressures began to rise. She immediately began increasing the infusion of fluids and vasopressor to support circulation and to give her the time needed to call the fellow for help and to order the necessary tests. Despite the patient's significant drop in blood pressure, the early diagnosis was life-saving because the rapid infusion of fluids and vasopressor sustained the patient until definitive intervention was possible.

Although there are standard ways of managing particular crises (e.g., the ACLS protocol to defibrillate in the case of ventricular tachycardia), for most scenarios, the protocols typically begin at the point at which the crisis has already ensued. The goal in excellent patient care is to recognize a problem and intervene before the crisis completely unfolds. Guidelines for care are often unavailable because there are more variations than can be accounted for in guidelines. Reasoning about the particular trajectory as it unfolds is required. The narrative accounts in this chapter will assist in making experts' practical knowledge and performance more visible. Their knowledge, however, cannot provide a "recipe" for care because their knowledge is context-sensitive. The skills that require development and the habits of thought and action that are pervasive in expert practice can however be pointed out, described, and better understood to help learners in their own development. These habits of thinking often overlap with clinical forethought (see Chapter 3).

Now, general acute and critical care classes and courses, which repeatedly review and rehearse standardized crisis interventions, prepare specialty nurses to respond to a particular type of crisis. For example, in the case of ventricular tachycardia, standardized responses to typical situations (such as preparing for electrocardioversion) prepare the nurse to act quickly in high time demand, high risk situations. However, standardized responses, while readily available, should not become rote or completely automatic because the particularities of a specific clinical situation may offer a less potentially harmful, more controllable, and less painful alternative, as shown in a pediatric nurse's story:

Nurse: The night before last, at 6:00 in the morning I was in this room helping somebody out and all of a sudden I heard the monitor clicking off at about 3:00 and I looked up and the kid was in V-tach [ventricular tachycardia] and I immediately ran out and pulled the code cart in because I figured we're going to cardiovert him . Supposedly kids don't go into V-tach, although every kid I've seen code up there has gone into V-tach. It's like an arrhythmia that kids supposedly don't have. They go right into asystole, they bypass it. Well, not the ones I've seen. But one of the other nurses who's been taking care of cardiacs (babies) for a long time, she turned on the pacer—he had a pacer but it wasn't on, it was off, and evidently by doing that she overrode the V-tach eventually—she had to turn the rate way up...

Because cardiac surgical patients typically have atrial and/or ventricular pacing wires inserted, overdrive pacing is a better and safer option for emergency intervention than is normally available in patients who develop ventricular tachycardia but do not have pacing wires available. Overdrive pacing carries the risk of inducing ventricular fibrillation but is superior in this case to the potential and unpredictable consequences of electrocardioversion which can lead to ventricular fibrillation, asystole, complete heart block, bradycardia, etc. or to antiarrhythnmic medications which can increase mortality rates. The nurse telling this story <u>intellectually</u> knew that the patient had pacemaker wires and had likely heard in a class that overdrive pacing was the intervention of choice (knowledge acquisition), but her limited experience in this kind of emergency and an over-reliance on a standardized response prevented her from thinking-in-action, using that knowledge, and reaching first for the pacemaker. However, the expert nurse's clinical judgment took into account the context of the specific situation (the availability of pacing wires and a pacemaker) so that she deviated from protocol in a way that best and most expediently benefited the patient.

In other crises, the nurse may have little to no prior history on the patient and thus the standardized protocols serve an important function for intervention. Guidelines are also immensely helpful in situations where the clinical picture is confusing or unclear. Some patient situations are unexplainable at the time of the crisis, as in the following narrative account, and one can only use collective judgment or the best judgment possible at the time:

Nurse 1: My [story] is that we went down to the [small town] area on the river, Meg and myself. Meg's been a Life Flight nurse for a pretty long period of time, and I had maybe been a Flight nurse for two years. It was an early March morning, and it was pretty dewy and kind of had that morning chill to it, and we flew down there and it turned out to be a traumatic CPR. And we got on scene, and the report basically was—it was a 60-year-old woman who was beaten and left for dead on a river road. A very <u>remote</u> river road. And we walked up, got report, and she was last seen crawling across the road by this person who just happened to be driving down the road, and she just literally collapsed in front of this car. And when the medics arrived, they found her still alive and got her intubated, and put her on a monitor/defibrillator, with the patches front and back just to get a quick look at her heart rate, and now if they needed to defibrillate her, they could just do that through the patches. And when we arrived, at that point she, according to the patches, was in asystole, and met our criteria for declaration of death. And I was the lead person, and Meg was the crew person, and everything else had been done according to the way it should be done and we looked at the medics and we will typically ask them, we'll say that this person meets protocol for declaration of death and we would like to go ahead and make that declaration. And we usually ask them if they're okay with that, because if somebody really feels uneasy about that, typically we will just transport the patient. And at this point, one of the medics said, 'She just went down right before we got here.' And I turned and I looked at the monitor, and she was still in asystole, and I said, 'I can appreciate that,' I said, 'but it is so hard to get these patients back.' And I kind of went through a little quick story about trauma patients in asystole and right at that moment, her left hand moved and she reached for her ET tube. And I looked at him, and I looked at her, and I looked Meg and I looked at the monitor, and she was still in asystole. And I said, 'Is there any way that [monitor] can be wrong?', and he said, 'No.' I said, 'Well, then we're going to have to go. We just can't leave this person in asystole moving...it's just...the picture doesn't fit.' So we loaded her up, put her in the helicopter, did all our usual ACLS protocols, including drugs and shocks, because she was in and out of V-fib, and amiodarone and epinephrine and everything we could possibly imagine to get her back here, and we got her back to the hospital, and in the hospital they opened up her chest, they did open-heart massage, and warmed up every orifice of her body, took her to the operating room, and put her on heart bypass, warmed her up, got her to the intensive care unit, because they got her heart back, and 15 days <u>later</u>, after admission, she was discharged from the hospital with full mental function. That's my story.

Interviewer: Well, I'm a little confused. (More laughter from group.)

Nurse 2: We all were.

Nurse 3: She was probably not in trauma CPR, she was probably hypothermic.

Nurse 1: She was probably hypothermic, and some people would argue that typically in [this county], because it doesn't get cold real fast, you don't get true hypothermia , is what the feeling is. But you have a person who, this lady was really cachectic and really emaciated, and there were a lot of other factors, probably, that led to her being able to survive this for whatever reason, I don't know. I mean, if I had to predict, I could predict probably within 99.99 percent of the time that this person would die. And this person was that 10th of a percent that would fool everybody, and she fooled us. Completely fooled us.

Interviewer: Now, I'm curious, when she moved, I mean it was purposeful movement?

Nurse 1: Yeah. Yeah.

Interviewer: And the monitor showed asystole. Was she pulseless?

Nurse 1: Yes.

Interviewer: She was pulseless. That sort of defies...

Nurse 1: Defies, that's exactly right.

Interviewer: My goodness. So did she respond to the—to ACLS...?

Nurse 1: We never got her to respond to any... I mean, the only thing was, she'd go into V-fib [ventricular fibrillation] every once in a while, but she was in and out of the rhythm so fast that all was did was chase her. It was like, as soon as you'd get ready to shock her, she's back in asystole and then you start to push more drugs, then she's back to V-fib, and you're trying to push drugs and shock her...we just chased her [physiologically] all the way back here [to the hospital]. And that's all we did. And I'd have to go back and look at the chart to see how much we actually got completed, but it was amazing how—how in and out she was and all over the place. And then to actually survive.

Interviewer: Wow.

Nurse 3: Well, hypothermia is what made her survive.

This situation raises multiple issues in managing a crisis. Such "exceptional" stories serve to keep the clinician open to possibilities in a clinical situation and clinicians tell such upending stories to foster openness. First, the patient's diagnosis of asystole seems as if it must have been erroneous. Yet, the clinician was very experienced and was as certain as possible about his observations of the patient's rhythm and the patient's purposeful hand movement. Further, multiple clinicians at the scene observed and concluded the same thing. Thus, the nurse's original judgment to stop resuscitative measures was reversed by the patient's surprising hand movement. It was only in retrospect, after gaining a clearer understanding of the patient's physiological condition by piecing the "facts" together, such as the hypothermia effect in the context of the situation, that the puzzling clinical findings made better sense.

Second, this nurse talked about the difficult situation of "chasing" the patient physiologically while trying to "manage" a crisis. "Chasing" conveys a distinctly different way of having to manage the patient's physiological responses rather than being on top of the situation or having a good clinical grasp. It refers to a reactive mode of intervention where, because of the rapidly changing, uncontrolled, and unpredictable physiological events, the clinicians must intervene with various therapies to treat ever-changing problems, yet they are not able to stabilize the patient's condition. In this situation, the patient was in and out of ventricular fibrillation and asystole, so therapies were rapidly changing in reaction to the patient's momentary rhythms. This patient's severely deteriorated condition made it impossible for the expert clinician to "manage" the crisis, which typically connotes being able treat the complication or crisis well enough to stabilize the patient. The nurse expression, "we just chased her all the way back here [hospital]. And that's all we did," captures his disappointment and a higher expectation of himself, since "chasing" the patient is exactly what critical care practices are set up to avoid. Developing clinicians will often find themselves "chasing" the patient condition until they learn how to quickly stabilize the patient and/or prevent foreseeable complications.

Third, this story illustrates how the declaration of death cannot and should not be determined according to a protocol alone. It shows how expert clinicians act as moral agents and also solicit the moral voice of others, such as the medic. In this case, the nurse acts as a moral agent who is equipped with a protocol to declare care futile, if that is warranted, rather than act as an implementer or instrument of the protocol. This is a critical distinction that renders protocols, guidelines, or clinical pathways safe in practice through the exercise of clinical judgment. The nurse's sense of agency is key in determining how the protocol is taken up in practice and whether it is used judiciously and flexibly. Declaring death is a solemn and moral judgment and the nurse acknowledges this by giving respect for each clinician's voice, so much so, that anyone's dissent can reverse the decision. This patient's life was saved because the nurse's and group's good judgment superseded the protocol for declaring death. A protocol can never include all the particularities and nuances of every situation as illustrated in this situation regarding the physiological effects of hypothermia. Further, this story demonstrates that ethical judgment is intertwined with clinical judgment in the everyday care of patients, and it is a mistake to teach students one in isolation of the other since a nurse's inability to eventually make this link by her or himself will hinder the development of expertise.

Fourth, the above account depicts how expert nurses reason-in-transition. "What to do" in a crisis is sometimes not as difficult as judging "whether or not to resuscitate." The nurse's initial sense was not to resuscitate and his judgment was strongly supported by current scientific evidence on the outcomes of resuscitation in the face of asystole (Martin et al., 1993; Robinson & Hess, 1994). The transition in reasoning arose when the patient moved her hand and arm because it shed new light that the patient was indeed holding on to life. Subsequently, we notice the nurse reason in a changing situation; that is, he reinterpreted the patient's physiological state, was turned around, and immediately began intervention. In clinical practice, expert nurses are characterized by an openness to reinterpretation of a situation and by flexibility and adaptability in their thinking and judgment when something significant presents itself or changes. This shift in understanding the situation causes the facts of the situation to take on different relevance. Recognizing changing relevance is central to expert practice (Benner, Tanner & Chesla, 2009; Dreyfus & Dreyfus, 1986).

Expecting and being prepared for the unexpected is essential in acute and critical care practice and is central to the attentiveness and vigilance of expert nurses because physiological transitions may occur rapidly without any warning. When caring for chronically critically ill patients who are relatively stable, the unexpected occurs less frequently so that sudden life-threatening transitions may bring greater surprise and stress:

> **Nurse:** I was taking care of the kid that had a trach. He smiles at you, he's going to Children's and he's so cute, and I was sitting in there on Friday night and he started to cough. And he kept coughing and he turned blue and he dropped his heart rate out and we coded him for half an hour. He had plugged his trach off and in the process of suctioning him, he flipped his head around and pulled his trach out. Because he had tracheal stenosis, we couldn't bag him. So that caught me off guard. That was one of the most horrendous nights I've ever had. And it was really stressful...you don't anticipate that kind of problem with a kid that's 4 months old and going to Children's [hospital] in a couple of days.
>
> **Interviewer:** So how did he do? Is he all right?
>
> **Nurse:** He did okay.

Here, the nurse conveys the conventional wisdom that long term patients who are ready for transfer typically do not arrest. So, the unexpected tracheal tube dislodgment caught the nurse "off guard" indicating that, because the infant was relatively stable, she was expecting a quiet and uneventful night. The stress of the unexpected was intensified by the inability to ventilate or re-trach the infant in a timely manner, resulting in a full code. The nurse indicated that smoother management of the life-threatening situation is linked with the ability to anticipate it. Had the nurse or anyone else been able to anticipate the unusual complication, the nurse could have better prepared the environment for the rapid intervention (see Chapter 3).

Because the infant went on to do well, one has the impression that the nurse and the team were able to provide the right interventions in a timely manner; however, this was not explored in the interview. Typical response sets to commonly occurring situations and anticipation of the usual course of events allow the nurse to read the situation rapidly and intervene appropriately. In high time demand situations, it is simply not possible to start from ground zero to build up an understanding of the situation element by element and still respond in a wise and timely manner. Identifying the most salient and urgent problems requires at least a tentative perspective on the situation and a repertoire of likely, effective interventions. But, rigidly holding onto initial readings of the situation and routinized responses generated by the slavish following of protocols create a significant risk for misreading or overlooking particularity and exceptions. Expert practice requires staying open to disconfirmation, unanticipated turns in the situation, and changing relevance as the situation changes. It is counterproductive to become hypervigilant, anticipating <u>every</u> possible eventuality (too much openness) and, likewise, counterproductive to rigidly hold on to expectations and set ways to act when they are no longer relevant (too little openness). This is illustrated in the following interview excerpt where a child's condition after surgery rapidly declined, requiring rapidly changing expectations and responses:

Nurse 1: This five-and-one-half-month old child had done quite well through the surgery considering that she had in essence a single ventricle, she only had a right ventricle and hypoplastic left cardiac chamber. And they were...creating a shunt to help her until they could do a Fontan[1]...and she did okay, and got back to the room and was in essence stable for that type of a child. She had a good heart rate, a decent blood pressure, her O_2 [oxygen] sat[uration]s were where they wanted them; she was there all of about 10 minutes, just in time for the surgeons to come in and the anesthesiologist to say, 'Everything's okay,' and then everybody left except for one of the residents. And then her O_2 sats started to drop. We tried bagging her, it didn't work. Then her heart rate dropped, then her blood pressure dropped, and she in essence arrested and we ended up working on her for over an hour. Opened her chest—she went down the hall to the operating room with one of the resident's hands in her chest pumping her heart....

Nurse 2: The parents hadn't even seen the kid after surgery, that's what's hard (talking together).

Nurse 1: They had sent her to the surgery that morning, and she was awake, healthy, I mean she was not a real tiny, emaciated little...

Interviewer: She was five and one-half months old... So what happened first?

Nurse 1: Her oxygenation decreased. Her O_2 Sats decreased. We could not ventilate her and consequently when we couldn't ventilate her, her O_2 Sats dropped down into the 50s.

Interviewer: And what was the immediate response to the desaturation? What was done first?

Nurse 1: Bagging with 100% oxygen...and then when her heart rate dropped and that didn't seem to help a lot. We tried to suction, tried repositioning to see if we couldn't ventilate her better. We were not able to ventilate her left lung that well. Then when her heart rate was dropping, we turned on the pacemaker. She didn't like that very much either. Her blood pressure continued to fall. Started with IV push epi, closed chest compressions. Dr. R. came flying in the room and we ended up opening her chest and then they went from there. They tried internally pacing her. That didn't work either. And you'd get a rhythm for a couple minutes, or a minute or two and then it would...

Interviewer: So the event really started off, do you think, respiratory?

Nurse 1: Oh, I know it was respiratory.

Interviewer: Rather than heart.

---

[1]A Fontan is a corrective cardiac surgical procedure.

Nurse 1: Yes. When they got her to the OR, they did a bronch[oscopy] and she had a mucous plug, for one thing. They had some kind of plug down there that was almost totally occluding that we could not get—I don't, I mean, I suctioned her and I swear that suction catheter just about went to her toes, and we were unable to get anything significant out... And what we also ended up doing—in the middle of it all, once the anesthesiologist arrived—we reintubated her, because they were thinking that maybe the plug was at the end of the ET tube, and it wasn't. They pulled the ET tube out and there was a little bit of blood on the end of it, but it was not occluded at all. But considering it all, it went 'well' for a code.

This excerpt illustrates the rapidly changing understanding of the situation as interventions failed and expectations were not met. The nurse later expressed remorse that "there was just nothing we could do to save her."

This story also emphasizes why rapid and effective intervention is imperative in a life-threatening situation in order to prevent the inevitable deterioration into an arrest. The nurse describes bagging the baby immediately after the oxygen saturation dropped. The inability to adequately ventilate the baby prompted the clinicians to suction and then reposition the baby, but without success. Finally, the baby was reintubated in hopes of removing the cause of the problem, but to no avail. At that point, a bronchoscopy was performed to identify a possible airway obstruction. Meanwhile, without oxygenation, the baby's heart rate dropped and multiple interventions, including emergency medications, CPR, open chest massage, and pacing were needed to sustain circulation until the mucous plug was identified and removed.

This situation highlights the clinical demands that a crisis places on the nurse for forethought, attentiveness, action, and mobilization of resources. In a crisis, instantaneous responses are imperative to treat the complication and/or prevent a cascade of devastating and/or irreversible events. When initial interventions are unsuccessful, clinicians must quickly make judgments about alternative actions and effectively pursue them within minutes. With each intervention, the nurse rules out the next most likely cause of the problem in that particular patient. Second, the rapid and intense actions demand the nurse's constant and undivided attention. In expert nursing practice, nurses are attuned, not only to the details of their own specific actions, but also to the patient's moment by moment responses, others' actions, and the ongoing team dialogue, all while anticipating what will be needed next. Clinical forethought (see Chapter 3) in a crisis involves anticipating the likely need for medications, procedures, equipment, other team members, laboratory tests, comfort measures, and family visits. These multiple demands contribute to making expert acute and critical care practice complex. Last, managing a crisis requires intense, effective, and often extensive mobilization of resources, such as calling in the anesthesiologist and operating team in the above story. The forethought, attentiveness, actions, and resources are not unique to crisis situations; however, the intense nature of all four simultaneously best characterize a crisis.

In addition to the clinical demands, crises commonly thrust many kinds of emotional demands on nurses. Even in expert critical care practice where crises are everyday occurrences, nurses can experience the fear of having someone else's life in their hands or of inflicting pain in order to provide treatment. In some crisis situations, particularly in trauma and flight nursing, patients are severely injured and often maimed or disfigured. If nurses allowed themselves to focus on the significance of the patient's injuries and suffering for the patient as a person while they provide life-saving interventions for the patient, nurses would be unable to intervene or help, but would instead be paralyzed by the horror of the patient's condition. A expert flight nurse describes a situation where the patient's unexpected plea leads the nurse to experience a momentary breakdown in his ability to function:

Nurse 1: We get to the scene of a bad accident—a big rig truck versus a van—where the man in the van was severely injured and pinned into the front seat. There is a fire-fighter in the middle seat of this van, and there is another fire-fighter in the front passenger seat, and we come up trying to find out where they're at in terms of getting him out because we don't want to get in their way. And he was tachypneic, he appeared to be hypotensive, his color was really bad, he wasn't breathing really well, and just looking at this guy...he had a business suit on. He just looked like a family kind of guy...that's the picture that you get from him. And they were trying to get him out of the car, and they were going to have to take him out through the sliding door on the passenger side, which is where we were. And at that point, [Nurse 2] looks at me and says, 'Do you think you can put a [ET] tube in where he's at?' and I said, 'Well, we can try.' And he was still awake, and I thought maybe he could help me, if anything. And the [fire fighters] said, 'We're about ready to come out,' and I said, 'Why don't we wait till we get him out?' So I helped the fire-fighters get set up with the long board and we start to pull him out, and he's a big guy; he's around 230, 250, somewhere in there.

Nurse 2: —about right.

Nurse 1: We pulled him out of the car, and [Nurse 2] was lead and I was crew and I went around to his head to talk to him, kind of give him an idea of where he was, and he was just...he wasn't talking, which is pretty typical when you pull these people out of the car. They just dump their pressure or they may go apneic on you or they just take a dump. Who knows why, they just do. So I took a quick look at him, he really wasn't answering questions very well, and I reached into my bag to get my stuff for a nasal setup, because he was breathing well enough at that time that I thought he could at least take a nasal tube, and it would be the fastest way to get him intubated and give him some oxygen. And I reach in and I grab my zip-lock bag and I begin to open it, and I look back at him and he opens up his eyes, just as clear as...he was just so lucid at that point, he looked at me—<u>directly</u> at me in the eyes and said, 'Help me.' I just stopped dead in my tracks and I was like...I forget everything that was going on. I just, I had no idea, nor did I care. And I just froze. And I called [Nurse 2] and I said—At that moment, time just stopped for me. He completely took me out of my element, because I've never had anybody with that much care in their voice say to me, 'Help me.' And we ended up intubating him and got him <u>out</u> of there, and got him back here and I think that he's still in the intensive care unit and he's just got so many injuries. He is so sick.

Nurse 2: The whole time, we could never get a pressure, we just had...femoral pulses...

Nurse 1: You know, it was just, 'Don't die on me today. No, not today. I don't want this today. Let's just get you to the hospital. Let's worry about all this stuff...let's just get there.' That's all I wanted to do. It just couldn't go fast enough. And we already fly at 150 miles an hour, how much faster you want to go? But it wasn't fast enough. Nothing was fast enough. You just can't move fast enough when they just look at you and just say, 'Help me.'

Interviewer: But patients typically are not aware when you pick them up?

Nurse 1: Yeah. Most of them don't even remember flying.

Nurse 2: Yeah.

Nurse 4: It's harder when they die if they talk to you beforehand... You get there and they're out, and you don't get to know them.

Nurse 1: Yeah, because you always want, you always want the family to be the last person to see them, last person to talk to them, I don't want it to be me.

Nurse 3: Did you nasally intubate him or oral..?

Nurse 1: Nasal.

Nurse 2: [Talking about seeing Nurse 1 intubate the patient] He nasally intubated him just like that (snapping fingers), too. Because I was trying to tie his hand down and turned around and he already had him tubed.

Nurse 1: It just seemed like it took me forever. It just seemed like I just couldn't go fast enough.

The breakdown in smooth practice illuminates several covered-over yet vitally important issues, especially for new critical care nurses. To perform well in a crisis, nurses typically cannot fully focus on (or closely empathize with) the patient as a person without the emotional weight of the tragedy impeding their skillful performance. When called into the crisis in a personal way, such as in this nurse's experience, one can lose the ability to respond. A life slipping away in an unexpected death makes a strong demand on those helping. To cope, it is commonly necessary to objectify the patient for the moment and become very task-focused. The momentary objectification sustains and protects the nurse from the unbearable emotional weight in order to perform skillfully throughout the event and therefore serves a good. It is this skill of directing one's attention and energy to the tasks at hand that sets limits on one's fear and is a kind of boundary work that must be learned over time. As Sallie Tisdale says, it is "a balance of pain and compassion" (Tisdale, 1986). Not to learn this skill can mean delayed intervention which can cost a patient permanent injury or death. At the same time, as illustrated by the nurse in the above situation, ignoring the patient is not a viable option either:

Nurse: [They] pulled him out of the car, and... I went around to his head to talk to him, kind of give him an idea of where he was, and he was just...he wasn't talking, which is pretty typical when you pull these people out of the car.

The nurse calmly, compassionately, and simply informs the patient about what is happening, what to expect, how he/she is doing, and then reassures the patient as much as is feasible. This situated possibility in a nurse's practice is a moral triumph, for it is a hard learned skill of involvement, which refers to the interpersonal engagement or relational connection between the nurse and the patient or family (Benner, Tanner & Chesla, 2009). However, once learned, the nurse is never immune from breakdown situations, as occurred with the above nurse. This very skilled clinician had intubated hundreds of trauma victims and was responsible for patients' lives daily, but for a moment, this patient shook the nurse out of his focused way of situating himself during a devastating crisis. It is a very narrow path one walks to be with and help someone suffering without becoming overly involved on the one hand or too far distanced on the other (Benner & Wrubel, 1989; Tisdale, 1986). This "lapse" shows that the nurse is still connected to the life-and-death meaning of rescuing trauma victims. Though usually submerged to do the task at hand, these strong concerns motivate and animate the work. Such work calls for self-forgetfulness in the midst of the urgent demands and for debriefing and working through the strong emotions after the event.

The path narrows even more when struggling to cope with strong emotions in extreme types of crises. For instance, within the first hours after admission, burn nurses are called to the do the unbearable; that is, to scrub and debride painful burn wounds, which further inflicts pain on the patient. To help the patient, nurses must develop some way of providing good pain management for patients while still coping with pain-producing procedures. Bearing witness to the patient's suffering induced by that care, rather than ignoring or denying it, is central to the moral art of nursing. This skill of involvement is learned gradually through many experiences of doing better or worse. In common types of everyday crises, nurses moved in and out of a protective mode invisibly. However, extreme types of crises challenged their ability to temporarily objectify the patient. Flight nurses talked about why and how they are able to intervene in horrible situations. During the dialogue, a nurse discusses the care of an extensively burned and severely disfigured victim just after a car crash. The whole account is not included to shield the reader from the suffering heard in the victim's moaning, the smells of gasoline and burnt metal and human flesh, and the picture of scant human remains of multiple victims, including the one who was barely clinging to life. However, this general description better situates one's understanding about how this nurse could provide care, after all other team members unexpectedly found themselves physically unable to help upon seeing the patient:

Nurse 1: I think I learned you can kind of be just about anything at the moment...

Nurse 2: ...that you have to...

Nurse 3: Yeah.

Nurse 1: Just get in there and do it and then deal with it somehow later. People ask me all the time, 'How do you do your job?' And you just kind of get blinders on and you just get in there and you do it. But as soon as you're done, if it's a really horrific, horrible, 'oh-my-god' flight, then you kind of get emotional about it.

Nurse 3: You sort of go into automatic.

Nurse 1: Uh huh.

Nurse 3: It's like flipping a switch. It's like turning off your emotional switch and just going sort of into in robot mode or something. That you just do what you have to do. And you wait to have the emotional part later, when you don't have responsibility for the person anymore.

Interviewer: Now, how is it that you went into automatic [regarding a burn victim] but Carol [another nurse] got sick?

Nurse 3: I don't know. Carol just got real nauseated. She usually doesn't. I don't know if it was the smell. The smell was really bad and she was pregnant at the time. So that might have been it. I mean, I've seen her throw up and still go on.

Interviewer: So whatever the situation demands, you pretty much, respond.

Nurse 4: I think at the time, [the patient] is not so much a person, either. It's like, 'I have an airway.' You know, it's an airway or it's an electrical activity that you don't have. It's not really a person. Not that you're um, meaning to mistreat them as a whole in any way, but you do have to focus to get your job done. Once you get back to the hospital and you stop taking care of them, well then they're a person again, and you can see them after.

Interviewer: Is that <u>necessary</u> in order to be able to do some of the things that you do?

Nurse 4: Yeah, I think that if you thought about this whole person when you were dealing with them at the scene, I think that would be too much for anyone to really deal with.

Nurse 1: Yeah, that really would be.

Nurse 4: Too much sadness, too much pain, too much frustration.

Nurse 2: And I think you can do that easier if you focus on, like you say, 'That's an airway I have to get,' or 'This I have to do, or that I have to do.' Especially when it's just the patient and there's no family around.

These expert nurses talk about their protective mode but acknowledge that they do come to grips with the emotions when the patient is no longer their responsibility. In fact, many nurses talk about specific ways that they deal with their emotions. Some find a nearby closet or utility room in which to sob, others discuss the crisis with peers, a few routinely set up team debriefings for any "out of the ordinary" or emotion-laden cases, and a few engage in all three ways. What is striking and crucial for developing nurses is to learn how to move in and out of this protective mode without getting stuck in or out of it.

The above skill of involvement, the balance between suffering and compassion, must never be mistaken as emotional disengagement or detachment, described by Rubin (1996), which prevents the development of expert clinical judgment and practice. These nurses are highly engaged in the focused "problems" of saving a life: getting an airway, a pulse, hemostatsis, et cetera. As these nurses indicate, in horrific situations of human tragedy, a moment of full engagement with the victim as a person can render the nurses extremely vulnerable to collapsing under the weight of the sorrow, leaving them unable to help. The temporary emotional withdrawal is distinguished from emotional disengagement to the point of no engagement with the problem at hand <u>or</u> the person that prevents ethical and clinical reasoning. Disengagement is a growing, disturbing, and often preventable problem in practice (beyond nursing) today. Kyriakidis (in progress) found an alarming rate of nurses who have been in practice beyond 5 years but who have not developed to or beyond the competent stage of practice, meaning that they are unable to respond to or meet the specific needs of the patient or family. The care provided is thus often inadequate. Their peers easily recognize the deficits in care, yet have little understanding or skill to help rectify and prevent the problem. Kyriakidis and Vitello (in progress) were able to show a remarkable rate of skillful engagement and performance development in new nurses over a 2-year period using expert narratives as a major source for developing a strong vision of excellent practice and transforming educational strategies to situated learning in authentic contexts.

For emotionally disengaged nurses, "clinical knowledge and ethical judgment play no meaningful role in their experience" as practitioners (Rubin, 1996, p.173). For instance, without noticing the ethical violation, one nurse told about managing a terminal cancer patient's life-threatening dysrhythmia, and repeatedly and successfully coding him, despite his clear DNR choice and orders. Without engagement, the patient's most important medical instructions, which the nurse conveyed during the telling of the story, played no role in guiding her ethical judgment or clinical interventions. The concerns the nurse had for the patient, which are good in most patient situations, were totally separate or disconnected from this particular patient's concerns and wishes. Although his multiple crises were managed effectively and efficiently, the care provided cannot be understood as ethical, safe, humane, or even competent. Articulating the role of both clinical knowledge and ethical judgment in this chapter and throughout this book is intended to assist clinicians in recognizing the foundational importance of engagement and the skills of involvement in varying kinds of situations to prevent the blunting of one's ethical perceptions which are essential to developing expertise.

Part of responding to a crisis involves coping with the outcome for the patient which is not always consistent with the nurse's hopes and efforts. In some institutions, there is no dialogue after an unexpected or tragic death, for instance, and nurses must learn to cope alone in the best way they can. In the best of practice, clinicians (including all interested disciplines) gather to debrief about the situation. Debriefing allows clinicians the legitimate space and support to grieve, review how the team performed, learn from situations where improvement is needed, appreciate other team members' efforts, and learn from others' experiences. Nurses also gather to cope with insufferable anguish. A nurse illustrates the importance that debriefing held in the team's practice after a tremendous team effort to extricate, stabilize, and transport a young trauma patient who unexpectedly died:

Nurse: We actually did a debriefing [conference] on this call with the medical staff and the fire department, because above everything else, I mean this guy died and they worked <u>so hard</u> to get this guy out of his car. I mean, you know this golden hour [for trauma victims] that they talk about is true. This guy <u>needed</u> the golden hour. He <u>needed</u> to get down here. We wasted so much time trying—not wasted. We—we—we killed so much time trying to get him out of that car. Had we gotten him down here in a reasonable amount of time, would that have made a big difference for him? And you have to believe that it really would have. And these guys really worked so hard. I called them back and I said, 'Well, it's hard to report, but he didn't make it.' And they're like, 'What do you mean he didn't make it?' They were just as much attached him as anybody else that was on the call. So we actually went back up there [to the scene]...

The nurse explains that he and his partner returned to the scene after the patient's death because the whole team had fought so hard and had given their best to save the patient's life. Because the patient was lucid and talking to them on departure from the scene, everyone had great difficulty accepting his death. The clinicians and fire department medics all found themselves emotionally rooting for this patient and had a fair amount of confidence that he would survive. Coping with this particular crisis is harder because the patient spoke to them. The verbal connection allows the nurse to get to know the patient as a real person for whom the nurse developed hope. A nurse in a previous story explains:

Nurse: It's harder when they die, if they talk to you beforehand... You get there and they're out, and you know...you don't get to know them.

Clinical and ethical practice are closely tied together. By that we mean that the <u>ethical</u> judgment is made about the clinical actions taken in a situation. Although diagnosing and managing a life-threatening situation may, at first, seem distinctly different from ethical expertise, moral action is central to learning and knowing: how to recognize "what is a good action" to take in response to the patient's physiological and personal needs; how to skillfully and compassionately respond in relation to an unfolding and changing crisis; and when to change the type of interventions provided (Benner, Tanner & Chesla, 2009, see "Agency," pp.157-160). The following story reveals the fusion of the two types of expertise:

> **Nurse:** We transported an elderly lady that got broadsided off of [a rural highway in the county] and she was really bad, a bad multi-trauma. Chest trauma, pelvis, everything. And, she was very, very pale. Her mucous membranes were as white as these walls, and we knew it was bad. We had intubated her and we had gotten lines, but we pretty much knew that she probably wasn't going to do that well... But, I remember when we started losing her pressure and we still had femoral pulses, we had asked her as we were coming in, 'Can you squeeze my hand?', and I remember her just giving me a little light squeeze. So I just held onto her hand because I knew she was going down. I just <u>knew</u> it. And I thought, 'I'm not going to let this lady lay on this gurney and die without somebody touching her.' And sure enough, as we're landing, she went under CPR. She coded. And she died (Choking up a little with emotion). But, that was important. I think... That was important to me.

Upon arrival at the scene, the patient's physiological condition calls for swift, life-saving technologic and pharmacologic interventions to stabilize vital organ functions. During transport, as the nurse grasps that the patient's vital functions are deteriorating to an irreversible point, her notion of what is good to do in this situation changes. Life-saving interventions are immediately understood as futile; yet the patient remains conscious. The patient's "light squeeze" of her hand claims the nurse's undivided attention. She holds onto the patient's hand during her last moments of life. It is, at once, a moral, spiritual and clinical act. Learning to identify what interventions are called for throughout an evolving crisis situation requires good ethical and clinical judgment and respectful caring practices.

DIAGNOSING, MONITORING, TITRATING, AND PROVIDING INSTANTANEOUS INTERVENTIONS TO MAINTAIN VITAL FUNCTIONS AND PHYSIOLOGICAL STABILITY IN UNSTABLE PATIENTS

This aspect of the domain focuses on care of patients who are highly unstable and whose condition could easily deteriorate into a life-threatening crisis. Nurses' clinical judgment and practice for these patients involve rapid and instantaneous interventions to stabilize the patient's physiological condition, ameliorate the cause of the problem if possible, and provide supportive technological, pharmacological, or physiological therapies that allow the body to recover. Patients require this type of nursing care when they are just beginning to physiologically decline beyond their compensatory capabilities, show the earliest warning signs of complications, or suddenly develop an unpredictable problem. In many of these situations, the best intervention is contextually determined and must be based on the particular patient's responses to treatment, the specific pathophysiological reason for the instability, the patient's history and prior complicating illnesses, and the clinical trajectory that similar patients typically follow.

It is not always easy to discern an unstable situation from a crisis. Some patients require such extensive and urgent care that it is indistinguishable from a crisis other than the fact that the patient has not "coded." A key distinction that orients the nurse's thinking and practice is whether or not the urgent interventional care that is needed is primarily resuscitative (as in a crisis or code) or if it is primarily care that supports and maintains vital functions to prevent partial or complete failure of one or more organ systems (as in unstable patients). An issue that further clouds the ability to make the distinction is the experiential preparation of the staff and the availability of appropriate and reliable resources. For instance, an unstable pediatric patient may seem routine in a pediatric ICU, whereas staff in an adult ICU may respond to a pediatric patient's instability as a crisis. Similarly, a PACU setting that typically recovers less acute patients may respond to a patient complication as a crisis if they are not accustomed to managing particular kinds of patient complications. The following example illustrates how the management of an unstable child's condition took on the characteristics of a crisis in an unfamiliar setting with staff who were unaccustomed to treating very sick children:

Nurse: I was assigned to go out on transport. I was told the child had arrested, was on dopamine for blood pressure support, but her main problem was her uncontrollable GI bleeding. With this information, I called the pharmacy for a two rounds of code drugs and drips of dopamine, epinephrine, dobutamine, isuprel and nipride. With a first transport already out I had our backup equipment and was just throwing what I thought I might need into a duffel bag.

   As we [pediatrician, respiratory therapist, and nurse] arrived to pick up this 5-year-old child, there was a lot of running around. My first impression was 'this child is really sick.' I noticed that there were three nurses at her bedside: one pushing FFP [fresh frozen plasma], another pushing PRBC's [packed red blood cells], and the third was continuously irrigating her stomach with normal saline. The child was tachycardic and hypotensive with a MAP of 35, bleeding profusely from her stomach, and in DIC despite all the coagulation factors she was receiving. As well as being hemodynamically unstable, the child was also ventilating poorly due to an air leak around the endotracheal tube. Her pulses were poor, she was mottled and pale with hematocrit of 20. We started her on dobutamine with no change in condition or vital signs. We then started her on epinephrine with a slight increase in her MAP but nothing significant. My first thought was that this child was a lot sicker than we had anticipated, though we had brought everything that we had thought of. My second thought, as all this was taking place and we were getting nowhere with this child was that we were way over our heads and how would we ever get this child back with the hands that we had and by ground at that! (instead of helicoptor) The pediatrician was getting ready to talk to the parents when I approached her to say, 'I am going to call our PICU attending because I don't feel comfortable with what is happening here and I don't know how we will get her back to [our hospital].' I called my attending physician and told him the history of what had been happening—that neither the pediatrician or myself felt, with what was going on, that we would be able to get this child back with just the two of us managing her medical status and the R.T. managing her ventilation. I told him she was bleeding approximately 500 cc every 30-40 minutes, and that they probably should have some uncrossmatched blood available because we were running out fast. It was decided with this history to send a second transport team via helicopter to assist us in the transport back.

Basically the remainder of the transport—while we awaited the second team—was to keep her MAP up by pushing [clotting] factors and blood and giving boluses of epinephrine and calcium each time she dropped her blood pressure. The second transport team arrived, only to be totally amazed at how sick this child was, and we continued our regime, as well as adding a few extra drips to maintain this child during the air transport. We continued all the way back to pull blood out of her nasogastric tube at the same rate as we were pouring blood in via her IV. We arrived back to the PICU to let the team take over with no major problems en route.

...This was the sickest child that I have ever transported, essentially coding her the entire time. The referring hospital was at a loss for what else could be done for the child and really wanted her out of there as soon as possible... As the child was decompensating my first thoughts were that I wish I had a stronger pediatrician with me. I knew I had to act fast in this situation and I could tell that she was very uncomfortable with the situation because she was not suggesting things to me but rather I was suggesting therapy to her and she was agreeing with me. The pediatrician was there but not acting on things that should have been second nature. This made me a bit nervous because I was hoping there wasn't something very obvious that I was forgetting or something I was unaware of.

The most demanding thing was not having the medical backup I needed in that situation. Being by myself to setup drips, art line, push drugs, and chart as well as assess the child's condition continuously, was quite demanding especially since I had to be quite innovative to run all the drips in with just four pumps. I realize at this time how much backup is there from nursing staff when a child goes bad in a PICU setting where everything is familiar. The child was so unstable that the nurses available were only pushing blood products and were unable to assist me with other things.

In this story, the nurse anticipates, prior to going on the transport, that the situation could digress into a crisis and prepared for that eventuality with extra equipment and drugs. The child's very unstable condition ends up mimicking a crisis for many reasons. First, the nurses at the referral hospital have little experience with sick children and therefore could offer only limited assistance. Second, the pediatrician also has limited experience which functionally shifts the weight of the diagnostic and treatment responsibilities onto the nurse. Third, the child's condition demands extensive, urgent, continuous, and multifaceted interventions and the nurse, by herself, cannot provide it all. Finally, in one's "home" ICU, there is typically at least one other team member who is monitoring and keeping track of specifics, as well as the situation as a whole, so that the burden of ensuring excellent care is shared and the risk of overlooking significant issues is minimized. Here, the nurse is challenged to perform with the added emotional burden of coaching the pediatrician while trying to keep track of all aspects of care until the second team arrives. Although this child survived the immediate crisis, she later died of complications.

This example also points out a challenging aspect of acute and critical care nursing and medicine. In unstable situations where the <u>cause</u> of the problem is unknown, clinicians must often intervene initially by treating the <u>symptoms</u>. The patient's particular responses to the initial treatments then guide subsequent interventions until the cause is discovered or resolved. The goal is to stabilize the patient by managing the symptoms while trying to identify the cause of the problem(s). In contrast, many unstable patient situations are familiar so that the intervention of choice is well known, as in the following situation where a patient has a low pressure hydrocephalus with pulmonary complications that continued over a long ICU stay. When the patient's level of consciousness deteriorates due to a non-draining shunt, the nurses urgently intervene:

Nurse: They put in an external shunt and we were draining his ventricles and gradually over the months—we had to put the drain 20 centimeters below the ear level and gradually tried to bring him up to ear level to see if they could internalize [his shunt]. When we did, he wouldn't do so well. He developed hydrocephalus and then we would have to drop the drain back down. So it's been going on for a good 9 months...

Interviewer: He has low pressure hydrocephalus. So that would mean...

Nurse: That would mean we were having problems where every time they put the drain up to ear level, his ventricles would just get enlarged. And whatever treatment that we did, he would always have an enlarged ventricle...but I guess every time they wanted to internalize it, if it was a <u>low</u> pressure, it wasn't enough (pressure) for it to drain by itself. This was about one and one-half to two months ago, before this last one that they did worked.

Interviewer: And so pumping his shunt, you mean when it was internalized that it was an internal CSF shunt?

Nurse: Yes.

Interviewer: And what does pumping mean?

Nurse: Because of the low pressure, the shunt wasn't able to drain <u>properly</u>, so the patient would get lethargic, sleepy, so what we would have to stand there and where the valve was, and we literally...had to pump his shunt 250 times every hour.

Interviewer: Pump the valve?

Nurse: Yeah. And that would drain the CSF and in a few seconds he would wake up.

The patient's low intracranial pressure (ICP) resulted in repeated cerebral spinal fluid (CSF) drainage failure which consequently raised the patient's ICP too high. Each time the ventricles enlarged from the accumulating CSF, treatment became urgent as the increased ICP threatened to cause ischemic damage to brain tissue. Although the procedure may have become "routine" in this patient's care because of the months it took to safely place a properly functioning internal or ventriculo-peritoneal shunt, the urgency for intervention became no less critical with each episode due to the threat of catastrophic consequences. As with many critical care interventions, physiological support via technological means offered this patient a life-saving option and he was eventually discharged.

In everyday practice, a rapid and accurate diagnosis is as important as the intervention itself since the diagnosis commonly determines the appropriate intervention (see Chapter 2). Despite an accurate diagnosis, intervention is, at times, delayed because of the difficulty in "giving" one's grasp of a situation to another person, as in the story below (Hooper, 1995). Here, an advanced practice nurse's consultation and diagnosis were prompted by a staff nurse's concern. The advanced practice nurse recognizes an imminent problem but is unable to get the resident or fellow to "see" the developing complication. Because the complication is in a very early stage of progression and the typical signs of this specific complication are not yet visible to the less experienced physicians, it is imperative that the advanced practice nurse alert the team in order to avert a life-threatening situation. Although the complication is not yet readily apparent, the advanced practice nurse's sense that something is amiss propels him to persist in getting a more experienced physician to recognize and respond:

Advanced Practice Nurse: A patient was admitted to the ICU with a status post cardiac arrest. The patient had been intubated, less than a day, and was on full ventilatory support. He did not appear to have any problems initially, at least in terms of ventilation and oxygenation, and ruled in for an MI. He was basically in a stabilization period of support. He was not instrumented with a PA [pulmonary artery] catheter, was awake and cognitively aware.

I remember getting a call late and the staff nurse asked me to come up and see the patient because she noticed, well she thought that the patient seemed to be working a little bit harder on the ventilator, and she had approached the intern and the resident. I work in a teaching facility, and they looked at the patient, didn't really notice particularly that the patient was struggling with his breathing, or that there was a slight increase in the respiratory rate that seemed to be sustained. The nurse also reported that the heart rate had been elevated, but the patient didn't appear to be hemodynamically compromised, but she was wondering if the ventilator settings were appropriate. So I went up and took a look at the patient and one of the first things that I noticed was that he wasn't breathing very rapidly, but was using a lot more respiratory effort on each breath, using more accessory muscles, and this patient was actively exhaling. The breathing appeared paradoxical, meaning, he wasn't using the diaphragm; he was using accessory muscles. But there really wasn't a marked tachypnea pattern. And, again, I looked at the ventilator sheets to see how long the patient had been on the ventilator and just wondering if it was just maybe an agitation situation, and maybe he needed some sedation. And she also remarked that in the last 20 minutes, the patient's mentation had deteriorated, where he had been a little more responsive, he was now less responsive than when she had called me, and so she was even more nervous.

So the three of us—the junior assistant resident, myself, and the staff nurse— were looking at the ventilatory parameters, and clearly the patient's mentation had deteriorated. Breathing appeared to be more labored. So I asked them if they had a recent chest X-ray, or if there was anything else new going on with the patient that was important, and they said, 'No, the patient had a routine chest X-ray in the morning.' I asked the nurse if there had been any change in breath sounds, and she said, 'No.' And the JR [junior resident] who was in the room said he had noticed no differences as well. So I took a listen, and the chest was really noisy, but I, I thought that the breath sounds appeared to be a little more diminished on the right side. So I asked whether or not there was any indication to repeat the chest X-ray, or if that was their finding as well.

Now, breath sounds often—there isn't symmetry necessarily but there wasn't anything outward in terms of chest excursion, and by visual inspection it looked like it would be symmetric. But nevertheless, I went ahead and looked at the ventilator parameters. The ventilatory support settings appeared to be appropriate. Possibly the back-up rate could have been a little higher, but the patient wasn't really assisting much over the control rate. The patient had a pulse oximeter. Those readings were fairly stable, in the low 90's, as I recall, and the patient was not hypotensive, was a little more tachycardic than what the nurse had led me to believe over the phone, somewhere around 120s, 130s, but the patient wasn't exhibiting EKG changes or hypotension associated with that. He was on no vasoactive drugs at the time. There was a slight increase in the airway pressures, but it wasn't high enough to really warn me that there was a marked change in compliance at that time. The patient appeared to be returning most of the tidal volume that was being delivered by the ventilator.

...So I stayed with the nurse, and we were talking and kind of going over what the plan was and things we might be looking for in the evening, because it was late afternoon, and I was getting ready to go home. The nurse had gone out of the room for some reason. But I noticed, and I wasn't sure if it was just the room lighting or if there was a true color change, subsequently there was a color change in the patient. But I noticed that the patient's upper torso looked a little duskier, especially the head and neck area. And I, I pulled his gown down. Again, the patient's mentation had not improved, and I noticed there was a clear demarcation and color, and this was sort of in the mid-chest area, up to the neck and to the head. Took a [listen] to breath sounds again and noticed that the breath sounds appeared even more diminished on the right side. So I was thinking that this was a pneumothorax. Now when I brought this up to the JR [junior resident], and actually the cardiology fellow was there as well, in the latter part of the afternoon, they didn't think it was a pneumothorax because the patient was returning most of the exhaled volume, and they thought, well, under positive pressure, this would be a tension pneumothorax, and we should see a decrease in exhaled volumes, or marked increase in airway pressures. And I know from the literature and from my own experience, it isn't always so clear cut like that. And certainly vitals signs are important, but blood pressure doesn't necessarily reflect cardiac output, nor does heart rate, and it just depends how people are going to respond physiologically. You know? So, I thought that this patient was developing a pneumothorax and it may be worthwhile to at least check another chest X-ray to see if there were any changes, even though I did hear breath sounds on the right side. They were markedly diminished, even more so than my first my assessment.

Interviewer: Which was about a time period of...

Advanced Practice Nurse: Within about an hour, maybe 45 minutes. Well, they didn't think that was indicated at that time. So, I actually caught the pulmonary fellow who was coming down the hallway to see somebody else and I asked him to come in and take a look—I really wasn't satisfied that's where we were going to leave things. And they [JR & cardiology fellow] just wanted to observe the patient, unless they felt he got into more trouble. But they didn't remark that they thought that the color really indicated much of anything. And I was kind of surprised because it wasn't, it wasn't <u>real</u> obvious, but it was a definite color change from before. But the nurse didn't see it, and the JR didn't see it, and so I felt like, you know, maybe it's me—it just seemed too different to me. He did appreciate—the pulmonary fellow, it was more of a curb side consult—there were some differences in breath sounds, and said, 'Well, just push him [JR] a little harder. I think you should go ahead and get one.' So, I talked to them, and encouraged them to go ahead and get one. So the chest X-ray was ordered, and not—probably 10 or 15 minutes from the time that I got this curb side consult with the fellow and even before [X-ray results] came up, this patient dropped his blood pressure, his heart rate went up. When we listened to his breath sounds, it was <u>clear</u> the patient's breath sounds had decreased even more. There happened to be an attending over in the MICU who came over and emergently inserted a chest tube and clearly it was a big pneumothorax... So we talked about it afterwards with the staff nurse, and I told her I thought one of the best things she did was that she, she picked up a change in status and that she reported it to somebody to look a little bit further. It may have been insignificant, but you know, this nurse was experienced. She had the sense [to know] that she was seeing something different, and just wanted another eye, another opinion to take a look at it. But it turned into a life-threatening situation. Fortunately we were there to intervene before something disastrous could have happened. Now, the color changes, I felt may have been—the reason I sort of suspected that that was a progressing pneumothorax was just a decreased venous return, and there was more venous pooling or congestion, and that was sort of the color change that I was seeing. I couldn't be certain that that was the case, but it was <u>amazing</u> that when the chest tube was inserted, how this guy's color came back.

Interviewer: Oh, my goodness.

Advanced Practice Nurse: It was so incredible...this guy just pinked up. But at that time he was very ashen, and <u>clearly</u> he pinked up pretty quickly afterwards... And I guess what stood out in my mind was that people were really looking at a lot of the classic parameters that they're taught that you should see. And I don't know if it was necessarily because of what I've read, or I think a lot of it has to do with what I've seen clinically, and I try to incorporate at least what I know, from knowledge, and what I've seen in practice, is that, it isn't always so clear cut. I mean, it just isn't. And sometimes you really have to kind of go on physical exam findings, and not necessarily—it's important to pay attention to the things you anticipate, but sometimes the things that aren't so obvious can be very clinically significant.

This story highlights the patient benefits and outcome of the expert clinician's fuzzy recognition and early detection of physiological instability. Without the advanced practice nurse's grasp of what was salient and knowing the diagnosis prior to the rapid deterioration, the patient would have suffered a greater delay in intervention due to the time required to call the residents, for the residents to exam the patient, and for them to make a diagnosis. The APN's perception of the slightest color change, the active exhalation, the use of his accessory muscles before actual vital sign changes were undetectable and indistinguishable when pointed out to inexperienced clinicians. As it turned out, once the patient presented with more obvious signs of distress, the advanced practice nurse made instantaneous treatment possible which averted a code.

A second essential feature which characterizes expert practice in the above story was the advanced practice nurse's ability, persistence, and courage to marshall necessary resources. Diagnosing the situation and bringing it to a physician's attention was not enough to prompt the needed care for this patient. The advanced practice nurse had developed the requisite confidence, courage, and persistence that enabled him to follow through on his reasoning-in-transition. Courage is gained as a clinician understands what is at stake for the patient, as one learns to negotiate clinical perspectives (see Chapter 10). Because this advanced practice nurse worked with the physicians smoothly and collaboratively, this aspect of his role remained fairly covered over. However, it is often no easy task to return to colleagues and try to "push" them to act when, by position, they have a greater degree of power and authority and have already disagreed with the nurse's suspicions. As in the above situation, making a difference in a patient's life fosters the courage and moral agency required for future challenges.

At the end of the story, the advanced practice nurse expresses two very important understandings. First, a complication (particularly early signs) does not always exhibit the clear cut, classic parameters. The best of science simply does not capture how different patients may present. Problem identification often requires honed perceptual acuity that includes recognition of nuances that can only be learned from experience. He points out that learning from clinical experience and incorporating what has been learned with one's previous knowledge is vital in diagnosing and managing unstable patient situations. The advanced practice nurse did not fault the resident and fellow for not "seeing" what he recognized. Expert clinical grasp is a developmental challenge and no clinician can ever be clinically wiser than her or his experience has allowed. We can never be beyond experience (Benner, Tanner & Chesla, 1992). After the crisis, the advanced practice nurse pauses and talks with the staff nurse to ensure that she understood how the situation unfolded and to point out the qualitative distinctions in the patient's presentation that informed him about the particular complication and compelled him to persist in getting help. In this way, the advanced practice nurse capitalizes on an opportune teaching moment for situated learning, a time when the nurse had noticed changes and could track the patient's transition.

The above story illustrates how difficult it can be to get another person to "see" or understand early warning signals. Some aspects of clinical grasp can be easily articulated; however, transitions are most challenging to convey because much of the understanding depends on knowing what the patient looked like and how he/she responded before. Articulating qualitative distinctions that are noticed in the patient's transitions can make a meaningful difference in another person's "take" on the situation. In the following excerpt, the nurse emphasizes the distinctions in an accident victim which assists the physician in grasping the urgency and significance of the patient's symptoms:

Nurse: I thought, that color goes with head injuries. Something is not clicking right. His color is—I know it's neurologic. It's not something else because I've been there. I've been working in the neurosurgery ICU and looking across the room and seeing that someone's color isn't quite right—about three years ago when I worked in the ER, this guy was in the top of the crow's nest, which is the thing at the top of an oil drill and he had been hurt. It took them a long time to get him down and he had a deformed ankle. Then he had a 45 minute transport time because it is the middle of nowhere and the paramedic said, 'he has a deformed ankle.' He's awake, he's oriented, he complaining of his—he fell up there and the paramedic said, 'Well now he's throwing up a little bit. Probably just the motion of the ambulance' and they bring him in and I just kept looking at him and looking at him and I thought, 'His color isn't right. No 30-year-old guy should have a heart rate of 38 when all he has is a swollen ankle.' And I went up to this near retirement aged general surgeon whose glasses are this thick (laugh) and I said, 'Mac, his color is not right.' 'Really?' 'No, Mac, his color just isn't right. There's something wrong with him. He threw up in the back of the ambulance and he shouldn't have. There's just no reason why he should have thrown up and he's thrown up again and his heart rate is 38. He's got something wrong with his head. I think you need to CT his head.' And of course, since we had a brand new CT scanner, 'Well sure.' So we CAT scan his head and he had an intracerebral bleed. It was big enough that he got sent to the referral hospital for observation and ordering that test was solely based on his color.

This nurse makes a distinction about the patient's color and his vomiting being disproportionate to and poorly associated with his ankle injury and these salient findings are strong enough to elicit further action from the surgeon. It is the nurse's ability to distinguish the neurologic nature of the clinical deterioration that is central to averting the unfolding crisis. As in this example, narrative accounts show how nurses are not ordinarily involved in compartmentalized attentiveness, thinking or performance. Rather they think and act across multiple domains simultaneously, as the situation demands. As in this situation, expert nurses also reason across multiple patient situations and across the responses of patient populations which is only possible from working with specific patient groups over time. It is through story that thinking and reasoning in multifaceted ways can be made visible and that the importance of teaching and learning this kind of thinking can be appreciated. In this instance, the nurse's ability to make qualitative distinctions and to also negotiate for that perspective are life-saving actions. Further, because this physician "knows" this nurse and her judgment, he is more open to her perspective.

Communicating one's clinical understanding is a distinctly different challenge and skill, particularly when the patient is unstable or there is a lot at stake for the patient. In the following exemplar, Andrea Edmands, a burn and trauma ICU nurse, demonstrates how her perceptual acuity is central to accurate problem identification (see Chapter 1), which then redefines the problem and enables appropriate, noninvasive management of the patient's condition. This story allows one to imaginatively experience the struggle and dilemma of diverse and consequential perspectives:

Nurse: Ethan was in his 60's and had a head injury from a motorcycle crash. He had an EVD (external ventricular drain) placed for a GCS (Glasgow coma scale) < 7 and the opening pressure was 16. I got to know Ethan and his two daughters (27 and 25) very well. His oldest was his health care proxy and 6 months pregnant.

Andrea immediately finds herself with a very distressed family (two daughters) after the neurologist surprises them about possibly placing a ventricular shunt in their dad. They are upset and feeling very out of control because the neuro intern, sent in place of the attending, failed to mention the shunt during the family meeting that they attended the day before to discuss the plan of care (POC). Andrea empathizes with them, obtains current information, teaches them about a shunt, and gains their trust by helping them understand it is only a possibility:

Nurse: They seemed calmer and felt comfortable but remained annoyed that it was not mentioned in the family meeting, which I knew translated into, "why aren't we all on the same page? I'm trying to trust you, but you're making it difficult." I assured them their dad was in good hands and that I would help guide them through this. With that in mind, I knew I was on for the next 3 days, so I signed up to be on the team of nurses to care for Ethan and his family. I would help figure it out with them.

The next day, the neurology team attempted a clamping trial, which Ethan failed, according to them, within an hour due to ICP's (intracranial pressure) > 20. Clinically, Ethan followed commands consistently for me and opened his eyes, MAE (moving all extremities), and PERRL (pupils equal round and reactive to light). The team felt very strongly that he should go for a head CT scan after failing his clamping trials, which reveal ICP's in the 30's. I wanted to see what was going on in his head too, knowing that ICP's in the 30's is really bad. They ordered Mannitol and off we went. The CT showed a clamped down ventricle on the EVD.

An hour later, the neurology attending pops by again to check in. Perfect timing because I had a few questions. She still felt Ethan may need a shunt if he continued to fail his trials. I needed more of an explanation. I asked, "A shunt is for draining a full ventricle, correct?" "Yes," the attending answered. "If the ventricle is clamped down, what is there to drain?" I asked. The attending answered, "nothing." "And if the ventricle is clamped down on the drain, then is it possible that these high ICP numbers are false?" The answer was "yes."

Despite this conversation, the neurology team still felt the tracing was accurate. They wanted to rest him overnight by opening the drain, and then do another clamp trial in the morning. Now at this point, I'm convinced Ethan has a brain tissue swelling issue, not a full ventricle issue. However, I'm not a neurology nurse. I'm a trauma nurse and I felt a lack of confidence in this field, but I also know my common sense is intact. At this point, I did not press them further, knowing they have locked out others when pushed. So I bargained with myself, "they will leave it open for tonight which is no different from the last three days and I will be back tomorrow morning when more action and trials take place. I will get my point across so that I feel confident about having the correct POC (plan of care) for Ethan and his family. I will not let something happen to him that I would not let happen to my own family," is what I thought before leaving for the night.

So I said to the neurology attending before she left, "Oh, before you leave, can you please speak to the family a bit more in detail about a shunt? Yesterday was the first time they heard about one, and it made them a bit nervous." She smirked, went in, and spoke with the family.

After reviving myself over night, I return the next morning, ready. "How am I going to present this?" I thought to myself.

The clamp trial began, ICP's rose >20 for a few minutes, then down to 12. The numbers were all over the place. I remembered from past experience the [pressure] waveform is supposed to have, for a lack of better explanation, three descending bumps. Ethan's waveform was not showing a good tracing, but the neurology intern was not concerned with that. She thought Ethan's waveform was okay.

"I don't know, maybe I'm missing something," I thought, so I started to do some research. As I read, what I remembered was correct, but these people were specialized in this field...ahhhhh! All along, the patient's neurology exam was beautiful! He's interacting, following commands, starting to speak, MAE, PERRL. This type of exam never buys an EVD or a bolt.

It's 9:00 am and time for the trauma ICU team (different from neurology, but consulting in trauma ICU) to round. At this point I'm frustrated. I have had open dialogue with the neurology team and got insufficient answers and plans. So as the ICU team rounded, I greeted them with a smile and "good morning." They went through the story and assessment and then came to the plan of care. I was ready to explode in frustration from the previous day and the lack of cohesiveness. I spoke up and told them that I was very frustrated with our current communication and it could affect the future POC for this patient. I have good rapport with the trauma attending and residents. They know I care about my patients, my work, and that my concern always comes from a good place. I stuck to the facts regarding findings from the clamping trial, the CT results, and what that meant regarding inaccurate numbers and the need for a shunt. They were now concerned as well. I also explained my view of the waveform and what I we should see if things were accurate. I pointed out his improving neurology exam. It was the best I had seem from him! They were unaware of how this was playing out, and the attending agreed that we needed a team meeting. "THANK YOU!" I screamed to myself.

The neuro-surgeon was away for the week so the neurologist filled in. He agreed that we should follow the neurology exam first and felt the numbers were inaccurate. He also felt this was brain tissue swelling, the inflammation needed time to decrease, and the patient may not need a shunt. "Great," I thought to myself... [Andrea and the team discussed the details of the new plans with the daughters.] This gave the daughters a definite plan and something to focus on. The ICU team, neurology, nursing and family were all on board and unified.

Now the only part that made me wonder was the patient. As we followed neurology exams, Ethan would only follow commands and interact with his daughters, myself, and the two other nurses that had taken care of him since arrival, which made us all look like liars to the docs. Ethan did eventually follow commands in front of the doctors, but only when I said, "Ethan, this is really important. I need to know you can hear me and follow these commands." Sure enough, he gave me a thumbs up. Seeing that, the doctors then felt confident about following his physical exam and were impressed in his ability at that point to form a relationship. Ethan continued to improve. He was up in the chair smiling and interacting with his daughters. Everyday he got better and better. So, after his EVD was removed, we watched him interact with his children, crack jokes, and witnessed emotion in his face. He was eventually improved and left the ICU.

Two of the greatest challenges in providing excellent care are embedded in Andrea's narrative account. First, even though Andrea claims not to be a "neuro" expert, she clearly knows all the scientific facts and has the practical knowledge to know that the neuro team's diagnosis is awry. Although she makes a strong and clear case, based on factual CT results and on Ethan's brain function as revealed by neuro exam, she repeatedly struggles to either have her clinical grasp understood or to understand how the neuro team makes sense of all the data. The exemplar details how to typically make a strong case that another could clearly grasp. Her questions provide a way of engaging the neuro attending to think and reason with her. Her questions also act as a kind of situated coaching to help discern what is salient in this specific situation. So, it is befuddling to learn that a shunt remains a possibility after the neuro attending agrees with Andrea about the ventricle clamping down on the EVD and the subsequent false ICP readings. Despite solid, corroborating data, the neuro team cannot "see" or grasp an accurate clinical understanding and persists with a possible wrong intervention. At the heart of good, or even safe, care is a good perceptual grasp, which always determines the preferred interventions. In the end, Andrea orchestrates the shared understanding among the whole team that protects Ethan from an erroneous shunt. Despite the emotional strain on Andrea, it is a good rescue.

The second greatest challenge is the moral dilemma, not just to act to protect Ethan, but to repeatedly take a stand on his behalf. Given her ethic of responsibility and moral sensibilities, Andrea is thrown into the situation in a strong way. Notice that this expert does not experience this moral obligation as a choice. It is not a "decision." Once she makes the right clinical judgment, her response is embodied. She is morally compelled to act, but timing is everything. So, she weighs the goods (the good of acting immediately versus acting when success may be more likely) and is poised the next morning for an inevitable opportunity to present itself to alter Ethan's clinical course. Rubin (2009) points out that nurses who do not experience the emotional engagement and therefore the moral struggles are unable to develop expertise, as they do not embody the moral imperative to act, are unable to distinguish what is at stake for the patient, and do not take a stand on the patient's behalf. Emotions necessarily accompany the moral press to act and are heightened when erroneous therapies are a threat. For expert nurses, the frustration is deeply seated, not so much at the unresponsive physicians, who are valued as intelligent and experienced clinicians, but in the whole team's inability to collaboratively make sense of substantial data and safely manage the patient.

For developing nurses, this narrative provides an excellent context for expanding one's clinical imagination as preparation for inevitable future situations. Reflecting on the puzzles and challenges in this particular context offers an engaged rehearsal for similar situations. It is a good example of the skillfulness required to make a strong case when communicating one's clinicial grasp, even though, in this case, it is missed by another. The skill of negotiating (see chapter 10) with multiple teams is visible and is easily appreciated by the trauma ICU team. In addition, Andrea describes her stress, worry, and unease about the possibility of Ethan suffering an incorrect intervention and the moral distress that she is responsible for preventing that insult. As hard as it is to cope with at first, clinicians can never escape the emotional engagement (that spawns worry) required if they are to become expert, for it sets up the moral imperative to strongly act on the patient's behalf, to courageously persist when needed, and to manage the breakdown situation (see chapter 11) until satisfactorily resolved. Emotions should not be dampened by others, as they play a strong role in clinical judgment, guide interventions, and compel development and action as a moral agent.

Experienced staff nurses, preceptors, advanced practice nurses, nurse managers, and nurse educators could greatly expedite the learning of less experienced nurses by role modeling, coaching, and mentoring excellent collaboration, negotiation, and situational leadership practices (see Chapter 12). Newer nurses would also immensely benefit from debriefing after clinical incidents and from role playing to practice newly acquired skills in multiple situations with various configurations.

Taking definitive action in a situation that is highly charged requires ingenuity and disciplined attention as the following example from a roadside accident illustrates. The nurse recognizes that the patient is at imminent risk of airway closure due to swelling. She rules out the unavailable options at the accident scene:

Nurse 1: The patient and her boyfriend were on a motorcycle on the river road when they crashed and she got thrown into a bush, down the side of the levee, and part of the branch of the bush impaled through her neck. And she had a head injury. So, when we arrived, we knew that she needed an airway, but, then [her teeth] were clenched because of her head injury. At that time we were not yet doing neuromuscular blockade on transport. Because she had a facial injury, we couldn't do a nasal intubation. So our only option was to do the surgical cric[othyrotomy] and we were sitting in the middle of the road. I'll never forget that. It was <u>really</u> hot. I was really nervous and the boyfriend was standing behind me yelling, 'Do something! 'You gotta <u>do</u> something to her!' He thought she was dying. Well, she was. And his yelling just made it worse for me and so the police made him stand back a little bit, but....

Nurse 2: That's what I remember about it. He was being so hostile when she was down the embankment. He wanted just to drag her up himself and not wait for us and the board to bring her up.

Nurse 1: Yeah, he wasn't hurt. He was just wandering around, yelling.

Nurse 2: And I remember I was fearful because of his hostility.

Nurse 1: She remained so calm. She was so good. I was responsible for the airway for that call. So, it was my airway, as we say (laughs). Yeah. But we always help each other.

Although this patient is breathing and alert when the trauma team arrives at the scene, her injury is sure to jeopardize her respiratory stability without a more secure airway prior to transport. The first nurse quickly recognizes the urgency of the situation and successfully performs her first surgical cricothyrotomy with assistance from the second nurse. Her problem solving is swift and definitive, as is her management of the unstable situation.

Although frightened about their own safety as the boyfriend is yelling at them, the nurses remain focused, thought clearly and swiftly, and continued to perform adeptly. Under considerable pressure, the only way to secure the airway was performing a cricothyrotomy, but notice the nurse's rapid thinking and reasoning through multiple less invasive contingency options first, guided by a notion of what was best for the patient rather than the fastest way to escape the hot, hostile situation. It is unclear how such courage and conviction develops, but we noted that these characteristics were common in the nurses who were regularly involved in rescue.

In the following example, the patient is in the more controlled environment of the critical care unit. The patient is not oxygenating well despite being ventilated on 100% oxygen. A very experienced, doctorally-prepared clinical nurse specialist (CNS) shared an example that is long and intricate and therefore provides a detailed illustration of clinical reasoning and puzzle solving:

Advanced Practice Nurse: A man in his mid 50's had just been brought to the ICU from a floor with extreme shortness of breath. He was emergently intubated, we had him on a ventilator, and we had just his vital signs and an oximetry. So his oximeter was reading in the high 80's and so we knew we were not oxygenating well and on a 100% oxygen. He was currently on assist-control, of ten, with a tidal volume of 800, but he was breathing in the 30's. Now, at that rate, we knew that he either had a large dead space problem or he was over-breathing. So, the initial blood gas showed, on a 100% oxygen, a PaO_2 of 67, his pH was 6.73, $PaCO_2$ was 113, and bicarbonate was 18. Now, based on this, it was immediately clear that we were not ventilating him well. And the question came up, 'What do we do for him?' Now, we put a capnography to try and track our progress, because we couldn't keep getting blood gases and the pH that he currently had was life-threatening. (This took place with 6 different physicians in the room, mostly interns or residents, a pulmonary fellow, the clinical nurse specialist, and the nurse taking care of the patient.) When we saw that the $PaCO_2$ was that high, that was just odd because his minute ventilation was really more than adequate to blow off the CO_2. He either had to have a huge dead space, or there may have been something with how the ventilator was functioning. It really wasn't clear as to why he was not able to blow off that CO_2 level. So, first thing, was, I said, 'We're going to have to take him off and bag him' just because it didn't make sense that he was not ventilating better. So when I took him off to bag him, I met tremendous resistance trying to inflate his lungs. The high pressure alarm had been going off often just before that. As I tried to bag him, he was very, very resistant, but as I bagged him, I could watch his end tidal level start to drop. It started off relatively high near 100, but as I bagged him, I could see it come down very quickly, and after a couple of minutes, it was in the 40's.

Now, the benefit was that I knew an end tidal would track the arterial gases. It doesn't predict it perfectly. On a normal person, the end tidal [ETCO$_2$] and the arterial [CO$_2$] correlate very well. But most people in ICU aren't normal, they've got a larger dead space than normal, so the end tidal-arterial gradient tends to be wider. So I didn't know exactly what the arterial level was, but I knew that it was coming down, and with that, I knew that his pH had to be getting better because the main problem with his low pH was the high PaCO$_2$ level. And so, at that point we decided to put him back on the ventilator to see what would happen. And again, the high air pressure alarm started going off, and the ETCO$_2$ level started to rise again. So this is at a point where, now clearly we're not ventilating him well with the ventilator. So we needed to make some respiratory changes... But we knew what we needed to do was try and make sure that we increased the mean airway pressure. Theoretically, if we could do that, then we might be able to prolong gas exchange. And so, we increased the inspiratory time and increased the inspiratory flow rate to see what effects that would have. With the increase in the inspiratory time and flow, I think we had a flow up to 120 liters per minute, we started to get a little bit better stabilization on the end tidal CO$_2$. The airway pressure was still going off but we couldn't quite get that down.

So, really, our options were pretty limited. We elected to try and reduce any respiratory work. So we sedated him first with fentanyl and a bolus of Versed, and then used ativan to act as a maintenance, and with that combination, the airway pressure alarm was not going off quite as often. I said, 'You know, we really still aren't where we want to be.' The end tidal was like around 60, the saturation—pulse oximeter's in the mid-80's, at times it had gone into the 70's. And we had checked any other thing that could account for that, like, a right main stem intubation, a pneumothorax, we got a chest X-ray and we knew that wasn't the case. So, clearly we figured that we were dealing a person who had a very large dead space. And, we weren't certain of the origin of that yet. That was going to take a little bit of time to try and resolve. But in the meantime we had to stabilize him, to get his pH back to a better level. About that time we got a second blood gas back, and his pH was up to 7.12, his PaCO$_2$ level was about 80, so we had an end tidal-arterial gradient of about 20. We knew we still had a way to go. We elected to go ahead and try to paralyze him as well, obviously making sure that his sedation was appropriate first and, with a paralytic, we started to get a much better response in terms of keeping his airway pressures down. And at that point, the saturation came up to the low 90's. His end tidal was about 50. Still not where we wanted it to be, but, it was better.

And the key thing was that the ability to make assessment of the person was enhanced by looking at the oximetry capnography. But one of the real important things was that we didn't have an SvO$_2$ level, so we didn't know what his tissues [tissue oxygenation] were doing, and the other thing is that the pulse oximeter probably improved, <u>not</u> because we did a lot to his lungs, but when you see an improvement in an oximeter reading, again you've got to analyze 'Why did the oximeter improve?' And the majority of times that's because the lung function got better. But in a person who is working particularly hard with his respiratory muscles, there is a small percent of blood that comes back to the heart, in the left side of the heart, in the pulmonary veins that drains the lungs. Most goes into the right atrium through the superior vena cava, but some goes into the pulmonary veins, and the pulmonary veins then empty directly into the left side of the heart.

So the idea is, if you improve the respiratory oxygen consumption, decrease that, which a paralytic would do, your pulse oximeter reading might go up. And so, we don't know what that answer was, although I suspect it was the reduction of oxygen consumption in the lungs that made the pulse oximeter go up. I think that our paralytic didn't do anything in terms of really improving his gas exchange. The capnography came down a little bit, like I said, to about 50, but still not as—if it really worked well, we would have seen the capnography come down to the 30s. So we still hadn't fixed his lungs and I think we just reduced the O_2 consumption of his lungs, but without a fiberoptic catheter in place, we really couldn't confirm that. And even that has some limitations because it doesn't measure the left side of the heart.....

So, the goal was, we were either going to ride it out or we were going to try and start nitric oxide on him, even though again, that's more of an oxygenation treatment than it is a ventilation treatment. High CO_2 levels are <u>extremely</u> resistant to treatment if the ventilator doesn't correct it. So we elected to just really try and ride it out. We didn't want to start nitric oxide if we didn't have any severe problems, plus his pulse oximeter is running the mid-90's. He was really not having any overt problems. Once again, we didn't have an SvO_2 level, so we didn't know what his tissues were doing. One thing I suggested and we did get was a lactate level. That was done later that day. And the lactate level came back 1.4, which is fine, normal. So, we use that if we don't have fiberoptic catheter in place. You can at least get a lactate to get an idea how well a person is doing tissue-wise... And so the normal lactate certainly was encouraging.

The above story, told in detail as the event unfolded, vividly reflects an expert clinician as a physiological knowledge worker who was thinking-in-action and reasoning-in-transition in an extremely complex situation. This CNS has extensive scientific knowledge of pathophysiology, diagnostic and monitoring equipment, pharmacology and the multiple available therapies. However, what is stunning is his flexible, adept, in-depth use of the knowledge acquired that is too simply referred to as experiential or practical knowledge. In this situation, the CNS's background,extensive scientific knowledge, and vast experiential wisdom made it possible to understand the patient's clinical presentation, determine what interventions could help, and then "read" the patient's responses which guided further therapies. He described what he was noticing, how that shaped his thinking, and how the patient's evolving responses altered or confirmed his reasoning and judgment about the situation. It simultaneously illustrates the complex problem search, identification, and logic involved when ruling in or out possible causes. Finally, this story demonstrates how an extensive and thorough understanding of physiology, pathophysiology, pharmacology, and technological interventions allowed the clinician to substitute one technology for another (that was unavailable or too risky) in order to "track" the patient's responses to therapy. Here, the CNS explained how he used capnography to estimate the patient's arterial CO_2 without continuously hurting the patient by drawing frequent arterial blood gases and without exposing a fragile patient to the risk of inserting a fiberoptic catheter. Similarly, without a fiberoptic catheter to assess tissue oxygen utilization, the singular lactate level was substituted as a way of evaluating tissue oxygenation (Ahrens, 1993a; Ahrens, 1993b; Ahrens & Rutherford, 1993). As this situation illustrates, managing an unstable patient situation to prevent a crisis can place as great or greater demands as managing a crisis.

Clinicians can be uncertain about whether or not to intervene during the early stages of the patient's unstable condition because the situation could possibly resolve on its own or worsen and demand intervention. Time and/or multiple patient responses may be necessary to determine whether intervention is required. Intervening too hastily exposes the patient to unnecessary risk and discomfort which violates the ethos of "First, do no harm." Here, making the distinction between an <u>unstable situation</u> and a <u>life-threatening</u> one is important because a crisis calls for immediate and decisive action, whereas an unstable situation may allow just enough time for the patient to turn around on her/his own, if possible. Expert clinicians are particularly reluctant to utilize unnecessary invasive procedures because every procedure carries some degree of risk (see Chapter 8). Any risk is undesirable if avoidable in such a frail population. The next two excerpts illustrate the distinction we are making between an unstable and an urgent, life-threatening situation. In the following excerpt, there is no doubt that the patient requires instantaneous intervention because there is no chance that his condition will spontaneously improve:

Nurse: There was a severe COPD patient. He was just transferred out of the CCU and he all of a sudden became very agitated. He was on a 35% [O_2 face] mask at that point in time. I looked at his fingernails—you didn't need an O_2 Sat monitor to tell you that his O_2 Sats were dropping below 60. He probably had a P[a]O_2 at that point of about 50-56... I walked into the room and said, 'Put him on at least 70% now—we'll get the order later.' He was really getting agitated, his nailbeds were blue, he was getting mottled—he obviously needed more O_2.

This patient shows physiological indications that he has exceeded his ability to compensate for his hypoxemic state and is now in a crisis. The situation requires immediate action. In this specific instance, oxygen is the best <u>immediate</u> intervention; yet, oxygen carries the dangerous risk of inhibiting the patient's respiratory drive which can, in turn, cause hypoventilation and exacerbate the situation. Thus, depending on the patient's particular context, oxygen may not be the long-term solution in this patient population. Risky interventions, such as this, require astute and continuous monitoring of the patient's responses to treatment to detect adverse effects as soon as possible. In contrast, the next situation from a clinical observation illustrates the indeterminate nature of early deterioration as a newborn baby showed beginning signs of retractions and color changes. It also conveys the caution used prior to intervening:

Nurse: 'His color looks dusky.' [The physician orders a 50% oxygen hood. After a minute or two the color improves, the nurse decreases hood oxygen to 25%.]

Interviewer: Tell me a little bit about what has been happening and what the priorities are now?

Nurse: Make sure he stays warm, and stays pink. And to make his assessments. She [other nurse] felt that on room air, his breath sounds were slightly diminished and tight. He was getting slightly dusky, enough that he might require some oxygen. So now he is on a 25% hood and we are going to put a line into his umbilical artery that will help us assess both oxygenation and administer fluids. And if he improves rapidly, then the line won't stay in long, maybe 12-24 hours. [Nurse gives meds, Vitamin K. Does reflex checks and assessment for physical maturity. Two nurses discuss that he seems stable 'for the moment'...] [ABGs done. pO_2 29, pCO_2 64, pH 7.16; O_2 hood turned up to 40% and the baby gets pinker but later worsens. The nurse calmly intubates the baby as the physician watches in the background]

Interviewer: Why was he being intubated?

Nurse: He got apneic and rather dusky. His pCO_2 was hovering in the 50s so he needed to be intubated but it wasn't an absolute emergency so I could take my time and really look before I did it. [Physician comments 'nice job.'] Let me fill you in... So the baby started out okay, was on a 25% hood, then went up to 40% and then was weaned back down to the 20's. The baby was only on 28% when we intubated him but twice he had gotten dusky with apneic episodes. He was beginning to have nasal flaring and significant retracting. It was anticipated he was going to wear himself out so we elected to intubate him so he could rest. Hopefully in the end he will wean faster than if we had let him get totally tired and then intubate. Usually then they end up being intubated longer. So this way he still has some energy left to help with breathing. That is the main thing with him. Otherwise, we proceed with our standards. He is on antibiotics and the usual blood work... (Observational Interview).

In this situation, the baby's responses conveyed a degree of instability but because he improved several times after increasing the oxygen by hood, there was no clear cut indication to more aggressively intervene. The nurse was aware that his condition could deteriorate or improve at any moment and therefore she monitored him very closely. The type of physiological transition became clear, as did the need for definitive intervention when the baby presented with apneic episodes, nasal flaring, and severe retractions. At that point, a gradual deterioration rather than recovery became evident. The nurse noted the changing context of the situation and intubated the baby to prevent exhaustion by supporting the baby's physiological reserves. At times, the type of transition in unstable patients is more subtle and can only be recognized by knowing the specific patient and comparing her or his responses over time.

It is not always possible to observe an unstable patient's responses over time in indeterminate situations. For instance, when a patient has sustained multiple injuries, the urgency to treat one of the injuries may limit the time needed to evaluate the need for intervention regarding other injuries. In those situations, an immediate judgment must be made and actions must be taken instantaneously, as demonstrated in the following story:

Nurse 1: I was on a call with Tina [a nurse]. And one of the hardest things to manage is if we get a gunshot wound to the face. The patient was lying on her side and she's leaning forward and she's got an airway, she's fine and she's responsive. But she's got this big dressing, bloody dressing to her face and her upper lip is hanging down by a string below the dressing. And it's like, 'Wow are you happy with that airway?' No. You're not happy. Tina's duty was managing the airway, and her decision was split second. She said, 'Does she have good lungs now? Yeah. Let's go.' I'm like, 'let's go??'

Nurse 2: Did you just fly her in—leaning against the—leaning over the wall?

Nurse 1: We did. And she was responsive and actually had no respiratory distress at all. Her airway was completely intact. And it would have been a miscall to interrupt that dressing and try to give her an advanced airway because she had intact airway— there were no bony injuries. It was all just tissue. She had just lost all the tissue. She had her eyes. But that was like, Tina just made the decision so quick.

Nurse 3: How long was your flight?

Nurse 1: It was fairly short. Probably about a six minute flight between here and there. Scary.

Nurse 4: I had a similar situation with Tina, too, a gunshot wound to the face but he had decompensated. He <u>was</u> maintaining his airway, but his blood pressure was dropping. He was really hypoxic so we had to do a cricothyrotomy on him.

In situations like this, the demand for clinical judgment is urgent and it is a hard call because a wrong call carries major consequences either way. The nurse, Tina, made the judgment call not to provide an advanced airway with the background knowledge and experience of the risks. A miscall from being too aggressive would mean further traumatizing an already severely injured patient and delaying treatment of the gunshot injuries. On the other hand, as occurred with a previous patient, the woman may have deteriorated in transport where securing an airway is much more difficult. Managing unstable patients places weighty demands on the nurse's clinical judgment abilities and, as reflected in the above story, one's skillfulness in making good judgments parallels the importance and urgency of skillfulness in performing the needed interventions.

In most unstable patients, unless the patient's condition has deteriorated into an irreversible state, there is something that can done to potentially help the patient. In a few situations, no technological or pharmacological intervention will help stabilize the patient's physiological condition. If the patient's unstable condition declines, the kind of care provided necessarily changes:

Nurse: A young man, in his 30's, had an arterial bleed in his throat, an aneurysm. And he knew that at any time that it might rupture. It was non-correctable. He was coughing up blood, and he couldn't control the cough. As long as he was coughing, he was going to continue bleeding. And it could rupture. Anyway, we had him in the resuscitation room and thank heavens I also had a very up-and-coming doctor with me. He turned to me and said, 'Get several vials of morphine; because if it's going to go, he's going to drown, and I'm not going to have this man conscious.' They were going to sedate him until he was comfortable, and we just sat there and waited and talked to him, and I think he didn't want his mom in the room when it happened, but he was really worried about his mom. He didn't even express worry about dying. He was like 33 or 34. He wasn't concerned about <u>dying</u>. He didn't like the idea of the discomfort of dying and Dr. D. told him, 'If this happens, this is what we're going to do. We're going to get out the morphine and we're just going to push it until we can make you comfortable. We are not going to allow you to struggle.' So that relieved <u>that</u> worry and then his only concern was his mom. He was single. And he stopped bleeding, thank God (quietly). I was just sitting there going 'Please stop, please stop, don't cough any more'. We were giving him liquids, anything that would soothe or numb the throat. [A number of interventions to suppress the cough.] Anything that we could titrate to help him so that he would settle down and quit coughing. But it was like an hour of anxiety, you know, 'Please don't do this.'

In this instance, because there was no physiological intervention to prevent or treat further instability, the clinicians were prepared to make a rapid transition into providing comfort care as needed. They remained present and vigilant to support the patient and they tried numerous options to soothe his coughing. This story points to an important issue when diagnosing and managing unstable patients. That is, it is crucial to the patient's well-being for clinicians to recognize their limits in some aspects of care and to know when comfort care is the best alternative (see Chapter 6). In this patient's case, the coughing eventually resolved and the bleeding ceased. However, clinical forethought and understanding the possibility of changing demands in a situation orients the nurse's thinking, practice, and preparedness.

DIAGNOSING, MONITORING, PREVENTING, AND MANAGING VITAL, BUT NON-EMERGENT FLUCTUATIONS IN PHYSIOLOGIC FUNCTIONS

In the two previous categories of physiological practice, patients' needs for care demanded urgent, instantaneous intervention due to critical fluctuations in their physiological conditions. All previously described patients were highly unstable, even if the instability was only temporary. In the previous categories, the patient situations required reasoning through rapidly changing physiological events within a very constrained time period, whereas here, the reasoning typically occurs during more gradual transitions or requires monitoring over time to determine if there is a transition. The levels of the nurse's vigilance and attentiveness extend to include other vital concerns such as the patient's nutritional needs.

Excellent practice in these patients requires constant and astute physical assessment and observational skills to detect the earliest and possibly unusual signs of a problem. An advanced practice nurse's observation illustrates this knowledge work:

> **Advanced Practice Nurse:** Well, certainly experience is one way you learn and you remember things. I'm always thinking about papers that I've read, or articles, [but there are] the variations from the normal expected findings—if you rely too much on that [articles] and not your clinical observational skills, you may miss things.

Detecting problems and intervening early carry significant benefits for patients. For that reason, the importance of ongoing expert monitoring is widely understood throughout nursing care of the acutely and chronically critically ill. During a clinical observation, a nurse articulated the essential nature of this category of physiological practice:

> **Nurse:** Most babies in here [intermediate care nursery adjacent to the Neonatal ICU] are just growing. Putting a little weight on before they go home. We tell the parents when the babies get to leave ICN and come to these rooms, it is a big step toward going home. Basically as a nurse in here, you want to watch for instability. These kids can start getting sick all of a sudden. For example, they can still develop feeding intolerance. I have seen several infants get really sick in here and develop a necrotizing bowel. They end up intubated and transferred to Children's for emergency surgery.
>
> **Interviewer:** From feeding intolerance?
>
> **Nurse:** Yeah, all of a sudden they stop tolerating feedings and they get an overwhelming infection in their bowels. If it is full-blown, they need surgery. The bowel is becoming necrotized. If caught early, at the first signs, it can be treated with antibiotics. It can go from almost nothing to the cause of death—really. It can be something as simple as temperature instability and they show no signs of feeding intolerance to all of a sudden they will just have one large bloody stool. By the time they have the bloody stool, it has already been going on. Or, they can progress very slowly; they may

have been spitting up and their abdominal girth increases very slowly. Catch it early and an X-ray will show a little air, stasis. Stop their feedings, keep them NPO for 10 days, watch them and rest them. Give them IVS. So basically these kids are growers. They are stable but you need to be watching (Observational Interview).

This nurse characterizes the nature of these patients; that is, they may be stable but they can change suddenly. In this category, the clinical judgment and practice differ because the physiological fluctuations do not demand instantaneous or life-saving intervention at the moment. The patient's condition could change rapidly and create urgent demands but the likelihood is less. However, the demands on the nurse involve closely monitoring for early changes and working to prevent changes that would make the patient more unstable. Patients may or may not be severely ill, but all have the potential to deteriorate very quickly. Here, patients have physiological fluctuations but these do not typically require emergent intervention. Many of these patients are stable (though fragile) only because they are being carefully managed on supportive technology, pharmacological agents, or other maintenance therapies. Thus, this category of practice differs in how the kinds of patient demands orient the nurse's clinical judgment and practice.

In these patients, the predominant focus is on a high level of vigilance and attentiveness: to monitor for changes in the patient's condition, to anticipate and prevent undesirable events, to keep track of the patient's responses in order to create new beneficial transitions, and to be prepared for emergent intervention as needed. These demands require good clinical grasp and forethought. Interventions aim to support and/or maintain the patient's physiological stability or to be as unintrusive as possible when interventions are called for. The demand to reason-in-transition is also distinctive. Constant and skillful watching is central to expert practice. Having an adequate mix of experienced nurses available to be at the bedside observing is crucial to providing early warnings. Barbara Hidde's expert surveillance in everyday practice provides the newer nurses a much needed safety net, as their grasp, judgment, and performance are not yet commensurate with the babies' needs:

Nurse: When I heard one of the cardiac/apnea alarms sound in the nursery, I headed over and saw a new nurse, still on orientation, at the baby's bedside. Not uncommon of a new nurse, Lucy was staring at the monitor. "Is it real?" she asked. "Look at the baby. Is she breathing?" I asked. Indeed, it was truly apnea and bradycardia (A&B) and I needed to intervene. "Give her a gentle rub on the back to stimulate her to breathe," I said. Baby Bailey's heart rate quickly increased from 62 to the 150's and she was breathing again. "What do you see, Lucy?" I asked. Although Bailey's heart rate was now fine and she had a regular respiratory rate, her color remained dusky and her O2 sat was 78%. Lucy noticed the monitor reading and validated its accuracy, but didn't notice the color change. "She's still desat[urat]ing, so we need to give her some oxygen." As I reached for the oxygen tubing to give blow-by O2 to Bailey, I explained my actions to Lucy. "You cup the oxygen tubing around Bailey's nose so she breathes in the concentrated oxygen." I handed the tubing to Lucy to hold and I walked her through the weaning process. Her hand was shaking as she held the oxygen. When I asked if she was okay, she said it was the first "real" A&B that she had seen and it scared her. I told her that Bailey was doing fine thanks to her quick response.

I asked Lucy if her preceptor had reviewed A&B's with her yet and she said "no." I reviewed how to assess apnea and bradycardia...

Together, Barbara took Lucy step by step though the criteria, the monitor's recall process, a return demonstration, the heart rate calculations, and related questions for documentation.

> **Nurse:** As we completed documentation, Lucy's preceptor returned from lunch and I updated her on Lucy's experience. Lucy eventually completed orientation. About 4-5 weeks after her orientation, I was staffing the nursery. Again, I heard an alarm and Lucy was there, giving mild stimulation, "Jason, you turn an ugly color when you do that," she said to a newborn. I asked if she needed any help. "No, we're good. He responded nicely to the stimulation, and I didn't even need to give any oxygen," Lucy answered with confidence. "Thanks for checking on me!"

As seen in Barbara's practice, the expert's watchful eyes and ears extend to include as much as can be seen, heard, or sensed within a unit. The same notion of good and ethic of responsibility are revealed in the way that Barbara gently mentors Lucy to enable her to develop the skillfulness and confidence to act independently. Instead of rescuing the baby from Lucy, she respectfully steps up to ensure that Lucy learns what is needed to safely care for a baby with apnea and bradycardia, leaving no stone unturned. This expert nurse represents the best of situated coaching and learning. She coaches in the moment when Lucy's learning is heightened and clinical knowledge and reasoning can necessarily be tacitly passed on. Barbara helps close the knowledge gap between having it versus learning to use it in a situation where Lucy can immediately see/think about the baby's responses and their significance. She hones Lucy's skills of attentiveness and discernment by pointing out the qualitatively distinct color change that Lucy easily missed at first, but practically learns for all future episodes. As importantly, Barbara teaches the ineffable habits of thought and action (clinical grasp and forethought) that are essential as one develops expertise. The rewards are abundant, for the future episode with Jason, for Lucy and for the mentor. For Jason's apnea and bradycardia episode, Barbara can now comfortably and confidently step back. It is a strong example of preserving expert practice and extending it into the practices of others.

All of the stories in this section highlight the importance and value of having a skilled clinician at the bedside by articulating the nature of physiological knowledge work. This illustrates the thinking and problem identification skills that only adept nurses at the bedside can provide and the dangers of replacing these nurses with unskilled workers. A thick background in the sciences, knowledge and experience with patients' trajectories, and expert interventional judgment and skills are required for early detection of changes in these stable but fragile patients. Below is an excerpt that highlights an ICU nurse's concerns and management of a sick patient who is teetering on the edge of physiological stability with the aid of multiple vasoactive drugs:

> **Nurse:** This patient had an MI about two years ago. She's had increasing coronary artery disease, so they decided to do a CABG and a mitral valve replacement. She had trouble coming off bypass in the OR, so they put her on the balloon pump but the balloon is now out. She was extubated about two days ago and she didn't do very well. She lasted for about an hour. She was real tired and her CO_2 was high, so she did get reintubated. Then she was intubated for a day and a half and this morning about 7:00 they extubated her again. Initially her gases were not that great. Her CO_2 was high again, but it was kind of borderline so I drew another gas and it was better.

Interviewer: Better is what?

Nurse: Her CO_2 was 46 as opposed to 57. So I'm a little bit more hopeful today that maybe she'll be better. I hope. She's really anxious and restless. Right now I'm kind of concerned about her heart rate because it's a little fast and a little irregular at times. I think it's because her potassium is low secondary to some Lasix she had right at 7:00. She's put out about 700 cc's from that, and the other day she had some rhythm problems when her potassium was low and we had to give her some verapamil and the whole bit. I would like to avoid that. I'm finding out what her lab values are now, and I've already given her 10 mEq. of K+ since that lasix. I'm waiting for the lab to call me back with the results. I don't want to give her too much more potassium until I'm pretty sure she needs it. I might end up giving her another 5 [mEq]. So that's kind of a concern, and her respiratory status is a concern, too.

Interviewer: And how about her cardiac status? I notice she's on several vasoactive drugs.

Nurse: Dobutamine and nitroglycerine. Actually they said we could wean the dobutamine off. I was just kind of waiting to make sure she was stable as far as her respiratory status before I started doing that... Uh, her lungs actually don't sound really bad. She's just been having a lot of difficulty breathing. She's just working really hard, and maybe she's just not really ready to do that yet...I have so many things to do, like changing the dressings and the lines, but I don't want to do them because Ms. M. is so tired and I don't want to tire her out any further or cause her to need to be reintubated. This patient is very, very tired. She's using abdominal and accessory muscles for breathing (Observational Interview).

The nurse's description of the patient's condition conveys how fragile the patient is and how even changing a dressing can tire the patient to the point of requiring reintubation. During the observation, the nurse kept the lights turned down low, whispered, and restricted any stimulation of the patient for hours, hoping to alleviate any extraneous stress. Her reluctance to begin weaning the dobutamine by even one drop is another indication of the patient's fragility at the time. As is common in critically ill patients, oxygenation is only one among many physiological problems. The nurse vigilantly monitors and manages the patient's electrolyte imbalance, fluid status, and cardiac rhythm. In addition, she recognizes the patient's restlessness and anxiety and responds by modulating her interaction with the patient and controlling environmental stressors as much as possible. The nurse's close monitoring and careful management of this patient resulted in the patient's gradual recovery without reintubation.

This aspect of practice is often the most covered over and misunderstood by non-practicing clinicians. An outsider observing this nurse may describe her as standing around and doing little for the patient. Yet, maintaining this patient's stability and preventing deterioration that would necessitate technological intervention required an understanding of the patient's complex and multiple pathophysiological conditions, keen assessment skills, good clinical judgment, wise restraint from providing routine care, careful management of multiple bodily systems, and management of the environment. Knowing when to act and when to stand back is a hard won skill and nurses often find themselves postponing interventions proposed by others who do not make these distinctions. For instance, this nurse postponed weaning the vasoactive drugs despite the order to do so in order to temporarily prevent any physiological disturbance that might destabilize the patient's ability to compensate.

The depth, timing, and demand of this level of rigorous attentiveness, moment-by-moment thinking, reasoning about how every physiological change affects the others, and continuous clinical judgments about the patient's condition, tolerance, progress, and interventions is rarely visible unless an experienced observer watches an expert in actual practice. Yet, one may easily notice in this nurse's "ordinary" account of care how impossible it is to capture the most important facets of care she is providing for this patient. The skillfulness in her performance simply defies being accounted for or quantified (the primary legitimate way practice is measured and reimbursed) despite being easily observed, described, and knowable (excluded from <u>measures</u> of excellent care that count and are reimbursed). Even if one "counted" the amount of time spent thinking, reasoning, and making judgments, or counted the number of judgments made in a patient's care, the numerical data would make no sense out of context. The sense of a clinical judgment, and therefore quality, is only understood in the context of a specific patient in a particular situation at a specific point in time. Narrative accounts make visible the links between thinking, reasoning, clinical judgment (means or process) and the ends or outcomes.

This is the means-ends issue, where the means (expert performance) disappear from notice while the ends (patient outcomes) dominate, for instance, the focus of quality improvement, outcomes management, and the like. With protocols, practice guidelines, and best practices in place, the assumption is that those are the means to the ends, overlooking the fact that a clinician with good judgment must recognize when they do not apply and can harm a patient if applied or when the patient is unresponsive to the protocol, indicating that interventions must change. To date, little progress has been made in the nation's elaborate quality and outcome tracking systems to account for the aspects of patient care that count the most, that is, HOW the outcomes are attained. Expert practice continues, by design, to be systematically ignored, discounted, and is therefore disappearing from view in favor of what CAN be counted and therefore reimbursed. Because developing and expert clinicians do understand what counts in ordinary everyday practice, for patients and their loved one, they strive to develop and be accountable for what seems to legitimately count so little. Our intent is to articulate the skillful performance of experts, which includes attentiveness and vigilance, and to close the gap in understanding the link between the means and the ends. The skill of knowing when to act is central to expert practice and is a pervasive theme in this aspect of practice. It is inseparably linked with vigilant monitoring. In another clinical observation, the nurse who is feeding another infant (Baby R), sees the heart rate of a fairly stable baby (Baby C) suddenly drop to 47 as the alarm sounds. The nurse describes her immediate understanding of the situation and goes on to explain her reasoning and accompanying intervention if the transition had evolved differently:

Nurse: That's unusual for him. [Calmly gets up from her chair while feeding baby R and gently shakes Baby C. Bradycardia resolves and the heart rate increases to 102.] He has not done that before. [Other nurse comments that maybe the monitor was inaccurate, not picking up all the beats.]

Nurse: No, the intervals on the monitor lengthened. It was a true bradycardia. [Keeping her eye on Baby C.'s monitor.]

Interviewer: What would you have done if it hadn't resolved?

Nurse: Well, as you saw, I lightly stimulated the baby. I could have been more aggressive if that didn't work. Shake a little harder, pick the baby up. If stimulation didn't resolve it, then I would give some oxygen. Drugs are a last resort if the bradycardia was sustained and the baby is not responding. But that is the first time in Baby C., so I will keep a closer eye on him (Observational Interview).

In this situation, the baby suddenly develops an urgent problem. Yet, the nurse calmly approaches the baby and observes him for a moment before gently intervening. She then lightly rubs his foot when the bradycardia does not resolve spontaneously. Although instantaneous intervention would have resolved the problem more quickly, this nurse waits to act in order to gain a sense of how the baby's own physiological mechanisms will respond. Nurses sometimes call this watchful waiting "following the body's lead" (Benner, 1994a). The knowledge and experience of knowing what to do and when to do it allows this expert nurse the flexibility of being guided by the baby's response and using the least harmful and most specific intervention.

In the above stories, interventions are being considered and/or implemented as the patient's changing condition demands. However, the nurse's judgment, attention, and practice is oriented in the same way when new interventions are attempted, when current interventions are titrated, and when interventions are being weaned. For example, during a clinical observation, a baby with a hypoplastic left ventricle, tricuspid and mitral valve atresia, and a severely narrowed aorta is being closely monitored to guide the titration of a vasoactive drug, prostaglandin E (PGE):

Nurse: He's on lipids, PGE....

Interviewer: And the PGE dosage is—do you titrate that at all or is that pretty much a set dose?

Nurse: No, we titrate it. He's on [dosage] nanograms/kilogram. We want to get it down to the lowest dose we can that will keep the patent ductus arteriosus open.

Interviewer: Okay, and do you have any way to monitor that? [The nurse reached for her stethoscope] Oh, okay, so you'll listen.

Nurse: You practically don't even have to listen. You can put your fingers on there (under the left clavicle) and you can feel it.

Interviewer: Oh, yeah. [palpating]

Nurse: But we monitor it every hour. We listen to make sure the murmur is still there.

Interviewer: Can you tell if the opening is getting larger or smaller?

Nurse: Oh, yeah.

Interviewer: Or do you just see if there's an absence or presence?

Nurse: Oh, you can hear it in his whole chest. I mean, you can tell by listening—like I'll auscultate his chest and find out where the sounds—first of all where his PMI is, his point of maximal impulse is, but when it's that large it's kind of hard to tell. I mean, it just feels like the whole chest—which is a good sign (Observational Interview).

In this patient, vigilant observational skills and diligent tracking of the murmur guide the level of pharmacological intervention. This infant is life-dependent on the Prostaglandin E to keep the ductus arteriosus patent. A patent ductus provides the only shunting of oxygenated blood into the aorta for systemic tissue oxygenation until palliative surgical treatment for the hypoplastic left ventricle is possible. Thus, in this situation, physical findings supersede advanced technology (e.g., echocardiogram) in providing the vital information required for good clinical judgment and life-sustaining therapy.

Similarly, when interventions are being weaned, particularly in very fragile patients, a skilled observer must continuously assess the patient's response in order to avert complications. In the following clinical observation, a neonatal ICU nurse details her observations, interventions, and their significance as a baby is being gradually weaned from ventilatory support and abruptly from sedation:

Nurse: This baby was born three days ago, has respiratory distress syndrome, RDS, and is 37 weeks which is kind of old to have RDS. The baby got sick and got transported to [this hospital] three days ago. Got Exosurf , it's a synthetic surfactant, and it's given to kids with RDS. He got two doses which is standard and was getting better. A couple nights ago he got real sick again.

Interviewer: Now by real sick, what do you mean?

Nurse: His pO_2 went way down and he got real acidotic. He was started on vasopressors and Exosurf and got a third dose of it. And since he got that third dose, he's doing better, although he's still fairly sick. He's still on dopamine and nipride. And fairly significant ventilator settings. He's still getting a lot of oxygen.

Interviewer: Like about?

Nurse: 45%, and rates of 20 and pressures of 34, which is a pretty significant pressure for a baby this size. He shouldn't—if he was ready to be extubated, he'd be down on pressures of 24 or 25. So he's got a way to go. I just pulled his IV, the IV was infiltrated and fentanyl was running for sedation, and they decided to stop it cold turkey. So we may have a challenge over the next couple hours trying to keep this baby calm, although we can always restart the IV and fentanyl if we need to. The first thing I need to do is check my drips to make sure they're going at the rate that they're supposed to be going.

Interviewer: Now he's on the dopamine for what reason?

Nurse: Usually we use it for perfusion. If a baby comes in and is really mottled and their feet and hands are cold, usually you start out by giving them lots of volume. Fresh frozen plasma is typically what they give and then you run a risk of fluid overloading them, and then you start with the dopamine and usually start at 5 mics per kilo. [Checks all the infusions. Prepares the baby's formula for the nasogastric feeding. After giving the feeding, she begins a detailed physical assessment. She talks as she's examining the baby and pauses when listening for various sounds.] (inaudible) on the right lower lobe, but I don't find them significantly different on either side. Pulses aren't very good. Sometimes on a baby like this that's real edematous, especially a big baby, it's hard to find pulses anyway. He's got good brachials, but his radials are kind of (pause as she assesses) poor. The various drips—it looks like they're going into a peripheral IV which is something that you need to check really frequently to make sure it's not infiltrated. Some babies are real sensitive to their drips and if it infiltrates then they can crash really fast. And then with dopamine, if it infiltrates it causes such nasty things to the tissue. He doesn't move around a lot on his own. For a baby this size, you'd expect him to be protesting quite loudly, although he wouldn't cry, but he'd certainly move around. He's kind of stiff (moving the extremity).

Interviewer: And why is that?

Nurse: Probably from the amount of fluid that's in his tissues. It probably hurts him to move a lot. He's really puffy. See that. His poor little hands are like marshmallow man.

Interviewer: So with this baby, what are your concerns for him tonight?

Nurse: What we'll work on is trying to wean his ventilator settings down as much as possible. He's got good air movement in his chest although you don't see his chest wall rise a lot. When you listen to him, he moves air really well, so we may be able to go down on his pressures some more. They tried to wean his oxygen a little bit earlier this evening, and he had to come back up, so I don't anticipate that we'll be able to do that much. As the fentanyl clears, although the half-life of fentanyl is fairly long in babies, he will need more support, ventilator-wise, he may need more oxygen or more pressure or more rate because he'll get a lot more acidotic. So you kind of walk a fine line between over-sedating him and then letting him wake up so they can start moving around. He needs to move to start getting rid of some of that extracellular fluid that he's got on board. I anticipate that for the first half of the shift anyway that he'll be pretty quiet. And we do have an order for Midazolam [sedative/hypnotic] if I need to sedate him further. And again, I can get that fentanyl restarted by putting another IV into him. I'll watch his perfusion to make sure that it certainly doesn't get any worse than it is. And if he gets too much more mottled or capillary refill time prolonged, then he probably needs some volume. And I'll watch his blood pressure (Observational Interview).

Unlike the care of a patient during a crisis which, by necessity, is very focused, this nurse is carefully watching out for the infant's multiple and complex problems as well as the confounding effects each problem has on others. The nurse describes a force field or network of concerns—sedation, over-sedation, perfusion, and volume overload—that guide her judgment and interventions. The nurse demonstrates that, with each problem, she has already anticipated what might go wrong and is therefore attentive to any cues that could indicate a transition. She also relates the possible interventions that can be implemented to manage each eventuality. This observational interview further illustrates how clinical forethought shapes ongoing perception and judgment, and reflects how expert clinicians think ahead or anticipate eventualities as they simultaneously monitor a patient's condition in order to detect early signs of trouble and are prepared to intervene immediately.

Specifically, this nurse knows that when interventions are being weaned, gradually or abruptly, the removal of supportive care will cause a physiological transition and place demands on the patient physiologically to compensate. While monitoring, she anticipates that the patient's transition can either be slight or significant. In this case, the baby's waking and becoming active due to the discontinuation of fentanyl are likely to increase the oxygen demand and utilization. Hence, the nurse vigilantly observes for signs of decompensation to determine whether or not the baby's damaged lungs can handle the increased demand.

Favorable or deleterious transitions may also occur when interventions are being introduced or increased. Because one can never confidently predict how a particular patient will respond to a specific therapy, attentive monitoring is called for until the critically ill patient's response can be evaluated. This was clinically observed when a nurse increased the feeding in a premature infant who had had a bradycardic event. The nurse describes what she is watching for and when the symptoms take on dangerous significance:

> **Nurse:** I started this [gastric feeding] about 5 minutes ago and it's already—I mean, as long as the baby's tolerating it, it's fine to let it go in fast, but...
>
> **Interviewer:** And you have her sucking at the same time?
>
> **Nurse:** Yes. That's called non-nutritive sucking and it helps the baby learn that she's filling her belly. And even though I'm filling her belly, she's sucking and she's getting satisfied. And she's getting a little sleepy now.
>
> **Interviewer:** And if she wasn't tolerating it, you'd see...?
>
> **Nurse:** She'd be regurgitating it.
>
> **Interviewer:** Spitting it up.
>
> **Nurse:** Yeah. She spit up a little bit the last time. In fact, she dropped her heart rate a little bit. But those things kind of happen... She's got a big tube in her mouth [intubated and on a ventilator] and sometimes it gags the baby. I think she's just beautiful. I just really love her. She's trying to get her fingers in her mouth. She likes that. I think she may be actually trying to swipe the tube out.
>
> **Interviewer:** Do they do that?
>
> **Nurse:** Yeah. Yeah, preemies have to have something to grab onto. It goes along the lines of keeping them flexed, and they love to have something to curl their fingers around. And if it's the tube or your finger, they'll grab onto it. She dropped her heart rate just a little bit, not what I consider a bradycardia, but she probably had that little mouthful of milk in her mouth.
>
> **Interviewer:** You were watching that monitor the whole time, I didn't catch that.
>
> **Nurse:** Yeah, I was watching the monitor, but I could tell she got pale and a lot of times babies do that.
>
> **Interviewer:** You knew before her monitor went off that she was going to brady.
>
> **Nurse:** Yeah, yeah. And we don't count bradycardia's during the feed, so I did pat her bottom, but if she was asleep, like if it was an hour after her feeding and she wasn't spitting or anything but she just dropped her heart rate and the alarm might have gone off, I would come over and I would look at her color, look to see if she's apneic and see if she comes up on her own before I patted her bottom. She's fine... (Observational Interview).

Here the nurse points out that, although a bradycardia during feeding is not expected, it is common enough and without consequence that "we don't count bradycardia's during the feed." Nonetheless, she is very observant and notes the baby's accompanying responses of pallor and possible apnea. She later draws attention to an important situational distinction. The same symptom (such as the bradycardia) under a different set of circumstances often indicates a different and potentially dangerous problem. This example highlights an essential skill of making distinctions that are qualitative in nature between a response that is a variance but within acceptable limits and a response that is unacceptable and requires immediate intervention. This skill is inextricably linked to the situational context and is dependent on the skill of knowing when to act and when to wait and watch.

In the everyday practice of expert nurses, it is not always so clear whether a physiological change is significant or not. The majority of acutely and critically ill patients have multiple and complex problems so that physiological changes (or the lack of) may not have definitive meanings in early stages of presentation. Similarly, a specific intervention does not always produce the physiological effect intended and may produce a negative consequence that is puzzling, as illustrated in the following excerpt:

> **Interviewer:** Now earlier you said that he's very edematous. How do you know that in a baby this age?
>
> **Nurse:** Well, the baby's eyes tend to become puffy very easily, and also the hands and feet are the first places that you tend to see the swelling occur. And—the baby's actually starting to get some generalized edema, but it's still fairly subtle at this point. Sometimes you can feel pitting edema, once a baby's very edematous, in the head—as you turn the head from side to side you'll see pitting edema, but I don't really see any with him yet. It's still pretty subtle at this point, and it's surprising because this baby has gotten a couple of hundred of cc's of colloid so far in his life and he has not made that much urine, so I'm—I'm worried... (Observational Interview).

Because a change (or lack of change) can range from being insignificant to ominous, nurses commonly experience a great deal of concern and worry when the situation has not yet unfolded enough to understand what is happening as in the above situation. The nurse is expecting to either observe more edema or a better urine output, given the type and amount of fluids infused. Not being able to better understand the causes of the baby's condition leaves her worried that something adverse may be evolving. For that reason, she continually observes the baby for any changes that might warn of a transition. Many nurses have witnessed a devastating eventuality in an under-determined situation such as this. For them, the weight of a potential crisis while waiting for the situation to unfold propels them to become astute and detailed clinical observers. Experiences where learners have detected early warning signals and saved the patient from needless suffering also contribute to their continued vigilance and attentiveness to early changes as being essential for averting a crisis.

Expert practice extends beyond monitoring for signs of physiological transitions and impending danger. At times, patients seem to be responding well or with no adverse symptoms from their current therapies. However, the ethos of "Do no harm" pervasively influences expert clinical judgment so that, when monitoring a patient's condition, these clinicians are ever aware of interventional options or changes that could be made to reduce the patient's risks for complications yet provide an equivalent or improved level of care. In the following account, after monitoring a patient's responses, the nurse speaks of her concerns that a few specific treatment approaches carry too high a risk of barotrauma and of dramatic swings in sedation:

> **Nurse:** He had amiodarone toxicity; he had a CABG; he had a couple of V-Fib arrests. This is a first line antiarrhythmic for ventricular arrhythmias. Anyway, it has a lot of toxicity, a lot of side effects. He now has hypothyroidism and most urgently this pulmonary fibrosis. That's the main problem. He had this internal defibrillator placed; he was out on the floor. He had a lot of abdominal pain. He perforated his cecum and

ended up with an ileostomy. Now he has resistant pseudomonas in his lungs, and he's been in ICU for 5 weeks due to his fibrotic lung changes and now worsening pneumonia... My number one priority was to ventilate him without causing barotrauma of his lungs. He was being ventilated on higher pressures than he needed to be. So we had talked a little bit about different modes of ventilating him. Sometimes for no good reason, other than it feels more comfortable to the patient, a particular ventilation mode works. So, it's delivering the same minute volume, you're getting the same amount of ventilation, but you can decrease the actual pressure it takes to give positive pressure ventilation just by changing the mode or the inspiratory-expiratory ratio. The vent and pressure alarms were going off a lot. So just as I came in, I didn't have a lot of time to make decisions other than to look at him, make sure the monitoring was right, because he was on a lot of vasopressors so I checked a blood pressure and made sure that the transducers were right. You just go over and look at that data and listen to his lungs and check out his ventilator, and then make changes from there because his PIPs (peak inspiratory pressures) were already 70, so I didn't want to go on that way for a long time if I didn't have to. That was basically where I started.

Interviewer: Now talk about what you were trying to do with his sedation.

Nurse: I was trying to give him a continuous level of comfort without having him snowed if he didn't need to be. If he needed to be snowed, I was perfectly willing to do it. I am willing to paralyze people if that is what is needed to protect their lungs. Anyway, just to figure out something else instead of bolusing him with fentanyl, versed, and morphine. We talked about his sedatives and narcotics. My idea was that if we got him on a drip, maybe he could be a little bit awake, look at what his ventilator was set on and what they had tried previously, because we go around and around with people like this. Sometimes, every eight hours, we are on a different mode. So I was going to try to start the drip, because I've had good success with having a steady state rather than letting them wake up and then needing twice as much sedation to get them relaxed, causing them to be comatose when they don't need to be [over sedation causes problems]. They're unresponsive and he's got a whopping pneumonia, and you want him to cough, and you don't want his endotracheal tube to plug, so get yourself into this whole other cycle. And he was massively, massively third spaced, and you don't want a person like that to be immobile if they can move. He didn't look good.

Interviewer: You started him on the drip [sedation] and how did that work?

Nurse: It did work, and he was not snowed and could move around.

Although the patient is tolerating the high ventilator pressures and the boluses of sedation, the nurse recognizes that the potential dangers of both are unnecessary. Thus, she works with team members to alter the modes of intervention enough to reduce the patient's risk of barotrauma and to find the delicate balance between a continuous level of comfort and a level of wakefulness that promotes activity and pulmonary toiletry. In the end, the patient experiences less air hunger, greater pain control, and greater satisfaction in being more awake and active. This story illustrates the significance of having a skilled clinician at the bedside to monitor and manage critically ill patients who are not necessarily "unstable." Additionally, it highlights a kind of practical technology assessment which is discussed in Chapter 8.

As alluded to earlier, because excellent nurses recognize the difference they make in critically ill patients, they are often reluctant to delegate the vigilance and attentiveness of maintaining life-sustaining therapies to under-skilled or technical workers. Financial constraints are currently causing healthcare cutbacks and resulting in an increase in under-skilled workers with a reduction in highly skilled clinicians. Without the direct access to closely monitor patient responses, nurses are often conflicted in how to provide safe care without continuous and focused access to patients. A flight nurse talked about this kind of conflict after having to repeatedly coach a resident physician to attend to an airway via cricothyrotomy because the nurse knew that airways are easily lost during transport. She and others recalled situations which supported their concerns about delegating observational responsibilities:

Interviewer: You said that once you get an airway, you don't want to leave it, and you feel like you've got to get over that.

Nurse 1: Well, airway's <u>everything</u>. If you don't have an airway, you haven't gotten anywhere. You can't even transport the patient without an airway.

Interviewer: But a resident would theoretically know that.

Nurse 1: Yeah, he did, but <u>usually</u>, the residents put in the airway and somebody else <u>manages</u> it. And in the hospital, everything's so controlled. You tape it nicely and restrain the patient and you've got your airway. Whereas here, you know how tenuous that airway is. You know you could lose it at any time. But at the same time, sometimes you are needed to do something else. That's really hard for me, because it's really hard for me to trust anyone else, except for my partner, like a pre-hospital provider even though I know they're terrific out there. And I <u>need</u> to learn to do that. To say, 'Okay, you need to hold this airway for me and bag the patient.' And to <u>trust</u> them with it.

Interviewer: Have you had a bad experience before?

Nurse 1: Well you <u>see</u> people treat airways differently. You see people bagging with the Ambu bag and looking somewhere, talking. Whereas, when I have my airway, I always hold the tube, and I hold their face, and I bag. It's just different—we're very compulsive about our airways. If we lose that airway, <u>we</u> lost the airway. Even if the fire fighter was bagging. We lost the airway. And people just don't understand how easily they're lost. I really know how <u>easily</u> it can be lost, so it's just a high priority.

Interviewer: But it sounds like a <u>good</u> one.

Nurse 1: Yeah. Oh I think it's a <u>very</u> good priority, but there are times where you have to trust somebody else and that's what I need to learn how to do. Because if you're stuck there, and you can't get the patient loaded in the helicopter because you won't leave your airway, well then you're prioritizing wrong.

Interviewer: [Nurse 2], you had said—you had mentioned that you remember how you learned that.

Nurse 2: Oh, just handing my airway over to somebody and turning my head and coming back and the airway's dislodged....

Nurse 3: Well, there was a car over an embankment. The patient was trapped in the vehicle, they still hadn't finished extricating him and I was standing on the embankment and they were using chains to hold this car secure. And I said, 'Do you <u>want</u> me down there?' There was somebody doing the airway. There was actually a couple of people and, I go, 'Here's a tube' and they're going, 'No, come with us,' So I said, 'Okay.' I get down there and they had lost the tube and I'm like, 'Okay, we need to...' and my [nurse partner] is up there on the embankment, handing me things. We get the airway and I checked placement and it was good. I'm getting ready to tie it and the guy doing the Ambu bag turns around with the Ambu bag, and takes the whole tube with it and it's like, 'Wait a minute you guys. It was a good tube. Then the patient had no pulses. [As ventilation was resumed per mask], I said, 'We need to put the monitor on.' They had stopped extrication. The patient was still in there, but they had to stop for us, and we put the monitor on. And it was asystole, and at that point, we discussed 'Do we proceed with extrication and continue CPR <u>here</u>? Or do we declare the patient?' The nurse on the embankment called medical control [talked to a physician] and we ended up declaring the patient there...it was a sad situation.

Accidents such as this make skilled clinicians reluctant to leave a worker with whom they are unfamiliar responsible for such vital interventions. For clinicians who understand what is at stake for the patient, conscientious monitoring and protection of a life-sustaining intervention like an airway can be as critical as the intervention itself. In settings where skilled clinicians are being replaced by unskilled technicians who do not understand how or what to monitor, the stakes for patients become increasingly higher.

As technology has become increasingly available and sophisticated, nurses have learned to use specific technologic interventions not only for the purpose originally intended, but also as a backup means of "observation" or as a reminder to check on a particular function or evaluate an intervention. Most pieces of equipment have alarms and these may be set to sound when there is a physiological deviation from a predetermined norm or when an infusion is completed. These alarms serve as a safety backup to alert nurses as they are constantly busy caring for another patient or engaged in multiple simultaneous interventions. This monitoring practice overlaps with other surveillance skills aimed at creating a safe patient environment (see Chapter 8). A neonatal nurse explained how vital these uses of technology are in infants where there is little room for error:

Nurse: This baby's heart rate was running in the 150s which is quite normal. Surprisingly, his heart rate has dropped to 140 in the last hour. At the same time, his blood pressure has been slowly dropping. You would expect the opposite. You would expect him to become tachycardic if he's becoming more hypovolemic, so we're just watching it. We do have an arterial line in the baby and the blood pressure you would normally expect in a full term baby would be in the 40s to 50s, mean arterial pressure. With this baby [premature infant]—with any baby with pulmonary hypertension—you <u>want</u> your blood pressure to be on the high rather than the low side of normal because more peripheral resistance means more blood is actually forced to circulate through the baby's lungs which, since pulmonary vasoconstriction is present, you want to facilitate as much blood flow through the lungs as you can. That's one of the reasons we try to keep the blood pressure a little bit higher.

Interviewer: What are you doing now?

Nurse: I'm setting the IV pumps forward. The baby's getting his maintenance fluid and his arterial line fluid. We keep the rate the same but we set an hourly limit just to check and make sure he's getting infused what he's <u>ordered</u> to get infused.

Interviewer: ...so it forces you to look at it every hour.

Nurse: Right. It just forces you to look at it and make sure that your IV fluids are on time and that the baby's gets what he's supposed to be getting.

Interviewer: So you reset it?

Nurse: I reset it every hour.

Interviewer: And that's very different with adults, isn't it?

Nurse: Well, because there are no small mistakes in infants. Any mistake that you make or any excess fluid makes a difference because they are so small. There's just very little margin for error. Even in pediatrics they're much less careful about keeping track of IV fluid infusions and things like that. And we actually account for every drop of blood that we take out of the baby, and for even the most minute amount of flush and medications and things like that. We keep track of all of that and take that into account as part of the fluid intake, which is pretty unheard of in adult care because it's such a small amount to them it doesn't matter. But it does to the babies. And it can add as much as—this baby is on 80 cc's per kilogram per day, which is pretty standard, but the medications and flushes and things like that that the baby's getting probably add another 20 cc's per kilo, and that's very significant (Observational Interview).

Because of the narrow margin for error, the vigilant safety work demonstrated in this example is crucial. Having a "backup memory" is critical due to three current trends: nurses face increasing workloads which afford less direct care time per patient for quality monitoring; patient acuities continue to rise and subsequently demand closer monitoring; and skilled nurse observers are being replaced by under-skilled technicians who are not educated to detect subtle or sometimes even blatant physiological changes. Although critical care nurses are commonly seen manipulating the bedside equipment, it is a misinterpretation to understand the nurse as nursing the equipment rather than the patient when the action instead serves as a means of preventing complications (see Chapter 8). Attentiveness to patients and equipment is required.

In this aspect of practice, excellent nurses not only monitor patients to detect early clues of problems, they also manage care in ways that conserve the patient's energy, reduce undesirable stimulation and discomfort, and protect the patient's desperately needed rest. Patients who are extremely fragile, sleep-deprived, or have increased intracranial pressure are at high risk for complications due to over-stimulation. A neuro ICU nurse identified the typical way that nurses structure interventions to control external stimulation:

Nurse: There are things you can do before you suction a patient like this to control their intracranial pressure. Clustering of nursing activities helps so that you're not always stimulating them. You do what you have to do and then you leave them alone. Also, really knowing what the effects of [Pa]CO_2 are on the cerebral circulation, combining that with increasing your osmolarity, and use of sedation.

The nurse points to how the clustering of activities is accomplished in conjunction with managing the patient's CO_2 levels and with other interventions, such as sedation. The specific way in which one balances these interventions is often determined by working with that specific patient and gaining a sense of that patient's particular responses. By clustering interventions, a nurse can typically limit the frequency, extent, and duration of adverse physiological effects on the patient. The same is true, for instance, in burn nursing where activities are clustered around the times that narcotics are given in order to reduce the patient's suffering and maximize the patient's activity levels. Many night nurses have mastered this skill of clustering interventions in order to minimize patients' sleep disruption yet perform necessary assessments and interventions. In each case, the nurse strives to protect the patient's ability to heal and recover through rest and comfort (see Chapter 6).

Finally, nurses try to protect patients from complications by monitoring their responses to learn what patients may and may not be able to tolerate. Observing the patient's responses over time helps the nurse judge how much, how long, and to what extent the patient can physiologically adapt to or endure the stress caused by many interventions. As illustrated in Chapter 3, a neonatal nurse anticipated a baby's potential response to the residents' "tinkering" with his ventilatory pressures. The example is worth revisiting because, even though the nurse knows that the pressures are high and risky, she is concerned about the baby's stability and ability to recover:

Nurse: Are you going to tinker?

Physician: Well yes. [resident leaves for a moment]

Nurse: Oh God.

Interviewer: What do you mean tinker?

Nurse: I think they're going to come in and play with this baby's ventilator. They're going to come play with the settings, try some different combinations to, I guess, see if they can get him [the neonate] to oxygenate better. I wish they wouldn't. It could make the baby better or it could start a downward spiral, and we'll spend the rest of the day trying to get the baby back to his baseline. I mean you do have to try things at some point, and preferably you try...

Interviewer: What are going to be your responsibilities if they start tinkering?

Nurse: Well, I'll watch his monitors a little more closely than I have and then watch his blood pressure very closely. Usually the standard is to get a blood gas about ten minutes after a ventilation change is made to kind of see which direction we're going. Sometimes babies will change dramatically. As soon as a change is made, sometimes they can take an hour or so before their lungs open up more. Or if the lungs collapse or get atelectatic, it might be awhile before you see it. So I'll really have to watch him closely for the next hour or so...[resident returns]

Physician: The important thing is to wean the vent.

Nurse: Right. So they're decreasing the peak inspiratory pressure (PIP). That means we're not giving the baby quite as big a breath. It could cause him to oxygenate a little bit less but it also hopefully will cause him less barotrauma, not to use as much pressure. Why are you choosing to go down on the PIP?

Physician: You know the chest movement is more than adequate and we've paralyzed the baby so that the breath rate is not that much of an issue, and we do want the CO_2 to go up so that the pH goes down a little bit. And that certainly will help the potassium, and it may also help with the blood pressure.....

Nurse: Well I'm just going to make the alarms a little more sensitive. We just went down on the peak pressure on the baby's ventilator and his oxygen saturation has definitely declined in response to that. Instead of being 97%, he's now between 96 and 91. And I'm willing to bet this is not going to be a very good blood gas and they're going to have to go back up on the PIP.

Interviewer: And why are you willing to bet that?

Nurse: Because a post ductal saturation of 91 on a full term baby probably isn't very good; it's probably not going to be a good PO_2 on this baby. It's probably going to be back down to 50.

Interviewer: Sounds like you've been in this situation before.

Nurse: Well, not on this particular patient. But, yeah. Generally on a full term baby with healthy lungs, you expect their oxygen saturation to be in the mid 90s, and if it's in the low 90s then something is wrong, and particularly on a baby like this where you want to keep them well oxygenated to sort of maximize pulmonary perfusion. The thing you <u>don't</u> want to do is have them start desaturating because that will start a downward spiral that will take them hours to get out of. His oxygenation would go down and just going back up to where his baseline was before may not fix it. Sometimes if you try to make one step forward you end up taking two steps back. So this baby could potentially end up on higher pressures than he was an hour ago because we tried to wean him and maybe the baby isn't going to like it. I don't think he's going to like it.

Interviewer: It seemed earlier when they were mentioning 'tinkering' you already had a...

Nurse: I already knew I didn't want them to do it. I mean you don't know until you try it. If they turned it down and he did very well and handled it, we would pat ourselves on the shoulder and say 'Good, he really didn't need that much pressure anyway.' If he deteriorates, then we say 'Whoops! Should have left him alone.' But the way you find out is by doing (Observational Interview).

This clinical excerpt presents a difficult situation for nurses to manage. In this instance, the nurse predicts that changing modes of intervention that should improve the patient's condition and reduce risks will possibly tip the patient into a "downward spiral." Going along with a clinical decision that does not match her judgment creates internal conflict and she has to stay open to the possibility that her judgment might not be correct. Stating her judgment clearly to the resident, while staying open to the resident's plan, could reduce her conflict and improve the collective wisdom about when to try weaning in the future. Because recent attempts to wean the infant had failed, the nurse was concerned that further attempts would set the infant back at this point. Recovery back to the pre-intervention point could take days and much of the infant's limited reserves. In fact, the infant's immediate drop in oxygen saturation supported her judgment.

The nurse was not reacting to weaning in general; her concern was that this particular infant was not ready to wean within such a short time period. She referred to this medical approach to management as "tinkering" which points out an important distinction in approaches to managing a patient's care. Tinkering in this instance connotes her appraisal that the resident's judgment is based on goals without necessarily taking the infant's specific responses and readiness for treatment into primary consideration. In contrast, prudent interventions are guided by the infant's specific responses and readiness for change with particular goals in mind. This excerpt highlights how patient-specific responses orient clinicians' judgment and practice differently than broad treatment goals.

Because the nurse did not anticipate that the infant would respond well, she immediately became more vigilant and attentive in monitoring his condition by watching more closely and by making her alarm parameters more sensitive. These actions convey the nurse's hope that she might detect a downward spiral very early and also illustrates judicious use of monitors. Despite her discouragement over the lack of a positive response, the nurse demonstrates her openness to being disconfirmed by admitting that "you don't know until you try it."

At times, there is little that distinguishes patients who are just transferred out of ICU to a medical unit from patients in the ICU. The patients' acuity, care demands, fragility and complexity often continue to warrant close monitoring and managing, not so much for life-threatening situations, but instead for life-incapacitating conditions. Transitions in levels of care create loss of first hand information of the patient's clinical patterns, concerns, preferences and so on (Naylor, 2000, 2003). As Foust (2005) notes: "Frequent transitions within a hospital, such as from the ED to an ICU to a step-down unit to a general medical–surgical unit, can have devastating effects on the health of older adults and the well-being of family caregivers. For example, serious medication errors are common during transition periods. Transitions during and after hospitalization often create anxiety for the patient and family members who have become accustomed and comfortable in the prior care location. Patient safety depends on allotting additional time in communicating between units, with family members and designing a new plan and style of care for the patient.

For acute care nurses, the demand is high, resources are few, nurse-patient ratios for even skillful nurses are questionable, and safety nets are scarce. Without the close proximity of other nurses to learn from, ask questions, observe, and model the habits of thought and action, newer nurses often find themselves doing the best they can. Susan Gagne Rego, a skin care nurse, points out the power an expert nurse, with a bit of coaching, can have on a less experienced peer's development and on the quality of life for acutely ill patients:

Nurse: Mary was admitted to ICU following a cerebral vascular accident (CVA). She was stabilized and transferred to the medical unit. After reviewing the patient's chart, I remember thinking, "This is going to be a straightforward consult." Mary had right sided paralysis, expressive aphagia, and failure to thrive, which required the insertion of a G-tube for nutritional support. Mary's nurse stated she was "becoming overwhelmed" with the amount of care Mary required." She was a new RN and explained why she was feeling so "overwhelmed." Mary's G-tube was draining gastric juices onto her skin, which required hourly dressing changes. Mary was agitated with each interaction, which was upsetting this nurse.

Upon entering the room, I introduced myself as the "skin care nurse" who was going to help with the leaking tube. The patient became agitated with rapid leg movements and attempts at verbal communication by moaning. I reassured Mary I was there to help her in any way I could without causing pain. I began my assessment by exposing her abdomen and G-tube site. I was immediately taken aback by the "raw meat" that had taken over her abdomen. The caustic gastric drainage had started to macerate her entire abdomen. My first thought was, "_____ [an expression of outrage], this has to hurt!" I was feeling the pain the patient so desperately tried to communicate. I wasn't prepared for the tears streaming down the patient's cheek.

I asked the nurse to join me in Mary's room to discuss my findings and formulate a plan of care. My first priority was to medicate Mary and provide her with the care she so rightly needed. I was [upset] at Mary's nurse, but I knew she was doing the best she could with her limited experience. I needed to use this opportunity to mentor her. I wanted Mary's nurse to feel like she could ask questions and not feel intimidated or belittled with her inexperience. I grew respect for her that day because she wasn't afraid to admit her inexperence and sought help to rectify the situation.

Once Mary was medicated, I felt comfortable enough to cleanse her skin, stabilize the G-tube, and apply a moisture barrier ointment to her excoriated abdomen. I made a mental note of a foul smell coming from Mary's peri-rectal area, highly suspicious of a yeast infection. I wanted to investigate my suspicions further. I replaced the Foley catheter and discussed the rationale with Mary's nurse, who agreed to obtain orders for both urine and stool cultures. We discussed the need for the gastroenterologist to reassess the G-tube and place a stitch for better tube stabilization. Together we formulated and implemented her treatment plan.

The nurse felt comfortable enough to ask if I wouldn't mind giving her suggestions on the pressure sore Mary had on her butt. I rolled Mary over and began to probe her sacral area. She had a dry intact dressing covering her sacrum, which I removed to evaluate the area. I looked at the nurse and [wanted to scream].... I needed to take deep breathes. I am thinking, "Susan, you were a new RN once." I began to explain that Mary had a 4 cm x 4 cm pressure ulcer over her sacral area, and she needed a pressure relieving mattress. I instructed the nurse to have [them] bring a Kin-Air bed. We discussed the rationale and once again formulated a plan of care. Mary was not going to tolerate any type of surgical debridement, so I chose a conservative treatment approach by using a dressing to aide in autolytic debridement. I don't believe I can heal the world but I do aim to make my patients more comfortable. I wanted to make a difference in Mary's comfort and would try all the methods of skin care treatments I knew of to achieve this goal. I was pleased with the progress the nurse and I had made in Mary's care and finished the consult by writing a care plan for every nurse to reference, with expected dates of healing. I was exhausted when I left the unit but I felt good about being nurse. I felt like all the work I put into the enterostomal therapy course was validated at that moment.

I went back two days later to reevaluate Mary's progress and revise her care plan. I was pleased to find Mary sitting in bed, peacefully listening to Mass on the television. I took Mary's left hand and asked her if she was feeling better. She responded by squeezing my hand and blinking her eyes. I looked and found "comfort" in her eyes, so I knew deep down, I made a difference in Mary's care. Mary was receiving pain medication on a routine basis and received antibiotics for a confirmed yeast infection. Mary was going o a long term care facility for additional therapies, but before she was transferred, I contacted the facility and made suggestions regarding her potential skin care needs. I thought as I walked away from the medical unit, "that was a job well done."

Mary's condition and suffering are unspeakable when Susan exposes both her abdomen and later her sacrum. Susan silently expresses moral outrage but moves on to the positive project of healing Mary and teaching the newer nurse. She gathers herself, modulates her interactions, relieves Mary's suffering, and ensures wound healing. Susan serves as a desperately needed safety net, unfortunately by chance rather than design, for Mary and for the nurse. The nurse has the benefit of situated learning about wounds, possible care alternatives, thinking and reasoning in the situation, and tracking the patient's responses and their meanings over time with coaching from an expert. Debilitating illnesses take days to months to improve, so the rhythm and tempo of monitoring and managing acutely ill patients differ from critical care, but are no less demanding of skillful thinking, reasoning, judgment and intervention, Susan takes the responsibility of helping this new nurse begin to develop the practical knowledge and skills that are the foundation of clinical wisdom.

This story is not unique in most acute care units where inexperienced nurses are assigned responsibilities that exceed their limited practical knowledge and performance, particularly when there are limited or no expert resources to monitor, mentor or intervene, for the patients or nurses. Despite the wide use of clinical and unit educators, the problem is not solved because most of those educators are directed to continuously teach in classrooms rather than teach at the bedside where situated learning is superior (Lave & Wenger, 1991). There are tremendous administrative implications for creating safety nets (meaning engaged, skillful, helpful nurses who are specifically assigned to rove and coach good clinical thinking and judgment), especially on evening and night shifts where the less experienced clinicians are relegated (Kyriakidis & Vitello, in progress). Orientation and even residency programs are simply not enough to prepare new nurses for the demanding and complex care they are made accountable for, particularly if their physician colleagues are residents who are just as inexperienced. It is imperative to rethink and redesign the work of skillful, clinically-proficient nurse educators or clinical nurse specialists are who committed to preserving and extending the skillful knowledge, judgment, and performance to those who are developing in practice (Kyriakidis & Vitello, in progress). We know too much to do anything less.

COORDINATING AND MANAGING MULTIPLE INSTANTANEOUS THERAPIES

In the previous three categories of physiological practice, we primarily articulated individual interventions as they are implemented in crisis, unstable, and stable situations and how they are intertwined with other areas of knowledge work, such as clinical grasp, forethought, negotiation, et cetera. In the education of most nurses, interventions are taught as separate, isolated treatments. In fact, in actual crises or unstable situations, therapies are not typically initiated individually and sequentially. Instead, numerous interventions are often needed emergently to reverse or sustain vital physiological functions, especially in patients with multisystem organ failure. However, it is rare to subsequently teach nurses how to implement multiple interventions simultaneously. Thus, in this section, we will illustrate the multiple clinical judgments and simultaneous interventions that the care of acutely and critically ill patients demands within constrained periods of time.

When learning to manage an urgent situation, students typically read about what interventions may be used. These are frequently listed, but a textbook "list" fails to provide the student with a sense of the complexity and skillfulness needed to perform several interventions regarding multiple problems at the same time as well as understanding of the relationship between the interventions. However, an ICU nurse details a clinical situation that she vividly remembers because she cared for the patient for a long time, and it is the first time she finds herself orchestrating a crisis. Although the story is long, the details assist the reader to imaginatively enter the situation as the nurse, and to learn and mentally rehearse for a similar incident. For instance, from this story, a developing nurse can gain a understanding about what interventions may be anticipated based on the patient's changing physiological responses:

Nurse: This gentleman, Mr. A., has been in the hospital for five weeks, had an appendectomy and then started to GI bleed. He ended up coming to ICU and was on pitressin for a couple of days. We were lavaging him, he was endoscoped, and they cauterized a couple of bleeders from an ulcer. He's had six surgeries for rebleeding and a cholecystectomy. Now this is a gentleman who believed that nurses save lives because we are the ones who are with him all day long... The physicians weren't really sure why he kept bleeding or from where. All they knew was that he just kept bleeding. So one of his surgeons came in one day and she gave him some xylocaine to numb the site and put in a triple lumen catheter. It didn't seem to help so she gave him a little more, more than we normally give. About 10 minutes after she finished, his heart rate went up to 150 and he dropped his systolic blood pressure to 80 and looked awful. So I put his head flat and he started to get diaphoretic and complain of chest pain. And I kept thinking, 'This guy's got something going on, cardiac wise.' I called his doc and he said, 'Just watch him.' And I said, 'I don't feel real comfortable with what's going on. I think there's something else going on.' He goes, 'No, no. Just watch him; he'll be OK. I'm going to call Dr. B (surgeon) and Dr. B will be in to see him.' And I said, 'What are you calling Dr. B for? This man's heart rate is 150, and he doesn't have a blood pressure.' He goes, 'Just watch him. It'll be OK.'

Well, he must have started thinking because shortly after, a cardiologist came in. The patient's blood pressure came up on it's own but his heart rate was still 140-150. I was feeling really uncomfortable. His chest pain was gone but he was still diaphoretic and I just kept saying, 'You know, Mr. A, hang in there. For some reason your heart rate's really fast and we're going to figure out why.' I said, 'Are you nauseated? Do you have any abdominal pain?' He said, 'No, I feel fine. I feel the best I've felt.' His NG tube was draining green stuff and I just figured the patient's not bleeding unless it is just so low, down in the stomach, that we just don't know about it yet.

So a cardiologist came in, looked at him, and talked to him. He didn't order anything [except] an EKG and an echocardiogram. But his heart rate was still 140-150. And this was maybe 45 minutes. And Dr. B came in and looked at him and said, 'Oh, he's bleeding again, huh?' I said, 'No. Look at his NG drainage.' He said, 'Well, why is he tachycardic?' I said, 'I don't know! You tell me. He was complaining of chest pain and he's diaphoretic. Maybe he's having an MI. With everything else, he could be having an MI.' He goes, 'No, he's bleeding again. He did this one of the other times he bled.' I said, 'Well, his NG tube—it's coming out green.' He goes, 'Well, maybe it's sitting too high. Watch this.'

Sure enough, he pushed the tube down an inch further and bright red blood just started pouring out. So, we just started irrigating and irrigating and I said, 'OK, do me a favor. I can't leave this bedside if you want me to irrigate this man. Go call Dr. S and let him know what's going on.' So he did and they immediately got the GI crew up there and scoped him. He had 2 bleeders but they couldn't really find out where they were. One was behind the stomach and one was in the stomach, but they didn't know if they were arterial.

So Dr. B leaves while they're doing this endoscopy. I had stepped out of the room for a minute and all of a sudden, Dr. B comes in and says, 'OK, I want him in the OR in 5 minutes.' I said, 'Five minutes!' That's not giving me much time for anything! I'll get him down there as soon as I can.' He goes, 'I'm going to go down and scrub and I'll meet you down there.' I said, 'Fine.' So we managed to get all his paperwork and preparation done. We had some stat blood work drawn and took him down to the OR. That surgery tied off a couple of bleeders and that was all they did. He came back to the ICU and stayed there for 48 hours, did well, went out. Started to bleed again on six NW. He hadn't even been out for 24 hours and when he started bleeding and then came back in. This was a daily reoccurrence...

One particular day, I didn't take care of him but I was orienting somebody. His heart rate went way high and he dropped his pressure again. I just said, 'Here it goes.' I went to the bedside and I said to the nurse, 'You know, has he been doing this all day long?' She said, 'No, he just did it.' I said, 'Does it seem like he's bleeding?' She goes, 'No.' And they had pulled his NG tube that morning and it had been out for about four hours. And I said, 'I hate to say this, but I know he's bleeding again.' She goes, 'Well, how do you know?' At this time he started saying he was nauseated. And I said, 'I think we need to put a tube in and I'll go call the doctor.' And then he started to retch and up came bright red blood in clots all over the place. He dropped his pressure and this was major.

I said, 'You get a tube in this man. I'll get the doctor on the phone.' So we got the tube in the guy and we paged his doctor stat. He came up and he endoscoped him. Said, 'He's bleeding but we don't know where!' They still couldn't figure out where this man was bleeding from. So they decided to take him to surgery. But, in the meantime, he started to put out bright red blood from the rectum and has got no blood pressure. But he's responsive the whole time. So I held his hand and I said, 'Jim, you're bleeding again.' He goes, 'Oh, my God. Not again. Will you call my wife?' I said, 'I'll call your wife but right now we need to get you stable. You might have to have surgery again.' He said, 'Oh, if it will save my life, dear. If it will save my life.' I said, 'Well, we're hoping that it will. You've been through so much. How much more can your body handle?' He goes, 'I'm so tired.' I said, 'I know you are.' I said something about his wife and he said, 'My wife would want me to have this done. I'll be OK.' I said, 'OK.'

So we got his wife on the phone and Dr. B came up and said, 'We've got to get this guy to surgery.' I said, 'OK, fine.' So I was cleaning him up and I said, 'Jim, are you OK?' and he said, 'Yeah, I'm fine.' So I finished cleaning him up and I said, 'OK, Jim, turn over And he didn't say anything. I said, 'Jim!' and I turned him over on his back. Mind you, he's in Trendelenburg. We're not talking slightly. He's almost on his head. At this time, we had 3 units of blood going in and 500 cc's of plasmanate at once plus his IVs, a liter of Ringer's and a liter of saline. So he's got all these IVs going; he's got tubes everywhere. So I roll him over and he's really agonal and he's gray and I damn near lost it. I said, 'This man is not breathing!' and I said, 'We better do something fast.' We just called the doc stat. I looked at his heart rate and said, 'OK, he's bradying down. Someone get me some atropine.' I just started calling out the drugs that I needed and we started to push these drugs in. In the meantime, I said, 'Can we have some more blood.' I was just barking out this stuff. I can't even tell you the sequence. I was saying, 'We need this.' I needed to anticipate what was going to happen because I had been through this a week before with this guy and knew what we had done. So, in the meantime, the anesthesiologist came strolling in and we had been bagging him. Dr. B. was up there and Dr. B. had intubated him; and though Dr. B. is a surgeon who doesn't usually intubate, he did a pretty good intubation...and he said, 'What kind of lines do we have?' I said, 'We have a triple lumen; we got blood. All ports are taken. We need another kind of line. He's got no veins left.' He goes, 'OK, fine, give me a cut-down tray.' He put in a cut-down line in his leg; R. was bagging him. I was pushing drugs and running this blood in. Then the anesthesiologist came up and said, 'What's going on with this guy.' I said, 'You know, Mr. A.?' He said, 'This is him?!' I said, 'Yeah.' He said, 'Oh, God, not again! Sounds like we need to open him up.' I said, 'It sounds like that's what's going to happen.'

He goes, 'OK, we need an arterial line.' He started it in his femoral artery... In the meantime, we're trying to get responses out of the patient. We couldn't get any responses and I kept looking at the monitor. And there was no doctor to really run what was really going on. The surgeon was busy putting in a cut-down and the anesthesiologist was busy doing something else. The nursing staff was busy just trying to get his chart and stuff together so we could get him down to the OR. So it was the first time I've been put into this situation where I've kind of had to call the shots. And it was really difficult for me because I didn't know. I guess I didn't think I could do it until I was in that situation. It wasn't as difficult as it felt like afterwards. But usually there are docs around and there were so many people, the last thing we needed was another doc or another body at the bedside.

Interviewer: Did you have somebody charting for you while all this was going on?

Nurse: Yeah, there was somebody who was recording, thank God. It was a good experience for her but it was the person that I was orienting that was charting. So afterwards she comes up to me and she's got three pages of code sheets and she's going, 'What rhythms was he in?' 'Well, that's a good question!' So everything was retrospective at that time with the code sheet. But it was a good experience for her.

So we managed to get him down to the OR. By that time he was intubated. He had an arterial line in; he had a cut-down in his leg; he had, if I'm not mistaken, he had four units of blood running, a liter of saline and a unit of FFP. We were bagging him. We had four people take him down to the OR. We let his wife come in and see him really quick before we took him downstairs... We got him downstairs. He was in surgery for four hours. They did a total gastrectomy on him. Found out that he did, indeed, have amyloidosis. The prognosis for that is not good because you can bleed at any time. They don't know why he had it. He had never had any kind of symptoms or signs of it before. When we got him the next morning, he was still unresponsive and pretty much maintained that the rest of his stay. He was on levophed. I think, initially, he was on both dopamine and levophed but managed to get the dopamine off. We had to keep giving him blood. He started to have like little tremors and seizures but nothing really responsive. Occasionally it seemed like he was responding but it was questionable. [Unfortunately, the patient later died from continued complications.]

In the context of a story, not only do the kinds of interventions needed in a specific situation become apparent, but also the logic of each as related to the patient's responses become understandable. Here, one can see that the Trendelenburg position and the rapid infusions of blood, plasma, saline, Lactated Ringer's, and vasoactive drugs are not only implemented but are required concurrently to keep up with the patient's hemorrhaging and to hemodynamically stabilize him until he is transferred to surgery. During the same time that the nurse is managing the numerous infusions, she continuously lavages the patient's stomach, communicates with the patient and his wife to keep them informed about the situation, monitors the patient's responses minute by minute to evaluate the effectiveness of the infusions, assists to some degree with insertion of the cutdown and the arterial lines, and then assists with the endoscopy. In each instance, the nurse's judgment and actions are oriented by the patient's responses and/or the demands of the changing situation. This is what we mean by a response-based practice. The nurse has the presence of mind and sufficient rapport with the patient to clarify that, despite previous ordeals, the patient and his wife are committed to further treatment because the diagnosis of amyloidosis had not yet been made. Although developing nurses need to learn to prioritize care, in situations such as this, few interventions could be labeled "low priority."

This story illustrates a central theme in the development of expertise. Although the nurse's suspicions that the patient may be having a myocardial infarction are understandable but incorrect, she immediately learns from the experience so that a week later, when the patient presents with similar changes, the nurse instantaneously grasps the significance of the evolving complication and calls for help. In the first instance, the nurse's initial judgment is influenced by only appreciating several of the patient's symptoms (chest pain, tachycardia) out of context with the whole clinical picture. Further, she counts on the nasogastric drainage as a reliable indicator that the patient is not bleeding. By the second incident, the nurse develops greater expertise by learning how to recognize this specific patient's subtle physical presentation of early bleeding. Learning to recognize the nature of a clinical situation is at the heart of all practical reasoning and therefore accurate judgment (Bourdieu,1980/1990). Her hunch is confirmed when the patient vomits bright red blood clots. In the second instance, reinsertion of the nasogastric tube is then needed to help remove the gastric blood to alleviate the patient's vomiting and to reduce the potential for aspiration. This story illustrates how effective situated learning can be; that is, teaching and learning clinical grasp can be when the learner is engaged in the situation. The nurse now understands the patient's particular modus operandi. After learning to grasp the presenting symptoms of this patient's GI bleed from the surgeon, the nurse teaches the orientee and another nurse the following week. The nurse describes a culture of community learning that extends the clinical wisdom of one to many. Thoughtfully nurturing a community of learning is a powerful and enduring way to continually develop expertise among clinicians.

This nurse's performance demonstrates another feature that characterizes excellent practice. In the midst of the crisis, she evolves as the clinical leader who orchestrates what interventions are needed and who needs to be called, despite the presence of two physicians. Because both physicians are deeply involved in urgent procedures, the nurse notices that there is no one other than herself to "call the shots." As in this case, the diagnosis and management of life-sustaining physiological functions in unstable patients regularly calls for the nurse to perform as the experiential leader. This aspect of excellent practice is further discussed in Chapter 5.

Managing multiple, simultaneous interventions extend beyond direct patient care and the management of various infusions. In the following account, the nurse was also responsible for assisting with the insertion of life-support equipment, an intra-aortic balloon pump (IABP) as well as a cardiopulmonary assist device:

Nurse: A 22-year-old patient had a residual ASD [atrial septal defect] after correction of his transposition of the great vessels. He had been having some problems and a little bit of dyspnea so they decided it would be a good idea to close the ASD off. It was probably compromising him a little bit. He got back [from surgery] in the afternoon and did okay over the night, but not great. He had a few pressure problems, was on some dopamine, a little epi[nephrine], and nipride—the usual. And that morning, he was awake and I said, 'Well, we'll see what we can do.' I talked to him, did my first set of vital signs and...everything looked okay. Then his MAP [mean arterial pressure] started to fall. I went, 'Oh, dear, I think we're going to have problems here.' So I got some residents in and Sam [physician] happened to come in at the time, and we titrated the drips and got the epi up. And it wasn't doing a lot. I got some gases, the P[a]O$_2$ was declining. I said, 'Well, we've got a little bit of a problem here.' So, Sam came in and he put the [intraaortic] balloon (IABP) in. And the patient just kept going downhill from there. The IABP helped for a little while. We still couldn't oxygenate him really well. And that went on all day, and then his P[a]O$_2$ really started dropping, down into the 40s. We put him on 100%, did this, that and the other, but nothing was working. Then they decided they'd try the Biomedicus [extracorporeal life support]. I'm going, 'Oh dear.' So Chris [perfusionist] came over with all the equipment, and we put in the Biomedicus, and then Chris hooked him up to it. We were able to oxygenate him for a while... [but he eventually died of heart failure.]

In the midst of trying to hemodynamically stabilize the patient's rapidly deteriorating condition by titrating several vasoactive drugs, the nurse drew blood gases to evaluate the therapies. After the balloon pump is placed, the nurse additionally takes over the monitoring and management of the IABP. As in many ICUs throughout the country, the nurse is later responsible for the management of the patient on the Biomedicus, as well as the operation and maintenance of the machine itself. These kinds of situations place weighty and continuous demands on the nurse's judgment and performance because these patients are already in a deteriorated, unstable state and any change in the flows and pressures produced by the equipment typically create the need to balance other hemodynamic interventions such as drug infusions. Skillful management requires a thorough understanding of the patient's condition, the meaning of the patient's responses, and the equipment and pharmacological agents used.

Physiological interventions necessarily take precedence when life-threatening changes occur. It is not unusual for a patient to remain unstable for extended periods of time or to have frequent episodes of instability which either delay routine care or completely interrupt it. Over time, however, many routine interventions must be completed in order to prevent complications and to provide meaningful comfort care to the patient when possible. The majority of the routine and non-emergent nursing interventions are performed concurrently with or in addition to those that are of higher priority. For instance, comfort needs and preventative care can often take precedence only after the urgent physiologic needs are managed. Although less urgent, comfort and preventative care are no less important, particularly from the patient's and family's point of view. There are some situations where the comfort needs are simultaneously the most pressing physiological needs. In the following exemplar, Jackie Cunningham, an ED nurse, details a poignant account of trying to provide instantaneous therapies in an urgent moment when meeting Martha's physiological need will also provide a vital element of comfort. She remorsefully remembers how unbearable it was to try to mobilize Tom, the physician's assistant (PA) to act:

Nurse: I can't remember all the details exactly, but I remember exactly how I felt. Annie, my very new orientee and I were in the ED. Not much going on at the time. Jack, one of our critical care floats had a busy patient, so I went over to see if he needed help. He was concerned and aggravated. He had a hypotensive patient, low EF (ejection fraction), whom he had been trying to get the PA and the MD to start pressors on. They had not been inclined to do so. "She needs to be started on something for her BP and I have suggested it at least 100 times, and they want to wait," he said with exasperation. I knew exactly how he felt, and I went back to my station, comfortable that he was an experienced nurse and would do whatever he had to do to get what he needed for that patient. Soon it was shift change and Dana, a new grad just off orientation, had the patient. I was nervous. Dana looked anxious, even though Russ is still there finishing up his paperwork, so I felt compelled to see what I could do to help. Dana called my name and asked me to come into the room. "She just almost went out on me!" The patient just had a transient episode of bradycardia and unresponsiveness, and was now waking, but anxious, dusky and hypotensive. Her skin was cold and clammy and there was almost a translucent quality about it. As I went in, I observed the patient's BP was in the 70's. "Okay, Dana, let's lower her head," and calmly lowered the head of her bed, while also instructing Dana to get the MD. Martha, the patient was awake, breathing rapidly but was non-verbal. Her blood pressure came up to the 80's with the head of bed lowered. Martha's daughter was at the bedside, smiled at me, seemed relieved to see me and took my hand. She told me I had looked after her mother a month ago, and that I had helped get her into Boston where she had a cath, and did I remember them. "Dr. Martin, right?" I said hurriedly and smiled at her. "Yes" she responded. By now the MD and Tom, the PA, caring for the patient were also in the room and giving orders. It was apparent to me that Dana was in over her head with this patient and 4 others in her assignment. I felt the daughter was so relieved by recognizing me from a prior episode that had a positive outcome. I had to get involved. I told Annie that we were going to take this patient. Dana was thanking me over and over again for helping her. "My pleasure" I told her, "We help each other." Inside I was thinking, "Okay, here we go." I took a deep breath. I was going to have to go after what Russ had tried to get earlier and, if he could not get the orders, I certainly was going to have trouble.

Martha was deteriorating but remained awake and alert, complaining of chest pain. Annie was looking at me for guidance so I suggested some tasks, "Okay, Annie, we are going to leave her hooked up to the Zoll. First, let's get her something for pain and then get a Foley catheter into her." I remember feeling the urgency to be able to have some idea of her renal perfusion after her prolonged hypotension. Tom was hesitant on the pain med as the patient remained hypotensive, and I told him then we WOULD be starting pressors AND medicating this patient. As I was talking to Martha and her daughter, I mentioned that we may need to go back into Boston to take care of her heart problems and it was then the patient and daughter informed us that she did not want <u>anything</u> done, even if it would save her life. I called for Tom to inform him of their wishes, and tell him again we needed pain med. I was frustrated at not being able to give her any sedation, especially now that the focus had changed from one of rescue to end of life care and comfort.

As we are waiting for Tom at the bedside, I talked to the daughter. Martha's husband had died many years ago. Since her father died, the daughter had never married and had devoted herself to her mother. Her daughter told me how beautiful her mother had always been, and how her mother was always so modest and careful about her grooming. "I was always the ugly one," the daughter said, "My mother was always such a dignified beautiful woman." I tried to keep Martha covered as much as possible throughout placement of the Foley catheter and positioning of equipment. As Tom entered the room, I informed him of the patient's and daughter's decision regarding resuscitation. In order not to discuss the DNR at the bedside over the patient, he takes the daughter out of the room where he goes over the DNR papers. The rest happened so quickly. Martha was hypotensive, and taking deep rattling death breaths. She kept saying how much it hurt and could hear herself breathing. "Why am I making this noise," she gasped. "I can't stop it making this sound." I do not recall any patient I had before or after being so close to death and so alert until the very end. I felt almost overwhelming desperation. I told Martha not to worry, we were going to take care of her and make her comfortable. Annie looked absolutely horrified. Tom was with the daughter STILL going over the DNR forms. I remember feeling so impatient as he is concerned about getting a signature from the daughter. I want pain med and the daughter at the bedside with her mother. Martha's heart rate started to drop again and I felt there was no time for further delay. I went to the door of the room and said firmly, "Tom, I need for her to come into this room RIGHT NOW and I am going to give this patient some Morphine RIGHT NOW." I had already asked Annie to pull some out. I felt I could not leave the bedside myself as Annie was obviously struggling with her own emotions. As Tom and the daughter entered the room, I told the daughter to take her mother's hand. I was desperate to give Martha back some of her control and let her go in peace and dignity. "I think Martha is leaving us," "Go ahead and talk to her," I said, as gently as I could to her daughter, as Martha started to fade. It seemed like forever before Annie rushed back with the morphine. As Martha took her last breaths, I desperately scrambled to give this dying woman some relief. But I could not give it fast enough. She died before I could do what would seem to be the simplest thing to help ease her into the next life. I will never forget her last final agonizing breath. The daughter was sobbing and Annie was trying not to cry. Tom looked sick, my eyes were welling up and I was mortified at the events that had just unfolded and my absolute inability to intervene. I stood there, holding Martha's hand, with the morphine syringe in my other hand feeling totally useless. I literally felt like I had the wind knocked out of me. I knew I would have to review this whole event with Annie to help her cope with this new end of life experience. Sue the advocate was staying with the daughter and I made sure that we called a friend or family member to come and be with Dr. Martin. I hugged her and told her that her mother was now at peace and that her mother was very lucky to have a daughter like her. I told her as we stood by Martha's bedside that when it is time to move on to the next life, one could not ask for more than to have the people you love the most with you when you passed, and that her mother must be very happy she had her as her daughter.

Outside the room I thanked everyone involved for their help. I knew later on, after I went to bed, I would be revisiting Martha and her daughter again, before I would be able sleep.

Jackie bravely tells a story of tragedy—not being able to do "the simplest thing to help ease" Martha's pain and suffering. She reveals being morally distressed, "mortified," by her failed notion of good; in this case, her lost struggle to mobilize essential team members leaves her unable to do what she believes a good nurse would do. Instead, her "absolute inability to intervene" leaves her distraught. Jackie does not lack a strong moral voice or the courage and persistence required of strong agents. Instead, Jackie tries to manage the patient's urgent needs while she simultaneously tries to wait, respectfully, for the emotion-laden, weighty discussion about the DNR to transpire. In this situation, the PA fails to fully grasp the urgent, competing goods and the precedence that the patient's pain, suffering from pulmonary secretions, and awareness of the closeness of death should have had over a long discussion about the DNR. At the end, Martha's timing outpaces Tom's, before the nurse gains access to the vital instantaneous therapies.

One of the most covered-over challenges, with ever-increasing workloads, is to accomplish everything that is important within greater time constraints. In the narrative, for the outside reader, the noise, demands, ambiguity and bustle of this ER's controlled chaos with patients lining the corridors are nonexistent. For the nurse, what MUST be done (includes documentation imposed by hospitals and agencies) and what is IMPORTANT to do (what patients need) are not always the same or clear but both compete for clinicians' time and attention. In most of the narratives and in almost all of practice, an invisible challenge is the very narrow window of time that a nurse is boxed into to meet a patient's changing needs. Moments, as in Jackie's case, can mean comfort versus tragedy. Few clinicians openly share the heartbreaks but most clinicians experience failed notions of good. Experienced nurses often say, "what doesn't kill you will make you stronger." Some mean "what doesn't kill your spirit will give you the courage to go on." Others indicate that what is learned will make the clinician better. For developing clinicians who struggle to cope with failed notions of good, reflection on what one might do differently in future situations and debriefing with experts who have learned good ways of coping can help foster the courage and conviction to learn what is possible and to come to terms with what it is to be human (predictably imperfect) in a human practice.

In retrospect, it is always easier to judge how close death was during the DNR discussion; however, if one imaginatively enters Martha's room without already knowing the end, she is fully alert and appropriate, indicating there is time. Martha's unusual alertness throws off skillful discernment, which is based on past and, what appeared to be, similar instances. Jackie ethically comports herself to wait respectfully. Had Martha's mentation deteriorated as expected, the competing goods would have disappeared in favor of the only good—comfort. However, instantaneous intervention with morphine is mandated once the death rattle is audible, as it a qualitative distinction indicative of imminent death.

In the midst of this high-demand situation, Jackie remains attuned and interpersonally engaged with the daughter, as the daughter talks about her devoted care for Martha and how beautiful Martha has been throughout her life. Although Jackie cannot sit down to be physically comforting, she provides the needed emotional comfort while trying to manage the patient's hypotension, chest pain, and physiological deterioration. In this case, there are no periods of lower demand which might have afforded the nurse an opportunity to complete other comfort care interventions.

However, during times of continuous intensive care in very unstable patients, routine and preventative measures cannot be neglected and nurses often find creative ways of working them into or between the implementation of more urgent treatments. In ordinary, everyday nursing practice, the physiologic practices are necessarily constant and pervasive, so much so that some are accomplished without conscious awareness. For example, when bathing patients, nurses often capitalize on that time to emotionally connect with them personally, educate them about their condition and their risk factors, or to physically assess aspects of their bodies that are not continuously visible. Although an observer may only notice the activity of bathing and educating of patients, this is also a time of assessment of the patient's tolerance level and reserves.

One of the patient situations with the highest-performance and high time demands—physically, intellectually, and emotionally—is the management of a patient who has become an organ donor. In many patients, once the brain is irreversibly damaged and begins to fail, all organ functions rapidly deteriorate and must be artificially supported to preserve adequate physiological function until the organs can be harvested. At the point that a patient becomes an organ donor, care provided by physicians typically ceases and nurses assume total responsibility for diagnosing and managing the patient's vital functions in conjunction with an organ procurement agency. The period of total body support can take hours before organ harvest is possible. Adequate care requires continuous, rapidly paced, and simultaneous monitoring, intervention, and communication. This is reflected in the following excerpt about a devastating injury that leaves a child brain dead and his parents decide on organ donation:

Nurse: This was a nine-year-old boy, involved in a skateboarding accident where he fell on his head. Severe edema affects the part of the brain where they just produce so much urine and you have to give them medication like DDAVP [pitressin] to turn it around and keep them from peeing out because it drops their blood pressure. But like multiple trauma patients, you're always doing something every minute...their blood pressure drops, you have to keep on top of their fluids. We have to give antibiotics and have certain labs drawn that the donor agency people want to know about, so that they can get the best match for the [recipients], like liver function tests, blood typing, electrolytes, CBCs, and [other blood counts]. Also, this particular patient was oxygenating, but his brain was so compromised that it was starting to compromise other parts of his body. So his lungs were in really bad shape and he was on 100% FiO_2 and his blood gases were poor. But they were trying to save his lungs so that they could use them, and so you needed to continuously draw blood gases, and you're on the phone with the organ donor people every hour, updating them, and they're telling you what to do and you're telling them what's going on and coordinating. That is hard.

Interviewer: At that point, are the residents on your unit totally out of the picture?

Nurse: Yes, and the status of the patient is changing almost every hour, so he's dumping out 2 L of urine every hour and you need to replace that with IV fluids, plus the maintenance fluid, plus blood, plus you're replacing KCl because they're peeing so much. There's always tons going on in the room—it's really hard....

Interviewer: How about keeping track of their potassium. Everything you hang has potassium in it?

Nurse: Right. But sometimes it will change from hour to hour, because one hour they've peed out 2 L. Next hour you give them four boluses of KCl. In the meantime, you've given them pitressin to stop their urinary output. The next hour, then their K^+ is 4.9 so then you have to change all your IV bags again. Their sodium is going up, their sodium is going down. It's always changing like that. And that's why you need to keep in constant contact with the [donor agency] people because they're really precise about the levels that they want. The margins that they allow on the patients are really narrow.

Interviewer: And so to do that, then you're also drawing stat labs, all the time?

Nurse: Yeah, all the time. Blood gases, I'd say about every four hours for sure, and often more than that... Once the process is started, there is no stopping it. Not literally, I mean the family could change their mind at any time and they have a right to. But once everybody, once it starts going, it gets really busy and it almost takes two nurses because there are so many different things you have to do. I don't think people understand how difficult it is to take care of a donor. It's almost as difficult, just as difficult as taking care of a multiple trauma patient.

The nurse intimated that "catching up" is never possible in these patients because their physiological conditions change so rapidly that infusion mixtures, flow rates, ventilator settings, et cetera must continually be modified to respond to the patient's needs. The patient's rapid physiological transitions and the necessity for multiple, simultaneous interventions tax nurses to continuously think-in-action as there is no opportunity to stop and think. Adept nurses with excellent clinical judgment are essential to provide the type and amount of care called for and to reason through the complex pathophysiological effects that one failing system has on others. Most of the knowledge gained about managing organ donors is experiential knowledge that has not been well articulated. More articulation and clinical research is needed in this area.

Patients with multisystem organ failure present with such complex clinical situations that it is often difficult for a single clinician to understand an evolving situation alone, especially when the confounding illnesses are undetermined. Multiple team members who are experienced and skillful are commonly needed to grasp a perplexing patient's evolving condition and to determine what interventions are most appropriate. At times, however, the situation is misread or not understood so that numerous interventions get targeted at treating the symptoms while the cause(s) of the complication continues to be unidentified and therefore untreated. Under those circumstances, each additional intervention carries the potential of either ameliorating or further clouding the situation. If the situation becomes too clouded and confused by the myriad of treatments, it is difficult to discern which patient responses are being created by the interventions themselves and which responses point to evolving complications. A neuro ICU nurse eventually found herself lost in terms of understanding the patient's complex and deteriorating condition when four residents and fellows began ordering multiple, simultaneous interventions to treat a patient's tachycardia, hypotension, and low cardiac output:

Nurse: This patient was a 79-year-old lady in a motor vehicle accident who sustained a closed head injury and multiple fractures so she went to the OR where they put in a ventriculostomy. I thought she was pretty stable last night with her ICP [intracranial pressure]. They had her ICP open to drain continuously and her ICP was stable, less than 25 today, so they decided to clamp her. She had a questionable X-ray, widened mediastinum, and so she was supposed to go to angio (angiography), but she became... very hypotensive and became <u>very</u> tachy[cardic]—as high as the 140s so the angio was canceled, and the physicians were at the bedside right away.They tried a couple doses of adenosine, so I guess she didn't really respond so they tried fluid boluses on her. She responded a little bit, like her rate dropped down into the 120s, but then she came back up again in the 130s, so they figured, 'Oh, maybe she's in a lot of pain,' so they tried fentanyl or morphine, but she bottomed her blood pressure. I mean <u>bottomed</u> her blood pressure. So they said, 'Oh, okay, I guess she's not in pain.' But they kept saying, 'Okay, it's okay, she's only in the 140s, but her systolic blood pressure is hanging in the 90s.' They said, 'Maybe she had an MI,' so they did cardiac enzymes, and then they said, 'We need to really go to angio, maybe she has an aortic tear.' So when I came on my shift, her heart rate was 150s, 160s, and her blood pressure bottomed to the 80s. So, they said, 'Oh, okay, we're not going to go to angio. Let's start boluses.' They decided to insert a PA [pulmonary artery] catheter and we just kept giving boluses and boluses. Then they said, 'Let's try esmolol on her', but have neo (phenylephrine) on standby because you know that's going to drop her blood pressure even further. She responded to the esmolol; her heart rate was in the 120s, but then I started neo and maxed out on neo right away, but her blood pressure's still 80. Her hematocrit dropped so we gave her two units of blood, too. We were just giving drug after drug and boluses and everything. The neo maxed out so they said 'Okay, let's do dobutamine.' Her cardiac output was five, but they said,'Maybe she needs a high cardiac output of 10 to sustain a higher blood pressure.' So we tried that, she didn't respond. And then they said, 'Maybe it's not that. So let's try milrinone. I said, 'Why are you using milrinone?' 'Maybe she needs a higher cardiac output.' So we tried but it didn't do anything. So we end up with Levophed and she didn't respond... I was just so lost. I felt like—I was getting frustrated. Probably because I was just doing things. Just doing. They were all at the bedside, you know, they were just hitting the buttons, touching the monitors, and the whole time they were saying, 'Oh, did you start this thing yet? Did you start that thing yet?' It's just like, 'You just told me two seconds ago,' you know? So I felt just like a robot.

This nurse tells the above story after also being clinically observed while caring for the patient 2 days prior. As mentioned, the residents called for one intervention after another and the nurse struggled to keep up with their requests and understand the patient's responses. She described the experience of losing her clinical grasp. She continuously titrated multiple vasoactive drugs and fluids to try to improve the patient's pressure and lower the heart rate. The nurse was surprised by some of the interventions ordered and she grew more concerned. At several points during the evening, she tactfully questioned the logic and treatment direction. She also requested that the fellow discuss the situation with an attending and even called a trusted physician colleague on the case herself. Nevertheless, treatment goals and logic remained unchanged and multi-directional without success. The nurse alluded to the fact that the residents lost their clinical understanding of the patient's condition and began to "chase" the symptoms of the problem as the patient's condition deteriorated beyond recovery. This clinical breakdown incident highlights that, although multiple, simultaneous interventions are commonly life-saving, they can further confuse the patient's clinical picture and dangerously contribute to the patient's demise. Hence, it is imperative for each clinician to realize that numerous, concurrent interventions are life-saving and life-sustaining only when patient responses are assessed and clinical understanding is improved rather than further confused.

As intimated, the clinical demands in this aspect of physiological care call for highly experienced and well prepared clinicians. One expert clinician can be sufficient if that person can take on the clinical leadership role of the team. Leading four residents and fellows is a challenge for even the most skillful nurse, particularly in under-determined situations. The above story is an example of how clear reasoning and understanding can be lost when the particular clinicians are not accustomed to working together and are in unfamiliar territory. The quality of care can be compromised. In contrast, the care of complex unstable patients more commonly is smooth and seamless when team members have experience working together and share common understandings about a patient's condition, therapeutic interventions, and expected patient responses (Hooper, 1995). Collaborative teams set up the possibility of sharing similar concerns, collective problem searches, the negotiation of differing clinical perspectives, and, in the end, the best clinical wisdom and patient care. Continuity in such teams creates the possibility of developing cumulative wisdom. As importantly, collaboration provides the best option for managing breakdown situations where team members can question, uncover misinterpretations, seek the help needed to enlighten the team's understanding, and withdraw confounding interventions that may be clouding the clinical picture. The management of breakdown is a crucial skill in the care of the critically ill and is further discussed in Chapter 11.

In contrast to the above situation, multiple simultaneous interventions are more typically wisely used by skilled physiological knowledge workers. Practice is smoother however when the patient's condition and complications are familiar. Clinicians are less likely to lose their grasp and the causes of adverse patient responses are more readily identified and remedied in familiar situations. During a clinical observation, an expert burn nurse details the patient's current condition and therapy. As in the preceding story, she too discusses a breakdown caused by small doses of valium and fentanyl but immediately recognizes the patient's adverse and unpredictable response to the two simultaneous interventions, withdraws both, and moves on to another pharmacological agent more successfully:

Nurse: His respiratory status is a concern and I won't give him valium again because I didn't trust his reaction to it. Basically the fentanyl took a long time to actually work, and then it caught up with him and then it took a long time for him to get rid of it. Hence, he oxygenated well, but his $PaCO_2$ was too high. It was 58, and he had severe sleep apnea. Severe. Even during the rest of the [scrubbing of the burn areas], we had to keep continually waking him up, and with the fentanyl, he just didn't wake up very well and we had to sit on him a while. In the process of all this, his blood pressure went really high, which is not usual. Systolic was 200 at one point, and his diastolic was 120 I believe. So I just put a bunch of pillows behind him to try to bring his chin forward. I talked to the doc and gave him some nifedipine. His heart rate went really high, 160 to 175. This was all happening at one time and basically I think that he was having sleep apnea, and he was very very groggy, and even though I kept asking him about his pain and he kept saying, 'No, my pain is fine,' I think he had underlying pain that he couldn't articulate because he was too groggy. Once I finally bugged him enough and his meds worn off enough and he started waking up a <u>little</u> more, he then could articulate that he had a little pain and I gave him just a <u>smidgen</u> of morphine, and his heart rate started coming back down again. And by that time, the nifedipine had assisted with his blood pressure, and I think he's doing better.

Interviewer: So, you think his hemodynamics were pain-related?

Nurse: I don't think they were all pain-related. I think probably the stress also [influenced them]. But I was concerned that we did have some deeper problems going on because I wasn't sure how well he was oxygenating. We had a blood gas and he was oxygenating fine, but because he has all four extremities burned and both ears, it's hard to get a pulse oximeter reading. Right now we happen to be lucky; it happens to be working. But it was really intermittent and I felt like I was struggling so, at one point, because there were all of these things happening, I was really unsure what was going on. And I didn't want to give him...I wanted to give him something to control his blood pressure because he kept denying pain to me. But I was also concerned, I didn't want to [vaso]dilate him too much, because he is a little bit hemodynamically dry. I'm not totally sure where we were because we were a little bit dry, although now he looks a lot better (looking at urine output in the urimeter). So, all those thoughts were going on and basically, once he woke up a little bit more and wanted something to drink, he realized, 'Oh, my hands are hurting.' So after giving him a little bit of morphine, his heart rate came down. His blood pressure had already come down <u>some</u> with the nifedipine. As far as his burn status fluids go, he is doing well... We're going to put him on a CPAP mask. I talked to him about [the sleep apnea] at home he said, 'yes,' his wife states that he does stop breathing during the night and that he is exhausted in the mornings when he wakes up. He said as long as he breathes in the morning—he always wakes up, so I said, 'Have you ever had it treated', 'No, there's no reason, I always wake up.' (laughs) Okay, there you have it. So, we're going to put him on a CPAP mask now, that's why I'm waiting for respiratory to call back. And we want to make sure we keep pulses in his fingers, and that's what she's (the orientee) checking right now. He doesn't really have circumferential radial or arm burns over here, but because of the edema that will be created with the fluids we've given him, we just want good circulation down to his fingers. And then he's got more burns on his right hand, so his right hand will be even more important to check on (Observational Interview).

Although the nurse was temporarily confused as to the cause of the patient's hemodynamic abnormalities, she was not "lost." The clinical importance of this distinction is that this burn nurse had a good idea about the physiological causes which permitted her to cautiously control the interfering interventions as she vigorously pursued the problem. As she probed, she discovered that the patient was recovering from drug addictions and he was extremely reluctant to allow the administration of narcotics. His denial of pain contributed to her initial difficulty in understanding his hemodynamic responses. As the situation unfolded, she confirmed her suspicions that the patient was very sensitive to valium and fentanyl. The two drugs "snowed" him and resulted in his extreme grogginess which was complicated by his sleep apnea, but had not sufficiently relieved the pain which he denied. His pain contributed to the hemodynamic abnormalities and needed to be treated in order to provide comfort and better stabilize his condition. In this situation, the nurse's wisdom in prioritizing the problem search over the interventions led to a clear diagnosis of the situation and effective intervention.

Here, this excerpt of the nurse's discussion focused on how the patient's pain, the pain medications, and his respiratory and hemodynamic status were interrelated and temporarily clouded her understanding. Not evident in the discussion are the other multiple simultaneous interventions in progress, such as the hours of wound scrubbing and debridement associated with his burn, application of dressings, ongoing fluid management, continual circulatory assessments, temperature control, history taking, emotional support of the patient and family, discovery of an undiagnosed sleep apnea as a contributing factor, and coaching and teaching the orientee. Although her attention was primarily focused on her verbalized concerns, the monitoring and multi-faceted management of this unstable patient required astute clinical judgment, continuous reasoning through multiple physiological transitions, and interventional adeptness.

COACHING AND ASSISTING PATIENTS IN WEANING FROM LIFE-SUPPORT TECHNOLOGIES

The management of life-sustaining functions in the critically ill commonly focuses on the implementation of therapies to stabilize and improve the patient's condition. Typically, little emphasis is placed on assisting patients to become independent of these supportive interventions. While some assessment technologies (e.g., pulse oximetry) and therapies may be instantly discontinued without destabilizing the patient, the majority of interventions must be tapered or weaned so that the patient can gradually adapt and compensate physiologically. Similarly, some interventions (e.g., anti-dysrhythmic infusions) may be weaned without a conscious effort or assistance on the patient's part; yet many require that the patient actively participate in some way.

Weaning patients who have been chronically dependent on an intervention or technology can require their full and sometimes exhaustive participation. A nurse-patient relationship that allows for attunement and expert coaching based on knowing the patient is required for a safe and successful transition. Therefore, nurses must keep patients and their family members well informed about forthcoming changes and the progress made during the transition. For some patients, weaning is work and can raise anxiety about their ability to again become self-sustaining; consequently, psychological support and reinforcement are essential to success. Not infrequently, patients must begin a weaning process while they still have pain, which can drain the energy needed to wean. Most patients become deconditioned to some degree while in the ICU. Severely deconditioned patients must work to resume physiological functions, such as breathing or moving, that were once effortless. Many patients are unaware of how they can assist in resuming full functioning and require coaching about how to gradually improve their tolerance and abilities. For the chronically critically ill who have been on life-support for extended time periods, coaching them in specific and individualized ways is central to restoring them to independent functioning.

Though essential, technological therapies are rarely benign and are therefore generally weaned and removed as soon as feasible because most can cause complications ranging from minor (e.g., skin irritations from EKG monitoring electrodes) to major problems (e.g., sepsis from central lines, limb loss from IABP catheter) (see Chapter 8). For patients who are very fragile, it is imperative to wean and remove invasive interventions at the earliest possible time because any complication can result in a downward and devastating turn. For instance, neonates in general are very fragile. Consequently, expert clinicians are ever vigilant about weaning interventions that place the infant at high risk. In the following clinical observation, after the nurse begins weaning ventilatory support and is evaluating a neonate's response to the change, she articulates how the risks at stake for the infant orient her practice:

Nurse: This baby was born three days ago at a local hospital, has respiratory distress syndrome (RDS), and he's 37 weeks which is kind of old to have RDS. So, the baby got sick and got transported here three days ago...

Interviewer: How do you know if you're weaning too quickly? Other than gases, can you tell?

Nurse: You mostly have to go by the gases. Sometimes you can tell if the baby's getting real tachypneic. If you've gone way down on the oxygen, obviously your oxygen sats aren't going to stay up as nicely. Or if you made a pressure change, then his breath sounds are going to change, he's not going to sound like he's moving enough air or his chest excursion isn't going to be as good. Mostly you have to look at gases and see what they do. And a lot of times the gases will be fine, and you've weaned for six hours straight and you've had excellent gases and two hours later you'll get a gas that's just the pits. So sometimes it just takes a while for the kid to catch up. And then you end up really having to escalate things. So, I never make more than one move at a time. And a lot of these kids—especially the really tiny ones—can't tolerate big moves. (Respiratory therapist came in). We can drop his oxygen down, maybe to 42, because I had a really good blood gas.

Interviewer: So what do you expect by looking at this baby?

Nurse: I expect his oxygen will be up in the 80-90 range. It will be interesting to see if his CO_2 will go up, his last CO_2 was 47. He's been hanging out mostly in the mid-40's. So he's got some leeway and they're going to allow his CO_2s to get up into the 50 range which is high for an adult. I know you wouldn't want to see a CO_2 of 50—we have kids with CO_2s of 50 and pHs of 7.28 where we accept that, but you get into trouble with these kids. You walk a really fine line between allowing their gases to be what an adult would consider a really poor gas versus leaving them on a ventilator and causing a lot of lung damage. So we try and get them off the ventilator with a minimal amount of damage to the lung as possible...for a baby that's really sick, he's been fairly stable.

Interviewer: What kind of lung damage do you mean?

Nurse: Well, it's not even after three days. Kids can get into trouble right away and develop PIE, pulmonary interstitial emphysema. We see that in the really immature babies where you'll look at their X-ray and it's just all cystic, and then they blow pneumo[thoracie]s, and then they die. You have a lot of stiffening of the lungs. A lot of fluid gets in there and then they get cystic changes and then they develop BPD [broncho-pumonary dysplasia] and chronic lung disease, so you really need to get them off the ventilator as soon as you can and if that means accepting borderline gases, then that's what we do. We'll even accept a PO_2 in the 40's, figuring the kids with cardiac lesions have PO_2s in the 40's and they do fine, so why not preemies with PO_2s in the 40's? But that's the exception rather than the rule. We accept, on most of the kids—we call them the 50/50 Club—they have PO_2s of 50 and CO_2s of 50, and we rarely go up into the 60s, but we will. We'll let them drift up a little. And I can see what they would do in an adult unit—they'd freak out. [The lab returned with the ABG results.] Oh, what an excellent blood gas! CO_2 only went up one, so that's okay, so we can probably either drop the flow, which we talked about, or just start weaning on his FiO_2 a little bit. When they came around on rounds and—(looking at the chart) he's on a flow of 14 which is a lot—14 liters per minute. That's a lot of flow, he shouldn't require any more than maybe ten... He was on an inspiratory time of .75 which is a long inspiratory time. I've seen chronic preemies on inspiratory times of 1 which is again really long. And again, that causes a lot of barotrauma to the lungs, so you try to minimize that by weaning that down. An appropriate time for him would be 0.6. I'd like to see his flow get down to 10. But you have a tendency, if you get these good gases then you wean and wean and wean. You do it too fast and then the infants crump, they just can't keep up with it. So you have to use your judgement and take it slow (Observational Interview).

Although the monitoring technology is changing, the skilled know-how of closely monitoring, keeping track of how the baby is tolerating the weaning, and constantly reasoning in the unfolding situation is essential. As the nurse points out, preventing unnecessary injury that technology can cause is a high priority in such a compromised patient so that wide swings in his PO_2 and CO_2 are potentially less harmful than the risk of barotrauma. Here, the nurse attentively monitors the infant's progress and is already thinking ahead about the next best step for weaning. At the same time, the nurse is equally clear about the risks of weaning too fast. She passes on two important maxims that express experiential wisdom gained from weaning. First, "never make more than one move at a time." As articulated in the previous section, the more interventions that are implemented simultaneously, the harder it is to accurately interpret the patient's responses. This maxim has been found to be pervasive in expert practice, both with weaning and adding or increasing therapies (Hooper, 1995). Second, "especially the really tiny kids can't tolerate big moves." Smaller, more frequent changes allow the very fragile infant a better chance to "keep up" physiologically than when big changes in therapy are implemented. Equilibration is crucial in preventing delayed deterioration.

Not all neonates in the ICU are as critically ill as the infant in the above story. Although some are less frail, care must still be taken to steadily but gradually wean them from technological support. As they are gently transitioned, their physiological responses serve as the primary indicator of their tolerance and their ability to reach a new level of equilibrium. If the neonate demonstrates no signs of decompensation, the weaning process can commonly follow a typical step-by-step course. In the following excerpt, the nurse articulates how she expects to progressively wean the infant from nutritional support and from the isolette:

Nurse: This little boy is a 34-weeker. Mom had pregnancy-induced hypertension. So he was intubated but not for very long. He has been extubated for several days now. So at this point he has to learn how to eat. He is being gavage fed and has a total parenteral nutritional (TPN) infusion because he is not able to take in quite enough yet. He is working on it though. He is taking in 23 cc now, and his TPN is at 4 cc. So if he continues to take in 23 cc okay, I will drop his TPN to 3 cc. So he is progressing nicely and he really doesn't have any other problems. He was initially on antibiotics but they have been discontinued... He is going to be here at least three weeks minimum and probably closer to his actual due date. We have to wean him off his TPN, wean him out of the isolette and begin nippling... Even though his TPN rate is only 4 cc, we drop it really slowly. 1 cc every couple of days. We will start weaning him out of the isolette slowly also. He is a good size baby for his age. Once we make some progress on those two things, he will be transferred to the intermediate side and we can really work on nippling and growing.

Interviewer: Talk a little about weaning from the isolette?

Nurse: Well first I'll put on a little T-shirt and a blanket and turn down the temperature in the isolette and watch his temperature. Then we will progress to two blankets and the isolette turned down farther. Working at bringing the isolette temperature down as far as it will go. Then we will bring him out and see how he does. Now depending on how well he holds his temperature and what he weighs by then, we will decide if he needs a heated crib or a regular crib. It just depends (Observational Interview).

Notice that the nurse repeatedly mentions, as she describes each step of the weaning process, that she will watch how the infant responds or tolerates the change. Although she has a step-by-step plan in mind, progression depends on the infant's responses along the way and she will follow the baby's lead. As is true throughout this domain, close observation and attentiveness characterize this aspect of expert judgment and practice. It also brings up the maxim of "following the body's lead" (Benner, 1994a). The next step is guided by the particular infant's response to the last step.

In each situation, excellent practice is guided by the particular patient's response to change. This infant's tolerance to the reduction in his parenteral nutrition infusion indicates that he is ready for another small transition. In contrast, adult patients can sometimes tolerate big changes that can safely be implemented without compromising the patient. Additionally, substantive changes are called for in situations where the patient is receiving a therapy that replaces a current, and more invasive or risky one. The following is an example of a nurse who is comfortably weaning two vasoactive drugs off the patient rapidly because oral medications were started:

Nurse: [Titrates the nitroglycerin down] So her pressure's fine. She's totally off nipride now.

Interviewer: And what did you do with the nitro[glycerin]?

Nurse: I brought it down about 20 mics per minute, from 130 to 110. And I did that because her [systolic] pressure's like 140, it's in a very nice range. Most people don't react to nitroglycerin dramatically in terms of blood pressure. Nipride is much more potent in that regard. But each person's different, and you have to see. And sometimes you can wean it down and all of a sudden find out, 'Oh, well! Guess they <u>were</u> sensitive.' But I'll be checking it...I've got to get some more nitro, it looks like. I'm not going to be able to wean it quite fast. [Getting another bag of nitroglycerin ready to hang. She's positioned the patient for rest and removed her glasses and repositioned her arm on the pillow. Later the nurse titrates the nitro again.]

Interviewer: So her nitro, you titrated down again to what now?

Nurse: I'm moving faster. She's not responding—it's not touching her.

Interviewer: Because you think her oral agents are kicking in?

Nurse: Yeah. I know what her pressure is and I know she's fine and I know that I can come down on it, so I'm going to do it. Her pressure's not budging much with what I've done so far, so I'm assuming one thing and that is that the amlodipine is working and we're seeing the effects of it, so I can come down, down, down (Observational Interview).

This aggressive kind of weaning is not typical, especially in the early phases. However, the patient's specific response, the lack of a hemodynamic change, guides this nurse's judgment in weaning two familiar medications. Because both drugs produce instantaneous responses and the patient's pressure remains stable, the nurse grows confident that larger changes are safe. Unlike ventilatory changes, these particular drugs do not tend to cause delayed responses. As she points out, each patient is different and one must start slowly to safely evaluate how the patient will respond. The nurse does, however, follow the maxim previously articulated, "Never make more than one move at a time." When one change is implemented at a time and the patient does not tolerate the change, clinicians do not have difficulty then identifying which change is associated with the patient's adverse response.

Weaning is commonly considered a physiological intervention and taught as such. However, when patients have been dependent on a therapy for an extended time and their active participation is requisite for weaning, the nurse's coaching skills are as essential as her or his weaning skills. After extended periods of of dependency on care, patients can become depressed, not solely related to the disease, but also due to a sense of hopelessness, failure, and a lack of control. Also, chronically ill patients commonly become nutritionally debilitated and are unable to tolerate the required work of taking on normal functioning. An ICU nurse describes such a situation where she and the healthcare team are able to coach and successfully wean a particularly difficult patient:

> **Nurse:** This 72-year-old guy with COPD came in, was put on the ventilator, and developed an acute abdomen with repeated complications...he had settled on the idea that he was going to be lung damaged forever—that he would be a respiratory cripple—so his motivation wasn't there. What we had to do was convince him that his idea wasn't true because of the new ventilators and how wonderful they are, we were able to keep his FiO_2 down to a more reasonable level where he didn't have permanent damage. We're always reluctant to turn up the oxygen...and so he didn't have a lot of lung damage and he had to be convinced that, yes he could get off the ventilator, and no, he would not be a cripple. He could be up walking and on oxygen at home and as soon as we convinced him of that—L. (attending) just came in one day, I was there and it was like, 'Should I believe it?' More or less after he asked the question straight out and she said, 'Oh yes, you'll probably be on oxygen for awhile but you'll probably be home.' By this time he was trached and had been on it for months and months but we had to convince him that he could be off the ventilator and the only way he could get out of here was to be off the ventilator and so that turned him around right there.
>
> **Interviewer:** How do you know that it turned around?
>
> **Nurse:** Because of the length of time he was willing to put up with the T-tube CPAP trials, and that takes [a lot of] effort. Sometimes we don't always appreciate how much work it is for these guys once they go more than a half hour not having a machine blow air in them. It really takes a lot of effort if you're willing to make that effort, and he did it... We told him, 'You've got to get off this ventilator or you're going to die.' If you work with a guy for a few months, you can tell it straight, making it short and sweet like that. You just make it very clear, 'You can get off the ventilator. You can get off the ventilator. And do it by getting yourself up, getting yourself around, and moving those muscles. You put yourself in a positive nitrogen balance,' and you just repeat this over and over. Because that's a big part of getting him off the ventilator is to have him in a positive nitrogen balance and you cannot get there, no matter what nutrition you give them unless you get them up and exercise them. Until we get them up and move them around, get them out of bed and walk them around, it doesn't happen and they don't get off the ventilator... [The patient eventually weaned and went home.] But I heard this guy is back to his writing.

Coaching patients takes on an individualized character. This nurse's approach could be criticized as harsh and this same style in another patient could be completely demotivating. Yet, this nurse has been his primary nurse for months and presumably the close working relationship conveyed her concern and allowed the patient to trust her judgment. The patient has not completely given up, but his fear is that he will be a "cripple." Given a new sense of possibility, he is able to do the work required. The challenge escalates when a patient gives up completely and prefers to die. The difficulties for this team are: 1) to convince the patient that he can wean and 2) to coach him to be involved in enough activity that he can eventually achieve a positive nitrogen balance, strengthen his respiratory muscles, and wean from the ventilator. Their close monitoring and physiological interventions are essential but, for this patient, the coaching and his subsequent determination make the difference. Nurses as coaches create imagination for what is possible based on their first hand experiential knowledge of seeing similar transitions in other patients. The patient is able to move into the next step often based on the confidence of the nurse's encouragement and even concreteness about the next step.

Coaching requires varying degrees of cheering, nudging or pushing patients to do more than they imagine they can. It is especially helpful that the nurse in the above story can empathize with the difficulty experienced by the patient. She expresses, "We don't always appreciate how much work it is for these guys." Sincere acknowledgment of the patient's labor and hardship is a core caring practice of recognizing the patient's plight. To ignore the patient's plight creates a false consciousness of control rather than care and solidarity with the patient. Her recognitional practice of the patient's plight orients the nurse to coach and encourage the patient in a compassionate manner. Although seldom assessed, patients commonly convey that the nurse's caring helps them persevere and make a difference in their ability to recover. When patients tell the nurse, "I couldn't have done it without you," it could not be more true.

Nurses have taught us that to best coach a patient for the work of weaning, nurses must first know the patient. Knowing the patient involves having a keen sense about what the patient views as a possible, realistic, and meaningful outcome. Knowing the patient also means that the nurses/healthcare team must recognize the patient's physiological capabilities and limitations so that the patient is not being encouraged to do the impossible. Second, to effectively help and encourage the patient, nurses must develop good coaching skills (Benner, 1984). Knowing what to do and say, when to act, when to stand back, how hard to push, and recognizing what the patient will interpret and accept as help are essential skills. Further, to help different patients, nurses need flexibility in their styles of coaching in order to best respond to the way that a particular patient is best encouraged. They must learn to "read" each patient and follow the patient's lead, even when nudging. Third, nurses need to develop the courage to skillfully push because compelling the patient on in the work of weaning and then having to witness their suffering as a result of weaning or complications can be unbearable. It is rarely clear how far to nudge, so expert coaching relies on full engagement and attunement to the patient's tolerance and limits. And, in some cases, the patient will target their frustrations at the nurse. Coaching a patient for weaning is difficult work that requires good clinical sensibilities, judgment, and interventional and relational skills. These skills are developed experientially, as nurses learn through trial and error in working with many kinds of patients.

Possibly the hardest skill to learn in coaching a patient for weaning is knowing how hard to push. When patients have complicated illnesses and express good reasons when they "cannot" do something, such as getting up to a chair, it is difficult to discern the cause of their resistance. Are they too fatigued and do not want to get up? Or is it a lack of confidence that they can actually do the activity? Or is their condition on the verge of worsening so that they cannot tolerate the activity? Moral tension is created by the fact that, if some patients are left to determine their own activity levels, many will never wean. Nurses are further encouraged to push because of their past experience with patients who did successfully wean and who later thanked the nurses for pushing. Fragile patients with multiple illnesses commonly present a daunting challenge in this arena of clinical judgment. To accomplish a tough wean, nurses find themselves having to coach or push patients to their maximum potential. The problem, of course, is that the maximum potential is often unknown until it is surpassed and the patient decompensates. As the ICU nurse in an excerpt from an account cited in Benner, Tanner and Chesla (2009, p. 139) explains, knowing the patient is crucial to being able to read how far to push:

Nurse 1: An adult patient had an abdominal aortic aneurysm repair, developed ARDS, developed pneumothoracies, and would become bradycardic if taken off of the ventilator. He developed ATN [acute tubular necrosis], required dialysis, and was tenuous for months...he also had three times when it looked like he was really moving along, and then something would happen. He'd get a mucous plug or pneumonia or something that wasn't picked up, and he'd be back. When he went backwards, he always took a giant leap backwards...it wasn't a small step backwards. It took a long time to get over those...

Nurse 2: Sometimes I just had to gauge what I was doing with him on how quickly he would become hypoxic, so it wasn't a matter of there weren't any numbers there because I would have to get a blood gas, take it to the lab, do whatever you had to do. You had to base a lot of what you were doing on what was happening with him right then. And rather than get a test to say, 'I've documented it,' you had to more or less look at him right then. And to know his fatigue, know just how much he could do. I was taking care of him one time and you had to really listen to him, not like ask him if he wanted to get out of bed or want to eat...there were so many things he didn't want to do after his [emotional] withdrawal period or he would only be selective with people that he was involved with. It was just a matter of why he resisted it, and did it mean to coax him or that you'd pushed him too far?

Nurse 1: And that wasn't always clear, because sometimes you'd push him and then discover that was the wrong thing to do because he would decompensate. I mean that happened up to a week before he left. Somebody got him up and tried to get him walking, which we were doing on a regular basis then, and he shouldn't have. He didn't want to do it and we tried to do it anyway, and it was like, 'Quick, get the chair under him.' He just couldn't do it.

These nurses gauged their coaxing on the patient's responses: his fatigue or hypoxia levels. This kind of observation requires that the person helping the patient be an astute observer and that they know the pathophysiological effects and clues to activity and overactivity. Even when careful, skillful nurses using their best judgment can push too far.

In the current healthcare climate, particularly given the current "fast tracking" of getting acutely ill patients out of the hospital quickly, patients must be mobilized within hours after surgery. The press toward cost containment has caused many interventions, such as early mobilization of patients, to be misunderstood as a mundane task. Once understood as mundane, it is easily delegated to unlicensed personnel who are ill prepared to interpret the patient's responses and to detect early decompensation. Nurses, advanced practice nurses, managers, and clinical pathway coordinators must make clinical distinctions in what particular patients need for skillful care and to not set up systems where skilled clinicians are delegating clinical judgment and skilled performance to technicians who are under-skilled.

At times, despite their most concerted efforts, nurses are unable to reach patients who have given up. No amount or style of coaching encourages the patient to engage in their own care and recovery. But, in a few of those cases, nurses occasionally stumble upon something and discover how to reconnect a patient to her or his world. The reconnection subsequently gives the patient the will to recover. An advanced practice nurse discusses such a situation in the following story:

> **Advanced Practice Nurse:** We were on rounds and we had a particularly young patient in his mid 30's, who, three or four days before he was admitted to the hospital, told his wife he thought he was going to die. And he was admitted and was in just unbelievable respiratory distress. He was in ARDS, was on reverse I:E ratio, was on maximum mechanical ventilatory therapy, and we were still not oxygenating this man. And he was [pharmacologically] paralyzed. We would let him wake up every once in a while, just to check his neuro status. When he did come up, he wrote a note to his wife, 'Let me die.' And this guy was in his mid 30's and had a 5- and a 7-year-old at home, and his wife was just devastated. Medically, we were just like, 'What are we going to do? We've tapped all of our resources.' And, so we had critical care rounds this particular day, and I had spent a lot of time reading about families and visiting and children, and was trying to make some changes in our institution as well, and so I talked to his wife and talked to the whole multi-disciplinary team and said, 'I'd like to have his children come to see him.' And so I talked to his wife, and she said, 'Okay, I'll bring the kids in.' We of course let him wake up a bit [by stopping the paralytic drugs], and I sat down and spent some time with the kids in the visiting room and talked to them about what they would see with their dad and what to expect. We went into the room and I let down the bed rail and, within seconds, all of a sudden his leg came flinging off the bed, and I thought, 'Oh my gosh! What I have done? He's going to try to extubate himself.' And a couple of seconds later, he took his toes and he started pinching his little boy and his wife, and we were all in tears by this. Well, she just looked at me and she said, 'He's in there.' She said, 'That's what he does all the time. He plays with the kids like that all the time.' And the little kid put his head on his dad's lap and his dad was stroking his hair and his face, and they brought in a picture, and they taped it on the ventilator and within 24 hours this guy was extubated! It was just, 'Oh my gosh!' It was like all of a sudden, like he just snapped (snaps fingers) and said, 'You know, I've got a reason to live.' And it was phenomenal, I mean, 2 days later he was out of the unit. It was unbelievable... After the children were there, we debriefed them a bit. They sedated him again for a while, but his pressures started to go down, he started improving, and overnight, he just had marked improvement, and the next morning he was extubated. This all went on about one o'clock in the afternoon, and by the next morning he was extubated. I couldn't believe it!

In this situation, not only had the patient given up on the hope of recovery, he had also given up the desire to live. Worse, the nurse stated that all possible resources had been tapped to try to improve his deteriorating physiological condition. Under those circumstances, it appeared as if there was nothing more that could be done to save this young man's life. In the care of the critically ill, the strong emphasis is on physiological interventions that are life-saving. Among expert nurses, there is also a deep and earnest respect for the power of care, concern, and connectedness in creating new possibilities (Benner & Wrubel, 1989). Being drawn back into one's world of concerns and meanings has profound motivating and healing powers. This intervention unexpectedly turned the patient around and helped him to reconnect to what was most meaningful and world-defining—his family. By the next morning, the patient was extubated.

When weaning patients from interventional support, nurses' concerns extend beyond the patient. Because various team members are involved with different weaning processes, excellent care involves collaboration and mutual coaching among team members. Collaboration and mutual coaching set up an environment of constant learning, as well as a safety net to prevent mistakes, correct discrepancies, hone clinical judgment, and take advantage of their collective wisdom (Hooper, 1995). The following excerpt provides a glimpse of how collaborative relationships set up the possibility for coaching and/or correction through collective reasoning-in-transition without disturbing smooth practice in a surgical patient who developed pulmonary edema, had to be intubated, was hypotensive, and complaining of pain:

Physician: [Nurse], I'm going to increase the PEEP a little more.

Nurse: To 10? Are we going to increase it to 10? Eight?

Physician: Eight to ten and see how close [interruption].

Nurse: Eight. You know what? Can I give him—I was thinking about ketorolac for his bone pain, but it's not a good idea with his bleeding. Does it make a difference?

Physician: The morphine will help his pulmonary edema.

Nurse: Alright. Well I was just thinking about using an adjunct now so I wouldn't have to use so much morphine so that we could get him extubated. I mean do you really want...?

Physician: So do you want to give him fentanyl instead?

Nurse: Well, yeah, I mean I think we should do something different.

Physician: You're right. You're right.

Nurse: ...because we've got to get him extubated, right? (Observational Interview).

Here, the patient experienced hypotension postoperatively, so the nurse is reluctant to use much morphine. She is also eager to get him extubated as soon as his blood gases improve. Yet, the patient is awake and needs pain medication due to his surgery and the multiple interventions that are needed (e.g., Foley catheter insertion, blood gases) to monitor and treat his pulmonary edema. The nurse's tactful coaching immediately alerts the physician that, in light of the patient's whole situation, morphine is not the best choice. She beckons the physician to more fully engage in the particularities of this situation and together, they reason through the best alternatives. The best combination of pain medications for this specific patient is then suggested and implemented.

This excerpt also highlights how the demands of the situation orient clinicians' judgment and interventions. In this case, the patient's pulmonary edema improves so that he is no longer in imminent danger. If the patient's next set of blood gases improves, the intent is to then begin weaning. The goal of weaning and extubation orients the clinician's judgment toward interventions that will not hinder weaning. If instead, the patient's pulmonary edema had continued to endanger the patient's life, morphine would have been the drug of choice and ventilatory weaning concerns would have remained secondary or even been placed on hold, depending on the patient's clinical condition.

SUMMARY

In this chapter, we have provided a thick description of the clinical judgment and skillful interventions of excellent nurses as they manage the physiological functions of acutely and critically ill patients. The narrative accounts from actual clinical situations, coupled with these descriptions, aim to uncover the thinking-in-action and reasoning-in-transitions that typify expert practice. This understanding, that excellent clinicians must continuously think and reason in constantly changing clinical situations, has strong implications for the way in which students and developing clinicians are currently educated for practice. Educating students in the best of the sciences alone is not sufficient because it falls short of teaching them what is central to expert practice—recognizing and responding to physiological transitions in the patient's condition. The kind of theoretical or disengaged thinking and reasoning that are commonly taught to students stand in stark contrast to the engaged reasoning of expert clinicians that is based on an historical understanding of the patient and the contextual and relational knowledge of the situation.

The thinking-in-action of expert clinicians also has important implications for those who develop, administer, and/or implement critical pathways, protocols, guidelines, or standards. These are, by design, decontextualized tools for guiding clinical interventions. These tools can improve substandard practice, but can severely constrain and discount the thinking-in-action required for excellent practice. Further, expert clinicians acquire cumulative wisdom over time by keeping track of context-sensitive knowledge, which depends on an ongoing collaborative dialogue with a team of clinicians and on the stability in the work environment. Enforcing the use of these tools can compromise excellent practice because they ignore the expert clinician's practical wisdom and essential habits of thought and, consequently, hinder a practice in which an expert clinician responds to the particular patient and the particular situation. Although studies reflect that critical pathways have improved outcomes in patients, the studies have not been designed to differentiate whether or not it is: 1) the tool itself 2) the wisdom of clinicians using the tools (or working around the tools) or 3) the combination of the tools and the clinician's wisdom that improves patient outcomes. These tools have an important place in updating and upgrading clinical practice, but care must be taken not to replace excellence with standard care and not to replace essential thinking and judgment with a tool.

REFERENCES

Ahrens, T. (1993a). Changing perspectives in the assessment of oxygenation. *Critical Care Nurse, 13*(4), 78–83.

Ahrens, T. (1993b). Respiratory monitoring in critical care. *AACN Clinical Issues, 4*(1), 56–65.

Ahrens, T., & Rutherford, K. (1993). *Essentials of oxygenation.* Boston, MA: Jones & Bartlett.

Benner, P. (1984). *From novice to expert: Excellence and power in clinical nursing practice.* Menlo Park, CA: Addison-Wesley.

Benner, P. (Ed.). (1994). *Interpretive phenomenology: Embodiment, caring, and ethics in health and illness.* Thousand Oaks, CA: Sage.

Benner, P., Tanner, C., & Chesla, C. (1992). From beginner to expert: Gaining a differentiated clinical world in critical care nursing. *Advances in Nursing Science, 14*(3), 13-28.

Benner, P., Tanner, C. A., & Chesla, C. A. (1996). *Expertise in nursing practice: Caring, clinical judgment, and ethics.* New York, NY: Springer Publishing Company.

Benner, P., & Wrubel, J. (1989). *The primacy of caring: Stress and coping in health and illness.* Menlo Park, CA: Addison-Wesley.

Bourdieu, P. (1980/1990). *The logic of practice* (Richard Nice, Trans.). Stanford, CA: Stanford University Press.

Corcoran, S. (1986). Planning by expert and novice nurses in cases of varying complexity. *Reseach in Nursing and Health, 9*(2), 155-162.

Corcoran, S., & Tanner, C. (1988). *Implications of clinical judgment research for teaching, Curriculum revolution: Mandate for change.* New York, NY: National League for Nursing.

Dreyfus, H. L., & Dreyfus, S. E. (1986). *Mind over machine: The power of human intuition and expertise in the era of the computer.* New York, NY: Free Press.

Foust J.B., Naylor, M.D., Boling, P.A. Cappuzzo, K. A. (2005). Opportunities for improving post-hospital home medication management among older adults. *Home Health Care Services Quarterly, 24*(1-2), 101-122.

Hooper, P. L. (1995). *Expert titration of multiple vasoactive drugs in post-cardiac surgical patients: An interpretive study of clinical judgment and perceptual acuity.* (Doctoral dissertation, University of California at San Francisco, San Francisco, School of Nursing.)

Kyriakidis, P.H. (in progress). Coaching skillful engagement; The foundational but often missing skill preventing the development of expertise.

Kyriakidis, P.H. & Vitello, J. (in progress). *Applying Benner's research to entry level registered nurses: An investigation of development and retention.* (Unpublished research, Nashville, TN. & Boston, MA.)

Lave, J. & Wenger, E. (1991). *Situated learning: Legitimate peripheral participation.* New York, NY: Cambridge University Press.

Martin, D., Gavin, T., Bianco, J., Brown, C., Stueven, H., Pepe, P., Cummings, R., Gonzalez, E., & Jastremski, M. (1993). Initial countershock in the treatment of asystole. *Resuscitation, 26*(1), 63-68.

Naylor, M.D. (2003). Nursing intervention research and quality of care: influencing the future of healthcare. *Nursing Research, 5*(6), 380-385.

Naylor, M. (2000). A Decade of Transitional Care Research with Hospitalized Elders. *Journal of Cardiovascular Nursing, 14,* 1-14.

Robinson, G., & Hess, D. (1994). Postdischarge survival and functional status following in-hospital cardiopulmonary resuscitation. *Chest, 105*(4), 991-996.

Rubin, J. (1996). Impediments to the development of clinical knowledge and ethical judgment in critical care nursing. In P. Benner, C. A. Tanner, & C. A. Chesla (Eds.), *Expertise in nursing practice: Caring, clinical judgment, and ethics* (pp. 170-192). New York, NY: Springer Publishing Company.

Stannard, D., Puntillo, K., Miaskowski, C., Gleeson, S., Kehrle, K., & Nye, P. (1996). Clinical judgment and pain management in critical care. *American Journal of Critical Care, 5*(6), 433-441.

Tisdale, S. (1986). *The sorcerer's apprentice: Tales of the modern hospital.* New York, NY: McGraw Hill.

5

The Skilled Know-How of Managing a Crisis

*C*risis situations are common in the care of acutely and critically ill patients. In this context, crises are typically life-threatening events where multiple, rapidly-implemented therapies and interventions are required to preserve the life of a patient. However, crises include dangerous conditions and dramatic emotional or situational upheavals. Nurses are typically the first health care providers to respond, diagnose, and treat, for instance, critically ill patients, by initiating resuscitative measures or emergent therapies (e.g., defibrillation, cardiopulmonary resuscitation or CPR, atropine, fluids). In contrast, a psychiatric crisis calls for de-escalation strategies, security personnel, sedation, and restraints. Often, the patient's response to treatment is immediate and definitive. In those situations, nurses stabilize them, consult with the physician, and then initiate follow-up care and mobilize resources as needed. When patients do not respond favorably or require further intervention to maintain stability, acute and critical care nurses rapidly mobilize assistance from other team members.

Because patients who are or become critically ill can present in any setting, nurses across specialties must be know how to recognize, anticipate, and manage serious situations that are common in their areas. For a crisis to be managed effectively, the nurse must skillfully: 1) respond to the patient's life-threatening condition and 2) facilitate resources and team members' efforts. Managing the physiological aspects of the patient's life-threatening condition was addressed in Chapter 4. However, the less-visible aspects of managing a crisis (e.g., environment, logistics, equipment) are the focus of this chapter, as outlined in Table 5.1.

During a crisis, in addition to providing direct care in response to the patient's urgent physiological needs for intervention, the nurse must also prepare, orchestrate, and coordinate multiple aspects of the environment. The environment must be planned and equipped; the logistics of rapid, multiple therapies must be properly sequenced and managed; the team must be organized to the degree demanded by the situation; the role and timing of various team members must be orchestrated; the social climate needs facilitation to maximize everyone's ability to function skillfully; skilled resources must be marshaled as indicated; experiential leadership is required in the absence of adequate medical direction; and necessary medical action must be taken until a physician is available. These skills are performed throughout daily practice but become most visible in crisis situations. Because acute and critical care nurses must assume responsibility for each of the above functions, nurses entering practice

TABLE 5.1

The Skilled Know-How of Managing Crisis

- Setting up the environment for the management of a crisis
- Sequencing and managing logistics of rapid multiple therapies in response to a crisis
- Organizing the team and orchestrating their actions during a crisis
- Exhibiting experiential leadership in managing the patient when a physician is present
- Taking necessary medical action to manage a crisis when a physician is absent
- Recognizing talent and skilled clinicians and marshaling these for the particular situation
- Modulating one's emotional responses and facilitating the social climate

should be educated for and prepared to skillfully manage the environmental and team-related aspects of common crises. Some of these responsibilities are assumed based on knowledge, skill, and experience; others are accepted or imposed based on necessity or a sense of moral obligation. To be performed adeptly, each function requires an integration of skilled know-how, experience, and knowledge about the type of patient crisis, the team members' roles and abilities, the available resources and equipment, and the illness trajectory.

SETTING UP THE ENVIRONMENT FOR THE MANAGEMENT OF A CRISIS

Acute and critical care environments are generally set up at all times for a possible emergency. The more specialized the area, then the more specialized and specific the set up. In situations where the nurse has some forewarning about an emergency admission, the nurse can prepare to better manage the crisis by setting up the environment. This involves gathering and drawing up emergency drugs, calculating drug dosages, preparing intravenous infusions, assembling and testing monitors and equipment, setting up for emergency procedures (e.g., chest tube insertion, thoracotomy for cardiac massage, endotracheal intubation, intra-aortic balloon insertion), strategically locating emergency equipment, mental preparation, and contingency planning. Thoughtful preparation goes beyond a routine laundry list of things to have available. Being prepared means knowing about the disease, the kind of crisis situation, and the likely complications in order to have the appropriate equipment, drugs, resources, and team members available to immediately respond, as reflected in this story about a burn victim:

Nurse: What I did was, before he [the patient] came up, I made sure that the room was prepared, like all the dressings and things I needed, so I didn't have to go out and pull the camera—a Polaroid camera—because it is routine to take pictures, and all the IV fluids. The amount of fluid to be given depends upon how much of the area is burned. So we were computing that with the intern... So the total of that would be given in the whole 24 hours.... All the dressings were ready, and the room was warm. The heater was on, and all the linens, and all the things we needed [in order] to debride. Because [the burn areas] have to be debrided—the blisters... And also the pain medications were already there. I made sure that a lot of morphine was there. So, I didn't have to go in and out of the room. Because once we start debriding and cleaning, the room is closed and everybody is with their own—the gowns and the masks and things like that. So, because I was well-prepared and I know what to expect, everything came out okay.

Knowing the team members who will be involved in managing a crisis is time saving since various people prefer specific kinds of equipment, drugs, etc. (e.g., a straight versus curved blade for intubation, levophed versus epinephrine, nasal versus oral airway). This kind of practical knowledge is gained only from experience and from the socially embedded knowledge shared by more experienced nurses. Knowing the team members and their preferences in crisis situations can assist nurses in best preparing the habitat, enabling themselves and others to act in concert without delay, and anticipating complications and probable interventions.

Preparing the environment also requires knowledge and experience in the particular specialty. Setting up the environment for a trauma patient differs from the preparation needed for a burn, obstetrics, or cardiac patient. Further, there are important differences in preparing the habitat for adult, pediatric, and neonatal populations. Within specialties, various sub-populations of patients (e.g., cardiac patients with congenital malformations versus acute myocardial infarctions) often require different interventions. The type of crisis and therefore equipment, drugs, resources, and personnel necessarily vary. The nuances are reflected in the following story by Barbara Hidde, a nurse working in the high-risk delivery area, who goes to the resuscitative room adjacent to the delivery room:

Nurse: I walked into report to hear, "Barb, you're on deliveries, and you're gonna have a bad one." A term baby with mom transferred here last night and diagnosed Diaphragmatic Hernia (DH). "Parents are still in shock," I heard her say. My heart sank because very few of these babies have good outcomes. The diaphragm is displaced into the chest cavity so the baby has little lung tissue.

I left to prep for the delivery. These (DH) babies often require aggressive resuscitation and I wanted everything ready. In addition to all the basics [code equipment], I drew up Epi, NS and D10W boluses. I had a 3.5 and 4.0 ET tube ready. I checked the battery on the transilluminator and prepared 4 needle aspiration sets with 20 gauge angiocaths. I pulled a chest tube tray and umbilical catheter tray for easy access.

OB called for the delivery team (staff neonatologist, pediatric resident, RT and me). We waited in the resuscitation room off of OB. My stomach churned. I took deep breaths. I said a prayer for this baby and our team, as we tried to help her.

The resident came in holding a lifeless baby girl. After drying and stimulation, still no respiratory effort. "Let's tube her." Our resident quickly intubated her. Initial heart rate was 50 and little change after intubation. I started chest compressions. After about 3 minutes of chest compressions and 2 doses of epi, we finally had a heart rate over 80. Although we had a stable heart rate, her color was still cyanotic with O2 sats in the 30's. Her eyes were open and she just stared at the ceiling. "Please let us get to Children's," I said to myself.

Then the door opened. "Is she doing okay?" asked this little girl's dad as his tears streamed. "Her name is Rachel," he added. We had needles in each side of Rachel's chest, in addition to the tube in her throat when her dad entered the room. The MD's gently explained what they were doing to try and help her. The tears flowed more rapidly. The room was somewhat chaotic as all of us were trying to work quickly, so dad left the room.

Once the chest tubes were in, I prepared for transport to Children's. Rachel was still quite labile and her HR had dipped a few times into the 70's. She was pale, her nail beds were cyanotic and her eyes were now closed. I placed her in the transport incubator. Usually, when we transport a baby to Children's after delivery, we stop in the mother's room so she can see the baby before we leave. In this case, the MD's wanted to go right away because of Rachel's instability. I explained that this might be mom's only chance to see Rachel alive and couldn't we just roll in for one minute. It was the quickest trip to a mother's room I've ever had. But, she got to see Rachel and that was important.

The team and dad immediately transported Rachel to Children's via a tunnel and upon arrival at the NICU, she sadly coded. With dad at Rachel's side, witnessing no response to resuscitative therapies after concerted effort, dad agreed to stop the code:

We all cried with dad. I moved dad's chair over to Rachel's bedside so he could hold her hand. I removed Rachel's monitors and tubes and bundled her in a blanket for dad to hold.

Dad was very worried about Rachel's mom. He wanted her to see Rachel and hold her too. I brought a bassinet and we bundled Rachel in it. Dad walked back through the tunnel to University Hospital with me and he pushed Rachel's bassinet to the door of mom's room. "Do you want me to go in with you?" I asked dad as he picked up Rachel. "No, I want it to be just us. Thank you for letting me stay with her."

In this kind of urgent situation, Barbara conveys how important the advanced preparation of the environment is to the infant's possible survival. Her experiential knowledge caring for neonates with diaphragmatic hernias enables her to anticipate "everything" needed in setting up the delivery room for the crisis. The skilled knowledge (thinking, foresight, and planning) needed to safely and thoroughly set up for specific kinds of crises prohibits routine and total delegation of these procedures to unskilled workers. Technical assistants can, however, be invaluable in a crisis by retrieving equipment and resources as directed.

The nurse's clinical knowledge in the above example points to how important the development of expertise in one practice domain enables the development of expertise in another. Setting up the environment is one of several skills where preparing to manage a crisis becomes inextricably linked with clinical forethought (see Chapter 3). For expert clinicians, understanding the type of crisis that one is preparing for means knowing what will <u>actually</u> be needed, but it also means developing habits of anticipating the risks and preparing for the most likely events that can possibly occur (Hooper, 1995). Hence, clinical forethought, which is a habit of thinking, sets up how clinicians prepare the environment.

Notice that Barbara anticipates, sets up, and manages, as much as possible, two kinds of crises. The most obvious is the physiological crisis of a listless newborn and the ensuing code, but the second is the emotional, social, and spiritual crisis for the parents—the actual death of Rachel. The clinical wisdom of a clinician who can skillfully manage a crisis includes a keen awareness of these likely eventualities. Recognizing that the lifeless infant foretold the future, Barbara is morally pressed to set up the only chance for mom to hold Rachel for a brief moment of her short life. Rachel's story reminds us about that attuned responsive nurses have the power to create worlds, in this situation, a brief moment of family. For developing clinicians, dialogue or simply just hearing narratives of expert caring practice can expand their clinical imagination for similar, future opportunities to recognize and respond to multiple aspects in a crisis.

Saving time and motion prior to and/or during a crisis, thus reducing chaos, is a common expert nursing concern because it often means the difference between, for example, tissue viability versus organ damage from ischemia. Preparation of the environment contributes to how smoothly a crisis is managed, as demonstrated in the following story about a very sick baby who arrests during transport by helicopter. The pediatric ICU is notified about the baby's arrival and condition just 6 minutes prior to landing:

> **Nurse:** We started really getting organized. We had all of our code drugs drawn up and we had mixed the dopamine and the isuprel and the dobutamine and just about everything we could think of. And we had the isolette set up and chest tube trays open and absolutely everything ready. Everybody had their task assignment. We had seven nurses lined up around this bedside waiting for this baby to come in and, sure enough, when he came in, he was coding and the physicians immediately started putting in chest tubes and the nurses were giving drugs, and it was sort of neat in a way...because you knew [the baby] was coming and everybody did really well, and everything flowed really smoothly.

Having advanced notice to set up the environment optimizes the management of a crisis, but often, crisis occurs without notice. Thus, nurses routinely stock equipment at or near the bedside and check it daily or ensure that someone else has done so. This is a form of safety work to ensure that emergency equipment and other life-saving technologies are accessible, properly working, and ready for use (see Chapter 8).

In the above situation, the nurse prepares specific vasoactive drug infusions and opens chest tube trays because the report she received prior to the infant's arrival alerted her to anticipate some very specific interventions. Her judgment and preparation cannot be generalized to other situations because each situation generates its own set of specific demands. Mixing infusions and opening sterile trays can be inappropriate in many situations and can lead to needless waste. However, this situation highlights how a good understanding of the clinical context and the habits of thinking ahead enables clinicians to prepare for particular kinds of crises.   In an previous exemplar (see Chapter 2, Making Qualitative Distinctions), when Judy Rumensky set up for a crisis, she was very experienced in the kind of emergency surgery that unfolded. However, when working with others and having responsibility for setting up the specifics they prefer, the nurse is positioned to set up everything that is needed, but nothing more, in order to avoid waste:

> **Nurse:** It was a night from hell in our OR... We had all 8 of our trauma rooms going with a wait list of urgent cases that every surgeon was clamoring to go next. The only people free were the anesthesiologist supervising the CRNAs (nurse anesthetists), the orderly, and me. I was in charge.
>
> I got a call from an excited resident saying an ICU patient was crashing, and they were coming to the OR. The few details I found out were that it was a 42 year old woman who had been on a motorcycle, wrecked and sustained multiple traumas. She's been in the ICU for a month with a trach and on the vent. That night she began bleeding profusely from around her trach and was getting a mediastinal shift...I moved to the biggest OR room. The surgeon was new in town (first night on call) so I opened every chest instrument pack I had...

In this crisis, without knowing the particular surgeon, Judy has no choice but to grab "every chest instrument pack" available. Further, because there is no time as the patient is hemorrhaging and there is no other help, Judy must open everything before the patient arrives in order to be ready in this extreme emergency.

In some areas of critical care nursing (e.g., flight nursing, neonatal transport units), details are unknown about the scene or setting where the patient is in crisis. In those situations, nurses must prepare in a more general way by taking all the equipment they anticipate needing at the scene and transporting it with them into the field. This preparation was observed first-hand as two flight nurses and a respiratory therapist (RT) prepared for an inter-facility transport of a baby from another hospital. The dispatcher conveys the call:

Nurse 1: It's a seven-month-old baby, apparently under CPR; they defibrillated the kid, had pulses, and intubated him. Dr. D. doesn't think that defibrillating him had anything to do with that. We think that something's kind of bizarre. Kids don't usually go into ventricular fibrillation. So we don't really know much.

Dispatcher: Okay. I just paged RT and...

Nurse 2: Respiratory therapy?

Dispatcher: Respiratory therapy. So I'll meet you out at the [ambulance] bay, right.

Nurse 2: Yes. Did you get a weight?

Nurse 1: Nope! He didn't know. [working on a computer] Oh, the computer's not up anyway. Oh, he's on his way there. [Nurse 1 and Nurse 2 quickly walk out of the dispatch area through the emergency department.]

Interviewer: So, we're going on a ground transport...

Nurse 2: Yeah, we are.

Interviewer: Can you talk about how those are different versus your air transports?

Nurse 2: This is closer. The only reason we're not going by air is because there's no place to land there and it's so close that we go by ambulance. It's just the same; we have the same kind of equipment. (To Nurse 1) Don't forget to change the monitor from the luggage cart to the ambulance. [We exit the ED and walk outside the receiving bay to a building nearby to a small storage room in the building near the receiving bay.] We're going to get our ground equipment. We have it all on a gurney that fits into the ambulance, the Panda, and we'll meet the Panda [the ambulance] out here.

Interviewer: So what do you anticipate about this baby?

Nurse 1: It'll be interesting to see when we get there if they have anymore history on what happened—why the baby coded, because Dr. D didn't have very much information. Usually on inter-facilities you have a little more information but sometimes you don't. (Nurse 1 is checking a portable monitor and continues to pack up the gurney.)

Interviewer: So, can you talk about what you guys are packing up?

Nurse 2: Let me just check to make sure this is the screen I wanted (turning on the monitor); yes, it is, okay (turning it off). We have a cardiac monitor.

Dispatcher: (over the 2-way radio) Okay, RT's been informed. D. is going to get RT down at the ambulance bay. M. is bringing down the RT's equipment bag.

Nurse 2: We have our IVAC pump for IV fluids. This is our airway bag [a big green bag] and that [another bag] has all our drugs and anything else we might need. This is our pediatric ventilator.

Nurse 1: Make sure we've got tubes.

Nurse 2: [Unzipping a bag and looking for supplies.] Yeah, yeah—it's an MVP10 [tube]. And then this is our bag with all our little odds and ends, whatever else we might need. Okay—and linen. I was going to say, 'Do you want to bring the child's seat.' But it was a CPR call so I don't think so.

Interviewer: Who is coming with us?

Nurse 2: Respiratory therapy, because we're going to use the ventilator. And even though the nurses have to know how to use the ventilator, because we don't always have a respiratory therapist that can come with us. When we do an inter-facility like this, if we can we'll take a respiratory therapist just because it frees us up to do other things. [An ambulance drives up and backs into the receiving bay area.] And, here comes our ambulance. So we're leaving to pick up the baby for transport. [The infant subsequently survived the transport and was admitted to the PICU] (Observational Interview).

Once the nurse arrives at the scene, particularly after a motor vehicle accident, the patient is not always easily or safely accessible. In many cases, the environment is dangerous (e.g., threat of gasoline explosion, extrication in progress) and therefore controlled by trained rescuers, often firemen. Nurses then enter the patient's environment after it is "set up" by others:

Nurse 1: I'm learning. I wasn't sure how much to get involved. When do you get in the car? I was hesitant. Getting in a...

Nurse 2: ...car over the embankment.

Nurse 1: They (rescuers) were so glad to have me down there [for the extrication].

Nurse 3: The fire department is always in control of who comes into the perimeter of the extrication. For safety reasons. And that's what we ask them to do when they do extrication training is talk about the tools and how to be safe around the generators and tools. And what's going to happen if you end up getting in the car? Because we don't wear all the equipment, we don't have all the heavy [clothes] and the gloves and the helmets. And so we always stand back and if they request us to come in and do something, then we do and they usually shield us and protect us. Sometimes they'll give you a helmet to put on too. It depends on what's going on...

Nurse 2: And I always have a tendency to ask. Because K. and I were on a car over an embankment, down on the river road a few weeks ago, and they were using ropes and chains and equipment like that...

For flight nurses and the patients, the care setting is commonly precarious, but as in all crises, time is of utmost importance in the patient's outcome. So these nurses adapt their care to the environments in which patients present in order to provide life-saving interventions, even inside contorted vehicles with little room to maneuver.

Flight nurses stress the central importance of preparation since every call for transport either is or has the high potential to be a crisis. Life-threatening situations, where the time spent at the scene and in transport means the difference between life and death, are the reasons that air transport is initiated. For anyone new to flight nursing and the transport of severely ill patients, preparation is the first and a crucial step in learning how to provide care for a patient at the scene. The following story where things did not go smoothly accentuates the significance of preparation and knowing the set up:

Interviewer: You talked before about how flying with residents was really hard. Can you tell a story about how that's stressful?

Nurse 1: Oh yeah. (Laughs).

Nurse 2: Big stress.

Nurse 1: Yeah. It's the emergency department residents, and they fly during their second year, and they have one month they call their emergency medicine month. And they ride along in the ambulance, they ride along with the fire department, and they fly with us. And they displace the [second] nurse. They get a didactic orientation. They get a little manual at the beginning of the year and that's just on altitude physiology, safety, and survival in the aircraft. Then the week before they start, they have to get their uniform and then they have to have their safety briefing with the pilot. We take them on a little test flight to make sure they don't throw up all the time and get sick. Or they're not scared to death... And then we go through all the bags and the equipment, but they're mainly [responsible for the] airway. And they have to follow our protocols. The nurse is in charge. So they're [residents] usually act as the crew nurse, meaning they're in charge of [securing the] airway. And they're supposed to go out and check the bags each time they come on so they know where things are. And some of them, they can be kind of cocky about it sometimes. 'Oh, yeah. Yeah, I looked at it. Yeah. Yeah.' So, I went out with a resident not too long ago and it was a scene call, it was a burn patient. This guy (patient) had gotten drunk and lit himself on fire. And...

Interviewer: Intentionally?

Nurse 1: Yeah they think so, yeah. He said initially that he was putting gasoline on some weeds that he was going to burn, and then he lit a cigarette and accidentally set himself on fire but we couldn't quite figure out how he got gasoline all over himself to light. So anyway, we got there and this guy was drunk, he was badly burned and he was <u>really</u> combative. And we got him in the helicopter and the resident was convinced that we were going to have to intubate this patient. And I said, 'That would be ideal, but he's like a little too awake right now.' We had <u>just</u> gotten an IV line in and I said, 'We need to give him some medication. We need to give him some morphine. We need to settle him down first.' And so we had loaded him up in the helicopter and we were leaving and it was a summer day. It was <u>hot</u>. I remember I was sweating really badly. [After some time in flight] I looked up at the resident, and I said, 'Get your stuff out. Get ready to intubate him.' And he's like fumbling around, he can't find his things, and he's got his equipment all over the place. And then, because I got a line in, I said, 'Give me some morphine.' And this guy [patient] was just fighting with me, and I was having to restrain him and try and keep him down. And the resident took the morphine out of the box and he hands me the little vial. And I'm fighting this guy [patient], leaning on him, and I just looked up at the resident and gave him the look and said, '<u>Draw it up!</u>' And then he didn't know what to do. He wasn't sure where things were... (Other nurses agree). It's like tunnel vision, 'I'm supposed to do an airway. So I can't do anything else.' So I'm fighting with this guy [patient], wishing my [nurse] partner was here with me. And so finally, I just took over and started giving him orders. 'Do this. Do that. Go in the <u>third</u> bag. Do this. Do that' till we got to the

> hospital and we got the patient in the resuscitation room and I went in the medication room in the ER and I was washing and sticking my head under the faucet because I was so hot. And he came in and said, 'I wasn't very much help, was I?' And I said, 'Well, no, not really.' He said, 'Well I'll try to do better next time.' I said, 'Okay, it would be nice if you knew where things were in the bags.' 'Okay, I'll do that.'

It usually only takes one such experience to learn the moral imperative for being prepared as a responsible member of a team. For these patients, time and stabilization are everything. Although flight nurses and anyone assuming patient care responsibilities at the scene learn the primary significance of adequate preparation during their orientation into this specialty practice, high-time demands and anxiety can interfere with performance. These breakdown instances re-emphasize the central importance of setting up and knowing the equipment and environment in order to facilitate rapid and pivotal interventions. Common adages have arisen through the years that emphasize this point. For instance, in cardiovascular nursing, a saying is, "time is muscle." In trauma nursing, "the golden hour" and "platinum 10 minutes" remind clinicians that avoidable delays can cause severe patient consequences.

As seen in the above excerpt, an experience of breakdown can be a strong and lasting lesson. As clinicians learn and develop expertise, the depth and quality of their cares and concerns grow, they more fully engage in what's at stake for the patient and family, their attunement and responsiveness extend to include the patient's emotional, social, and spiritual need, and their anticipatory and preparatory practices mature into habits in their everyday thought and actions. For expert nurses who manage a crisis, what is at stake physiologically is only one of the concerns they anticipate and prepare for. Because they commonly have a strong understanding of what outcomes are and are not possible in particular types of crises, they can foresee, and therefore develop preparatory practices around emotional needs. Tracy Davis, a pediatric ICU nurse, shares Gabriel's story, which opens up thinking about how families often cue our judgments about how to set up environments to help them better cope in and through a crisis:

> **Nurse:** Two things went through my mind the first time I saw Gabriel: what a beautiful child and how would this family ever survive this tragedy? Gabriel was a 2 year old, blonde-haired, blue-eyed angel admitted following a near-drowning. His family went to a nearby lake and Gabriel got out without his life jacket. As his family busily unloaded the boat, he wandered off. They found him facedown near the water's edge, blue and lifeless. From report, his extremely prolonged resuscitation did not go well. His pH was 6.91, temp was 84 degrees, and pupils were fixed and dilated. He was already instability, as we were barely maintaining his blood pressure with epinephrine and norepinephrine drips. What a profound tragedy. My heart positively ached for his parents, whom I had yet to meet....
>
> It seemed that nothing could be done for Gabriel that would improve his chances for survival. I knew my job would be to provide crisis intervention through emotional and spiritual support to these parents. It was truly all that could be done.
>
> When I met his parents, their devastation was readily apparent. It is a challenge to find any words of comfort that do not sound hollow and meaningless. I introduced myself, and told them how beautiful I thought their son was. I then gently told them about Gabriel's condition. I knew they would not be able to fully process a lot of technical terms, so I was as direct as possible. This is so hard when all of the things you are saying are the most awful possible words any parent can ever hear. They had a

few questions for me, but did seem to understand his grave prognosis. I then let them just be with Gabriel, talking to him and holding his hands.

Gabriel's condition continued to worsen throughout the day.... I noticed that his Dad was especially quiet, and had isolated himself from other family members. We have an ICU brochure that we give to families. I realized that his Dad had been "reading" it most of the afternoon. I walked over and sat down next to him. As I told him how very sorry I was about Gabriel, he began to cry. He then explained that it was his job to make sure the kids were in their lifejackets before they got out of the truck. He had forgotten on this trip. His guilt was beyond measurement. A few quiet moments passed while he cried and I put my arm around his shoulder. There were no words to make this man feel better or less guilty. So I just sat there, with tears in my own eyes.

After a while, I asked him to tell me about his son. He started telling of a lively, happy, joyful child. His love for him was immense. He spoke of their routines, as Gabriel was a typical toddler and "set in his ways" as to reading, bath time, bedtime, and prayers. He was very close to Gabriel. One of their favorite rituals was bedtime. Gabriel would get in his Barney pajamas and slippers, and his Dad would rock him and read him a Barney Bedtime Story before bed. It was their special time together. As he told me this, he began to cry again, saying he just could not believe he would never be able to do this again. We talked for quite a while, as he was eager to talk about his son.

The next day, after a series of tests, our Neurologist told us what we already knew, that this sweet angel was brain dead. Gabriel's aunt was a nurse. She had asked me if there was anything she could do to help his parents. I decided to take her up on her offer. Knowing what was coming, I asked her to go to their home and get Gabriel's pajamas, slippers, and storybook. I imagine she thought I was nuts, but I had developed a good relationship with Gabriel's family, and she trusted me. After telling Gabriel's family the news that their son's brain was dead, we went through the agonizing tasks of discontinuing life support. All of his family had the opportunity to hold him, and they did. After all of his grandparents, aunts and uncles held him, I spoke with his parents. I told them I was going to clean him up so they could hold him one last time, and asked if they wanted to help me. His Dad spoke right up and said "yes." This was when I showed him Gabriel's pajamas, slippers, and book, and told him that I had asked his Aunt to bring it from home. I explained that I thought he might want one last opportunity to go through their bedtime ritual together. He cried very hard, but nodded his head yes. Together with his parents, we got Gabriel dressed, and carried him to the Quiet Room. I had already put a rocking chair in there, and he and his dad sat in it. I told them I would be in the hall if they needed me. I could hear his Dad reading to Gabriel as I stood out there. It was quite emotional. Both of his parents were very grateful to me for helping them. I told them it was the least I could do, and that I wish it were more.

I will never forget the image of that sweet little boy being carried by his Dad in his little Barney pajamas and slippers. I know that the pain and guilt that Dad felt will never go away. In an otherwise hopeless, tragic situation, I believe I gave his Dad one last memory. I hope it was the start of his recovery.

Tracy tells us that she did not know what say; yet, what she deeply embodies is the meaning of another's tragedy and loss. Her way of being with and supporting dad reveals a kind of recognition practice of who Gabriel is to his parents and of the joy they hold on to. Tracy's ethical comportment and inquiry about Gabriel, born of her genuine interest and reverence, were exactly the "right thing" and allowed dad to share his most cherished memories. Their bedtime routine struck this expert nurse's keen sensibilities and notion of good to respond by setting up the world dad held dear one last time. Dreyfus (1990) talked about nursing, and the expert caring practices embedded within, as one of the last saving practices in our Western culture. Tracy's world-preserving practices exemplify what he was referring to. In our high tech culture, which all but ignores the most demanding yet incredibly human aspects of care in its view of "legitimate" science, "experts are an endangered species...while we still know what expert judgment [and care are], let us use that expert judgment to preserve it" (Dreyfus & Dreyfus, 1986, p. 206). Narratives like Gabriel's story define the best of expert caring practices. When shared in a community of learners and developing nurses, these saving practices and expert judgment can be preserved for and extended to generations of caregivers to come.

The above examples point to the extensive amount of practical knowledge that expert nurses gain over time in order to effectively manage whatever type of crisis may occur. Articulation of these invisible preparatory practices highlights an essential aspect of nursing that can make a crucial difference in the nurse's and team's response time and subsequent patient viability and outcome. This taken-for-granted knowledge needs to be incorporated into orientation, classes, and curricula to nurture the development of clinical imagination. Further, financial resources should be budgeted for the learning of this skilled and world-preserving knowledge.

Preparatory practices become a part of the nurse's habits of thought. When nurses are "floated" to unfamiliar settings or to work with unfamiliar patient populations, skilled performance is disrupted. Without knowing the patient population, the team members, the available resources, or the setting, the float nurse cannot safely prepare the environment for an actual or potential crisis or access things that have already been prepared. This is seen in the following interview excerpt where a neonatal ICU nurse agrees with other nurses on this issue:

Nurse: I had to go down [to the delivery room] a couple of weeks ago and I hadn't been down there in years. But we had a diaphragmatic hernia baby being born. I was taking the patient, so [an experienced nurse] set me up to go down there. In anticipation of not knowing where everything was, I had put everything I thought I would need on my bed. Well, that bed wasn't for [the delivery]; it was for the baby in the isolette. And then they said, 'Sorry, you've got to go down there now and that's not the bed that you're taking,' so I didn't have all my supplies.

The lack of preparedness can predictably compromise patient care and create anxiety for the nurse. A more inclusive orientation for nurses who float can assist not only in improving the nurse's ability to provide safe patient care but also in alleviating the degree of stress. A neonatal ICU nurse suggests how to better orient nurses to a new area:

Nurse: I think that people are overwhelmed when they go down there [delivery room] for the first time and I think the reason is the logistics of just trying to know where everything is. Because you have to be able to work quickly and like working in any new environment, the first step is just learning where everything is. And so you bring people down there and you make them the back-up person for awhile and they just get your supplies and they chart. There's a rhythm that, no matter what's wrong with the baby, certain things happen in a certain rhythm and sequence, and once you get that down, you're able to anticipate what the next stage is, what the next equipment needs will be, and what the next procedure will be. That's about 75% of the battle.

This nurse articulates that there is typically a rhythm in each situation, a sequence, that is foundational for new nurses to learn because familiarity with the rhythm (the typical trajectory) sets up their ability to anticipate what will be needed, when, and by whom. This ability to anticipate and be prepared can reduce delays and duplication. Collaborative relationships can contribute to creating a rhythm. A nurse cannot skillfully manage a crisis without gaining the skilled know-how of sequencing and anticipation. Paying attention to team members' responses, as well as the unfolding crisis, requires "time on task" and there is rarely sufficient time devoted to teaching these skills in most orientation and cross-training programs.

What is easily missed about the importance of setting up the environment is an understanding of the time required to do it. Because setting up the environment is not simply a technical task, the nurse must think through most situations as they present. This thinking-in-action occurs <u>as</u> the nurse is preparing. For instance, a burn nurse knew the weight of a patient to be admitted to her unit. On the way to prepare the medications, she was thinking out loud about the various narcotics (e.g., fentanyl, morphine) she would need and also about how much of each she should have readily available at the bedside. Another form of thinking-in-action ensues when nurses handle some types of equipment. The specific piece of equipment often reminds the nurse about other associated equipment that is needed (e.g., gel pads for the defibrillator, saline for wash basins for scrubbing and debriding a burn wound). Thinking-in-action, thus, enables the nurse to think <u>through</u> the anticipated patient situation, set up the environment, and mentally prepare for action. Each of these preparatory tasks takes time, as does the thinking for the preparation.

SEQUENCING AND MANAGING THE LOGISTICS OF RAPID MULTIPLE THERAPIES IN RESPONSE TO A CRISIS

In a crisis, numerous interventions are needed rapidly, often by a variety of people. To prevent chaos and ensure therapeutic effectiveness, the rapid, multiple therapies need to be sequenced and managed logistically as much as possible. A key factor in accomplishing this is grasping the <u>cause</u> of the crisis, the underlying pathophysiologic problem, and responding to the cause rather than the symptoms alone. For instance, in the following story, a critically ill pregnant woman in the coronary care unit (CCU) prematurely delivers before reaching Labor and Delivery because her condition rapidly deteriorated. The baby is in distress and immediately rushed to the ICU nursery. The neonatal ICU nurse clearly understands that the infant's primary problem is respiratory and rapidly intervenes:

Nurse: They handed me this baby—a 26-weeker. And we don't have beds set up for admissions because we don't get emergency admissions. We usually have an hour, right? They bring the bed up and they handed me this baby that I'm supposed to do something with. It's not breathing, its color is totally horrible and the mother had leukemia [with multisystem complications] and had a whole bunch of things going on and so you can guess the baby wasn't doing very well. I fortunately had one bed empty, but not set up, that we could [put] the baby in and the next thing is the baby's not breathing. I need to get a mask and a bag from somewhere. There's one on the next baby's bed, so I quickly take the one on the top. It was a clean bag and we had the code cart there and we were going through the steps and another nurse is attempting intubation and then the doctor walks in and he said, 'The baby's heart rate is 110!' and he's getting all excited and I go, 'The heart rate is [not the major problem]. Hush.'

He did. We had things under control by the time the physicians came back for the baby. The infant survived the immediate crisis; however, the mother was too sick to survive.

In this case, the nurse has the advantage of "knowing the baby" from the time of birth and being involved in the situation as it unfolded. Thus, the infant's respiratory distress stands out as the salient problem, not the heart rate. For this reason, the infant's airway and breathing take first priority in sequencing and managing this crisis. Not infrequently, as in this situation, nurses must rapidly manage interventions in a crisis while additionally assisting others in their understanding of the crisis and the emergent interventions.

During many crises, physicians enter in the midst of the emergency and commonly request a list of things to be done. Nurses are left to prioritize the interventions and procedures that need to be done so that technicians and nurses are not converging to do the EKG, X-ray, and blood gases at the same time. Prioritizing care is more important in ensuring that the therapies that are needed urgently are completed first and, whenever possible, appropriately clustered to minimize patient discomfort. Skilled clinical knowledge about the patient, the disease and complications, and similar situations are critical for a nurse to adequately prioritize and stage care. Experience is needed to teach a nurse what things must be done immediately versus what can wait or be left out, based on the ramifications to the particular patient (e.g., danger, infection). For instance, when a patient becomes septic, a physician may request numerous interventions at once, such as a levophed infusion, a fluid infusion, laboratory tests, blood cultures, and antibiotics. The list of tasks must be prioritized and implemented in the best sequence. For instance, the blood cultures must be requested and drawn prior to the initiation of the antibiotics. Allowing these to occur out of sequence can prohibit the culprit organism from being cultured, identified, and treated. While all of the tasks have a high priority, they must be performed in a logical sequence and in response to the patient's condition.

Sequencing and managing particular kinds of interventions require close attention, such as the infusion of multiple pharmacologic agents. For instance, acidic agents such as epinephrine, levophed, or amiodarone must <u>not</u> be infused in the same line with sodium bicarbonate or aminophylline to avoid precipitation. Additionally, care must be taken not to bolus an IV drug (eg. Lasix, morphine) through the same infusion line with a potent vasoactive drug like levophed, labetalol, or amiodarone to avoid a bolus of the infusing drug which can cause deleterious hemodynamic effects. Thus, the nurse must be ever cognizant of what other team members are doing since few may be aware of the potential logistic hazards. For instance, expert nurses always look and ensure that the respiratory therapist does not continue to ventilate the patient during defibrillation since the electrical shock can be conducted to anyone touching the patient when the electrical current is delivered. In each of these instances, safe management of additional interventions must take into account other ongoing therapies which can jeopardize the patient's condition.

Nurses must also sequence actions whenever a patient is to be transported or a major procedure is to be done because the completion of legal and administrative papers is often required. Anytime consent is granted for organ donation, particularly for vital or multiorgan donation, the viability of the organs harvested is dependent on swift, accurate, and careful logistical management of the patient's care, the OR teams, and organ transport. For emergency procedures (e.g., surgery, catheterization) that require transport, it is imperative to sequence who has to be informed, who is to be called and in what order, who needs to sign consent forms, what preliminary tests or procedures are needed, and how long various things will take. Skillful logistical management prevents unnecessary delays.

Expert nurses have heightened awareness around logistics in specialties where patients travel far for care or the procedures causes great angst because delays or cancellations are so expensive, both in financial but also emotional resources and the patient's physical stamina. Stacy Steuerwald, a plastic surgery OR nurse, highlights this level of attentiveness in a child who has gastroschisis (abdominal wall defect where organs develop outside the abdomen):

> **Nurse:** A child was having combination Pediatric [and Plastic] Surgery for Alloderm placement and Cultured Epithelial Autograft biopsy....The process involves the surgeon taking a small diamond shape piece of skin from the patient. That piece of skin is divided into two pieces and sent off to the company to grow this patients own skin cells to cover his abdominal wound. This is a very expensive process and every step has to be done correctly or the process and grafts will be ruined.
>
> Earlier in the week I saw this child was on the schedule for Alloderm placement. With no communication from the surgeon on the amount of Alloderm needed, I guessed on the amount to order. Since I had never seen this patient, it was just that—an educated guess. There are many types of Alloderm, not all of them are routinely stocked. This patient needed the type suitable for surface wound grafting. During the procedure we realized that we didn't have enough Alloderm to cover the large wound. These are the moments that it is important to maintain your composure and act like it's no problem and rack your mind calmly for Plan B. Plan B was to call University Burn Unit. They were helpful and loaned us two pieces of Alloderm.
>
> I assisted the people in OR about how to prep the area for the CEA biopsy and the size. After the biopsy was taken and secured in the culture medium, I then had to complete all the necessary paperwork. Following the paperwork, the company was contacted and sent a courier to pick up the biopsy and ship it to the company. I had to let purchasing know that we sent a biopsy and needed a PO # in the near future. I then waited to hear from the company to coordinate the date of the surgery.
>
> The company called...The rep gave us two dates that allowed at least two week notice to finalize the grafts....[After some confusion], the surgeon confirmed the date. I explained there was no changing the date [to the surgeon, secretary, and OR]. The grafts will be completed, flown in on that day by a courier, and must be grafted onto the patient. If cancelled, we pay the full amount, which for this child would be $20,000. Everyone was in agreement.
>
> As the day drew closer, I contacted the company, got them a PO# to ship the grafts, made sure we had all necessary supplies, and informed them of the time of surgery. As I investigated what the time of surgery might be, I saw that this patient WAS NOT on the computerized schedule. PANIC! Everything I had tried to avoid by explaining the situation to everyone was happening anyway. When I called the secretary, she acted like she had no idea what I was talking about. I reminded her of the situation and told her we had to find a way to get this child on the schedule because this surgery had to take place on the scheduled date. If it didn't, it would not only cost us the $20,000 for this set of unused grafts but also another $20,000 for the next set of grafts. It took a lot of coordination from the surgeon, the OR, the scheduler and myself to pull it off but we managed to get the child on the OR schedule in a way that fit everyone's needs. The child did fine. Most of the chaos was invisible to everyone but me. To others, it seemed like this case went off without a hitch.

For patients like this, managing the logistics requires keeping track of this child and all the sequencing over weeks, not just a day. As seen here, excellent planning and communications is sometimes not enough to avoid every glitch. However, the collaborative bonds formed within and across teams over time matter when situations like this emerge so that problems are resolved almost seamlessly.

Sequencing interventions appropriately can minimize discomfort to the patient by preventing duplication of therapies. For instance, an expert nurse often ensures that all invasive procedures (e.g., chest tubes, pulmonary artery line) requiring an X-ray are completed prior to calling for the X-ray to be done. Developing nurses may learn this sequencing, in part, from experienced physicians who reflect the logic of practice in the way they write their orders. Teaching students and new nurses how to sequence and manage the logistics of frequently occurring crises make the experiential learning less hazardous to the patient and the nurse.

In the current climate with fewer experienced nurses to manage the care of more patients, prioritizing and sequencing interventions is a growing challenge, particularly when the nurse must manage a crisis while simultaneously managing the ongoing care of other patients. After one such day, a nurse explained, "There were just too many things to do all at one time that became equal priorities with not as many resources... Controlled chaos, that's what it is..." Educating administrators and decision makers to understand this important and skillful aspect of patient care can assist in rethinking staffing ratios and skill mix. As described above, without skilled nurses, costly duplications, expensive delays, patient discomfort, patient complications, and lengths of stay rise.

ORGANIZING THE TEAM AND ORCHESTRATING THEIR ACTIONS DURING A CRISIS

An organized team effort significantly affects the smooth management of a crisis. This is a broad category of skilled know-how that most immediately involves assigning roles in the emergency, designating staff not involved in the crisis to cover other patients' care, assigning specific tasks, moving alert patients away from direct exposure to the crisis, matching clinicians' skills/talents with therapies to be implemented, and determining the mix and number of team members needed (those who grasp what needs to be done versus those who need learning experiences). In one situation, the nurse describes how she involves the medical student:

> **Nurse:** ...a medical student was there and I said, 'Would you kindly go back to the nursery and tell them to open up the OHIO bed, the intensive bed. Open an umbilical catheterization [kit]. Call the respiratory therapist for the ventilator.' So when we went there, basically everything was set up...

Despite the fact that nurses are rarely described as the team leaders, it is rare that anyone other than a nurse organizes the team in a crisis. Experienced nurses are best positioned for this role for several reasons. First, as direct care providers, they are always involved in the patient situation and are thus in a position to anticipate what may be needed, as in the above example. Second, they are hospital employees and are typically familiar with the "appropriate" procedures and chains of command for mobilizing resources. Third, they work with all other team members in various types of situations and recognize individuals' potentials and limitations. In addition, as coordinators of patient care on a daily basis, nurses gain experience organizing the team in everyday practice during noncrisis situations.

Organization of the team is not necessarily a formal effort. When people work together for a long period of time, they tend to gain a sense of who needs to do what and simply organize themselves in response to the situation, the patient in crisis, and to the demands of other patients. For instance, if a nurse has a very critical patient, he or she will commonly stay with that patient and cover for other patients rather than participate directly in another patient's crisis. Experienced healthcare providers commonly notice what other team members are doing and immediately fill in. A nurse with a stable patient is likely to do much of the "running around" type tasks in a crisis to allow the primary nurse to remain at the bedside where needed. This organizational knowledge is socially embedded in the history, lore, and norms of those working in a unit. However, the less familiar that team members are with each other, the more they need a leader to organize the team's efforts. Because many of these skills are subtle, they are easily missed by learners. Leaders could assist in the development of nurses by verbalizing their thinking-in-action and the eventualities they anticipate in particular situations.

Once the initial organizational work of collecting the team and reassigning priorities is completed, there is an ongoing need to <u>orchestrate</u> the team's management of the crisis to maintain coordination and smooth flow. Without skillful orchestration, it is easy to overlook or delay needed interventions (e.g., the timing of a second dose of epinephrine, starting CPR when pulseless electrical activity is present), unnecessarily duplicate actions, fail to evaluate crucial treatments and patient responses (e.g., the effectiveness of CPR), lose track of what has been done and what is still needed, and miss recognizing when resuscitative efforts become futile. A skilled clinician plays a central role in orchestrating a crisis because, at any point, unorchestrated team efforts can move in an inappropriate direction or slip into chaos. Although the clinician orchestrating the team may also be the team leader who specifically manages the patient's immediate care, a skilled physician is often the team leader and looks to the nurse to deftly orchestrate overall team functions.

During a crisis, additional team members often become available. Frequently, so many people arrive at the bedside that few can see what is actually being done and some may have difficulty getting to the patient to do what is called for in a timely manner. Also, team members or a designated but inexperienced team leader may not grasp what needs to be done and when, as demonstrated in this story:

Nurse: They were arguing so nothing was happening. No epinephrine was being given, no atropine, nothing was happening and no chest compressions were being done. I asked the anesthesiologist—when she finished intubating and the baby was being ventilated by the therapist—I asked her to do compressions because she was at the bedside and she looked at me like, 'I only do airways.' I asked somebody else to start doing compressions because the kid had a heart rate of 30 which, in an infant, is not compatible with life. She had no blood pressure. The CT guy [cardiothoracic surgeon] is really the one that should be giving the order. I asked him, 'What do you want me to do?' He tells me. So we give epinephrine and then the therapist can't ventilate, so the anesthesiologist tries and they say the baby is having a really bad bronchial spasm. A lot of times with these kids, if you give them a lot of sedation, they are a lot easier to ventilate. I asked, 'Can we give some [ativan]l or can we paralyze her or something to make it easier?' The CT surgeon said, 'Give [ativan].'

In this situation, the team initially looks to the surgeon for leadership, but without his direction, "nothing was happening." As the baby rapidly deteriorates, the nurse sees that the team clearly needs orchestration and leadership. By delegating responsibilities and asking questions (which can be a form of leading), she begins orchestrating the team's actions to respond to the crisis. Experienced nurses must often orchestrate and informally lead, coach, or take charge of the team, despite the hierarchical tradition, in order to ensure patient safety and quality care. Expert nurses respond to a moral press to take a leadership role in situations of confusion. Orchestrating involves recognizing who is needed and delegating responsibilities, identifying who is not needed and asking them to leave, noticing what needs to be done and ensuring that someone does it, keeping track of what has been done, anticipating what will need to be done and who else will be needed, prompting or coaching others in order to avoid or correct breakdown, noticing what and when support services are needed, designating who is needed to run blood samples to the lab or retrieve blood for transfusions, and recognizing and responding to the family's need to be informed and/or at the bedside. Leadership during a crisis also involves recognizing the effectiveness (or lack) of therapies and evaluation and management of breakdown situations where therapies are inappropriate, ineffective, or untimely.

The skilled know-how of orchestrating the above activities during a crisis depends on experiential learning. It is from actually being in situations that one gains a notion of what constitutes a "good code." Expert nurses describe a good code as one in which the team's familiarity in working together fluidly results in little need for formal orchestration in order for things to flow smoothly, rapidly, and effectively.

In flight nursing, where the central role of the nurse and the whole team is managing crises of all types on a daily basis, the individuals and the team as a collaborative unit have the opportunity to develop an extraordinary level of team expertise. As a team develops expertise, the organizing, orchestrating, and supportive roles are assumed by many so that each person's contribution complements the other and allows the nurses at the scene to have more complete attention on the care of the patient(s). A nurse in an interview tells the following story about a family that is involved in a catastrophic propane-related trailer fire in a national forest. It points out the excellent teamwork among the nurses, helicopter pilot, ground dispatch, and the local volunteer rescuers:

Nurse 1: Robin, [another flight nurse] and I went to [a rural community in the hills]. That was really good team work. It was the middle of the night and we landed in the lumber yard in [that community] because of the fire that was in the national forest at a campground. And Robin and I decided to take the pilot [Nan] with us too. Got in a squad car that we took back into this campground, way down this fire road. And a family, a mother, father, and a little baby, had been in a trailer that had caught on fire. And they were all badly, badly burned. Really badly burned. And we got there and there was only one first responder there. It was, what's his name?

Nurse 2: Willis?

Nurse 1: Willis. He was the only one there. And he had intubated the father and we went to the baby and looked at the baby and the baby needed to be intubated. There was no way around it. And we got an IV in the kid, gave succs (succinylcholine) to the kid, and intubated him. Well then [because Willis stayed with the father], that left me to go look at the other patient. So Robin basically ended up being dedicated to this kid. She couldn't leave the kid after we intubated him. So I went to the father, and he had an airway in, and there was the first responder there, ventilating him. And so I went on to the mother. And Nan, our pilot, was with me. And the mother was badly, badly burned. And there were no IV sites. There was no way I was going to get an IV into her to succs her and she was very awake, so I couldn't orally intubate her. So I tried to nasally intubate her several times. And I couldn't get the tube in her nose. It just wouldn't go in. <u>All</u> these people were like 80-90% burns. So they all had to be intubated. There was no way around it. So, I proceeded to do a cric [cricothyrotomy] with Nan, the pilot. And we always do crics with the other nurses. And I just told Nan, I said, 'I got the kit out. As I ask for things, just give them to me.' And, we cric'd this lady. And there were a couple of firemen there to help us. I incised her neck [for airway access]...and we ended up getting airways in all three of these patients. And then we put them in two ambulances. And we went back to the [helicopter] landing zone, which was like a 20 or 30 minute ride. And by then, the teamwork at this end was working very well too. Because our dispatch center had called in two other helicopters. So we had three helicopters in the landing zone when we got there, one for each patient. So we gave report to the other two helicopters. We kept the baby and I turned over the mother to one helicopter and the father to another helicopter and we all flew in to the [hospital] and off-loaded all of them. It was a horrific flight. It was just surreal, it was in the middle of the night... Robin and I talked a lot about it. Because it was dark. It was middle of summer. Out in the middle of nowhere. I was just <u>so</u> glad when I looked up and saw the hospital. And we got in here like around 6:30. The day crew was just coming on, so they were helping us and we were just <u>stunned</u>.

Interviewer: From?

Nurse 1: Just the hurt. Three horribly [burned] patients and getting out there and not having all the equipment that we really needed and not having enough resources. All three people needed so much care, and just not enough people to go around. But it was just really, we went through CIS [critical incident stress] debriefings over that. That flight still bothers me a lot...

Interviewer: Now, you said, part of it being horrific was that you didn't have what you needed. What did you need that you didn't have?

Nurse 1: More ALS (advanced life support) providers there. At least an ALS prepared person for each [patient]. A <u>couple</u> of ALS people for each patient. And they just weren't there. And these volunteer firemen, as great as they are, they were just stunned. They had to be told, 'Do this, do that,' otherwise they just were standing there. When I walked up to the mother, she was just laying in the dirt. Nobody knew what to do with her. You know how people are with burns, they just kind of go (demonstrating a horrified look)... And we were at scene for awhile. And then another ambulance had to come in so we had enough ambulances to transport all these people back. We had the mother and the baby in one ambulance. And Robin and I were in that ambulance with Nan. And Willis was with the father. But when we got back here, as soon as we got into the [trauma] room, after we gave a report, Robin and I went into the utility room and started crying. (Silence).

Interviewer: What happened? To the patients?

Nurse 1: Both the parents died. The father died early on. The mother died in a few weeks. The little boy is still alive. Actually <u>Heart Beat</u> [health TV show] or somebody here did a story on him. Yeah, his aunt and uncle are raising him. But they were all horribly burned... But, as horrific as it was, it was very good teamwork at both ends, at dispatch and the nursing end.

Nurse 3: With your pilot?

Nurse 1: Yeah. And Nan, absolutely.

Nurse 3: She won an award for that, [Nurse 1] nominated her.

Nurse 1: Yeah, I did. Robin and I nominated her for an award, which she won.

In this situation, the needs of these severely burned patients are too demanding because the two nurses cannot adequately or quickly manage the crisis and transport all three patients without assistance. The volunteer rescuer's assistance with the father's airway frees the nurse to attend to the mother. When the mother can not be nasally or orally intubated, it is the pilot, who does not typically participate in patient care, who assists and enables the nurse to perform the life-sustaining cricothyrotomy in the dark. The pilot's spontaneous and smooth performance is so needed and appreciated that her colleagues nominate her for an award. Without discussion, the dispatcher self-organizes by anticipating the need for another ambulance and two additional helicopters. His timely actions avert a critical delay in transport. With a bit of orchestration from the flight nurse, the stunned volunteers are able to respond as needed. Although not his typical style of orchestrating team members, the nurse recognizes that the volunteer rescuers are too stunned to act independently and therefore gives directives, "Do this, Do that," in order to initiate a response.

Learning to organize and orchestrate team members during a crisis involves risk and can be intimidating. At an unpredictable point and time, critical care nurses all find themselves in the position of orchestrating, whether by plan, by default because they are the most experienced person in the situation, or by being the first person to recognize orchestration is needed. A nurse talks about finding herself in this situation for the first time:

Nurse: I really hadn't been on too many scenes where the first responders and the fire fighters—by the time we got there—they were overwhelmed. They just didn't know what else to do, so they were all just standing there or sitting there or watching me... And I just remember when I bent down and we realized he [the patient] was esophageally intubated and his Glasgow [coma score] was so low, I just remember looking over at the helicopter thinking, 'I wish I was in that going to the hospital' because it was like a fraction of a second of panic. 'I'm in charge here,' you know? But then it's like, 'No one else is going to step in. There's absolutely no one else to step in, so you might as well just move on.' And it was a good feeling because that was the first time I had to do that... I learned so much from that one call.

Interviewer: Tell me what you learned.

Nurse: I learned to prioritize; I learned that I <u>could</u> make those decisions. I knew when it was time to go to a cric [cricothyrotomy]. I learned and I did orchestrate the care, but I still need to improve. But you've just got to start dealing out tasks. At first maybe you feel, 'Gosh, I'm being bossy,' but it's not that at all, if that's your position. You need to orchestrate. You need to help people because they want to help. They're there. They're waiting to help. You just got to learn how to do it. How to facilitate some helping. And I just learned all that in one call.

The nurse points out the role of emotion and moral agency as she recognized the press to take on the role as orchestrator during the crisis. Her flash of "panic" is from fully understanding that the patient is on the verge of coding (and did within moments), that she is the primary person responsible in the situation, and that absolutely no one else is going to step in. It takes courage, particularly when the other team members, such as the volunteer rescuers, are not familiar. With this leadership role, the nurse extends her understanding of being a good nurse to someone who can orchestrate others who want to help in the situation.

EXHIBITING EXPERIENTIAL LEADERSHIP IN MANAGING THE PATIENT WHEN A PHYSICIAN IS PRESENT

Experiential leadership is seeing what needs to or must be done before or during a crisis and doing it, even though a physician is present. When the legitimate leader is inexperienced or unable to provide appropriate or adequate medical direction or skilled know-how, an expert nurse typically feels morally compelled to take the lead in managing or coaching the management of the patient to ensure safe, timely, appropriate, and quality care. Experiential leadership is also exercised to ensure that medical management is not contrary to the patient's wishes or directives.

Taking the clinical leadership role in a crisis (diagnosing and treating) when a physician is present can go relatively unnoticed if the physician is open to clinical learning and values other team members' input and capabilities. The following situation involving a 40-year-old patient, who is admitted from the operating room post-thoracotomy, reflects the ease with which the nurse takes the leadership role without question from the physician. The nurse is precepting two other nurses in the care of this patient who is initially stable, but suddenly deteriorates while the anesthesiologist is giving report:

> **Nurse:** ...about a minute into the report, the patient's heart rate slowed down and I looked at the monitor and it was '50,' and then I looked at the MAP [mean arterial pressure] and the MAP was '50,' and sinking. Both of them were just—the numbers were going down, down, down. I looked at the patient and he wasn't breathing. And so I just said, 'He's not breathing,' jumped up, ran across the room, got the Ambu bag, and the other nurse in the room, she came over and straightened his head out and that still didn't work, so we bagged him immediately. And then the anesthesiologist said he needed the chief there to intubate and then I realized that he was a junior, he was orienting too. So we had all these orientees and the experienced people were the ones that had to react so fast. And the others, they knew to step back and let us do our thing... The nurse in the next room went and got the [emergency] cart, so everything was ready for him (the chief) when he got there. But you just go into that mode of acting regardless of who's there. If they're going to react, they're going to react, but I wasn't waiting for them.

Despite the anesthesiologist's primary role in airway management and maintenance, he is in an unfamiliar setting. He sees the nurse act immediately, and steps aside for her to respond to the crisis. In this case, the nurse's rapid intervention initiates a successful resuscitation.

Another story points out how fluidly and expediently a crisis can be managed when the team works synergistically, complementing each other's strengths, and power issues are nonexistent. This level of collaboration and synergy enables clinicians to fully focus on the patient and to respond to the patient's and family's needs. In the following account that was cited in Benner, Tanner & Chesla (2009, pp. 149), a flight nurse arrives to transport a very sick 7-year-old child with several congenital anomalies. The child is only two and one-half feet tall. She is not doing well, is tachycardic, and the previous team could not start an IV:

Nurse: ...this little kid was way too pale, way too tachycardic, and yet the referral physician and the parents were both saying, 'Well it's not that bad; why don't you just take the child back in the helicopter' and the physician said [to the transport nurse], 'Well, do you think we can go ahead and transport?'...and I was saying, 'No, no, no, no.' And actually within about 10 minutes of being there, we had to intubate the child. She had rapid breathing; and heart rates normally stay in the 120's and 130's; hers is now in the 160's, 170's ...They were wondering if she'd blown out something in her gut or was septic. But she was pale, her respiratory rate was maybe in the 60's. Just too fast, not real hard, but she just wasn't responsive. She just didn't respond no matter what I was doing... Even though this child was really developmentally delayed, she would still normally have pulled away or whatever. I asked the parents, 'Does she usually do something if she doesn't like what you're doing?' 'Yeah, she will try to pull away.' And she didn't and that was when I said, 'I think we need to get her intubated now.' And I took her blood pressure and it was only 38 [systolic]. And children typically keep blood pressures until the bitter end. And this is a child with no IV and whom, I just got told, it took them seven hours to get an IV in the last time she had to have one. So needless to say, my confidence going into this wasn't great. Anyway it turned out to be one of those miraculous things where we end up remembering it forever and a day, just because of the sheer luck. I found a vein and I got an IV in and I'm like, 'Oh, oh!' It made my week, but anyway, it was great from the physician's standpoint because this was a physician who worked really well with us. We stood there and said [to the physician], 'Okay, we need to intubate and we need to get in a line, we need to get in 10 cc's per kilo[gram] boluses of fluid'...[The team work was] just where everybody was willing to play together and just get everything done because we didn't waste time fussing with physicians and trying to see whose ego isn't going to be stepped on. Then I can spend some time, after [the resuscitation and after the child's] physical needs had been taken care of, to actually talk to the parents.

In contrast, other situations show that doing what needs to be done on a patient's behalf can be one of the greatest challenges for a nurse when power and authority issues take precedence over the nurse's clinical knowledge and experiential wisdom.

Stories about experiential leadership typically involve life-threatening situations or moral dilemmas. In each story, the leadership and team skills are as important, sometimes more important, in managing the crisis than the actual clinical expertise, as seen in the following story:

Nurse 1: ...they had to take a patient down to interventional radiology. What had happened was that this patient had a liver transplant and had several complications afterwards. He had this triple lumen catheter. It's an IV catheter that goes into the subclavian, right into it, and you have three ports to it, because he was getting different IV fluids, TPN[total parenteral nutrition], etc. Well, it was time to change it, and the resident was teaching the medical student how to change it over a wire. So, the medical student was doing this, and the resident was supervising. What had happened was when they rewired it, the wire was in, but the medical student didn't hold on to the wire, which he was supposed to, and it slipped under the skin, and we lost the wire.

Interviewer: You mean, in the patient?

Nurse 1: In the patient. Traveling, we don't know where. I looked over and this resident was white. He was absolutely pale. I said, 'What's going on?' He said, 'We lost the wire.' I said, 'What? OK. You want a chest X-ray? Call for the chest X-ray, first, and don't move the patient, please. We want to know where it is.'

We had to figure out how we were going to get the X-ray film underneath the patient and, unfortunately, we had to tip the patient over which I think helped the wire to travel. But we got the X-ray done. The whole time, I explained things to the patient; he was with it. He was kind of slow, but he knew where he was and what was going on. He could feel pain. I kept asking, 'John, are you okay? It's really important that you stay still and not move around' because he liked to move around and turn a little bit. I said, 'John, it's so important. Please. I'll be here the whole time. You let me know if you hurt anywhere. You let me know if you're uncomfortable, but don't move.'

Interviewer: Did he know that the wire had slipped in?

Nurse 1: I told him that we have a problem... I didn't tell the patient that the wire was possibly in his heart, and as it ended up, it was in the right ventricle. This patient has a history of arrhythmias, so I was thinking that we could have complications, major complications (nervous laughter). So, I knew we had to go downstairs. There was no other way.

Interviewer: Downstairs where?

Nurse 1: To Interventional Radiology. It was either that or the OR. We had to get the wire out. You couldn't let that thing sit in his right ventricle; there would be major problems. The first thing I did, I told the charge nurse, 'Look, this is what is going on. I need to get the transfer equipment ready.' I had somebody get the RT, get the oxygen tank because he wasn't intubated. He was breathing fine. He was talking to me, thank goodness. Call the resident. I want him to know what was going on because it's the ICU team that does the rewiring.

Interviewer: Call the resident on the service?

Nurse 1: The service resident. So I talked to them. I said, 'I just want to let you know, this is what happened. We have to go down to Interventional Radiology. You don't necessarily have to go down with me because the ICU resident is here. But please, let your attending know what's going on. And that news traveled really quickly up that ladder. Apparently the resident arranged for Interventional Radiology to go retrieve it. We were all ready to go, and I said, 'Wait a minute. Are they ready for us?' Because we were about ready to roll. So we called down there and they said, 'No, an hour.' It was a good thing that I checked those things because the resident just assumed that we could go down there right now... They couldn't get to us for an hour. So we had to literally sit on it for an hour. Otherwise we would have been sitting in the hall for an hour down there, and we wouldn't have been able to monitor the patient as closely.

By this time, I had everything on the bed ready to go, my code box, and everything. And I kept the patient real calm. I said, 'John, are you okay?' Then, I noticed that he had this huge stool. I said, 'Wait a minute.' I can't move him. I can't roll him over but I can't leave him like this, because he is really uncomfortable with it, and he was going to start moving around more, and that's going to make things worse. I just did the best I could. They said, 'No, don't move him at all.' I thought, 'Wait a minute. Let's try at least to clean him up because it's just going to get worse.'

I kept thinking, 'You [residents] don't want to move him off it, but when you move him on to that gurney downstairs and into the Interventional Radiology, you're going to have a mess galore and things are going to get contaminated galore.' Because it was all over... Actually what I did was, I pulled the sheet out from underneath him slowly and it worked. Everyone couldn't believe I did this, but I was glad I did it because the mess was not there anymore.

We finally got down there and the whole time, I kept asking, 'John, are you okay? Do you hurt anywhere? Please be still, we're almost finished.' I had to keep talking to him.

Interviewer: How did he hold up for that? How was he?

Nurse 1: He was doing okay. He had no arrhythmias, thank goodness.

Nurse 2: She was a wreck.

Nurse 1: (laughter) I was a wreck. An ICU resident was having problems too...because he knew it was his fault. I also knew he [patient] had to have his antiarrhythmic medication before he went down. I didn't want him to have it delayed. I kept thinking of all the medications that I needed to give him. But most important was, let me give him his antiarrhythmic before we go down. And it actually went really smoothly. We went down and they fished it out with no problem... and the patient was fine, had no complications, and we got him back upstairs. And also before we went down, I said, 'Can somebody please call the wife, just to let her know what's going on, because I think it's important for her to know.' She was a person who was very well informed. She knows what's going on, had gone through a lot with her husband because he had this liver transplant. She would definitely like to know... That transition, I think, went really well, going down and coming up without any patient complications. Because it could have been disastrous...

Interviewer: What happened to the medical student?

Nurse 1: He was there pretty much the whole time, but he felt terrible, like 'There goes my medical career.' I had to reassure him that things like that happen. It was an honest mistake because he held a part of the catheter that he thought was connected to the catheter but actually wasn't. It's hard to explain. But he was holding the wrong part, and the other part slipped in. He felt absolutely terrible. He will never forget this, I know. It was trying to make him feel better and more confident because you need confident people.

In this story, the nurse emerges as the team leader in both the orchestration of the team and the clinical management of the patient. Seeing the resident's face turn white, the nurse immediately suggests the course of action and the resident follows her lead even though neither of them have ever experienced a similar situation. Simultaneously, she anticipates what is needed in the ICU to prepare for a code, equipment and the personnel needed for transport, and the people who need to be notified. She then solicits help from colleagues to initiate the necessary preparations. During the whole crisis, she remains calm outwardly, modulating her emotional responses to facilitate a climate in which she and others could maximally function. Her utmost concern is for the patient—so she stays at the bedside continually to keep him calm, reassuring him in a soothing tone while vigilantly monitoring him moment to moment. The nurse specifically points out how modulating her responses prevents the performance of team members from becoming chaotic.

This nurse also stands out as a leader in her ability to blend comfort and care for seemingly less urgent patient needs while tending to the patient's emergent care. Had this been a case study instead of a narrative account of a real event, we would have left out the inconvenient timing of the patient having a stool. But the narrative keeps us honest and points out that crises too come with the mundane and inopportune timing of the body. Contamination, comfort, and dignity are at stake and one more contingency is managed. During the crisis, the nurse's concern also extends to the wife and the medical student who is devastated by the mistake. Throughout the situation, the nurse's leadership is as important to the patient's outcome as her clinical expertise. In addition to being an excellent exemplar illustrating experiential leadership, this story demonstrates the nurse's thinking-in-action as it unfolded. It also shows how the numerous aspects of managing a crisis are not discrete and separate, unlike a procedural account of expert practice, but rather flow and overlap as the situation demands.

When nurses take or are given the clinical leadership role in a crisis, physicians may step back in and take over once they are comfortable with the situation. This alternating role of leader is exemplified in the following story about a nine-year-old child who is the only survivor in a big car accident in a small town. Flight nurses arrive at the emergency department to transport the child to a trauma center:

Nurse 1: They'd had him intubated. He was looking pretty awful when we got in there. And almost as soon as we got there, his heart rhythm changed. He started going bradycardic and the ER doctor was pretty overwhelmed. And I was standing at the bedside and I noticed that he was arresting, so I started CPR. And the ER doctor just stood back and we (flight nurses) ran the code. And I told him, 'You know, we need to put chest tubes in. This is a trauma, he's now arresting, so the algorithm is chest tubes. And he didn't know how to do that. And I got out our Cook catheter chest tubes and I showed him how to do it.

Nurse 2: Nurse 1 walked him through it. He just did an excellent job of walking the doctor through it.

Interviewer: Now do [flight nurses] insert chest tubes?

Nurse 1: They're like 12 gauge trocars, Cook catheters. So it's not huge, it's not a size 36 catheter. But it's about like this [showing the group].

Interviewer: But do you guys usually insert those?

Nurse 1: Uh huh. Yeah.

Interviewer: Now tell me why you deferred to him [the physician].

Nurse 1: Because this was an inter-facility transfer. So we were in his realm and he was in charge and we were actually working under his orders, basically. But he did not know ATLS (advanced trauma life support), you might say. And so, I got out our Cook catheters, we continued CPR, we put chest tubes in on both sides of this kid. And we still didn't get him back. And we gave drugs, we did everything. We gave fluids and the kid was, I think, in an asystole and there was no response, and the doctor didn't want to give up. And he said, 'What should I do now?' And I said, 'Well, if we were at the medical center, we would open his chest, because he's arrested in front of us.' But I said, 'We can't do that here. We have no place to take this kid if you crack his chest. I think you have to declare him [dead].' And he couldn't do it.

Nurse 2: He <u>wouldn't</u> do it. He just could not. We went on coding the child for another ten minutes?

Nurse 1: Awhile. Yeah. And we finally called med control [a physician at the medical center]. And gave report, and we had him talk to the physician and say, 'You've done everything you can. You need to declare this child,' and then, even <u>then</u>...

Nurse 2: He was <u>really</u> hesitant. Really hesitant. I had gotten on the phone with the doctor and I said, 'This is the situation. The physician here does not want to call the code. It's pure asystole, it's not going to change.' And I said, 'I think you need to talk to him and tell him that it's okay.' And he did, or I assume that's what he did. He was on the phone with him for awhile. And the doctor still could not do it.

Nurse 1: He called the family in while we were still doing CPR...

Nurse 2: ...that was another side of the story then, with the aunt coming in.

Nurse 1: The mother, father, and sister were all dead in the car...and the family had all been to the accident and knew there were fatalities, but nobody [at the scene] would let them look. And they knew one person had made it to the hospital. So they didn't know which one was alive and who was dead. And so, they finally got in and saw, they knew he was alive and everybody else was dead. And then they <u>came in</u> while we were doing CPR.

Nurse 2: The doctor let the aunt in. And she did not speak English, so that was difficult as well. But the physician spoke a <u>little</u> bit, I believe, so he tried talking to her and he told her then that the little boy was dead. And we stopped... Nurse 1 did an excellent job with that physician. He just did <u>wonderfully</u>.

As the child arrests, the nurse unobtrusively begins managing the code when the physician pulls back. Although the nurse knows when and how to insert the chest tubes, he later explains that he respectfully re-involves the physician because the nurses are in the physician's facility and he is ultimately responsible. The physician resumes the leadership role when he disagrees that further intervention is futile. It is only in the primary role of managing the crisis that the physician understands that no further treatment is available or promising. The nurses go on to describe that the first nurse removed himself to the corner of the room when he became overwhelmed by the tragedy and sorrow in the situation. The second nurse intervened to assist the family and other nurses as they realized that the child had died. This tragic example shows how leadership is assumed and can alternate as different clinicians respond to the changing demands of the situation.

Because crises can be the most stressful of all situations in clinical practice, how nurses comport themselves as they take on the leadership role can strongly influence other team members' ability to function optimally. Depending on the type of situation and the experience of those involved, experiential nurse leaders will often facilitate the work of the team by asking questions rather than giving directives. One nurse explained that she typically asks questions like, "Have you given this? Have you done that? Do you need to give some more bicarb? Did you see the last gas? Does the baby need to be baptized?" while she avoids saying, "Do this! Do that!" Questions can be effective in focusing efforts and improving responsiveness without underestimating others' abilities or setting up power struggles. There are, however, situations when directives like, "Do this" are appropriate and helpful in re-engaging a stunned clinician to assist in a crisis. The context of the situation guides the style of interaction, and interactions are interventions.

It is not uncommon for the nurse to disagree with the physician's response to a question. For instance, the nurse asks, "Do you want to give this medication?" The physician responds, "No." If the nurse disagrees, it can be helpful to ensure that the physician has sufficiently updated knowledge of the situation by mentioning the salient aspects and again asking the question, "Are you sure?" New information that the physician was not privy to can alter the course of treatment.

Asking questions stems, in part, from the nurse's understanding that "they [physicians] get very focused during codes—very focused on procedures—and sometimes they miss the whole management piece of it, especially if there's difficulty with access." Here, the nurse respects how totally absorbing a challenging, life-sustaining procedure can be and the impossibility of keeping track of the "big picture" when the patient's life depends on securing the airway during a difficult intubation or getting a IV access on a patient who is coding. This nurse further explains, "I've never been told to hush by suggesting different medications. If they say 'no', they say 'no', but for the most part people appreciate it all." Although expert nurses commonly develop facilitative communication styles that respect and, when needed, protect team members, their first and foremost concern focuses on responding to the patient's immediate needs. A smooth functioning team can best provide that care.

TAKING NECESSARY MEDICAL ACTION TO MANAGE A CRISIS WHEN A PHYSICIAN IS ABSENT

Nurses routinely find themselves in the position of being the most experienced or qualified healthcare providers in an emergent situation where there is no physician. Patients' lives depend on nurses taking necessary medical action in order to manage the crisis until a physician is available. Managing or preventing a crisis often depends on the nurse recognizing the subtle changes that indicate imminent deterioration in the patient's condition. These crisis situations all demand diagnosis and treatment. In many sudden, life-threatening situations (e.g., bradycardia, ventricular fibrillation, cardiac arrest), standing orders or emergency protocols are commonly pre-approved for implementation by nurses as needed. However, there are numerous types of "pre-code" and unexpected emergencies in which nurses must act, where no protocols or guidelines cover the particular situation. They must use their best clinical judgment for each specific situation. A nurse explains, "Well, we have certain parameters that we go by. We have standing orders on some things, but other things you just do..." In the following situation, Clara Reagan illustrates taking necessary life-saving medical action which, in this situation, is addressed by a policy that blocks the oncology nurse's expert judgment and definitive intervention in an elderly gentleman who suddenly and unexpectedly deteriorated:

Nurse: The nursing aide rushed in and said, "Clara, I can't wake up Mr. R and he doesn't look good." I had learned that when <u>this</u> aide says you better come, that is a guaranteed transfer to the ICU, or a death by the end of shift in DNR patients. I quickly recalled details about Mr. R as I went to the bedside. Yesterday, he was alert, oriented and sitting up in a chair. I knew he had metastatic prostate cancer, but this admission he was in for unrelated problems and was certainly expected to survive the hospitalization. He had cardiac history and diabetes. I was his primary nurse and cared for him all week. Before I got to his bedside, I thought, "It's Father's Day." I dreaded having to deliver any kind of unexpected bad news to his family on Father's Day.

I called Mr. R's name and he clearly tried to respond, but his speech was slow and garbled. He spoke only Portuguese, and although I speak enough of the language to get by, I am not fluent, so it was more difficult to understand him. His arms were flaccid without grasps and he couldn't follow commands in any language. It appeared that he was losing consciousness. I immediately thought of a hypoglycemic reaction, but certainly other diagnoses could not be ruled out. We didn't have glucometers on the unit, so the lab performed all blood sugar testing. Also, we needed an order to administer boluses of dextrose for hypoglycemia—a policy my colleagues and I had argued about many times.

Fortunately, Mr. R had lab work drawn an hour ago, so I raced to grab his results. His blood sugar was 226. I was puzzled because I really felt he was hypoglycemic. As I picked up the phone to call to his physician, I scanned his lab results. I immediately dropped the phone. His labs didn't make sense. Yesterday, his potassium was 5.2 and his digoxin level was 4. His physician felt his chronic renal failure was the cause and had not treated Mr. R aggressively because he was asymptomatic. He had simply placed the digoxin on hold and repeated the labs the next day. Today, the potassium level was 3.0 and the digoxin level was < 0.3—the value one gets when a level is ordered on a patient who doesn't take digoxin. I knew these results could not possibly be his and my heart sunk. Even though Mr. R had a DNR order, I couldn't let him die from a potentially reversible metabolic problem. I paged a lab tech stat and told him that I suspected a lab error and I needed someone right away because Mr. R had all but lost consciousness.

Two daughters arrived to spend the day and obviously stunned by the unexpected and profound change in his condition. They began to cry as they tried frantically to arouse their father. Fortunately, the lab tech arrived minutes after my call, and as he prepared to check a fingerstick glucometer, I prepared the D50 I grabbed from the code cart. I asked another nurse to call the physician for the order, but I was giving it with or without the order. The lab tech nodded to me that his sugar was indeed low. I saw the reading—18—as I simultaneously began to push the dextrose bolus and explain to his daughters what was happening. I prayed silently that we weren't too late to reverse his somnolence. I just kept thinking how awful it would be for him to die so unexpectedly on Father's Day. As I proceeded to draw serum to repeat all his labs and confirm the error, Mr. R opened his eyes and said "Happy New Year" in English. His daughters laughed and corrected him by saying "Happy Father's Day." I breathed a huge sigh of relief. I was then paged for a call from his physician. I explained the events and obtained orders for IV fluids and glucometer readings for the rest of the day. A few minutes later, the chief lab tech called to tell me that they had blood typed the specimen drawn earlier and that it was not Mr. R's. There had been a labeling error, and they would investigate.

Mr. R spend the rest of Father's Day enjoying the love and company of his family. Shortly after, each unit became equipped with a glucometer…We can perform a stat glucometer when hypoglycemia is suspected and we can treat it.

The pre-code crisis management practices of acute and critical care nurses fall into a "gray" area of practice. Gray areas of practice are those which are not yet legitimately or formally recognized as being within nursing's domain of practice, but present a clinical and moral necessity to act independently and expediently. Trying to cover all these eventualities by specific protocols is not practical or possible because the "emergency" is contextual. In the example above, if a physician had been available, the nurse would have immediately obtained a blood sugar (glucometer or lab) order and secured an order for the dextrose to cover her actions. In fact, had a physician been available, a bolus of dextrose would likely have been given empirically. In this situation, Clara is not only faced with an avoidable crisis and death, but also with a clear and controversial policy. But in the face of imminent death, coupled with a glucose of 18, Clara acts on the moral imperative and takes the immediate action that is necessary. No one would advocate medical therapy without a physician's order or without a laboratory assessment; however, the risk is prudent in the above situation. In this particular organization, administration heeded the incident as a warning, learned, and intelligently responded with a policy change and the needed equipment.

To date, the expertise in critical care nursing has been better explicated than other areas of nursing practice so there is greater awareness about their skillful management of urgent and crisis situations (Benner, 2000, Benner, Tanner & Chesla, 2009, Benner, Hooper-Kyriakidis & Stannard, 1999, Hooper, 1995). However, crises occur throughout acute care areas where nurse-patient ratios do not afford close monitoring, few extra skilled clinicians are available to help, fewer nurses know their patients due to inconsistent and heavier assignments, and the occasion to manage a crisis (incidence and rapid response teams) and therefore hone one's skills is infrequent. Given the current environment, the ability to avert a crisis in many acute care areas is truly remarkable.

In the face of current regulatory laws, nurses take great risks when managing some types of crises since they necessarily function outside the legal boundaries of nursing and cross over into what has traditionally been the domain of medicine. Yet, patients' lives depend on nurses taking necessary medical action in pre-code emergencies and in emergencies where the time demand requires immediate action. The lack of legitimacy contributes to these practices being covered over and remaining invisible; yet, the logic of acute and critical care demands that nurses continue to have the latitude to manage pre-code emergencies and prevent fatal outcomes. The following clinical incident, cited in Benner, Tanner, and Chesla (2009, pp. 344), demonstrates the nurse taking swift, life-saving medical action in the midst of a crisis after her early forewarning and coaching of the resident fails. An orientee is caring for an elderly woman who had bilateral femoral-popliteal bypass surgery, complicated by a critically high blood pressure that is not being controlled on oral medications. There is also no standing order for a vasodilator infusion. The physician fails to see the imminent danger, leaves the unit, and the inevitable occurs:

> **Nurse:** ...her blood pressure was, on her first full day post-op, was 190/110 and that's just too high. Anybody else would have been on nipride to keep their blood pressure down, otherwise [the high pressure) could blow her graft. I remember being very concerned about this lady's blood pressure and her being fairly refractory to any of the [oral] agents that they were using on her. [After nitropaste] she was still sitting 170/100 and the third year resident came by...and I said, 'This lady's blood pressure is [190/110] and we can't get it down. What would you like us to use to get it down further?' 'That's okay,' he said, chewing his gum. And I said, 'Well, as a rule, vascular patients are not allowed to have a blood pressure higher than this.' He goes, 'We'll go with that'...'Well, we should give her something for pain.' [The resident did not change orders and left.] I should have fought harder. I should have gone up [the ladder] because a few moments later, I was helping another nurse when the orientee said, 'C., come here.' I go whipping around the corner and the patient had blown her graft. She had an artery pumping from her groin into the bed with a thigh this big around... We started doing all the appropriate things—dipping her head down, [putting] her oxygen on really high, going ahead and calling for blood, calling over to the OR, calling the physicians...

Here, the patient's situation demands that someone respond to her bleeding. So, the nurse, the only skilled clinician at the scene, orders exactly what is called for in this crisis—the urgently needed blood and the patient's return to surgery. Unfortunately, the patient did not survive the surgery. When seconds count, waiting for a physician to arrive to prescribe the same interventions can further delay treatment and possibly have devastating ramifications for the patient.

In acute and critical care nursing, the above instance is one of many common and highly predictable situations that result in crisis when rapid and appropriate intervention is not taken to prevent complications. Recognizing these emergent and predictable patterns in rapidly unfolding patient situations requires the development of perceptual acuity which is the sense or ability to notice salient aspects in the situation. It is an embodied and practical skill, experientially gained through the senses (e.g., seeing, touching), that scientific knowledge can strengthen but never replace. This recognitional ability is gained from being fully engaged in practice, with attentiveness to and learning of clinical distinctions and similarities in patients' responses. The nurse recognized and was concerned that the patient might rupture the surgical graft. Her concern served an important role in orienting her perception to the situational urgency, her clinical judgment that action was needed, and her actions to warn and coach or nudge the resident.

To best respond in an emergent situation, perceptual acuity must be accompanied by appropriate and timely action. In this situation, the nurse discusses her concerns about the patient's blood pressure with the resident, but later feels remorse about not having "fought" for her perspective and the needed intervention so that the crisis may have been averted. Skilled know-how, knowing how and when to act, is developed by learning from such experiences. In this case, the nurse learns that she must "fight" or take a stand for her clinical perspective for the patient's sake, particularly in preventing a crisis. What she learns is transformed into a commitment for what she will do in future situations. The nurse's commitment to act as a strong agent is essential for developing expertise (Rubin, 2009). As the nurse's reflections illustrate, she will be more forceful in the future (also cited in Benner, Tanner & Chesla, 2009, p. 344):

> **Nurse:** ...I just killed myself over that. If I had fought harder, maybe that wouldn't have happened...and I just felt really bad about not going with what I felt was right and so since then, when I'm fairly convinced about something, then I'll fight for it.

It is from situations like this that nurses commonly learn they must go up the chain of command to elicit necessary help and interventions. Sharing narrative accounts such as this can assist developing nurses in recognizing what to do and how to "fight harder" in pre-crisis situations.

Because all crisis situations cannot be anticipated, nurses draw on past, similar experiences when managing emergencies. The medical action taken is not necessarily prescribable; it is often determined by unpredictable changes in the patient's response during the crisis, as demonstrated in the following story about a patient with congestive heart failure (CHF) who is admitted into an amiodarone research study due to dysrhythmia problems. He is in the CCU to adjust his medications in hopes of improving his activity level. A pulmonary artery (PA) catheter is inserted and a chest X-ray is done. Two nurses involved in his care discuss his situation:

> **Nurse 1:** Before we had the results of that [X-ray], I went in to see the patient. Even though I had never seen him, I knew something was not right. He was talking. He was on nasal prongs. He said he was not short of breath, but for some reason, and, thinking about it, I still can't put my finger on why I knew something was wrong. His blood pressure was fine. His pulmonary pressures were actually normal, even for a CHF patient. They were probably better than mine. His heart rate was fine.

Interviewer: Why did they put the PA line in?

Nurse 1: For the study, and then they realized that he was on antiarrhythmics and for tuning up purposes, they left the line in just so they could see exactly what the medicines would do hemodynamically. Within, I'd say, 15 minutes he was in pulmonary edema. He was really short of breath. His lungs were full of fluid and I had called the intern to see [the patient earlier] and said, 'Something is wrong. Somebody needs to see this man. You've seen him more than I have. I have no baseline to base my judgement on. I'd like to have your opinion.'

Interviewer: And you called the intern before the pulmonary edema set in?

Nurse 1: Right, as soon as I came on. Just to say, 'Look, you've seen him. Is this his normal? Or is my worry legitimate?' But [the resident] didn't show up.

Nurse 2: Was the X-ray showing pulmonary edema?

Nurse 1: It did. But it was not diagnosed until afterwards. That was about an hour after I started the shift. So, finally the resident did come. I had given the patient a nitroglycerin, sublingual, which eased the pulmonary edema to a certain extent before I had any orders to do anything.

What medical action is necessary may only become apparent as the situation unfolds and new or unexpected possibilities present themselves. In this case, the flash pulmonary edema in a patient with little cardiac reserve demands prompt intervention to avert a code. Nitroglycerin provides a readily accessible and rapid-acting treatment that temporarily alleviates some of the ventricular overload by reducing cardiac preload until more supportive therapy can be prescribed. Just prior to the crisis, this situation is filled with ambiguity for the nurse because, although the patient's objective findings are "normal", she perceives that "something was wrong", is unsure about what was needed, and calls the physician to examine the patient. As the crisis unfolds, the nurse gains a clearer understanding about the patient's evolving condition and knows how to best intervene until the physician arrives.

Despite the fact that these kinds of medical actions fall outside the traditional boundaries of nursing, nurses do and will continue to find themselves in these positions. Because nurses are typically the first responders in a patient crisis, acute and critical care nurses will continue to have a clinical and moral mandate to act in response to the emergency needs of the patients.

RECOGNIZING TALENT AND SKILLED CLINICIANS AND MARSHALING THESE FOR THE PARTICULAR SITUATION

Recognizing clinical talent and skilled clinicians means that nurses recognize the clinical knowledge, skilled know-how, and embodied intelligence of colleagues. This recognitional skill almost always depends on past experience in situations with the particular person. Marshaling skilled clinicians means eliciting help or initiating an appropriate response from a clinician who can recognize and manage a real or potential crisis. Nurses typically turn to experienced clinicians for help because of their ability to grasp the significance of a situation.

Recognizing clinical talent and marshaling skilled clinicians requires astute clinical judgment and skill and is a pervasive aspect of caring for critically ill patients in crisis. The need for these skills and judgment commonly arise when there is a breakdown in smooth taken-for-granted performance of the nurse or the team. Breakdown is experienced and can be identified when what is being done for the patient fails or will predictably fail to meet the patient's needs. Breakdown may also occur in a situation where the nurse does not yet know the patient and the patient's particular pattern of responses, which may or may not be an early indicator of an impending crisis, depending on what is "normal" for that patient. The following expert neonatal ICU nurses describe how they enlist the help of peers who have gained socially embedded knowledge about a particular baby in order to judge the likelihood of an impending respiratory crisis:

Nurse 1: Sometimes these kids, they get to a plateau where their $PaCO_2$ is 80 and it's not coming down, but it just stays there. It's like, 'Well maybe I should leave him alone.' You call somebody and say, 'What do you think about this kid?' What I usually ask is, 'Have you taken care of this kid before? Does he do this?'

Nurse 2: That's the other thing. Sometimes, if it is a kid that you don't know very well and it's the beginning of the shift, it's easy to say, 'Does anybody else in the room know this baby? Does this kid do this all the time?'

Nurse 3: They say, 'Oh yeah.' Then you can calm down.

Nurse 1: Or you can always get the doctors and say, 'I have never taken care of this kid before. You've been here for two weeks. Does this kid do this all the time?'

In situations like this, understanding the responses of a particular baby is needed to guide the nurse's timing and type of intervention in the crisis. Consequently, gaining historical knowledge about the patient from someone experienced with that particular patient can greatly assist and influence the nurse's clinical judgment.

The necessity for recognizing and marshaling skilled clinicians varies in different situations. When breakdown occurs in an actual or imminent crisis situation in which rapid intervention is needed, nurses often need a physician to "see," to understand, the clinical situation and its gravity and to initiate treatment. This nurse's story reflects the ease of involving the resident because he grasps the situation as a crisis:

Nurse: Somehow the [endotracheal] tube got dislodged... And thank God. God is listening to me. A third year resident, who I know is really very good and clinically skilled, came in the unit. He said, 'Do you need some help?' And I said, 'Of course! Come in!' And so he was trying to intubate the baby. He had difficulty intubating the baby but finally the tube went in.

Marshalling help can occur instantaneously when clinicians know each other and understand the other's bodily signals of distress without verbal communication. When distress is recognized, help is commonly offered. In this excerpt, the resident happens into the ICU at an opportune moment. He reads the situation, immediately grasps the nurse's need for help, and asks, "Do you need some help?" Because of the limited verbal exchange, this way of marshalling help often escapes notice.

In another crisis, an Advanced Practice Nurse who is called to consult on a patient recognizes that the patient is rapidly developing a life-threatening complication, a tension pneumothorax, that requires urgent intervention from a physician:

Interviewer: When you realized that the patient's pressure started dropping, you said that the attending physician happened to be in the unit.

Advanced Practice Nurse: Yeah. He just happened to be over on the MICU side.

Interviewer: So tell me what happened.

Advanced Practice Nurse: It was real fast. The patient dropped his blood pressure. The breath sounds were markedly diminished, heart rate really increased, airway pressures were increasing, it was a combination of a number of things. The nurse was in the room and [I decided] 'I'm going to get some help.' So I just walked across to the MICU and said, 'I think this guy's got a tension pneumothorax and we've got a chest X-ray ordered, but we need to get somebody in there <u>now</u>.' There really wasn't a discussion, and he didn't question or challenge it. He said, 'Get a tray, get a chest tube up here.' Then I returned, and when he came in, he didn't even ask. He did listen to breath sounds, but I think the combination of all the other information helped him. I really wasn't feeding him information because I was probably helping set up a chest tube tray, as I recall.

Interviewer: But you initiated the intervention.

Advanced Practice Nurse: Oh, yeah! Yeah.

Interviewer: And is that common? Do you commonly go outside the specialty and recruit in a consult?

Advanced Practice Nurse: In our unit, not always, but in certain situations, especially where I feel like I'm not being heard, or where I feel like I had to, in terms of that specific case. I don't have any problems. Talk to them. And sometimes it's informal, sometimes it's formal, it depends on the service and situation behind that. Politically, in certain units you might have to follow a chain of command. But my office is up in the ICU and so I've been up there long enough that I think there's just acceptance of me. It worked out well. If it had been another area, I probably would have had to go through a different chain of command. [This patient survived the emergent situation.]

In both of the above stories, marshaling experienced clinicians immediately saves the patients from further danger and from arresting. Recruiting the physicians is possible because the team members in both instances know and respect each others' practices and judgment. Other team members know that the expert diagnosis and judgment of these nurses warrants immediate attention and action and simultaneously prevents undue delay and costly additional interventions.

In contrast, eliciting appropriate assistance can be very challenging if the clinician with authority either does not grasp the significance issues or is not fully engaged and responsive. In the following story, an 88-year-old woman has a non-survivable injury of 80% second and third degree burns. Her family does not want her to needlessly suffer. During the day, the management of her fluid resuscitation is questionable. The resident wants to insert a pulmonary artery catheter for research purposes and the nurse finds the intervention unconscionable since the patient is on the verge of death. To prevent unnecessary suffering, a decision needs to be made about further treatment in an unfolding crisis:

Nurse 1: [The nurse noticed the physicians standing outside the patient's room.] 'I pounded on the glass door. There were two teams of physicians watching the patient's pressure drop from outside the room. I just pounded on the door and I said, 'You need to get in here now.' And I opened the door and I looked at the plastics attending, and as this woman started to go in and out of V[entricular]-tach[ycardia], I said, 'You better make a decision [about DNR].' [Her sister was] saying, 'Don't let her suffer.' But no [decisions] were made.

Nurse 2: I said, 'You have to do it NOW.' So we started the fluids. We increased her pressor. We had [put her into] Trendelenburg and I looked at him and he said, 'Okay, don't start any amiodarone. Don't go any farther than you have. Just support her enough for her sister to come in and say goodbye and do what she needs to do.' And the sister wanted the priest to come in. So it resolved okay, but I felt like I wasn't aware enough in the beginning to really have fought, and then finally when I did, it was like, 'You cannot go beyond this. This is unconscionable and against everybody's wishes. Don't tell me you're going to treat this.' It was really frustrating in a lot of ways and ethically I had some problems with it. I even brought it up at the American Burn Association meeting.

In sharp contrast with the previous example, this situation calls for the nurse to be very assertive in order to elicit a clinical decision regarding this patient's continued care. The kind of comportment needed in this type of situation is often developed in conjunction with a strong sense of moral agency. Pointing out excellent role models to less experienced clinicians can be helpful in their development of these ethical notions of good and skilled performance.

This story and others throughout this section highlight how the clinicians' grasp of the situation and their skilled know-how influence the need to recognize and marshall other resources. In the above situation, although team members have a good clinical grasp that this patient has a non-survivable injury, the physicians' hesitancy in making a decision about the patient's code status causes confusion and delay regarding immediate interventions and the course of action needed (e.g., to prevent suffering, to provide life support). A decision not to continue resuscitation is made after considering the patient's best interests. In other instances, team members have a good clinical grasp and intervene, but lack the skilled know-how or knack to perform what must be done in a timely manner or at all. Coaching and role modeling commonly help clinicians to more adeptly perform. However, the high-time demand of a crisis often requires that a more skillful clinician be solicited for assistance because the patient's care cannot be jeopardized in favor of teaching. In other situations, the team members may question their grasp of the patient's responses and desire another colleague's impression to validate their clinical understanding in order to determine the appropriate interventions.

For less experienced nurses, the ability to marshal more expert clinicians and the availability of those clinicians is crucial to the safety of the patient as well as to the quality of care and the nurse's clinical learning. Talented clinicians are sorely needed when the patient's clinical or perceived condition outstrips the clinical judgment and performance of less experienced nurses. Some hospitals have responded to this need by creating rapid response teams, which are only as effective as the expertise of the responders. The first step in eliciting skilled assistance is carefully attending to one's typical responses in ambiguous situations, such as sensing confusion. For example, a beginning nurse is caring for a post-cardiac surgical patient with COPD who was just transferred from the ICU and is experiencing mild respiratory distress. He has received no lasix, is 10 pounds over his pre-op weight, and has 1+ pitting edema:

Nurse: ....and I can just remember being so scared thinking, 'Oh, my God, what do I do?' So my first reaction was, go get help, go find someone, go get some help.

The role of emotion in a crisis situation compels nurses to either push until appropriate action is taken or to subtly involve experienced clinicians who can help but whom the nurse cannot formally or legitimately ask to consult on the patient. Foreboding or a sense of urgency may develop well before the crisis. Sensing a dangerous or potentially dangerous situation and the significance of the situation become embodied. The embodiment is reflected in nurses' comments, such as "I just pounded on the door and I said, 'You need to get in here now.'" Or "This is unconscionable and against everybody's wishes." Or "Thank God. God was listening to me."

In many situations, before one can marshal specific team members for a particular situation, nurses must have already developed prerequisite skills. Clinical forethought is essential to grasp what needs to be done and who is needed for assistance. In the following example, an experienced neonatal ICU nurse goes to assist with a 'routine' delivery. While suctioning the baby, the nurse has difficulty clearing the airway. She is able to get the physicians to admit the baby to the neonatal ICU for observation. This situation points out how clinical grasp and forethought are essential in order to recognize clinical talent and successfully marshal skilled clinicians to avert a crisis:

> **Nurse:** And she [the baby] started having trouble breathing so we started her on some oxygen via a hood. The physicians still wouldn't admit that her respiratory distress had anything to do with her secretions. They thought something else was going on. Well, Dr. S., the pediatric surgeon, happened to walk into the nursery and I said, 'Oh, Dr. S., I think I have a TE [tracheal-esophageal] fistula baby for you.' And he looked at me and he goes, 'How do you know?' So I told him and he turned to the doctors and he goes, 'Get a chest X-ray, what can it hurt?' They did. The baby had a really bad H-type TE fistula and they operated on her like two days later. She did really well because she never got fed. With a lot of babies, you don't know. They get fed and then they get aspiration pneumonia.

The nurse recognizes that a skilled clinical person, the pediatric surgeon, is available. She is able to make a case for her clinical perspective by sharing her grasp of the situation in a way that engages the surgeon to see and understand the situation and potential crisis accurately. Because of her adeptness at marshaling assistance, she is able to judiciously involve the surgeon without creating tension among the other physicians. Marshaling skilled performance further involves engaging and prompting others to take appropriate action, as reflected in the example.

In other situations, it is necessary to marshal resources for transport to the scene of the accident. Flight nurses must frequently be innovative in marshalling resources because it is an area of critical care practice that presents unusual challenges in gaining access to patients since accidents often occur in remote places. Depending on the terrain, the helicopter may not be able to land in close proximity to the patient. At times, getting to the patient requires hiking down a ravine, crossing a river, or hiking into a wooded area. A flight nurse describes this in a memorable incident:

> **Nurse:** We flew to the river and it was in a very remote area. It was a guy who dove off his boat and had some paralysis. And I'm thinking, 'This isn't good.' But we had to land far away from the scene, we were in high brush, there were trees <u>all</u> around, and we had to get on the back of a brush truck. So we threw all of our equipment in the back of this brush truck, and we were literally sitting on top of the brush truck, going through the bushes and trees, and these trees were smacking us in the head, and we're trying to dodge them and we <u>got</u> there, and this guy is <u>still</u> in the water. And I looked at my partner and I immediately thought, 'Oh my god, we're going to have to get in our skivvies and get in the water.' Fortunately, by that time, one of the medics was

already in <u>his</u> skivvies and he was able to pull the patient into the shallow water. So I took my boots and socks off and pulled up my pants... It was just one of those unique situations where you have to think, 'What am I going to do?'...Because there was nobody there.

Once at the scene of an accident like this, the major difficulty becomes transporting patients out while trying to physiologically stabilize them. In remote areas, whatever resources can be marshaled are often needed, not only to get the nurses to the patients, but also to get the patients back to the helicopter for transport.

On occasion, nurses may persist in trying to marshal any one of a number of clinicians, but be unsuccessful in recruiting anyone to act appropriately or in a timely manner. Experienced nurses commonly find themselves morally and ethically in the position of recognizing and diagnosing the patient's clinical condition and advocating for treatment on the patient's behalf in order to manage the crisis. The following story, cited previously by Benner, Tanner, and Chesla (2009, p. 228), demonstrates an expert nurse's leadership and persistence in trying to marshal help from a clinician who would take appropriate action. Although the vasoactive medications used in current practice may differ, this exemplar reflects the challenges nurses still confront. Here, an experienced nurse enters to assist a new nurse who is struggling to keep up with the care of a patient:

Nurse: This patient had an abdominal aortic aneurysm repair...and had come up from the operating room during the night. She (the patient) was intubated and on a ventilator, had a big fluid requirement, and had a metabolic acidosis. I guess she wasn't doing too well. Everyone (the physicians) just kept saying that she had a big operation; it's just taking her time to warm up, and once she does, then all of these things will correct. The patient's systolic blood pressure was very labile, going from 180 to 40 mmHg, and they were playing the nipride game. I had a sense of what was going on and I looked at the patient and there were two things that I noticed right off. One, her abdomen was very large and firm, and two, her knees were mottled and I said, 'She has dead bowel.' And they (the physicians) said, 'She doesn't have dead bowel.' Trying to back off a little bit, I said, 'Would you consider that maybe she has an ischemic bowel?' And they said, 'What makes you say that?' And I said, 'You can't maintain her blood pressure. We're playing nipride/fluid, nipride/fluid. She's acidotic as all get out—she's had a pH of 7.26 for hours. She's hypothermic and tachycardic. Her legs are mottled and her abdomen is taut and firm. This nipride game has got to stop. This is ridiculous. As soon as you put the nipride on, she drops her pressure. She's cold, she's clamped. She needs to be warmed, she needs fluid.' They (the physicians) wrote for lactated ringers. I said, 'Wait a minute, she's got a lactic acidosis—the last thing you need to do is to throw more lactic acid into her with the ringers.' And they said, 'Oh yeah...hang some saline.' The SICU house officer was there, the intern on the service was there and he just had no clue. So, we finally paged the senior person on the team and he was unavailable. He was in the operating room but the patient's attending was in-house, so he came up. The attending felt the patient just needed a few more hours to warm up and that would clear the lactic acidosis and then she would be fine. He left and was out of the hospital and beeper range for some time. Meanwhile the surgical attending walked into the unit and said, 'What's going on with so and so?' I was right there and I said, 'She really needs to go to the OR. Someone needs to look at this belly. I really think it's ischemic.' I'd stopped with the dead bowel trip; that was too fine a dance for them. I called it ischemic bowel and I said, 'The only thing that's going to save this woman's life is to get to the OR in a hurry.' And she said, 'Dead bowel!' and I said, 'Yeah, I've been trying to tell them for 3 hours.' She'd been following the patient's blood gases through the computer. So without even seeing the patient, this woman knew. So she came into the room, looked at the patient and she was like, 'Oh, my God, this patient's got to get to the operating room. It's definitely dead bowel.' And I thought, 'Thank God'...but everyone [wanted] to wait for the attending. I said, 'This woman is going to die... Someone better go talk to the family now.' The patient was starting to get less tachycardiac. The blood pressure was starting to slowly drop off. And we had the fluid wide open. And I said, 'It's even too late. She's going to die. So someone better go talk to the family to see if we can not code this woman because I know she's going to die.' And the resident said, 'K., keep your pants on. What are you getting all in a wad for?' And I said, 'Excuse me, I'm going to get the emergency cart, if anyone cares, and put it at the door.' And he said to me, 'You're crazy.' I said, 'She's going to arrest.' I went to get it. As I brought it to the door, she arrested [and was unsuccessfully coded]... On autopsy, they proved it was dead bowel.

The nurse goes on to explain that she "gave them every clue but they either couldn't see or didn't want to believe it." Once they did recognize the problem, "they just didn't see the end as imminent...or didn't have the same urgency "as the nurse did. This story points out the crucial role that nurses play in marshaling skilled clinicians in order to manage a crisis. This role is invisible to nurses, physicians, and managers, in part, because action is more readily noticed than the background skills that initiate and formulate action. This societal bias makes learning these background skills difficult. Without visibility or legitimacy, some crises will not be managed optimally or even satisfactorily.

What holds significance, what claims attention, and what nurses care about shows up in the way the nurse tells a story. An exclusive focus on outcomes that ignores the means or separates the means or actions from the outcomes is also a problem because the effective outcomes are, in fact, generated by the actions. With a singular focus on outcomes, the effective actions that generate the outcomes get lost. Yet, clinical and moral concerns constitute what must be told in order to give another person access to one's own understanding. In the study data, often what does not show up is the means; that is, marshaling of clinicians in situations when other team members are immediately responsive. Because of the immediate response, the momentary breakdown is covered over or goes relatively unnoticed. In these situations, only the outcome is alluded to. For instance, an elderly patient is admitted to the ICU because the lack of proper care at home created a crisis. He has several decubiti and requires a special bed to enhance healing. The nurse relates the outcome so simply that one may easily overlook the skilled know-how in marshalling the resources needed for this patient's complex care:

Nurse: He had a bedpan decubitus, so they [his family] must have left him all day on the bedpan. His whole back was covered in this rash that looked like scabies. We found out later it was not. He was covered from waist to knees in stool. He was just an unbelievable mess and it took three nurses working on him for an hour and a half just to make him presentable. We had to shave him because there was no other way to clean out his beard. We got a [pressure-relief mattress] because he had decubiti all around his buttocks and he had another one in the middle of his back... One of his toenails came off with his sock, so Podiatry came in and cleaned up his nail. Three days later, he was fine.

When team members are immediately responsive, smooth, fluid flow is minimally disrupted so that intervention is initiated without noticeable pause.

However, as the current health care climate changes and fewer skilled clinicians are available, marshaling expert clinicians is a growing challenge. A neonatal ICU nurse highlights her concerns about floating and replacing nurses with unlicensed assistive personnel or patient care assistants (PCAs). In this situation, a post-cardiac surgical neonate begins crying and turning blue. The nurse informs the fellow that something is wrong and tries to initiate therapy, but the fellow disagrees and leaves the unit. Few nurses are available in the unit as the crisis unfolds:

Nurse 1: So I said, 'I need help over here,' and I wasn't familiar with the north side where the code button was. I yelled, 'I need some help over here.' [But no help arrived.] I went to give code medications. At the moment the infant was arresting I yelled to a PCA, 'My baby's arresting. Get me the charge nurse.'

She (PCA) was new at her job. I guess she didn't know what the word 'arresting' meant, because she continued stocking the shelves, the supplies. Now this is all, mind you, happening very, very quickly.

Nurse 2: And this was not Nurse 1's home unit, so she didn't...

Nurse 1: Right! I didn't know names, I didn't...

Nurse 2: You didn't know people, you didn't know how to get things done exactly.

Nurse 1: And I already had this interaction with the ICU fellow where he didn't believe what was going on and then, I said, 'She's not <u>breathing</u>!'

This nurse goes on to describe that, with no response to her call for help, she had to initially manage the code without much assistance because the nurse next to her was caring for a very sick child. She talked about yelling for help and, in the above excerpt, directs the PCA to get the charge nurse (whom she perceives may be more help than the physician who left) and later to get the code cart. Not knowing which clinicians will help, or even their names, leaves this nurse struggling alone in trying to manage this crisis until the charge nurse arrives. Although she tries numerous times to marshal assistance, no one is notified until after the charge nurse assists. After a prolonged and difficult resuscitation, the baby dies.

As the health care climate changes, we must not lose sight of what good care is and the kinds and mix of care providers necessary to sustain good care. Patients must have experienced, skilled clinicians and support services available to provide their care and available to be marshaled to assist in an emergency. Articulating the clinical judgment and skills in practice is the first step in preserving this aspect of critical care nursing practice and sustaining good patient care.

In situations like the above story, family members and sometimes clinicians need additional support or assistance in dealing with a particular situation. Marshaling assistance from the clergy and/or a psychiatric clinical specialist can help an individual or group discuss their concerns and explore ways of coping. People from these support services can be particularly helpful in assisting others to work through the crisis. At times, instead of breakdown arising in a specific situation, a unit or team of clinicians will get stuck in repeated patterns of breakdown. Naming these breakdowns, raising consciousness about them, and engaging in collaborative problem solving can interrupt the patterned repetitive breakdowns. Psychiatric clinical specialists may also serve as an invaluable resource in facilitating the group process of problem solving.

MODULATING ONE'S EMOTIONAL RESPONSES AND
FACILITATING THE SOCIAL CLIMATE

Another aspect of skilled know-how required for smooth management of a crisis is modulating one's emotional responses to assist others in their ability to function well. This relational skill is emotional labor which can be very demanding and requires sensitivity and attunement to one's own and other people's responses in the situation. Being able to keenly read others' responses in a situation enables nurses to sense what might be helpful and respond accordingly. In crisis situations, this emotional and social labor can be life-saving. But the first focus must be on the good of the patient and family, not on the protection of healthcare team members as a primary goal. Modulating one's emotional responses is a way of facilitating the social climate in order to maximize everyone's ability to function during a crisis. Tone of voice, pace, and manner of directing others varies, depending on the situation:

> **Nurse:** I am not excited. I am so calm. And I keep saying, 'Okay. Go ahead and bag the baby... Somebody has to try and get a blood gas...'

This nurse points out how calm she remains as she talks herself through a crisis. With experience in crises, this response often becomes reflexive, out of habit when experts recognize how calm enables others to respond more smoothly and effectively. Expert nurses commonly talk about how projecting a calm demeanor helps to settle others down:

> **Nurse 1:** I think a lot of times that an experienced nurse's [presence at a crisis] is really important. Sue is a classic example of just having a <u>really</u> calming demeanor. You walk in there and settle everybody down that's bouncing off the walls, and I think...
>
> **Interviewer:** So you <u>run</u> [to the crisis] until you get to the door?
>
> **Nurse 2:** That's right!
>
> **Nurse 1:** You really try to project calm if the situation is looking out of control.
>
> **Nurse 2:** And the worst it gets, the more calm you have to be, I think. I think it works better than anything.
>
> **Nurse 3:** Sue was saying if it happens, you go into a situation very calm and you think, 'That's alright, they're jumping around and I'm going to look at the situation and I'm going to help out.'

Knowing that a calm demeanor can assist others in functioning better does not ensure one's ability to comport oneself calmly in the midst of a crisis, particularly when the crisis occurs suddenly and unexpectedly. It is not natural for many clinicians to remain composed and thus it is a skill that must often be developed over time. Expert nurses are compelled to develop this skill when they see that a nurse's comportment strongly influences the effectiveness of others' actions and, in turn, the patient's outcome:

> **Nurse 1:** This story is about a young GI bleeder. The intern did not know what to do. I almost had to direct things for him. 'Call your attending now, he's bleeding out.' 'I can draw these. Just because we're down in Angiography doesn't mean we can't do labs.' We intubated him. I had the suction and watched the monitor. Nobody else knew the patient. We didn't have a history. I had to be the spokesperson for the patient until the

attending came, who also knew the patient... You feel very responsible and you have to make sure that you stay calm and know what you're doing.

Interviewer: Kind of sobering?

Nurse 1: You have to watch how you say things so that they're communicated in the right way, so that people don't mistake something you say as something else. You have to be very direct about things... Like, in one case, the light wouldn't go on [on the laryngoscope when the intern was trying to intubate] and I said, 'Screw in the bulb, make sure it's in' and then it worked. Most of the time it's something simple like that but I was like, 'Where's the extra battery? Wait a minute check the bulb first.'

Nurse 2: That intern was probably scared to death. If you're very prepared and you're calm and you're not screaming in his ear but say, 'Here's your stylet.' He'll say, 'Oh she knows what she's doing.' He'll think, 'We can handle this.' He stopped shaking and screaming and he was able to look down and concentrate on the landmarks and what he was going to do. So it [being calm and instructive] can slow down the action to where you can concentrate.

With the nurse's assistance, the intern is able to calm down, get the equipment to work, and the patient is successfully intubated quickly and survives the crisis. At the same time, skillful clinicians do not calm everyone in every situation to the point of neutralizing all tension because a degree of tension heightens vigilance, sharpens the senses, and stimulates responsiveness.

There are times, however, when particular team members do not respond to calmness. Allowing team members to release their anxiety (which can take many forms) can facilitate smooth management of a crisis when it does not interfere with others' abilities to function well. Two nurses discuss this:

Nurse 1: But after many years, I ignore most of the screaming that goes on because it's just their (physicians') way of handling...

Nurse 2: Newer nurses couldn't have handled this though. They probably would have been blown away by it.

In some situations, calm or accepting behaviors permit others to grow more and more out of control, reducing their ability to function and hindering the performance of other team members. Thus, a more assertive approach is needed. A more assertive approach may also be necessary when it is imperative to get others to focus their attention on what is salient in a situation in order to facilitate a more appropriate or timely response, as demonstrated in story cited in Benner, Tanner, and Chesla (2009, p. 112):

Nurse: We admitted a man who became very sick very quickly. He had a huge infarct. About 2 hours after he was admitted, he had vomited and obviously had aspirated his vomitus. He was hypoxic. He was blue and crawling off the stretcher. He was a huge man. I said to the intern, 'You need to draw a blood gas.' And he said, 'I drew one when he came in.' I looked at the resident and I tossed him the blood gas syringe and said, 'Could you please draw a blood gas?' His PaO$_2$ was 30 or something like that. He had to be intubated. I said, 'You know, the situation changes often [in critically ill patients], and you can't say, 'I drew one.' I said, 'Look at him. Take a gander. Does this look like the same patient you drew the blood gas on?'

Facilitating the social climate further includes how and what to say when a team member's interventions are ineffective. For instance, when someone is doing CPR but no pulse is palpable, pointing out the observation to that person quietly and calmly, "There is no pulse with compressions." More directly, one can instruct, "Try compressing deeper," for instance, to clarify the change needed. If the person continues ineffectively, immediate action must be taken. This can be stated kindly but definitively, with as little friction and disruption as possible, in order to maintain the team's focus on the patient and to keep each clinician open to learning in the situation. For example, "Joe, could you give Kathy some relief and do CPR for a while?" Creating interpersonal conflict could derail focused attention on performing CPR adequately.

Another example of modulating one's response while preventing conflict and defensiveness is to request the person's assistance in an area where the person's strengths better match the patient's needs, "It would be helpful if you could assist with..." After the crisis is over, it is essential to provide debriefing that can highlight and clarify the lessons to be gained from the expensive experiential learning during a crisis. Emergency department nurses talk about how an exceptionally good ED physician debriefs the team on a daily basis. Given his interest in improving as a clinician, he welcomes corrections when called for, as one nurse describes:

> **Nurse:** He was very nice about it, and he said, 'It [the nurse's concern] was a good call and you're right,' and as we talked about it—he debriefs like the military does, you know? He sits down after the shift and debriefs about everything on the shift, 'This is where I did this wrong. I did this okay. We did this okay,' and he's very good nurse advocate, very much so, and very much of a team player.

The ethic is to learn as much as possible from each crisis situation so that individual and collective team functioning is improved for future crises. Through the process of debriefing, strong clinicians and excellent role models can stimulate others to learn and become more attuned in their own practices.

Because each crisis situation and each team differs, there is no specific technique or prescription for facilitating the social climate. The skilled knowledge is highly relational and situational. One must gain a sense of what team members respond to favorably. The responses thus cannot be formalized, but must be learned experientially or from observing skillful role models. Care must be taken to keep the primary goal and communication focused on the good of the patient. This creates the possibility of solidarity around the most important issue. It is a disservice to the team members if they do not receive direct, clear, and tactful feedback about their performance in a timely manner. The skilled knowledge of coping with a crisis in such a way that facilitates the high functioning of others is a complex interpersonal skill that requires understanding the demands of the situation.

In expert practice, skilled nurses modulate their emotional responses daily in non-crisis events to calm tempers that may flare, soothe anxiety, and break or reduce tension in challenging situations. They can therefore serve as strong models for learners because this skillful daily activity parallels their modulating skills in a crisis. A group of operating room nurses discuss a common modulating response in their setting:

> **Nurse 1:** We're all there for the same reason. We want what's best for our patients... And you never can reprimand them when they're in that situation [referring to a surgical case]. It's just not the right time. You can't [say], 'Now stop that...' It's using your common sense. It's not a good time.

Nurse 2: It's not only that, you can lose a lot of your credibility.

Nurse 3: Yeah. By the same token, I think we all have a really, very strong and unique sense of humor in the operating room. I think that it aids in the cohesion of the team. Of course, you have to know when it's appropriate and when it's not. But I think it really holds the team together for people to have a real strong sense of humor...

Interviewer: It changes the energy in the room.

The nurses point out that the context of the humor, the type of modulation, is central to its effectiveness. It is important to stress that knowledge about what to do and when to do it is not prescribable since performance during a crisis is not simply an intellectual task. Expert nurses develop the know-how, the relational skills, of reading the situation and grasping what response will be helpful at that moment. As a situation or the team members change, the same intervention may not work. The social skills require the development of perceptual acuity, skillful comportment, and teamwork that is socially embedded and learned.

There are some crisis situations that are highly charged because of the potential for violence. For those who have been injured, spat upon, or have had objects thrown at them, violence is a very real threat. For nurses working with potentially violent patients, the threat is strong enough that many complete a course with certification that focuses on coercive physical and pharmacological management as a primary intervention (Binder & McNiel, 1999). Although the whole team must be astute and well-prepared to avoid injuries, Binder and McNiel (1999) report that there are a few emergency rooms that only use restraints or IM medications rarely. Instead, "the few" care for these patients through connection and skillful involvement (eg., knowing the patient). As seen in the following exemplar, the power of a skillful blend of excellent attunement, an ethic of care, the ability to modulate one's responses, and engaged, skillful involvement can avert some crises and/or transform the patient's and others' responses in some situations. Gary Dang, a psychiatric nurse, grasps and responds to the patient as a person who is worthy of remembering and respect. It is a powerful reminder of the primacy of caring:

Nurse: Peg, my clinical leader informed me that there was an emergency, a potentially violent patient in the ER. The same patient tried to strangulate Peg during his last psych hospitalization on our locked psych unit. According to her, he had particular aversion to white blond females. She gathered three of us to go to ER. As is customary, we took our restraints box. In the elevator, Peg explained that we knew the patient as he had been with us two or three times before with the same presentation of hypomania, but this time he seemed worse. The patient, Richard Barton, had bipolar disorder. He would stop taking his meds at home and become hypo maniac, slowly become hostile and then full-blown violent. During his last hospital stay, he tried to attack Peg so she was apprehensive that he would be worse this time.

Last evening, Police brought an agitated Mr. Barton to the ER, but after a few hours, he refused to take any treatment and escaped. Later, the police brought him again for disturbing the peace by making hostile gestures in public. According to Peg, Mr. Barton was getting increasingly agitated, refusing meds and had the potential of being violent. As a precaution, she assigned each of us a limb, if there was any need to restrain the patient physically. We were all tense. There was a high risk for a grievous injury to either the patient or the staff during the restraining process. I was still trying to place Mr. Barton, but was unable to connect his name to his face.

On reaching ER we found Mr. Barton lying on a bed, completely covered by a blanket. Three security guards, with latex gloves on, were around his bed. Stacy, the ER nurse was preparing injections to be given to him as a chemical restraint. At that point, Mr. Barton removed his blanket and we were able to see him. An unkempt man mumbling profanities was sleeping on the bed with his shoes on and had a vacant look in his eyes. He was staring at us and still not seeing us. Because of his long beard and long hair, it took me a moment but then I remembered him!

Instinctively, I said "Richie Baby," the name he liked me to call him during his previous stays in our hospital. Peg always insists that less experienced nurses stand back while she talks to the patient. She decides when to "take the patient" for four point restraints after all other measures have failed. So I was "out of line" to speak or act. I was to stand on guard for any instruction. But, my uttering his name was just a reflex action resulting probably from the typical increased rush of adrenalin. For a brief moment, it seemed that my voice reached his inner mind as he shivered slightly. The fog in his eyes lifted and the profanities stopped. Encouraged, I again said "Richie Baby" loudly. Now he looked at me and a flicker of recognition crossed his eyes. In a pressured voice he told me, "these people are poisoning me. The police arrested me and now they are forcing meds. I did not sleep the whole night." Softly and gently but firmly I told him that I wanted to help him and that he had an alternative choice—to take his meds by mouth and come with me to the psych unit.

Richie thought for a moment (a moment which seemed like a year during that tense time) and agreed to take the meds by mouth. He paused and looked at me and said "OK" with a nod. I knew I had risked acting on my own judgment by taking over the situation myself. If Richie had become violent, my actions would have been viewed as inappropriate. Not only did Richie take his meds but walked, with me by his side, to the psych unit on his own. He got more medications and slept peacefully for next six hours. All of us were jubilant at the outcome. Peg told me that I had performed a "psych" miracle. Richie spent two weeks in our unit without any incident and was discharged.

The whole incident was gratifying to me. It confirmed that if you truly care for your patients, they recognize it and remember it, even in the deepest of their turmoiled minds.

Because of the transformative effect of Gary's interventions, Mr. Barton did not seem violent and Gary did not appear to be "managing a crisis." Yet, Gary's skillful involvement in this psychiatric emergency literally averted the crisis, particularly for Richie who was rescued from the harsh, unnecessary control, the tranquillisation typically imposed, and four point leather restraints. The ethical understanding and judgment embodied in Gary's actions reflects what Taylor (1995) refers to as a strong evaluation. He makes a strong, and some would say risky, moral judgment. Gary acts as a moral agent, taking a stand for a person who is worthy.

Expert psychiatric nurses have taught us that the violence and hostility they witness often stems from fear. The first thing Richie says to Gary upon recognition is, "these people are poisoning me." Gary shows that a calm, respectful "meeting of the other," as a worthy person, can tame the fear and literally usher the patient back into the world. This "meeting of other" as a person describes a "recognition" practice and is world transforming when a frightened or lost patient realizes that a trusted and/or trustworthy clinician can be counted on as safe and caring. In a practice, any practice, where beneficence trumps control or domination, fewer patients and families are violent, hostile, difficult or challenging.

When this story was told in an interview, a few ER nurses who experienced this situation with Gary were quite animated as they described the danger in the room. One of them had been injured in a prior altercation with Mr. Barton. She could not help telling, with amazement and passion, the stunning change in the patient's mental and emotional states. The established caring relationship revealed in a few gently spoken words, "Richie Baby," reveals Gary's deeply rooted notions of what it is to be a good nurse and what it is to care for and about another. The ER nurse shared that "everyone in the ER who witnessed the episode learned" the power of connection and compassion.

It is not by happenstance that Gary is able to rescue Richie from a worse outcome. It is by habit. Following this incident, the ER specifically requests Gary to intervene in psych emergencies because he habitually respects and gently interacts with patients that he understands as frightened, alone, and mentally dwelling in unspeakable worlds that most clinicians have not considered. Rather, clinicians are typically socialized to "see" crazy, dangerous, monstrous beings to be avoided. Clinicians embody their views and these views are sensed by patients, even those who are severely troubled like Richie. In crises, patients may not, at first, be able to make sense of the words they hear, but expert psych and ER nurses have taught us that patients do make sense of how words are spoken, how they are approached, comportment, and whether a clinician can be trusted. They sense good.

Many clinicians are never coached to develop these transformative human skills, rendering control/coercion as the sole mode of engagement with potentially violent patients. Nurses who routinely respond to psych emergencies may welcome a more balanced education and preparation that includes skillful and genuine engagement and involvement. The opportunity to witness how an expert nurse like Gary modulates his responses in a dangerous situation can tacitly convey (nonverbally pass on) the kind of interactions desired. A adept role model can exemplify how to comport oneself in a compassionate, respective way and open up the possibility of the same in others. As recipients of care and compassion, patients strongly sense the distinctions between care versus control and/or domination. Feeling known and cared about as a person can have a strong influence on the extent, nature, and intensity of care required as well as the care accepted, Dialogue around narratives such as this can strengthen the clinical and moral imagination of developing clinicians and, subsequently, their notions of good and ethic of care and responsibility.

Nurses, at times, find themselves in the midst of a crisis but unable to help without violating a good, which may be legal, moral, spiritual, physiological or combination. Regulatory agencies impose rules that are intended to protect patients and their privacy, but can instead give rise to moral dilemmas for nurses who are positioned to help and simultaneously committed to protect. Cindy, an oncology nurse shared such a narrative in which she modulates her response to resolve a crisis:

> **Nurse:** In this story, I bent the rules, just a little, to give a family peace. Sophie was 53 years old and admitted with pneumonia related to her advanced lung cancer. She had new brain and bone mets. Her care was complicated, as she weighed close to 400 lbs and had some psych issues. It always took 3 or 4 of us to roll her and give her personal care, as she was grossly edematous with huge blisters on her legs that made it very painful just to turn her and caused her skin to tear.
>
> She was with us for months. Special bariatric equipment was rented to care for her. We could not send her home with hospice as her daughter, Carly, had psych issues and had already stated that when her mother died, she was going to take her own life to be with her. We were worried about Carly, as her mother was now a DNR and on

comfort measures. Plans had been made so that when Sophie died, Carly would go to the ER to be committed for her own safety. Carly stayed nightly with Sophie on a cot.

One night near the end, Carly left abruptly. Her mother's boyfriend stayed instead. When I came on after report, I went to see Sophie. She was still arousable. As I touched her cheeks, she opened her eyes and smiled at me saying "Hi!" Her boyfriend Judd sat in a recliner across the room. He was not a healthy man either. I asked Sophie if she was comfortable, as she was now on an air bed with a dilaudid PCA running continuously, and she nodded, yes. I checked her Foley and saw that her urine was scant and dark, a sure sign that her kidneys were shutting down and the end was coming soon.

Judd followed me as I left Sophie's room. He looked very worried. He had not heard from Carly in a few hours and it was not like her to not be at her mother's side. He left to go drive around the streets to look for her, but he was torn, so he returned after a few hours. He wanted to stay with Sophie. Carly did not answer her cell phone when Judd tried to call. He had also called several friends and relatives to see if they had seen her. I listened to him and held his hand. I said, "Sophie needs you right now." He went back in the room and sat with Sophie. I was worried about Carly, too. Where was she?

I went back to the desk and the supervisor came up on her rounds, notifying me that Carly was in the ER for treatment. She told me no details because of patient confidentiality. Now I had a dilemma. How could I let Judd know Carly was safe in the ER when HIPAA regulations forbid me to say anything. I went back to Sophie's room and Judd had left. Sophie was sleeping peacefully, but I worried that now Judd was out looking for Carly again. He came back an hour later. "I've looked for her everywhere and I can't find her. I'm worried she'll hurt herself if I don't find her." His expression mirrored his fear.

I knew I had to give him peace of mind, so I looked him in the eye. I said, "Judd, you trust me when I tell you that Carly is safe, don't you?" "I'm so worried that she is out there alone," he said, wringing his hands. I, again, gave him a clandestine look, raising my eyebrows and holding his gaze. "Look at me and trust me when I tell you that Carly is okay. She is safe." He looked at me differently, then, like I was telling him a secret. He said, "You know she's okay, don't you? You just can't say it, right?" I just smiled and winked. He looked so relieved. He went back in with Sophie. I called the supervisor and asked her to ask Carly if Judd could be made aware that she was in the ER. She had been sedated at that point, so I was unable to tell Judd that she was in the ER.

Sophie died late that morning after I went home, and Carly was committed to a psych hospital for her safety. After Sophie's funeral, Judd was admitted for cardiac issues to the telemetry floor.

I know there are privacy issues we face with patients every day, but I couldn't let a father worry so about the welfare of his daughter. With his trust, I helped relieve his heavy heart. And I know I did the right thing.

In this situation, Cindy clearly acts in the patient's and family's best interests, or on what is good for them, without violating HIPAA regulations. There is leeway for interpretation (thinking and understanding the meaning in a context) of these regulations, but there is additional flexibility to use good judgment when the patient is incapable of giving consent. The moral dilemma confronting Cindy in the moment is, should she do what's right or do what's good? What is striking about Cindy's comportment, her raised eyebrow and "wink," is that it is both ethical and moral. She is able to quell the crisis of the father's frantic worry about Carly's safety; yet, does not give even the slightest hint about Carly's health information. Dad still has no idea where to start looking for Carly, but he is comforted and can turn his attention and heart to Sophie.

At the expert stage of practice, the ability to modulate well becomes intertwined with becoming very skillful in one's involvements with others. Modulating one's responses is one of the many skillful ways of being involved and eliciting particular ways of being in others. Used in this context, nurses have taught us that modulating one's responses to facilitate improvement in the social climate embodies the intentions and notions of good and reflects a strong ethic of care. In our fast paced, high-demand health care settings, this will continue to be an essential skill in managing the multiple types of crises that unfold in everyday practice.

SUMMARY

In a crisis, providing timely and appropriate emergency interventions is life-saving. Because many crises demand multiple, simultaneous interventions from various team members, these must often be organized and orchestrated to be effective. Nurses with a strong sense of agency and with situational leadership skills were able to smoothly facilitate a team's activities under stress so that team members could function skillfully and so that necessary resources were available when needed.

The tact in managing crises is an example of the skilled know-how and embodied intelligence vital to expert critical care nursing. This skilled clinical knowledge is founded on and organized by the clinician's perceptual acuity and those recognitional skills must be linked with a rapid and apt response. Skilled clinical know-how, clinical wisdom, and good judgment are linked in the process of becoming an expert clinician.

REFERENCES

Benner, P. (2000). *From novice to expert: Excellence and power in clinical nursing practice.* Upper Saddle River, NJ: Prentice Hall.

Benner, P., Tanner, C. A., & Chesla, C. A. (2009). *Expertise in nursing practice: Caring, clinical judgment, and ethics.* New York, NY: Springer Publishing Company.

Binder, R.L. & McNiel, D.E. (1999). Emergency psychiatry: Contemporary practices in managing acutely violent patients in 20 psychiatric emergency rooms. *Psychiatry Services, 50*(12): 1553–1554.

Dreyfus, H.L. (1986). *Mind over machine: The power of human intuition and expertise in the era of the computer.* New York, NY: Free Press.

Dreyfus, H.L. (1990). *Philosophy 185: Heidegger.* University of California, Berkeley. Berkeley, CA.

Hooper, P. L. (1995). *Expert titration of multiple vasoactive drugs in post-cardiac surgical patients: An interpretive study of clinical judgment and perceptual acuity.* (Doctoral dissertation, University of California at San Francisco, San Francisco, School of Nursing.)

Rubin, J. (2009). Impediments to the development of clinical knowledge and ethical judgment in critical care nursing. In P. Benner, C. A. Tanner, & C. A. Chesla (Eds.), *Expertise in nursing practice: Caring, clinical judgment, and ethics* (pp. 171-198). New York, NY: Springer Publishing Company.

Taylor, C. (1995). *Philosophical arguments.* Cambridge, MA: Harvard University Press.

6

Providing Comfort Measures for the Critically and Acutely Ill

*C*entral to good nursing practice is providing comfort and psycho-social support measures for patients in the midst of technological interventions and suffering. Comfort promotes the sense of well-being of patient and family. To comfort means to strengthen, aid, and encourage as well as to soothe and console. Our everyday understanding of the word "comfort" acknowledges the inter-related mind-body-person-world spheres. Comfort measures and life-saving, instantaneous interventions are related because discomfort and anxiety influence patient responses to therapies, and patients' level of comfort and well-being are critical indicators in most clinical judgments. Patient comfort and well-being are central notions of good that guide the patient-nurse relationship. Clinical judgment and action are based upon taken-for-granted understandings about physical and emotional comfort of patients. Comfort in one sphere influences all the others. This chapter will illustrate how comforting patients forms a backdrop for clinical judgment and care of acute and critically ill patients, whether they are in the hospital, in transport, or at home. Knowledge and skills related to comfort must be integrated with highly technical care that is often intrusive and even pain inflicting. It is a mistake to overlook the clinical imagination and knowledge-skill required for offering as much comfort as possible in the midst of an acute illness.

Central to nursing practice are many "comfort measures." Nurses use the phrase "comfort measures" to describe a myriad of comforting practices such as physical touch, holding the hand, being visible, wiping tears, providing a warm blanket, soothing talk, a cup of tea, and providing for bodily comforts with smooth, dry bedding, movement, light, warmth, color, distraction, and that which is familiar to the patient. The phrase "comfort measures" occurs naturally in nurses' accounts of their work and was pervasive in taped interviews. Nurses were not asked specific questions about comfort measures unless they used the phrase. Then, probes were used to elicit more concrete descriptions of actions. Comforting is occasioned by distress, loss, or suffering, and is dependent on timing, trust, relationship, and the patient's openness to comfort. Sometimes suffering is inconsolable and comfort measures may feel like an affront to a collapsing world that will not sustain comfort. One is hesitant to promise to comfort or be comforted because comfort is never fully born of choice and freedom. Because it can mean so many things to different people in different situations, this broad term and ambiguous practice does not easily find its way into technical and scientific discourse.

The capacity to comfort and be comforted lies neither fully within the nurse nor the patient. It is relational and housed within the experience of embodiment. Comfort measures are most often distinguished by nurses as a way of being with patients. It is impossible to spell out or formalize all forms of comforting, its occasions, and responses. The limits to formalizing comfort in terms of isolating procedural steps and establishing principles may explain why nursing literature and public discourse are so silent on comforting practices. We typically write about what we can standardize. Comfort measures can appear trivial, homey, ordinary, and somehow less legitimate and less important when compared to powerful technological interventions that "fix" or "cure." To comfort, one must acknowledge loss or suffering and admit the limits of protection and immunity. Comfort calls for solidarity and connection rather than distance and control.

Offering comfort measures requires the nurse's perception that comforting is needed, a recognition practice that is dependent upon attentiveness, noticing, and presencing as illustrated in the following researcher's description of a nurse who is trying to understand the patient's discomfort:

> **Interviewer:** While she [the nurse] was talking with me [the researcher], the patient became restless [I don't think he could hear us]. She tried to determine what he was upset about. She asks if he can write, and then says 'it is worth a try.' She gives him the paper and pen, but he couldn't coordinate his hand movements enough to write legibly. Without finding out specifically what his restlessness is about, she repositions pillows, talks with him, 'Let's get you more comfortable here.' He seems to settle down. The nurse doesn't seem satisfied, looks like she's still trying to figure out what's going on... She suctions him intermittently when he coughs, and says she's trying to get him more comfortable. She pulls him up in bed. She seems to still be trying to get a sense of him, how to get him comfortable. She hasn't worked with him before, she tells me (Observational Interview).

The nurse is trying to find comfort measures that work for the patient. One does not often think that comfort measures require puzzle-solving, but finding the sources of the patient's discomfort and what promotes comfort require problem identification, clinical judgment, and skilled know-how. As illustrated in the observation note above, the problem is solved only when the patient is resting comfortably. Listening to and observing the patient who cannot talk in order to make the patient more comfortable complicates the puzzle solving but as an intensive care nursery nurse describes in an account cited in Benner et al. (2009, pp. 164), she has learned to "listen" to an infant:

> **Nurse:** There is something about listening to the patient. This particular patient I'm thinking of wasn't speaking, but was getting his message to me—as if the baby was saying: 'I'm not doing much of anything, so everyone better leave me alone.' So, once people started leaving him alone, his own systems, for whatever reason, started to function again... It's like when the baby seems to be saying, 'No, we're not going to do it that way—I can only eat so much, or I can only tolerate so much.' So we try to find out what the baby seems to wants to do—I know that sounds strange—but letting the baby guide his/her care a little bit more directly rather than putting them into the mold we think they should be in. This holds true for feedings and oxygen... This one infant started to come around once we put him on his tummy and started feeding him.

With experiential learning the nurse reads bodily responses and patterns. Without attunement to bodily rhythms and needs one cannot comfort or be comforted.

Comfort is central to healing practices because comfort and reassurance (the opposite of fear, distress, and anxiety) offer the person space to regroup, to allow the body to recover, heal, and grow. The nurse above goes on to say:

> **Nurse:** Ordinarily, we don't feed babies when they're on ventilators, but this baby had tolerated everything else, was getting older, and needed to start feeding. So, we started feeding him and we found that he responded very well to the feedings—and that he wanted to stay on the ventilator—so we accommodated him. And he began to get better, and within two weeks, we were actually able to get him off the ventilator and put him on a nasal cannula.

In addition to the perception that comfort is needed, the nurse must understand the situation and be able to imagine what would be experienced as comforting. The nurse must experientially learn what touch is comforting, what talk is soothing, what sources of support work for particular patients and families, what closeness or distance is comfortable, and what demeanor and gestures convey understanding and responsiveness. Because these skills are experientially learned within particular relationships, they can never be adequately formalized or turned into prescribed techniques or procedures. Comforting skills exist in relationship with the other person and require trust, openness, and acceptance. Attunement to both the patient's needs and responses to the comfort measures offered are crucial to becoming skillful at comforting others and to being comforted.

Comfort measures, as nurses talk about them, are integral to setting limits on technology use, though a tension exists between searching for a technological fix that may bring comfort and the need to comfort in the face of the limits of technology. The ethical claim is that self-nurturance and human dependency on others for help and comfort are more basic and sustainable than technological dependency. Comfort measures defend against unnecessary discomfort. Nurses offer comfort measures in the midst of doing painful procedures, therefore inflicting pain presents a moral and coping challenge to clinicians who provide comfort measures (Madjar, 1991). Comfort measures are seen by some nurses as a first response before medical interventions so that sedatives and paralytic agents are not used as substitutes for everyday comfort measures. This leads to an ethical discourse about the dangers of substituting drugs for human solace and physical comfort, and also about the dangers of giving insufficient pain medications or over-dosing patients with pain medications.

The capacity to be comforted, consoled, and soothed is a socially developed capacity that nurses seek to foster and protect, particularly neonatal and pediatric nurses. The challenge for a neonatal or pediatric nurse is to develop the infant's or child's ability to be comforted by human connection in the midst of highly technical environments, where it is possible to offer sedation and pain medication in lieu of human comfort measures and at the expense of ushering an infant into a human world. The infant must learn self-comfort as well as be comforted by touch, motion, and holding. An infant who has not learned to find sufficient comfort in the human world is indeed handicapped. This challenge calls for astute attentiveness and judgment since the equal danger is to provide insufficient pain medication and sedation for infants who cannot discriminate and communicate the sources of their pain.

Pain and suffering shatter the familiar world such that patients must learn how to comfort themselves and be comforted in the context of an unfamiliar body and situation. The challenge in caring for adults is to co-discover what is comforting, since one's comfort is dependent on past socially-learned, embodied responses and these must be called upon in a new context. For the adult who typically prefers control and fears dependency and helplessness, comfort measures may entail creating small spheres of possible control to stem the tide of fear of dependency and helplessness. But all human dependency and helplessness cannot be masked. To be able to receive comfort in the midst of dependency can help one confront and accept inescapable dependencies with solace and perhaps connection and security. Laurie Foran, an oncology nurse, understands patients who are fiercely independent and need to maintain control. She engages with them in the fight they define and comforts them in ways that best enable them to cope with pain, dependency, and receiving help, as seen in the following exemplar:

Nurse: I cared for a patient named Amy who had rectal/colon cancer. She weighed 90 lbs. soaking wet, not much for her 5'8" stature. Her port [portacath] protruded like a doorbell from her bony chest. You could count each rib. She was also tough, street-wise, 60ish, and tattooed across her arm was her name. You could tell that she had earned each line across her face.

She took to me and I took to her. Upon meeting her, she was very anxious, hands shaking and very leery of being touched. This included her port. She did not like people to touch her port. Throughout the hospital she would only allow two people to touch her port, Mary, my clinical leader and myself. So much that if she were admitted through the ER and we were not available, she would make them place a peripheral line.

On first impression you would think she liked to complain. "Oh, I had to wait" or "They didn't send mustard, I don't want to be here." But soon I realized she was just trying to maintain control. Her disease was running rampant; she did not have much control. She was young, and time was running out.

She was an avid reader; we would exchange books and stories. She forever reminded me when I was setting up supplies of her allergies—broccoli and raspberries. To the point that I pretty much put on her identification and allergy bands before saying "hello." I'd say, "I know, I know broccoli and raspberries." This would make her chuckle. I think it almost became a game to see who would say it first.

She was going to fight this disease. She had more determination and will than most people could dream of having. She was by all means failing; her weight was down to 84 pounds. When she demanded treatment, she never complained of any pain. She silently winced as she shifted position. She never so much as let her eyes fill, let alone cry....she kept up every front to prove she could do it.

Sometimes while receiving her chemotherapy, I would swaddle her in blankets, her Ativan would kick in, she would fall asleep and look so peaceful. I wondered if she ever felt this peaceful in her life.

One day she came into the Clinic somber from the MD's office. The Doctor came and whisked through to drop Amy's record and told me that "she needed to be banded"—as a DNR patient. I was at a loss for words because of her strength and her will to live. Any other person would have already succumbed. All 82 lbs. of her, I had to place this ball and chain [DNR band on her]. I regrouped, and I closed the curtain around us and began. She looked at me—her eyes filled. My heart broke. At first silence was our only communication. But we were speaking volumes. I embraced her and she openly sobbed. Her tears were on my neck. I felt hopeless. I held this frail, skeletal woman who had been filled with so much strength.

She thanked me for being with her, "that if anyone had to do this for her, she was glad it was me." She said, "I decided to stop treatment. I can't do it anymore." She admitted to having increased pain. Her rectum was continuously seeping.. If you read the reports, you would wonder how anyone could have survived this far, let alone get up and come to treatments alone. She lived with her daughter and son-in-law. They would leave her home without dinner on their "drinking nights." I was forever sneaking her [food] for the evenings. At her weight, she could not afford to skip a meal.

Her hands were shaking as I placed her bands. We each knew what these meant. We locked eyes, held hands; she calmed and folded her hands. She was in control. I told her that I enjoyed caring for her. I thanked her for wanting me to be her nurse. I told her I was proud of her that she put up an incredible fight. For once there was no joking over the broccoli and raspberries. How I wish I were putting those bands on instead.

I hurt for what was and for what wasn't. She did not really have anything in life and each line on her body proved it. She was weathered and beaten. But she always had a smile. She had a grandchild and talk of that baby would make her eyes light up. Somehow, through it all she saw the goodness in life.....

When I think back on Amy, I have mixed emotions. I am saddened and yet I chuckle at so many different moments we shared. What I learned from her was strength, resilience and mind over matter. To appreciate each day, never dwell on what could be, see life as it is and appreciate it for just that. There is good all around and in each moment, a reason to go on. She instilled in me the importance of my profession—the impact that we have the honor of making as Nurses, in so many lives. How fortunate we are to be part of their journeys.

When a patient seems difficult to comfort or the patient's condition deteriorates, and he or she becomes more and more challenging to comfort, it is tempting to imagine that the patient is just being difficult. But Laurie connects with Amy, accepts Amy's way of coping and holding her emotions at bay, discovers how to joke with her, finds their common interests, and develops a rich relationship—all of which is comforting. It is heartbreaking for both Laurie and Amy when it is time to let go of the fight. What is sustaining for expert nurses who have learned to engage with patients (challenging or not), become skillfully involved with them, and comfort diverse patients and families is the rich and mutual nature of comfort.

Comfort is associated with the Nightingale imperative to put the body in the best condition for self-repair and healing (Stretkowicz, 1996). In Table 6.1, eight major kinds of comfort care were pervasive in the narratives of nurses we studied. Comfort care offered to the dying and their loved ones raises distinct ethical and clinical issues and is presented separately in Chapter 9, however, we offer an example of weighing the issues of providing pain relief and managing the risks of respiratory depression through human presence and gentle stimulation in this chapter to highlight the ethical role of providing human solace and comfort.

TABLE 6.1

Providing Comfort Measures for the Critically and Acutely Ill

- Caring for the body as a source of comfort
- Providing adequate stimulation, distraction, and rest while limiting disruption
- Taming the technical environment
- Comforting through connection and relationship
- Being available without being intrusive
- Weighing the ethical tensions of pain relief, sedation, and comfort measures
- Limiting the impact of painful procedures: relaxation techniques, visualization and distraction
- Comforting through familiar rituals and routine

CARE OF THE BODY AS A SOURCE OF COMFORT

Many examples are provided in this chapter about the everyday comfort measures of caring for the body: grooming, shampooing hair, positioning, range of motion exercises, and back rubs. The nurses dismiss these routine ways of caring for the body as inconsequential when the patient is stable. We suspect that these acts of "routine care of the body" are not inconsequential for the patient. They are noteworthy acts central to the nurse-patient relationship that help a critically ill patient feel refreshed and more comfortable in the midst of a labile physical condition. Care of the body, as the lived social and personal body, is given in between critical interventions and subordinated to them. It is a cultural achievement that practices of caring for the body are maintained in the midst of caring for unconscious, sedated, and/or unstable patients. In many cases, critical care nurses' practice is similar to that of the anesthesiologist who is in charge of maintaining the patient's vital functions in the operating room—managing a sedated, paralyzed patient—except that nurses attempt to keep the patient in the social world through caring for and presenting a groomed, cared for person.

Nurses often link their own comfort with the comfort of patients. This is evident in the everyday embodied experience of unwittingly mimicking another's discomfort, such as the fidgeting of restlessness, where an uncomfortable person or a relaxed comfortable person are mirrored in one's own physical comfort. It is hard to feel comfortable in the face of an uncomfortable other. Nurses note that grooming and bathing a patient can make both nurse and patient feel more comfortable:

> **Nurse:** I made sure that he was clean. And it felt good to know that when the mom came in, she said: 'Oh, you washed him up. He looks good. Oh, thanks...' I always try to make them look comfortable and I always make sure that I'm explaining everything [to conscious or unconscious patients]... I'll tell them, 'I'm going to open your eyes, and I'm going to check your eyes. I going to be suctioning you. I'm going to be bagging you. It's going to make you cough. I'll be turning you, and I'm lifting your head.' Whatever it is that I'm doing, I tell them. It comforts me because you never know what patients can hear.

Here, the nurse explicitly links her comfort with the patient's comfort. This illustrates the relational aspect of comfort work. That there are links between patient-nurse-family member comfort is an embodied moral source and demonstrates a relational ethic. The mother feels comfortable if the child looks comfortable. The nurse feels comfortable if she has connected with the patient by explaining what she is doing, even if it is not clear whether or not the patient can hear or understand her.

In contrast, over-identification such as reading one's own physical comfort onto another is a source of humor about mistaken boundaries as illustrated when a parent tells her or his child to put on a sweater because the parent is cold. Even though the physical-embodied links with another's physical states can be distorted by one's own physical states and projection, these directed sense connections remain a source of relatedness and moral imagination. A human connection is made with the patient through concern for well-being and comfort of the other. Patients link their own sense of identity, control, well-being, and continuity with grooming, such as having clean hair that is combed or for men, being shaved in their usual patterns:

> **Nurse:** The house staff were reviewing his condition [the patient's] with Dr. S., the director of the unit. It was decided from his X-ray that he needed to be intubated. I remember feeling so bad for him; this was yet another set back for such a nice man. I went in to tell him what would happen. He was looking at me with wide eyes, shaking his head that he understood. Then he asked if he could shave first. I told him there was no time at the moment, but that I would be sure to shave him afterwards. I prepared him for the intubation, medicating him well so that it wouldn't bother him. I held his hand through the whole thing, and soon after gave him the shave he wanted.

The shave is symbolic and forms a sense of continuity with his usual self.

Comfort is related to developmental and physical capacities. For example, there are important distinctions between care of infants and premature babies as illustrated in the following two examples. But care of the physical sentient body is crucial to both:

> **Nurse:** Babies are not small children, they're not small adults, babies are newborns, ...they need TLC, they need touching, they need someone to nurture them a little bit and to, you know, balance [the treatments] with kindness...
>
> **Interviewer:** Tell me what you did.
>
> **Nurse:** I turned the television off, I turned the lights down (laughter), I took the restraints off the baby; I bent her little arms—her first name was Cathy. And I stayed in there and I talked to her and I washed her hair, which is the ICN [intensive care nursery] thing, you know, the first thing we all want to do is wash that hair. (Laughter) I nested her; I rolled some blankets up and put them around her. She's a term baby; she didn't need anything like premature babies need but—I just spent those hours that I could, touching her and talking to her...

This kind of comfort care through caring for the body is a common nursing practice, and when it is overlooked, the necessary treatments are not balanced with soothing, comforting touch, or in the nurse's words "balanced with kindness." Even in the midst of intrusive interventions, comforting and respectful handling of the body is crucial.

In the care of premature infants, nurses confront extreme demands for creating specialized care of a body that is not quite ready for the physical world of intrusive touch, light, or sound. So, care of the body is indissolubly wed to creating a safe and comfortable environment:

> **Nurse:** This baby likes a pacifier and I wipe his face with a wet cloth and put him back on his tummy and then, if I have to do something like draw blood, I open the isolette all the way out and I put a blanket over his tummy so he doesn't get cold, also he probably feels more secure having something on top.

Bundling babies and attending to their immediate physical environment are crucial to comfort for the neonate who is used to a tight bounded space and to muscles that have been buoyant in utero. In another example cited in Benner, Tanner, and Chesla (2009, p. 254), two neonatal ICU nurses discuss approaches to handling premature infants:

> **Nurse 1:** You're prepared when you go in; you have everything lined up that you need at hand, so that you're in there for the shortest possible time.
>
> **Nurse 2:** Turning them. You don't turn them over; you bring their knees into their chest and hold their arms at their sides so that they don't turn their back on you when you pick them up off the bed. It's reflexive that when you startle them, they are going to do that. It makes them very nervous. So you get them contained when you go to turn them. In fact a lot of times when I first go to do vital signs, first thing I'll do is put the kid's feet inside his diaper to get small enough. You just diaper them entirely up to their waists and get their legs inside. They can't kick around and it makes them much happier. A lot of times I'll wrap a diaper around them or a blanket for the entire vital signs as much as I can so that they don't flail around and they feel secure. It's just—it's making them feel secure, that's all it is. It's so easy. [laughter]

Simulating conditions in utero, these nurses provide comforting boundaries for developing neonates. Earlier this same nurse "2" describes working with a particular preemie. Note the particularized language and the perceptual-recognition skills that allow the nurse to know the extreme sensitivity of the premature infant:

> **Nurse:** If a shadow falls across her face she desaturates [oxygen levels fall]. She cannot stand knowing there is anyone else in the world, but I found I was able to suction her. This baby has terrible bradycardia and desaturations when she gets suctioned. And I was able to suction her by myself and keep her saturation in the 90's just by being slow and careful. And, it bugs me because it's real counter-productive to those babies when people get in there and throw covers off and have them lie flat on their back, and they're flailing in the breeze and they're handling them efficiently but not particularly gently. And I just think it's really bad for those kids. I think their intracranial pressure probably goes sky high because you get them upset (Benner, Tanner & Chesla, 2009, p. 226).

This is an ethical language of gentle touch over "efficient" touch. Tones of moral outrage and anger can be heard over the mis-handling of infants. The particular infant is brought into human existence through response, recognition, and touch in ways that make moral claims on the nurse to be observant and gentle. In the following excerpt from a clinical observation, the particularized skillful observation of an infant's feeding capacities are evident:

Nurse: The other thing with this baby is—you develop a lot of feeding techniques to feed the baby. Some of these babies are not well coordinated. They need to get a little help pacing (talking as she feeds the baby). She is starting to slow down a little. She is taking a few breaths. See. I am also feeling her back move as she takes these breaths; I feel her back expand. But some babies are so excited about feedings they will just gob on to the nipple and suck and suck. They will start to choke right in front of you. They won't stop and breathe. That is not a problem for her.

Interviewer: Is that related to maturity or not?

Nurse: No, it really just is individual babies. Two babies with the exact same maturity. One might never pace itself but gulp if you would let it and another one which would never forget to breathe. Now sometimes this baby will put her tongue up to the roof of her mouth so I have to make sure the nipple stays in the right place.

Observational Note: Although this baby is new to this nurse (she has only fed her once before), she is noticing all the individual aspects of feeding this baby. While talking with me, her eyes and other senses have not left the baby.

Interviewer: How much are you giving her?

Nurse: 45 cc. Usually we start babies at about 25-30 cc. That's after they have been getting that amount by gavage. Now look again. She is taking a little break and resting. Let me see if she has a burp. I like to try and burp them about half way through, about 25 cc. She is doing well. She is pacing herself. She is also fairly rested so she is not tiring yet (talking to baby, calling her by name). The other thing with these babies, besides finding out the best way to feed them, is also how to burp them. Some require lots of patting. Others require no patting and it is strictly positional. No success with her yet. I have not figured out what works best for her yet. I start with very gentle pats at first (rubbing back).

Observational Note: Baby beginning to dose off, eyes closed.

Nurse: Now she has slowed down her breathing a little. Notice how she is a little dusky around the mouth?

Interviewer: It is very subtle.

Nurse: Yeah it is. Right around the mouth. So I am watching her to make sure she stays pink. If I stimulate her a little she will take a big breathe and pink up. (repositions her, baby awakens, dusky color improves).

Observational Note: The nurse begins to feed the baby again. The head nurse enters and asks nurse about the schedule for inservices she is going to be giving related to drug screening.

Nurse: She seems to be a little pinker now.

Interviewer: You know it is very subtle to me. It is not like adults.

Nurse: Yeah, you would have to compare her to other babies. The color around the mouth is a little different but also the extremities. It is not that they are blue but if you look at some of the other babies when I unwrap them you can see they are not as pink. And not quite as warm either. Now watch her eating. She is needing to take more frequent breaths; she is getting more tired as the feeding goes on. Her suck was stronger at the beginning of the feeding.

Note: Again she is getting to know this baby. The subtlety of this baby. She is totally engaged with this baby (Observational Interview).

The above observation reveals the particularity of the infant's feeding patterns and illustrates the nurse's experiential learning about many particular premature infants. Comforting touch, gentle physical handling, and skillful knowledge about the preferred handling and touch of these premature infants characterizes expert neonatal critical care nursing practice. The above example demonstrates a relational, response-based ethic that acknowledges the way tension, abruptness, and lack of skillful touch is transmitted, creating a negative a response in the infant. Being gentle and comforting are notions of excellence that are internal to these nurses' practice. This nurse understands her work as creating a secure and responsive baby through concern, gentleness, and skillful touch.

Comfort measures change as new patient populations develop and interventions evolve. For example, in the past 20 years neonatal critical care nurses have had to learn how to comfort the neurologically sensitive infants whose mothers were addicted to crack cocaine:

Nurse: I took care of a 37-week-old infant named Tim, with gorgeous eyes and hair... And he was absolutely frantic, just berserk every time he woke up. He would sleep, maybe one to two hours max—and that was after he had been medicated. If you didn't have the bottle ready when his little eyes popped open, he became so agitated that he really lost his ability to get it together with sucking, swallowing, and breathing all at once. We used to have to wrap him very tightly—and it got to the point that you couldn't look at him. If you engaged him too much, it was just too much for him to handle, so you had to sort of look out of the corner of your eyes at this very attractive baby when feeding him. You could feel his little body tense up and you can hear his cry escalating.

Comforting a premature infant is a hard won skill that requires attentiveness and responsiveness, but even the best comforting practices may not bring comfort. To comfort requires knowing the particular patient's responses. The natural inclination is to engage eye contact with an infant and the nurse acknowledges that this inclination had to be quelled for this very attractive infant because he could not tolerate the stimulation of that much engagement. The infant must be able to shape the nature of the comfort measures and the nurse learns the infant's preferences by feeling his tense body and noticing the infant's response to the comfort measures offered.

In the following excerpt, two neonatal ICU nurses are clear about their gains in skillful knowing and comfort practices, but they are also clear that this is a fragile practice:

Nurse 1: But after they get older, a little bit older, when they're a month old or so and they're sort of into the chronic stage, they start developing their idiosyncrasies. You know whether they're going to tolerate suctioning well or twit out for half an hour. Things like that. Whether feeding them makes them feel better or feel worse.

Nurse 2: Yeah, which comfort measures work and which don't. Do they like to be bundled? Do they like to suck their fingers or does that make them have bradycardia. That sort of thing. You learn about each kid. I think you learn it really quickly though. I can go in an take a chronic preemie that I don't know and by the end of the 12 hours I know exactly what works.

Nurse 1: Yeah, because you know what to try.

Nurse 2: Yeah.

Nurse 1: That's the most likely thing to work and you go down the list until you find something that does.

Nurse 2: It took a while, it took years probably to get to that point. That I could get in there, try all my little tricks, figure out what works and what doesn't and get the kid squared away. Although sometimes they don't and sometimes nothing works.

The last sentence points to the response-based nature of comforting. It is simply not always possible to comfort. Comfort is embodied and relational. These nurses have increased their repertoire of comfort measures—"they know what to try"—but their expertise lies in reading the infant's responses and tailoring their comfort measures to those particular responses. The fact that this skilled know-how is transactional and response-based, rather than general, timeless, and located in specific traits or techniques, should not disqualify it as knowledge. One of the nurses showed us "the small baby bundling protocol" which was an illustrated description of bundling or "nesting" premature infants so that they felt secure in their environment. The nurse, pointing to the illustrated procedure at great length, was oblivious to how little of the skilled know-how could not be captured in the written document. The procedure requires skilled touch and a knowledge of particular infants along with much practice in handling such fragile, variable bodies.

This skillful practice is also elusive because the most skillful, attuned nurse cannot promise that comfort measures will always work. Comforting or any mutual, response-based knowledge and skill cannot meet the traditional criteria for knowledge claims of prediction and control as measures of efficacy. But observations of deft handling of premature infants and observed differences in oxygen saturations dependent on skillful touch leave little doubt that this is indeed knowledge and skilled know-how despite its variabilities. Comforting practices, like judgment and craft, have inherent uncertainties. A situation can look impervious to comfort and yet comfort can be found. On the other hand, as the nurse above says, "sometimes nothing works."

Pediatric nurses talked about giving extra cuddling and attention to children who did not seem to have adequate parental attentiveness and especially in cases where child abuse or neglect was suspected:

Nurse 1: You see such a void in them. You want to fill it for them if they have a lousy mother.

Nurse 2: So, you cuddle them a little more at work, you hold them. When you're not busy, you carry them around, you take them off the monitor and carry them around with you. Or, you sit them up on the desk with you. I don't know if you do this on your unit—put the baby in the infant seat? We take them for walks in the stroller or something like that because babies aren't meant to be in cribs 24 hours a day.

As illustrated above, these nurses offer heightened attentiveness in order to get the child to respond and to overcome the separation and void created by an unresponsive abusive and environment.

Reassuring touch is essential for infants and children, but also for adults. Comfort measures for adults are often related to physical care of the body, with cleanliness, stimulation, relaxation, grooming, and keeping the person looking as close to their usual self as possible:

> **Nurse:** I just did things like playing tapes and washed her hair a lot and kept her pretty and clean, did her nails—all the usual kind of nursing things. But I think I did a little extra for her. She was given a lot of one-to-one care when I had the time to do that. We prolonged it a lot because she seemed to show that she needed it more... But we did all these things even while she was asleep because her mother felt like it was important, that she really liked it. And it turned out she really did. And so we were always doing something to make her feel nice and we tried to make lots of space for her husband.

Grooming for this young woman was a major source of comfort and security. Being groomed, as she would do for herself if she were able, allowed for a sense of continuity in her identity and world. When she was sedated, the ordinary grooming, "making the patient look as much like herself as possible," was a source of comfort for the family and was a way of preserving personhood.

Care of the skin in critically and chronically ill patients is vital and complicated due to immobility, poor perfusion, poor nutrition and hydration, and the high risk of infection, so many nurses take on skin care as a point of expertise:

> **Nurse:** Well, my expertise is skin care. I mean, I really excel in that area—I just love it. I took one look at that skin and told them no more salve on her skin; she doesn't need it. If anything, it is holding in a lot of perspiration which is making her rash itch more.

She goes on to describe her specialized care plan and the debridement of the patient's broken down skin. Skin is the locus of many comfort measures—a point of connection. Care of the skin, preventing pressure sores, is central in the practice of nursing. Nurses describe the vigilance required in the midst of high care demands to take simple precautions such as preventing pressure sores on the patients' heels by floating the feet in heal protector boots, especially when patients are at great risk due to poor peripheral perfusion. Preventing pressure sores prevents patient suffering and prolonged hospital stays that are no longer reimbursable under changing regulations. In our observations we have detailed accounts of specific problem-solving associated with dressing wounds and with providing skin care for patients with stomas. This requires knowing the particular patient's wound size and response to various products. It requires keeping track of how the patient responds and adjusting the available products to the changing needs of the patient.

Sociologists point out that care of the skin and body are not high status work, nor are they likely to be in a society that avoids images of dependency and the need for care. Providing comfort through care of the skin can appear less significant than more pressing life-saving measures, yet, if the simpler measures of mouth and skin care are overlooked, they can lead to complications that prolong hospitalization, patient suffering, or even trigger a cascade of untoward events that eventually lead to death.

COMFORTING THROUGH CONNECTION AND RELATIONSHIP AND RECOGNITION OF THE PERSON

Comforting another person through connection and relationship refers to meeting another in ways that sustain a sense of trust and being cared for. Connection with a patient or family first requires meeting or engaging with them as persons rather than as diseased or damaged bodies. In a highly individualistic culture Charles Taylor (1989; 1991) has pointed out the centrality of being recognized and known by others as a source of identity and feeling of belonging rather than that of an isolated individual (Taylor, 1989; 1991). Nurses meet the patient and families as persons, for instance, by being physically comforting through touch, in their style and tone in talking, and through their comportment (way of being or demeanor) which put the patient and family at ease. Connection and the development of a relationship with another person sets up the possibility of comforting. Whether in the midst of a crisis or not, meeting the patient and family as persons presents the ethical demand to respond to the other person's suffering:

> **Nurse:** . . . the patient could get lost amidst the tubes and the excitement and the chaos going on around. And so I was trying to really know about the patient, about what he means to the family... Because this wasn't necessarily a patient that you were going to be able to save, but you could help the family and the patient as a person, and do the best you could with the pure physiological needs as well. It was very important for me to get that across to this less experienced nurse at the time...I just feel so focused on not forgetting about the patient under there. They are a living, breathing, human person with thoughts and feelings and how the family relates to them despite what all we may be doing to them...

During a crisis, nurses focus on the physiological problems and the treatment needed, but it is an ethical issue to meet the fearful patient and family as persons during the crisis (see Chapter 4). A large share of the emotional work of meeting the patient is done by the nurse, as illustrated in the following small group interview excerpt:

> **Nurse 1:** I think it's important to talk to your patients, especially in crisis situations. I think all of us have had trauma experience and when a trauma patient comes in, there's so much going on and everyone has their little task and their job, but a lot of times no one ever get's in their face and says, 'You've been seriously injured and this is what we're going do, and try to stay with us and tell us what's going on.' And I think a lot of times people forget or they figure, 'Oh, they're so dramatically injured and they're so messed up, there's no way they can hear you or understand...'
>
> **Nurse 2:** But you never know.
>
> **Nurse 1:** But you never know.
>
> **Nurse 3:** I typically notice that it is nurses who keep an eye on the patient. The doctors come in looking at the wound, looking at what they're looking at—look at all the numbers and the physiological aspects of the person, but I think for all of us...
>
> **Nurse 1:** Yeah.
>
> **Nurse 3:** We're the ones who were actually talking to the patient, saying, 'you're okay,' and finding out what's going on with them and remembering that they're a person...

Fear of the unknown, harm, loss, damage, and dying may be foremost in patients' thinking, but they may not be able to speak their fears, or, if spoken, their fears may go unheeded. Escalating fear and panic may be a significant factor in their physical well-being, but well-being as a person is equally relevant. Not everyone can focus on the patient/family's emotional state, but it is an ethical breach of practice if no one does.

Meeting the other as a human being, as in the case of premature babies, before they are able to respond, provides a bold example of the non-reciprocal demand of meeting the other (Logstrup, 1971):

Interviewer: What is it that you love about preemies?

Nurse 1: I think the fact that you see them. I mean—they really don't—you can bond with them but they don't bond with you at all for the first month. I mean they just don't—they're not neurologically there enough to be able to do it. They don't know you from Adam, they don't like being handled, they don't—they send you so many negative signals.

Interviewer: And this was why you like them? [Chuckles.]

Nurse 2: Well, but I think it's when they stop doing that and when they sort of get to the stage that A.'s at where she'll open her eyes and suck on her pinky and just do cute little things that. It's seeing their progression.

Nurse 1: I think full term kids kind of spoil you because they do that stuff right from the start—and I—I just really like seeing how preemies evolve. And the fact that also that they're here for months, you know, the really small pre-termers. They're here for three months and you really do get to know the parents and you get to just enjoy the babies a lot.

Interviewer: Mhum. That's a good point. That's something that is very different from the pediatric intensive care unit. I was up there recently and those kids are in and out and there isn't—I notice that you don't have the opportunity to build those types of relationships...

Nurse 1: They're in and out. They don't have the relationships. Although they do have relationships with the parents because they get repeaters.

The nurse describes how she works to create a human world for the premature infant to join. It is one sided, unreciprocal at first, but the nurse describes the intrinsic rewards of watching for the first relational responses from the infant. Whether in infants or adults, being in a "comfortable" relationship implies a basic trust and a sense of being cared for. We frequently heard phrases like [the patient] "felt comfortable with me" or [the spouse] "felt comfortable when I took care of his wife":

Nurse 1: I had one patient, she was 25, had just got married, and was diagnosed with ovarian cancer, which is the worst. She had just gotten her teaching degree, so that was very sad. She was with us for four or five months, I remember her husband; he was <u>so</u> devoted. I worked second shift at the time, so every time I worked, I <u>had</u> her for a patient. And [I tried] just to make her comfortable and even the husband said, 'I'm going to leave early and go home, because I know you're <u>here</u>,' he'd always say that. 'I know you're here, I know she'll have a good night.' So that made me feel good.

Interviewer: What was it about your being there that made him comfortable?

Nurse 1: I think because I always addressed her needs, like if the pain medicine wasn't working, I'd call the physician right away and say, 'You know, I think we need to go up on the pain medicine,' or any little thing—like I'd do mouth care as often as she needed it, instead of saying, 'I don't have time, you can do it,' I'd take the time to do it. I got so attached to her, probably because she was young and I was there the first time she came in, so I think that's why he felt comfortable with me. But I think I made a difference.

Interviewer: In what way? Can you talk more about that?

Nurse 1: Well . . .

Interviewer: What is the difference that you think you made?

Nurse 1: I think because the husband saw that she looked more comfortable maybe. You know specifically . . .

Nurse 2: It probably eased his mind a lot. . .

Nurse 1: Yeah,

Nurse 2: they need that break in order to be able to support her the next day. Probably seeing you, that relieved him, I would think.

Nurse 1: Yeah, I think so, because sometimes there's some patients that you know, you make them comfortable and then okay, they're happy. But I <u>think</u> in her case, I was <u>very</u> consistent and, I was honest with them, and I think I worked extra hard with her, too. I gave her special attention, too. I think that's one reason why the husband felt really comfortable with me, and so was the patient. She was very comfortable with me, so...I think that's how it was.

A comfortable relationship is in itself a comfort measure, and nurses talk about recognizing when a patient/family is or is not comfortable with them or with other nurses.

Critical care nurses face the challenge of the technological imperative to efficiently intervene and save lives and this imperative causes families to be separated and distanced from their loved one's (Koenig, 1988). Some nurses work at overcoming these barriers and incorporate family members into the care of the patients, allowing family members to do routine care and to facilitate bonding and comforting touch (Chesla, 1996; Stannard, 1997). Nurses coach family members, helping them overcome their fear and anxiety in face of a seriously ill family member:

Nurse: I think some of the most valuable things that I've done with parents is to take them in that situation and put their hands (starts to cry) on the baby.

Interviewer: Tell us about that please?

Nurse: And be physically...comforting. Because they can't. And, it's that thing I like about nursery too, that you can be physically comforting in situations that are outrageous.

Finding ways to help family members care for and bond with their premature infants requires inventiveness and commitment to the parents as well as to the infants. The ability to find ways to help requires attentiveness and openness to possibility. For instance, a mother is observed in practice standing by the baby's isolette with her hands on the baby's back and legs. The advanced practice nurse comes and turns the infant's head toward the mother. The nurse then points out to the interviewer:

Nurse: Her mom has a little tape player in bed [with the infant] which I assume [looking at the mother] is your voices.

Mom: It's both my husband's voice and my voice (Observational Interview).

A number of Intensive Care Nursery Nurses have adopted a practice of "Kangaroo Care" or skin to skin holding for the baby and parents (Affonso, Bosque, Wahlberg & Brady, 1993; Bell & McGrath, 1996; Bosque, Brady, Affonso & Wahlberg, 1995). In the following excerpt the nurse captures the change in family participation over time:

Nurse 1: We're talking about skin to skin holding with that preemie, and when I started here twenty years ago, babies who were under a thousand grams never ever came out of the isolette to be held by their parents. Even if they were extubated they were just not allowed because it was felt they'd lose too much heat, and we never allowed intubated babies of any size to be covered because it was felt they were, you know, it was too risky, that they would lose their endotracheal tubes. And now it's so taken for granted, even with fairly ill babies. Some real long-term chronic babies—the parents come in, they hold them as soon as the art line is out—that's sort of a safety risk. But we progressed from just having the parents hold the baby, to the now doing skin to skin, which is where the mother or the father—and actually A.'s parents have both held her skin to skin where they will basically open their shirts up and the baby has no shirt on, just a diaper, and you just put them skin to skin. And it's very nice stimulation for the baby and it also helps to keep the baby warm. They almost never get cold, even if they've just got a blanket draped over them, they get so much heat from the parent, they just soak it up like a furnace, and....

Nurse 2: Well we know this is what it does.

Nurse 1: I know, I know. The mothers sit there with their breast—. But it's—it's a <u>real</u> important bonding thing, we really encourage parents to do it.

Interviewer: Who initiated those changes? Was it the medical staff or the nursing staff?

Nurse 1: Oh! The nursing staff. But there's been a lot of literature to support it and there actually wasn't a lot of resistance over the years. It's come a long way in terms of being willing to try new things.

In this group discussion, there is a fragile dialogue between the technical system world and the lifeworld (Habermas, 1984/1987; Ihde, 1990). The rationale can be made from a technical, physiological perspective, but this is not enough to capture the significance of the practice of skin to skin touch and human closeness between the parents and their infant. The practice is shaped by notions of good about human connection, comfort, and development and notions about physiological and psychological well-being.

PACU nurses use their voices to help focus and organize the patient awakening from anesthesia. To the interviewers and observers they demonstrated an encouraging style and tone of voice as they described their practices of affirming that the surgery was over and that the patient was safe. The tone and style of voice changed during the emergence phase of recovering from anesthesia and during the excitation stage in response to the patient's level of awareness. As one PACU Nurse describes:

> **Nurse:** You speak softly, slowly but reassuringly... I usually touch them and say Mr. So and So, your surgery is over. You are in the recovery room right now. Things are going well. You are just waking up. And then you go over verbal cues, especially if they are thrashing around... With kids, you say: 'Oh, surgery is over. You've been so good, and you've been so brave. You did a great job. Do you want Mommy? I'll get your mommy for you.'

The style and tone of voice changes as the patient becomes more awake and able to communicate. The nurse's sound and tone and style of voice creates the initial environment for the patient. Nurses use their voice to help organize and focus the patient.

When patients is dehumanized and labeled as a difficult or challenging, or "spoiled" demanding patient, it is often because they have not been recognized as persons. They have not been "met" and recognized for who they are as a person. Recognition practices (Taylor, 1991) are particularly difficulty in critical and acute care units because patients are very ill, stripped of most of their identifying cues in terms of how they are in their lifeworld. In the following intricate story, Michael DeMello meets and genuinely likes John and his family. The family feels cared for because they are known, and John's care is tailored to his tastes. Outsiders might think that the nurse would not have time to know about the whole life of a patient as a person and they would be right. The patient has usually lost his identity conferring job, social context, and often his or her ability to express himself. Yet, it is relatively accessible to identify John as a "hard working family man," who is loved by his family. In the following story, Michael DeMello uses simple accessible knowledge about John and his family. He engages in learning Portuguese with John. He finds out his favorite dishes....and that he has a love of the taste of Coca-Cola. These small aspects of the patient's identity, revealed in a stripped down, clinical hospital context are sufficient for John and his family to feel "recognized" and valued as a person and family. There is no evidence of "over-involvement" in Michael's story. One might say that it is an expert skill of involvement as a nurse, because the nurse greets the patient, comes to know the patient and family members and adjusts his care appropriately:

> **Nurse Michael DeMello:** John was well known for a few things. He was a family man, a hard worker and a comedian of sorts. John loved Portuguese food, particularly chicken, and he thoroughly enjoyed the taste of coca-cola. It was sort of his signature drink. He loved it so much that whenever they would come by his visitors would bring him Coca-Cola bottles to drink.
>
> John became my patient pre-operatively, before his carotid endarterectomy, a surgical procedure commonly performed to prevent strokes in patients with significant plaque formation of the carotid arteries. John had so much plaque that he was already having TIAs. If he didn't do something to increase the circulation to his brain, he would eventually have a stroke. His only hope was this surgery.
>
> The procedure is one in which we surgically go into the blood vessels and literally clean out the plaque. Metaphorically, it is like going to the dentist for a

cleaning. They use instruments to scrape off the hardened junk. Like any surgery, it is a risky procedure, but many elect to have it because the untreated consequences are much riskier.

John walked into the hospital and had his surgery hoping to prevent a stroke. I did his admission, his pre-operative checks, and his surgical preparation. I reserved an ICU bed for his post-operative care and monitoring, and I educated both him and his family around what to expect post-operatively. During the process of preparing him for surgery, I became particularly fond of John and his family. After shaking John's hand and wishing him well, I escorted him to the surgical suite. I offered a prayer and some good luck. I told him that I would see him later in his admission, after his stay in the ICU. I looked forward to it. Two days later while working, I was asked to take an ICU transfer. I had hoped it was John and sure enough it was. We are not always fortunate enough to have this kind of care continuity and I remember thinking how lucky I was to get John back as my patient. I called the ICU to get report and when I did, I heard some very upsetting details of John's postoperative course.

While in the ICU, John suffered a massive CVA (stroke). My eyes welled up a little when I got report because this man's procedure was meant to prevent a stroke. How could he be experiencing the very thing his surgery was designed to avoid? It was an awful and extremely ironic complication of his surgery. Through report I learned that JOHN was completely paralyzed on one side. Functionally, John was severely limited and his vascular surgeon felt as though this residual was permanent.

John was transferred back to me and I assumed his care for several days. Every body system and every aspect of John's life was affected by this stroke. Despite all of the efforts we made, his health deteriorated horribly. His activity was severely limited and he was left bed or wheelchair bound. PT/OT worked with John routinely in hopes to preserve the little muscle strength and integrity he had left. His skin began to break down, his muscles weakened, he was in pain more and more frequently and he even developed pneumonia…all of these, consequences of the stroke and it's sequelae. John needed a PICC line for IV antibiotics, aggressive decubitus prevention, and meticulous nursing care to maintain his already compromised state of health. I remember once watching John in bed and thinking that he resembled an injured animal or bug; on his back moving, struggling and fidgeting to get somewhere but completely unable to make any progress at all. It was mortifying, and such a trauma for both the patient and his family.

Nutrition was also a huge issue for John. He was unable to chew or swallow regular foods or fluids. Everything had to be cut up, and all of his liquids had to be thickened so he wouldn't aspirate. Someone had to be present during all meal times to feed him to ensure his safety. He was no longer allowed chicken unless it was pureed and he was no longer allowed coca cola unless we added a thickening powder to it. While this powder didn't alter the cola's taste, it certainly made the texture intolerable for John.

As the days passed I took care of John routinely. As he declined, I supported both him and his family through some really significant moments. There were times when his wife or one of his children would just weep, and I would sit with them to offer support or a listening ear. I found myself constantly updating them on the plan of care, teaching them about the new medications that were added to his regimen, and coordinating his lab and diagnostic times around visits with family because I knew how important these times were to John. At one point I even had to sit with John and his family and discuss changing his status to DNR. It was emotional, provocative, and very difficult sit and talk about such issues, but it needed to be done and I am blessed that I could be the one to facilitate the process. John and his family ultimately agreed on the DNR order but I don't think they ever would have, if it weren't for our in depth conversations about what "do not resuscitate" really meant.

As time passed, John became severely depressed. He was trapped inside a body that refused to coordinate with his mind. His pneumonia progressed, likely due to aspiration, and so his diet got downgraded to ice only. As health care professionals we are taught to always examine the bigger picture; in this case the picture was so grim. John had lost many of the things that he enjoyed. He lost his ability to talk and joke, his communication with family and friends had been compromised, his mobility was extremely limited, and now he couldn't even enjoy his chicken or coca cola.

One night after my shift, I really marinated myself in John's situation. I thought of the multidisciplinary interventions we were doing for John but felt as though something was missing. Despite everything we were doing, I knew I needed to do more to comfort John. I prayed for an idea. Suddenly, it hit me... What if I froze the coca cola and then broke it into ice chips? Technically, I'd be following the doctor's instructions while still giving John something he's always loved... Hmmm. Could this work?

The next day when I went to work, I did just that. I remember the look on his face as I approached John with this idea. He was reluctant, but wanted to give it a try. The moment the chip was in his mouth, I could see this man's eyes light up. John loved his coca cola ice chips. He could only articulate a couple words at a time when speaking but he always mustered up enough strength to ask for "Mike" or "coca cola ice chips." John would ask everyone who walked in the room for one of the two, and if they couldn't get the first, he would ask for the second. I smile as I write this because I think of him so fondly. Often the staff would get frustrated with these requests; one even said I was "spoiling him."Tell me, how can someone who has just lost everything be spoiled? If the one thing this man looked forward to was a couple ice chips, I was happy to provide. I would bring in the ice chips at the beginning of my shift and give him a little bit each time I went into the room. I remember how he would purse his lips around the spoon as the ice went into his mouth. He savored each drop, each and every drop. In exchange he taught me his native language. Each day he would teach me one word and quiz me on it the next time I entered his room. After I had mastered it, he would teach me the next. He would joke with me, and gave me the nickname "Galinha" which is Portuguese for chicken. Only after he was discharged did I realize the significance of that nickname, considering how fond he was of that dish...John ended up stabilizing to the point where he was able to go to a nursing home for the remainder of his life. I think of John whenever I take a swig from the cola bottle. It makes me happy to know that he is in a better place and that while he was in his time of need and asking for a lot of things we couldn't give him; there was always coca cola ice chips—and they made him smile—a crooked but really excited happy smile.

Last month, John's wife Emily was admitted to my floor with a kidney stone. I was assigned to care for her. As I was writing down my assignment, I realized who she was and I ran into the room. She lit up when she saw me, as did I. She reminisced about the days when her husband was on the same floor and all of the care I had provided. She told me John had passed away at the nursing home. She continued to tell me that I was one of the most influential people in John's care and really helped to make such an awful situation so much more tolerable and a little easier to understand. We talked about the coca cola ice chips and "galinha."

PROVIDING ADEQUATE STIMULATION, DISTRACTION, AND REST WHILE LIMITING DISRUPTION

Discerning when patients need stimulation, distraction, or rest is a complicated and subtle clinical judgment based upon knowing the patient and/or family, having a good understanding of the sciences, and having experiential wisdom. Science informs a nurse's clinical judgment when the patient's specific physiological condition is known to worsen as a result of increased stimulation. For instance, in the acute phase of a head injury or immediately after cardiac arrest (causing localized or global brain injury, respectively), studies show that stimulation, necessary or not, often increases cerebral oxygenation (Henneman, 1986; Mitchell, 1986). In pathophysiological conditions where science specifically guides practice and experience confirms scientific findings, clinical judgment is not as complex.

Similarly, science and clinical experience have taught nurses that neonates commonly deteriorate after unnecessary, prolonged, or sudden stimulation. Thus, knowing the neonate may be less influential immediately after post-delivery. However, science does not inform clinicians about when neonates become less neurologically sensitive so that clinical judgment or discernment skills are essential. A research assistant who is an expert neonatal ICU nurse wrote the following observation note after watching an expert clinician care for a premature infant over the course of a morning:

> **Inte**rviewer: [During this observation, very little hands-on care was done by the Neonatal Intensive Care Nurse, and, consequently, there was little to observe. However, leaving the infant alone was in itself a crucial intervention that demonstrated the nurse's expert assessment of a potentially very labile and brittle infant who could easily fall apart if bothered. Leaving the infant alone was the indicated therapy, but it required restraint and planning. The Nurse seemed confidant of her ability to use visual skills, the monitors, and her prior experience with similar infants to guide her assessment of the infant's status and needs.] (Observational Note)

In this situation, knowing how most neonates respond as they grow and knowing how this particular neonate continues to respond informs the nurse that this infant continues to require rest with minimal disruption. Critical care nurses who have cared for labile neurological patients develop a similar practice of limiting stimulation. The skill of providing comfort care which in interspersed with periods of respite is seen in the following clinical observation:

> **Nurse:** I'm trying to do things pretty much in stages and not get him too excited about...
>
> **Interviewer:** So that's why you bathed half his body and came back to that?
>
> **Nurse:** Yeah, and I gave him a little bit of rest and then chest physical therapist came in and saw him, and then he had a little bit of rest after that, so now I'll do this side.
>
> **Interviewer:** Where did you learn to bathe a little bit, and then go away?
>
> **Nurse:** I definitely learned it with neuro patients, I know. With neuro people, they really can't tolerate any big type of changes. A lot of activity in a head injury isn't good. You don't go in there in the morning, wash, weigh them, do everything at once,

and let them sit for two hours. You go in, do a little, and come out and a lot of times people who are very bronchospastic when you do a lot of things to them... they'll get agitated and they'll start to cough because of the tubes and they get more bronchospastic. So I learned the lesson: once they start getting agitated, you stop, back off, do some paperwork, clean them up a little bit, and when they calm down for a little while, you come back and do a little bit more. So you sort of plan your day according to how they're doing.

Note: The Nurse is going to start bathing this man, and she's trying to do this, providing very little stimulation to him. And again as she bathes him and cares for him, she looks at the monitors and oximeter and all his pumps and is carefully evaluating his IV sites, all the while talking to him and telling him what she's doing. She's removing his gown, as she does that she speaks to him and says, 'I'm taking off your gown.' She very gently lifts up his arm with support to his wrist, looking over at his oximeter. Now she is about to carefully bathe him...

Nurse: Yeah. I'm going to wash you up here. (break)

Note: The patient seemed to have a bronchospasm. The nurse stopped what she was doing and talked to him a little bit. As she's bathing him, she puts the basin of water on the bed and soaks his hand in the water. While she's doing this, the ventilator alarm goes off and she very skillfully turns and adjusts the ventilator. The Bio-dyne bed that this man is on has the capacity to gently rock the patient side to side within the time cycle and it's selected carefully by the nurses in this unit for anybody with severe pneumonia, with blood gas changes which obviously this man has. As the nurse bathes him, she's just giving him range of motion to his arm. I'm really most impressed by Nurse's great skill with basic nursing care, bathing and range of motion, coupled with her extensive and expert knowledge of this patient's medical condition (Observational Interview).

Stimulation and rest are adjusted according to the patient's response. The nurse carefully observes the patient's responses during the bath. The stimulation the nurse provides is also orchestrated with other disciplines to ensure adequate rest.

Critical care nurses discuss the problem of waking patients minimally every 1 to 2 hours to do vital signs, and of giving patients ICU psychosis due to sleep deprivation. In critical care units, the intensive nature of the therapy and the instability of the patients collide to make sleep and rest a difficult therapy to introduce into the cure-oriented system. In the Nightingale Tradition (Stretkowicz, 1996), sleep and rest are understood as reparative and central to putting the body in the best condition for self-repair and healing. This creates a dilemma for critical care nurses who try to cluster their care and sometimes skip or reschedule some of the vital signs or delay routine treatments to allow for the competing goods of rest and sleep:

Nurse: All I know is when I saw him (a child), he looked like someone who hadn't had enough sleep, was extremely tired, and was just worried to death. And so as soon as the father came in, I did the bit of introducing myself. And then I just basically told him what I planned, what my care was going to be... And he started telling me that yes, that he felt that his son wasn't getting enough sleep.

The nurse goes on to describe the plan to allow for uninterrupted sleep for the child. Since the care goes on 24 hours a day and the patient's sense of days and nights can get mixed up, ICU psychosis due to overstimulation and sleep deprivation are common. Allowing for adequate rest and sleep takes planning, active intervention, skills of unobtrusive assessment, and clarity in resisting the social pressure to do unnecessary disruptive vital signs and treatments as illustrated in these excerpts from different nurse interviews:

Nurse: And I think, again, it's one of those things that comes with experience and knowing what's best for these poor chronic patients is to let them get the sleep-rest cycle and leave them alone for at least four hours to sleep and maybe even heaven forbid, six hours (laughter). And for people to learn that they can assess a patient and know that the patient's okay or not okay without touching them. Going into the room, observing them, watching them breathe and looking at their monitor and kind of looking at their skin...

Nurse: You know most of these patients still have arterial lines six months down the road and I think it's just one of those things that come with experience and time, but it's almost like no matter how many times you say to people, 'It's okay not to have something down on the chart every two hours,' they still feel that. You know, who is that for? Who are those every two hour vital signs for? Certainly, in my opinion, not for the patient.

Neonatal ICU nurses cluster their care by grouping stimulation and painful disruptive procedures to limit periods of discomfort and stimulation and allow for rest. They must learn to physically handle the body in gentle ways that do not unduly startle the infant:

Nurse: We do try to ...get a rhythm about it so that we are not constantly handling the babies. In other words, either every hour or every two hours, or every three hours, depending on the baby, you do all of the tasks that need to be done, and the rest of the time you try to keep your hands off the baby and let the baby rest, let the baby sleep. We try to coordinate this also with the physicians and with respiratory therapy and blood gases. Anybody who needs to put hands on the baby, we try to coordinate that so that the baby is not being constantly disturbed every fifteen minutes (Observational Interview).

This nurse's notion of good practice and comfort extend to coordinating her interventions with the team. This orchestration of care takes planning, judgment, and skillful handling.

Nurse: She came back from angioplasty to CCU around 7:00 p.m. with only fair results. She was just worn out...so my approach to her was to get her comfortable and to make sure she got a good night's sleep. She'd been on her back with a sandbag because her groin had been oozing, but I took the sandbag off and I put on a pressure dressing. Then I turned and repositioned her...I told her that a little bit of morphine would take the edge off of the groin pain and that I would also give her a sleeping pill and that the combination of the two medications usually work very well for people, and that she could get a good nights's rest and wake up in the morning and not feel drugged...I asked her if she and any objections to my combining the medications...I gave her some choice.

These last two excerpts illustrate how much skill and thoughtfulness are required to provide comfort measures in a highly technical environment. The third excerpt illustrates the integration of comfort measures while enlisting the patient's expectations and consent for the planned rest and sedation. Responding to the pain and preparing for the rest are dependent on the nurse's recognition of the patient's fatigue since, in this situation as in many, the patient is unable to advocate for needed rest.

The struggle to create a quiet environment is at odds with the light and noise in critical care areas, and is at odds with the intensive therapies. A pediatric ICU nurse describes one approach for limiting stimulation:

Nurse: My approach was to attempt to group his activities, to leave him quiet in his environment. He has tapes with really soft music. We put that on. We pulled a blanket over the top of his crib, like a tent you used to climb into when you were a little kid (laughs). But, he sits there in his tent awake! I sedated him, but because of how easily he gets agitated, a wet diaper wakes him up, and even though he's sedated, once you change the diaper, it's as if he never got the sedation. So, it's really important to group his activities, and then, additionally, he spiked a fever of 40 degrees last night so we had to draw blood cultures. He's a really hard stick. It took over an hour... I don't know what was happening in the lab last night, but one of the blood samples that we sent hemolyzed and we had to draw again, because he had a low K+ during the day. We'd given him K+ supplements, and we had to find out what had had happened. It was something that we definitely had to send again. So, I was trying to make judgments about what labs had to be drawn and not drawn and I talked to people about that and decided because of his K+, the labs needed to be re-drawn... And then I just talked with other nurses about what can be done here. How can we group his activities?

The major strategies are to cluster activities to limit disruption, do necessary procedures in the least disruptive way, create as normal conditions for day and night distinctions as possible, and give sedation with judicious timing in relation to disruption:

Nurse: We had a child in for his second cardiac surgery. He has Down's Syndrome. A lot of children with Down's Syndrome are difficult to comfort anyway, then these cardiac and respiratory complications made it much more difficult for him... When I took care of him two weeks ago, he was so agitated that I had to sedate him heavily or he was going to pull out his endotracheal tube. Now, he's not agitated like that. He's just awake. So, we're working with him and tonight I'll try to reinstitute days and nights and try and give him chloral hydrate [sedative] at night and have them not do it during the day and try and get [a support service] involved where they come in and play with him during the day to keep him awake and stimulate him.

This, like the other examples of the work of trying to provide for rest and sleep show the centrality of this taken-for-granted source of well being, (Bruyna, 1981; Daiss, Bertelson & Benjamin, 1986). Hospitals are notorious for their noisy and unaesthetic design. The struggle to humanize an uncomfortable, hostile environment is a pervasive theme in the interviews.

In contrast to trying to limit stimulation, the combination of the patient's illness and critical care units as they are currently designed create disturbances in the patient's world, for instance, by blocking out needed and rejuvenating stimuli. Institutionalization (Goffman,

1961), a phenomena of all total institutions, is even more extreme in critical care areas. The patients' world often shrinks to the center of their specialized beds. There are many examples of broadening the patient's perspective to extend their sense of possibility and future through changing their location and thus their horizons:

> **Advanced Practice Nurse:** This patient had a big MI. He had cardiac surgery, and now was ventilator-dependent and a chronic wean. He had gone through ICU psychosis and had all kinds of problems. And I could say I offered one suggestion... we wanted to get him out of the unit to take him for a ride in the hall. He was an ex-police officer and he was real depressed. And what we did, the primary nurse thought I was insane, I said, 'We could take him out, we could do this.' The nurse caring for him said: 'No, I've got the vent and I've got the tube feeding, and all this stuff.' It wasn't an easy task, but it really was a simple task, just needed some people to help get him in a big Geri chair, and about four of us wheeled him down the hall. And the first time we did it, I stayed with him. And when I needed help, I called on people, brought in help and brought him back. And it was actually kind of nice, he ended up being in our unit probably two more weeks, and he probably made about six or seven more trips down the hall... His is a pretty simple example... of helping nurses to see different things that they could do to help the patients make it through the experience...'

This is a good example of judiciously opening up the patient's world by changing the patient's position and view. The sensory deprivation of a technically equipped brightly lighted room closes down a comfortable, familiar world. But an intervention like mobilizing the patient down the hall requires timing. Sometimes a trip out of the room and a safe return has a symbolic impact conveying to the patient that they can "move." They can leave and safely return (Holden, 1992). This gives them a sense of direction and progress.

TAMING THE TECHNICAL ENVIRONMENT

Critical care units have been designed much like operating rooms, with little attention given to the aesthetics of the environment. There have many studies of ecological and environmental problems in critical care units that range from irritability, fatigue, and anxiety to ICU psychosis from over-stimulation, disruption of circadian rhythms, and noise. But in all of the critical care units observed, the technological imperative was dominant (Koenig, 1988). In addition to the ever-present disturbances created by technology, other patients in close proximity may require resuscitation, creating a sense of dread and sorrow. In pediatric units, children's crying may disrupt sleep. These are the environmental challenges to providing rest, sleep, and comfort. Thus, the nurse's attempt to alter the environment through controlling the noise, light, and emotional climate at the bedside is always against great environmental odds (Thollaug, 1991). In every aspect of the caring practices presented in this work, nurses work in inhospitable environments. Sometimes it is a heroic act to procure a quieter room for a distressed or dying patient. This working against the odds is evident in the following example:

> **Nurse:** Throughout the day the child kept telling me how tired he was. 'I'm so tired, I can't sleep in here because it's noisy and can't I have a quieter room?' The room that he was in is always noisy... I felt bad for him because he really needed his rest. He

hadn't slept for a couple of days and so I asked the charge nurse and she didn't want to do it because of the staffing... I said, 'Well, let's move both of the kids over'... I stood up for him and was finally able to do it.

This is indeed a fragile practice in an environment that is hostile to solace, familiarity, aesthetics, and silence in favor of efficiency. Procuring a private room for a chronically critically ill patient is often crucial for patient and family well-being and recovery:

Nurse: We were always doing something to make her feel nice and try to make lots of space for her husband... We moved her to a single room because I felt like she would be better in a single room and the family should have more time with her. We weren't sure she was going to make it, but that wasn't the reason we moved her there. We started putting up pictures. We had pictures all across the whole place. People would stop in that hallway to see the pictures on that wall. We put pictures of herself and her husband around and tried to open her eyes so she could see them. We'd have her husband sit in the bed with her and hug her. We did a lot of those kind of things. We really personalized the room for her and spent a lot of time with that kind of care. We talked to her. That was the big thing.

Interviewer: You have a very soothing voice. I think that would work for me as well.

The environment of the room is personalized in order to encourage the patient to rejoin a more familiar and safe world. The researcher notes how the nurse in the above excerpt was highly skilled at creating an environment in the small ICU space around the patient. The arrangement of the bed, chairs, table, equipment, the use of lighting, managing sound as much as possible, and orchestrating the traffic and access to the patient all have a calming effect in the patient's immediate environment. This skill of taming and domesticating the patient's immediate surroundings stands out in critical care areas that have been designed more for the most efficient use of technology than for soothing patients.

Parents understandably do not want to see their infant crying and interpret the nurse's checking on another baby prior to their crying infant as indifference and lack of concern. Family members often become angry as a result of their sense of helplessness to intervene and provide what they see as basic care, comfort and above all, a human comforting response to their infant's crying. It is always possible that an angry parent will become violent in a desperate attempt to get the care he or she feels is needed by their infant. In the following example, the clinical leader is called to work with an angry father, whose anger and fear escalates when the pediatrician explains that his child will need to be transferred into a higher level of care due to symptoms of withdrawal from the Mother's methodone prenatal program. The nurse judiciously aligns herself with the Father and avoids escalation of his anger.

Nurse Luigina Maniscalco: I received a phone call from one of our pediatricians letting me know that she had just had a verbal altercation with the Father of one of her patients (babies). One of the staff nurses felt she, the pediatrician, should let somebody know that this Father was rude to her and that someone needed to do something about this Father: as the weekend Clinical Leader I was "that someone." The pediatrician stated to me that the Father became verbally abusive to her when she made it known that, because of the baby's symptoms, he would most likely be transferred to the Level II nursery on the fourth floor and that Dad was told by the pediatrician that Phenobarital would most likely be started. I immediately went to the Newborn Nursery to meet this Father who would not leave the bassinet of his son. "Leo" (dad) informed me that "he was going to get a new pediatrician because he did not like the one he had now for his son."

I calmly approached Leo and asked if there was anything upsetting him about the care his son was receiving. Leo immediately became louder (verbally). Leo informed me that through the night, "he observed many of the nurses in the nursery ignoring crying babies." I asked Leo if he could be more specific and he stated that he was "watching the nurses and he knew the nurses knew they were being watched and he insisted that when his son was crying, they purposely ignored him." They would "go over to other babies and walk past his son." He told me that he thought "this was unacceptable" and he "REFUSED" to let his son stay in the newborn nursery. He "wanted his baby to spend all of the time in the Mother's room (rooming in) where HE could watch his son." I made eye contact with Leo and I did agree that from the outside looking into the nursery, I could "see how he might misinterpret a nurse caring for the crying infants. Not every crying infant can be the first one attended to." My hope was to let Leo know every baby was important to the nurses and I intentionally maintained eye contact and stayed calm. My hope was that by agreeing with him, he would calm down. Leo really did not seem to accept this rationale, he was talking loudly, pointing his left index finger to my shoulder as if to "drive home his point and his right hand was clenched (at his side). We only had the baby's bassinet between us. My nursery staff, behind Leo, kept motioning to me if I wanted them to notify security. At this point, I did not feel I needed any security back-up and felt I could help Leo become calmer by talking calmly to him and maintaining eye contact. The louder Leo got, the softer my tone of voice became. I asked Leo again if there was anything upsetting him in particular. Leo proceeded giving me the story of why he was so upset and why he wanted a new pediatrician.

Leo's significant other, the Mother of his son, was in a Methadone treatment course and throughout her pregnancy she was on increasing doses of methadone (for her drug history). When she delivered by cesarean section (C-section), she was receiving 95 mg of methadone twice daily. Leo informed me that "he had done his research and he knew that methadone was metabolized differently in every patient and that babies especially metabolized methadone differently and that his son might not have any symptoms of withdrawing." He also stated that the pediatrician told him his son was "jittery and irritable" but that Leo did not see that in his son. I first commended Leo for being proactive in the care of his son. I told Leo that "as the baby's Father, he should know what to expect about his son's behavior and I thought it was good that Leo researched the effects of methadone on babies." I also told Leo "I have been doing this type of work, working with babies and babies of moms on methadone, for 17 years and that in my experience, and what I have seen, babies born to Mom's who have been on methadone throughout their pregnancy DO show signs of withdrawing and that these babies do spend time in the Level II nurseries, and his son may not be discharged home with Mom on her discharge date." Leo looked somewhat confused when I mentioned "withdrawing", I tried to make it very simple and told him that the pediatrician and the nursing staff would be looking for his baby to have "shaking of his arms and legs as though he were shaking a rattle," not the type of shaking a baby would have if he just woke up and had a startle effect. I also explained we would be looking for the irritable crying, the crying that IS NOT controlled by feeding him, changing his diaper, wrapping him in blankets and talking calmly to the baby. This type of behavior would indicate to the pediatrician and the nursing staff that his baby was showing signs of withdrawing. I explained to Leo that although he wanted to change pediatricians, right now the doctor on record was the doctor whose orders I had to carry out. Leo and I spent several hours together and I kept making eye contact and talking calmly. Leo initially was loud and pointing his left finger at me, however, after our time together, Leo seemed more relaxed with me and my explanations. He now stopped pointing at me and would talk softer. He would still try to avoid my eye contact, but I was persistent.

I knew that Leo's son would be transferred to the Level II nursery. I spoke with the Neonatologist, informed him of the potential transfer and I filled him in on Leo. I told the Neonatologist about the Pediatricians interaction with Leo (because I did not want to alienate the Neonatologist and Leo). I also informed the Neonatologist that Leo felt he was "very knowledgeable about methadone withdrawal" and that Leo needed to be in-control of every situation (this was my impression of Leo). I asked Leo to come to the Level II nursery and "see" where his son would be staying and to talk to the Neonatologist. As soon as Leo entered the Level II nursery, he became loud and verbally aggressive with the staff. His back seemed to get very straight and there was a definite sense that Leo was feeling out-of-control in this unit. He stated very loudly, with his right hand clenched and his left hand pointing: "I DO NOT want my son on Phenobarbital if he begins to withdraw." The Neonatologist stated, "That is really interesting, because on Phenobarbital your baby can go home. If we start him on Neonatal Morphine, he has to remain an inpatient." (My impression was that Leo reacted aggressively when he was TOLD what would be done and that he had a misunderstanding of the purpose of Phenobarbital and withdrawing infants). I took Leo aside at this point and calmly told him that "there is no reason for me to lie to you. Your baby will get the best care we can offer and he will recover as soon as possible from HIS methadone exposure." Leo looked at me and said, "I think we're going to be OK. You and I get along, so I think we will be alright." I understood that to mean that Leo felt comfortable with me and my explanations. In addition, my colleagues would tell me that Leo would cross his index and middle fingers and say, "me and Gina are buddies". This was interesting to me because, I felt Leo and I were miles apart.

Since I am the weekend Clinical Leader, I was not there when Mom was discharged, however, I was told Mom was discharged from the hospital on the Monday (day 4 post C-section) and the baby was discharged from the hospital Level II nursery the following Thursday (day of life number 7). To my knowledge, there were no further issues with Leo.

Nurse Luigina Maniscalco aligns herself with Leo, and listens carefully to his concerns. She hears and understands his distress over his child crying. Based upon what he has read, he does not think that his infant is experiencing Methadone withdrawal. Nurse Maniscalco gives him a way to read his infant's signs of withdrawal, and to understand the proposed treatment. She recognizes and respects the Father's knowledge and fears, and learns about his perspective and interpretation of the chaotic and seemingly callous environment.

She acknowledges the Father's knowledge and builds upon it, expanding it rather than dismissing it. In contrast, when a situation is reduced to a power discourse in response to a patient's or family member's anger, the situation almost always escalates. Understanding the Father's perspective and acknowledging it, opened up communication so that the Father's concerns could return to a discussion of what is best for the infant, We have numerous exemplars of nurses de-escalating anger episodes by aligning with the patient or family member's concerns about the efficacy and quality of care the patient is receiving. Until the family member can understand the reasons and purposes behind nurses' and physicians' actions, they will understandably feel frightened and even distrust the safety of the environment.

The Father's behavior might have been labeled "ineffective coping" or as a "difficult, unreasonable" parent, however once Nurse Luigina Maniscalco understands what the Father is actually "coping with" nurses' seemingly inattention to his infant's crying, and an unreasonable desire to sedate his infant when he did not believe that the infant was exhibiting withdrawal symptoms, his fears and anger become understandable, and amenable to coaching and to interpreting the care being given to his infant.

One of the costs of the invisibility and devaluation of the helping work of the nurse is overlooking the healing powers of comfort. If care were valued in its own right as essential to cure, then the design of the acute and critical care areas would change drastically. Patients' rooms could be designed for both cure and comfort. At fault seems to be our cultural blindness to the importance of a comforting environment, the powers of the family's comfort measures, and the comfort measures of nurses for the efficacy, safety, and humaneness of highly technical cures.

For the researchers entering critical care areas with only the task to observe and ask questions, the noise of the equipment, the moans and cries of patients and families, the maze of technical equipment, the communications among clinicians, and the sounds of ventilators, monitors, and alarms come in with near equal force on the senses. In fact, parts of the verbal data were often obscured on the tapes by environmental noises. Critical care areas were not designed for rest and comfort. The challenge remains to design patient rooms that meet basic human needs to physically and relationally domesticate the critical and acute care environments to the extent possible.

BEING AVAILABLE WITHOUT BEING INTRUSIVE

Providing care that comforts, strengthens, and protects depends on well honed skills of involvement, so that patient and family are given the space they need to experience their own ways of comforting. Discerning how close and how far away to be with patients and being available without being intrusive are critical distinctions in learning to be comforting.

Nurse: I stayed just outside the room most of the time, but I'd come in to see, just to touch her and put a wet washcloth on her forehead. She had asked that the rest of the family come in but not to stay so I went to get them and brought them and asked them not to stay for too long because she wanted this time pretty much alone with her husband. Yet once they got there, it seemed like the proper thing to do. They didn't want to leave right away, so they stayed longer. But they finally pulled themselves together and went out and left her alone with him. But then they came back and they hung out in the hallway. I was always within sight of her and sound of him. And I'd come in and out... She had a lot of support, but she wanted a lot to be alone with him so people just sat back and were quiet mostly until after he died... If we can, we create nursing time to be able to do that [on our unit], which to me is real important. It's just as important as a code or anything else. It all goes together. I don't know how to explain how. I just know that she didn't really want me there all the time at the bedside, but that she appreciated that if there was anything she needed I would have gotten it for her.

Interviewer: It just seems to be a tricky clinical decision to know where the line is between being intrusive, but also being available.

Nurse: There are times when you know that you're being intrusive and you stay out of the room. As much as you can, you go away, further away. I stayed just outside the curtains most of the time and I came in. But even then I still come in just to see if they were OK. You never completely leave them alone, even when I think I should, I still don't. Usually I have to check up on them. But I give them a lot of space. You try and make sure that your alarms aren't going to ring or something's not going to freak them out. It's the little things of trying to make them comfortable.

Comfort, in this sense, allays anxiety and attempts to breach the terror of loss in a strange environment. Care of the body is a culturally sanctioned task for nurses in a culture where there is little language to describe the sentient, lived social body. Care of the body is fraught with tension, taboos, and status issues. Dependency is feared in the Cartesian Tradition where the body is considered that which must be controlled by the mind (Benner & Wrubel, 1989). In the body lies our vulnerability, the personal mentor for the limits of control in a culture that seeks to master uncertainty, risk, and vulnerability. Sexuality, desire, and intimacy are embodied. As Foucault (1973) points out, our power and control discourses are located in the body where we live out the direct, immediate understandings of domination and subordination in our stances, our gestures, expressions, distances, and proximities. The body is politicized and gendered. Vulnerability, weakness, finitude, suffering as well as desire, skill, strength, and pleasure are bodily integrated and bodily sensed. Ultimately our ethical comportment with others is embodied in our stances of closeness, distance, gesture, gentleness, roughness, attentiveness, carefulness, or carelessness. Being available without being intrusive requires that the nurse judge the patient's response and that any sign of retreat or withdrawal be honored. This requires careful skill of involvement and boundary work as illustrated in the following exemplar cited in Benner et al. (2009, pp. 317-318):

Nurse: I could just tell that he was winding down away from me, pulling back. I'm like, 'O.K., calm down, this person isn't going to talk to you. I overstepped my boundaries by probably talking too much....'

Interviewer: His response was kind to pull away and so you thought?

Nurse: Yeah, he's had so many different nurses that he doesn't need to keep getting close to each one that comes in and talks to him. He has his primary nurses and he can be close to them. But for somebody that fills in for four hours, he didn't want to interact with because he doesn't have that much energy to bond with me, which is fine.

This new graduate nurse had been caring for unconscious patients and was looking forward to caring for a patient who could talk to her. She describes her experiential learning and corrects her relational stance by pulling back in response to the patient's need to conserve energy and retreat. The beginning nurse is learning both timing and attunement. Talk about the patient's more ordinary world and using humor can help distract the patient during times of waiting, but distraction has to be used judiciously.

WEIGHING THE ETHICS OF PAIN MEDICATION, SEDATION, AND COMFORT MEASURES

Pain and anti-anxiety medications work best if reassurance, the nurse's presence, and other comforting practices are provided with the medication. Alleviating pain is a moral mandate. Too little or too much pain medication present both ethical and clinical problems. Using pain medication or sedation in the absence of basic comfort measures decreases the effectiveness of the medication and may entail a disregard for the person's total well-being. Comfort measures assist patients in weaning from pain medication. Decreasing another person's level of consciousness or mobility makes them vulnerable and requires attentiveness to the patient's safety and well-being. This ethical and clinical judgment is illustrated in the following interview where an emergency department nurse talked about a young man who was injured in an accident:

> **Nurse:** ...He was painting trim on a house, fell off, and went through a tree on the way down. I told him he was trying to eat a tree limb, because that's what caught his mouth and ripped him open through here (motioning from her mouth to her cheek). So he had a significant injury, and he was a young man in his 20s, so I know in the back of his mind he's thinking that he's scarred and all those kind of things. You just kind of make it light. 'I'm going to give you a little nerve medicine, calm you down, and let them irrigate you so that you don't have any trees growing out of your face later.' You know with the tree limbs,... and it relieved some anxiety, it made him voice... 'You know, I was drinking last night, and then I didn't eat this morning.' I said, 'Yeah, those stupid things we all do. We shouldn't go drinking the night before we decide to climb on top the house and not eat anything.' And [I] just kind of let him voice his own stupidity and get it out (laughs) and have somebody say, 'Well, yeah, we don't always use the best judgment in the world. And you're fine, you're going to go home.' You know, 'You're going to get through this just fine. Just don't climb on the house again real soon.' That's what I said.

> **Interviewer:** Was there anything in particular that you did that he recognized...?

> **Nurse:** I think I just, I took _time_ just to stay with _him_ for a few minutes. I didn't just give him some morphine and walk away. You know, I explained that I was giving him some versed this time, and I was going to give him some morphine, but not as _much_ as the last time, since it did irritate the other IV site, and he, didn't complain of any burning [this time]. I gave him versed first, though, so, I made him a little goofy before I gave him the morphine and it worked really well. And it calmed him down, and brought down his anxiety level, because I think without him ever saying anything, then numbing up his face, and suturing and everything was he was in his twenties, it doesn't mean he's going to like it any better than somebody younger. And I think

about the versed, because we use it so much with the children and it brings down the anxiety level. Because you're not going to remember quite so much, now that we're giving this, too. You know, 'This will kind of help you. So it's not so uncomfortable.' I didn't get to see him before he went down. But I did get to see the repair job. It was going to be a dandy...

There is much human contact going on in this interaction. The nurse gathers the patient's story of his fall, his remorse, and acknowledges his current anxiety. In addition to pain and anti-anxiety medication, she comforts with her presence, humor, and encouragement. She is justly proud that she didn't just give the medication without also providing human comfort.

The nurse acknowledges a common temptation to provide comfort through sedation without or instead of physical or emotional comfort measures. This is named by expert nurses as an ethical breach of the notion of good that pharmacological agents should supplement but not replace ordinary comfort measures. The flow of the following small group dialogue that was cited in Benner, Tanner & Chesla (2009, p. 216) is fluid and animated as nurses complete each other's sentences. This demonstrates the engagement and shared ethic and practices among these expert nurses:

Nurse 1: I think that sometimes we sedate kids because the nurse doesn't want to be bothered with them. I think that's the bad side of that situation, that this kid's twitting out so I'm going to hit him with some morphine or some nembutal. Rather than changing his pants or...

Nurse 2: We see that a little more than we'd like.

Nurse 1: Or putting a cover over him, or putting him on his belly, or ...

Nurse 3: Or sometimes, they can just leave them alone. Sometimes their twitting out because you've been messing with them for 20 minutes.

Nurse 2: Or it's time for them to have a temper tantrum you know.

Nurse 1: Yeah, yeah and you can leave them alone.

Nurse 2: He's not desaturating, nothing's happening to him; he's just mad. You don't want him to extubate himself or pull out his lines but as long as he's safe let him have his temper tantrum. I think that's the down side of it, that people do forget to wean kids off of narcotics or barbiturates. Because they'll say hold sedation before they'll extubate and then they'll just stop. Then you're peeling the kid off the ceiling, you're going 'What's wrong with this kid?' 'Can't handle him.' 'Have you ever heard of withdrawal?' [laughter]

Nurse 3: It really bugs me. A lot of times too, people don't try comfort measures. I think they're a little too fast with the sedatives sometimes and they don't do basic things, like when people go to start IVs in these kids. They just throw them over on their backs, grab an extremity, start sticking, and the kids' screaming even if they're intubated. And there are things that you can do to prepare the baby and get it comfortable, get it sucking on something, bundle it up so it doesn't flail around when you first stick it. They tolerate it so much better. And it drives me crazy because people...they say well this kid's desaturating horribly and he needs a spaghetti line...[laughter]

Nurse 1: I wonder why?

Nurse 3: You didn't have to get this kid into this state, you know. If you had taken it a little more slowly, and done a little preparation, the kid would have tolerated it fine. That really bugs me. People aren't really conscious of comfort measures.

Nurse 1: Well it takes time. Before, you use that kind of tunnel vision where the task is what's paramount and not the kid. Where getting that IV in is really like the only thing in your mind.

Nurse 3: There are people that have worked up there as long as we have who do that when they start IVs.

Nurse 1: I'm sure that's probably true.

Nurse 3: And, it would never occur to them to bundle the child and give it a pacifier before they start. Never occur to them.

Interviewer: Why?

Nurse 3: I don't know. They don't think it's important. They just figure the kid's going to cry and there's nothing you can do and...get it over with. That's exactly it. 'Let's do this and get it over with.'

Nurse 1: Do it as fast as you can and get it over with.

Interviewer: How do you make that judgment around sedation vs. comfort measures?

Nurse 3: Well, some kids end up being sedated pretty much around the clock. If they're chronic kids who been stuck a lot and cry as soon as somebody in green approaches, you do sedate them pretty much around the clock. But, I always try other things first. Even if somebody tells me this kid has to have or really needs his sedation at such and so point, when he starts this behavior, you need to sedate him. I never believe that.

Nurse 1: You always try once.

Nurse 3: I never believe them. I know it makes the primary nurses so mad. You know it's like we know this kid and he needs this, this, and this. And, but when they're not there, and it's my kid, I try comfort measures first.

The tension between the technical interventions and the possibilities of non-technical comfort measures are apparent. These nurses refer to the beginner's tunnel vision, where trying to master the technical skills takes precedence over the more subtle ones and, in many respects, more difficult to learn response-based comforting measures. The dialogue can be seen as an ethical enterprise to maintain the human world of connection through comfort. To recover, the infant or child must be weaned from the sedation and pain medication, and the directive to "try comfort measures first," aims for the earliest possible transition to occur.

Response-based comfort measures are best learned in practice, while being attuned to the patient's physical needs but also to the emotional state. As pointed out by the nurses above, pain-inflicting procedures make a moral claim on expert nurses for even mundane, routine interventions. It takes time to convey respect and compassion that can calm and reduce the patient's tension so that the pain inflicted is not exacerbated by undue fear and particularly by an unknown person. Sandra Kennedy, a transport nurse, embodies the ethic of care and comfort that expert nurses so strongly embrace and advocate for. She is frequently serves as the "last ditch" person to start IVs after multiple clinicians cannot:

> **Nurse:** The needle stick with an IV or a blood draw is probably one of the most memorable bad experiences a pediatric patient has. I consider [IV starts] a great responsibility....In addition to the physical procedure of the stick, there is the emotional side. It can be a very traumatic time for the child. Children differ in their reactions depending on their developmental stage but all dread the procedure. I am responsible for helping the child through this period with as little stress and painful memory as possible. This takes the form of having a comfort object for the toddler to joking for distraction with the teen. Every child is different and is approached as a unique individual with his own needs and fears.
>
> An example was a child who had already been stuck at least four times since admission to the ER. When I entered the room, the thin, frail-looking 3 year old child was snuggled on her mother's lap. I introduced myself and spoke with Mom and the ER nurse, Jane, and they said the IV's all blow with and without a tourniquet...I pulled a chair up beside Mom's and examined Rachel's arms and legs. She snuggled in to Mom. If at all possible I like parents to remain at the bedside during painful procedures. Rachel was very thin and had many visible veins. I told Mom and Rachel what I was doing and proceeded to spare the tourniquet and stick a hand vein. I try to avoid foot veins in walking children to continue to allow their greatest mobility. Rachel cried but didn't fight the stick. I blew the vein. I was very disappointed. I could feel the resignation in the room. One more person had tried and failed. Rachel needed her lab work and IV access. There was another reasonable vein in her foot. I didn't want to remove Rachel from her mother because she was the only person in the room who wasn't doing something painful to her. I moved to Rachel's level so I sat on the floor and put her dangling foot on my knee to stabilize it for the stick. Again, she was accepting of the stick. Success! Rachel kept asking with worry if we were going to do it again. Over and over we reassured her it was "all done." After we drew labs and secured the IV with tape, Rachel realized there would be no more sticks. "Yeah" happily came from her lips. That exclamation of excitement broke the stress in the room.
>
> I know with each call will be a new challenge...a challenge that always causes pain and distress. The reward is being able to look into a child's eyes and truthfully say it's "all done."

The nurse's non-intrusive stance of sitting next to mom, of keeping Rachel next to mom, and of getting down on the floor reveal a way of connecting that is received as comfort. For Rachel, Sandra's comportment is more comforting than verbal interaction. In turn, Rachel's delight when it is "all done" rewards the expert nurse. Meeting the challenge on the toddler's terms counts as a job well-done.

The following bedside observation illustrates assessing a premature infant's capacity to be weaned from the ventilator:

> **Nurse:** She hated the tube [endotracheal tube]. She really wanted it out. In fact we were kind of joking about it at the beginning of the shift tonight, because she really hated it. We weaned her [from the ventilator] in record time. She got back at midnight, and was extubated at 4 a.m. She was doing really well, in terms of oxygenation, hemodynamics, temp. I knew she could do it (Observational Interview).

This candid interview at the bedside reveals the thinking-in-action and skillfulness required in helping infants make the transition from technology dependence to self-regulation. The nurse makes qualitative distinctions about the infants color and confers an intentionality to the infant's embodied responses by observing that the infant "really wanted it [endotracheal tube] out." The infant is granted moral stature by the nurse's careful observation and response to the infant's capacities. The infant's human capacities and struggle for life are given the stature of desire and choice. It is choice born of relationship and the one-sided ethical demand for the infant's growth and safety (Logstrup, 1995).

This same ethical demand can be seen in the care of adults, where the adult's human dignity and comfort set limits on the technology used:

> A few times he saw the patient take off his oxygen mask—usually in his sleep. The nurse would go into the room and tell the patient very matter-of-factly that he was putting his 'oxygen back on,' and that he should try to keep it on because it was good for his heart. The nurse said to me that if he were going by the book, he'd tape the mask to his face, or maybe restrain him. But, he explained, that didn't make any sense. It would just backfire—the patient would get angry and upset. After a few attempts to keep the mask on, the nurse mentions to the resident that he's going to try a nasal cannula, which delivers less oxygen per minute, but the patient will actually get more oxygen with the cannula because its more comfortable, and the patient will leave it on. He did this, explaining to the patient that it would be a lot more comfortable, and that 'we'll try this to see if you get enough oxygen this way.' The patient agreed. The nurse explained to me that the whole strategy, as far as the cardiac system goes, with this patient, is to reduce the demand or need for oxygen in the cardiac tissue. We know he can't deliver the oxygen very effectively to his heart muscle. We know we're doing everything we can—'he's maxed out medically.' We know from his numbers—his PA line and his blood pressures—that he's in a good range. If the patient is very anxious, or angry, or combative, the heart is stressed. This means reducing sources of conflict, such as the face mask, if possible. (Observational Note).

Here, the nurse favors a more comfortable alternative for supplemental oxygen delivery rather than using restraints to continue using the oxygen mask. The patient's physiological condition does not warrant more extreme measures so the nurse tries comfort first. There is much controversy about the problem of providing adequate pain medication, especially in babies. There have been past notorious incidents of babies undergoing cardiac surgery without pain medication, only neuromuscular blocking agents. A group of intensive care nursery nurses discuss this as a past controversy, but also in terms of discerning whether comfort measures are sufficient or whether pain medication or sedation are needed:

> **Nurse:** I don't think there's controversy that babies feel pain. There's just controversy about how to manage it, or whether it's more important to give them drugs first and ask questions later or whether it is worthwhile to try other things. Sometimes it is not worthwhile trying other things. I mean sometimes comfort measures really don't work and you find out very quickly that maybe they need sedation. I would say at least there are many other times you find out, no, the kid really didn't need pain medication right now.

Pharmacologically-induced paralysis is used in critical care settings so that the patients' own respiratory efforts do not interfere with or preclude ventilation. The use of paralytic drugs also prevent movements which can disrupt delicate surgical repairs. Drug-induced paralysis raises its own specter of ethical questions (Vitello, 1984). Nerve and respiratory paralysis calls for pain medication and sedation because the normal bodily signs of discomfort are absent and the nurse can no longer be guided by physical signs of discomfort. Also, the human experience of paralysis is terrifying. Because of the patient experience and safety issues with muscle paralysis, neuromuscular paralytic drugs are now used less frequently, primarily in cases where there is little or no choice. The following dialogue is a continuation of the earlier conversation about judging when to use pain medication and sedation and when to use comfort measures:

Nurse 2: Anyone who is paralyzed needs to have sedation.

Interviewer: Because?

Nurse 2: Because you can be paralyzed and wide awake. That will be very frightening.

Nurse 3: It's frightening, causes anxiety, and they cannot tell you if they're in pain. They've talked to adults that have been paralyzed and they say that they hallucinate. They can hear everything that's going on, but they come in and out of reality and they're never sure when. And, that they feel much better when they are just asleep. Because it was just too frustrating to be...

Nurse 2: And, they still have sensations. So it's skeletal muscle paralysis but you're not anesthetized so sometimes your arm is just tired from being like this but you can't lift it up and you're intubated. So, you can't tell the nurse 'Can you move my arm?' Even people that haven't had surgery so that they shouldn't have pain, need to be sedated. So that they are a little more asleep. But, also, if there's a reason, like some of our post-op heart patients have pulmonary hypertension. And because they've patched their VSD [Ventricular Septal Defect] or fixed their truncus or whatever, so if they're pulmonary pressures really go high, they don't want patients to get to the point where their pulmonary pressures are going to exceed their systemic. Their cardiac output is going to decompensate. Those kids need to be sedated. And, another thing is kids that have been sedated because we have a baby that's being very well sedated because he's had a lot of abdominal surgery. They don't want him to dehiss because he did that after his first surgery two months ago. So, he's getting a lot of sedation. Or kids that have tracheal reconstructions that are going to be intubated for a month, they don't want them to move because the ET tube can rupture the suture line. But those kids need to be weaned from their medications because if you stop them cold turkey because you're going to extubate them, or whatever, they really wig out. So, even those kids that don't need to be paralyzed because they are getting better, need to be weaned off the sedation.

Pharmacological paralysis is a drastic measure with physical and social dangers and is now used far more sparingly than it was 10 years ago when we wrote the first edition of this book. We leave the example above in, even though it now sounds out of date, because of the historical significance of developing clinical and ethical knowledge around the practice of neuromuscular blockades, and of course, their use varies in different regions and countries.

Neuromuscular blockades are now avoided whenever possible. One of the patient issues is that when patients with neuromuscular blocking agents get accidentally disconnected from a ventilator, they are not able to breathe on their own and their life depends a well-functioning ventilator alarm and on someone noticing and responding immediately to the disconnection or to the alarm. Nurses in this study gave "the danger of the loss of respiratory drive" and "the horror of being paralyzed" as the primary reasons for curbing the non-essential use of paralytic agents in critical care. In the dialogue above, the horror of paralysis without sedation provides a moral imperative to sedate. To be fully conscious and paralyzed captures a modern vision of torture, helplessness and the loss of the ability to communicate even the simplest needs and discomfort. Nurses worry about the practice of using paralytics and talk about the difference in the patterns of use:

> **Nurse:** There are places where every post-op heart patient is paralyzed when he comes out of the OR. Because Dr. A. didn't believe in that, our open heart patients do not get paralyzed unless there's absolutely no other way to control the pulmonaries [pulmonary artery pressures]. For those kids with really bad pulmonary hypertension, there is no other way. Or the kids that have ARDS [Acute Respiratory Distress Syndrome] that are on really high ventilator settings, we paralyze them. Or, some of the surgical kids, abdominal ones that gain like about five pounds and they started out at three and you know that they have these big incisions that they don't want to open up and then we'll paralyze them.

Technology assessment and control (see Chapter 8) are warranted because of the differing patterns of use of neuromuscular blockade observed in the multiple critical care units in the 11 hospitals of this study. The ethics to prevent harm, prevent suffering, and provide comfort are the only defense against the mindless increase in the use of paralytic agents. As the nurse above indicates, therapeutic paralysis is a life-saving and humane intervention in particular pathophysiological conditions. The struggle is to keep its use limited to essential instances. Besides the human terror of complete helplessness and the threatening possibility that the paralyzed patient might experience respiratory arrest should the ventilator be accidentally disconnected, neurological damage and the hazards of immobility are also concerns. Positioning the paralyzed patient requires gentleness since the patient can feel painful movements. Attentiveness is required to render paralysis less hazardous.

These qualitative distinctions require attuned situated clinical reasoning as evident in the following narrative by Beth Baldwin, a medical Nurse:

> **Nurse:** This woman came in with this new diagnosis of lung cancer, older woman, in her mid 60s. She was as really struggling with breathing. And I was doing what I could,to make her more comfortable. Sitting her up, we got her in a chair, she didn't like the chair. Different oxygen masks, didn't like constraints of the face masks. So we changed it to a shovel mask, so we tried a couple of different oxygen delivery systems, and she still was struggling. Her husband was at her bedside, and he was *so in tune* with how she was doing. And I immediately bonded with the both of them. And really, I kind of felt like if this was my family member…would I want to be seeing someone who was just so uncomfortable? And as the pain and palliative care service came in, we met before we went back into the room, we all went in together, they were interviewing her, trying to figure out what would work. And she basically understood

that her prognosis was very poor, and she really was ready to die. She said, she really wanted to die. And not as a, (hushed voice) suicide, but she was just at that point, where she was like, "I know that I'm sick. This is really hard for me, and I'm ready." So we put into place medications to help with her air hunger, you know, just trying to do some comfort measures for the two of them. So, I'm on a twelve hour shift, and it's around 6 o'clock at night, and the patient says she's feeling a little bit better, the medication seems to be helping, and the husband, who came in with her overnight, had been up for about 20 *hours,* was just *exhausted.* He was just done. We kind of all sat down, and he's like, "I think I want to go home and get some rest." I said, "I think you need to do that. Can you get home safely?" He said, "Yes, I can get home. I just want to go and take a nap." I said, "you go home," I said, "just give us a call when you get in to make sure everything's okay." Well, of course he leaves. And all of the medicines I seem to have been giving her, I walk into her room, and she's breathing... I counted a whole minute. She had two breaths. I said, "oh my goodness." I said, "This is going to happen soon." And I kind of stirred her and she woke right up. And I said, "you know, you're really not breathing as often as I'd like to see." I said, "you know, are you in pain?" She said, "no, no I feel comfortable." I left the room briefly to call the doctors, because, this was—this was close. And I learned that there was actually a scale that you use for patients who are—comfort care—whether or not you need to give them medication to reverse their narcotic use. And I specifically asked her, I said, "I think you've got a little extra medication in your system. Do you want me to give you something to reverse that medicine? I can do that. It will help you breathe more regularly. But, you might be in more pain," I said, "these are the things we have to weigh." "Absolutely not. I don't want the pain again." When I would wake her up, she would be okay. I could talk to her and she understood, but if I stopped any stimulation, she would just about stop breathing. And I said, "what can I do?" She said, "I want—I want my husband here." I said, "ohh." So I call the husband back, who's barely walking in the door—and I said, "things have changed since you left." I said, "she seems to have a little extra medicine on board, and she's not breathing as regularly, and I *have to* just stimulate her to keep her awake, and she wants you here." He said, "oh. I'm on my way. I'll be there in 30 minutes." And I spoke again with the pain and palliative service, and they said, "if you can stimulate her, and she can wake up, and say that she doesn't want this narcan medicine, to reverse, that fits into the realm of this protocol, that you don't have to give it to her." So I sat with her. The next shift came on and I said, "I'm not leaving! I CAN'T leave her in the middle of this right now. I'm going to sit with this patient and wait until her husband comes." So I sat there and I was holding her hand, and I'd let her kind of doze off, and when she'd get really slow breathing, I'd [wake her], and she'd go, "oh oh... is my husband here?" She kept asking if her husband was here. And I offered her whatever I could, and she said, "no, I just want my husband."

Interviewer: Offered her what?

Nurse: I offered her ice chips, I offered her, you know, "are you comfortable? What can I do to make you feel better right now?" And it was one of the first times I asked one of my patients this. I asked, "are you scared right now? And she looked at me and was like, "No. No. I'm okay." And we just held hands. There was a lot of eye contact. When she woke right up, she would smile. It was almost like, "I know, I'm just waiting." And I sat with her until her husband came in. trying to be really strong, "Honey,

I'm here. I'm here. What is it that we can do?" She just reached out her hand and took his. And it was at that moment when I was like, "okay, now I can go. [Voice is breaking slightly, trying not to cry.] Now I can, I felt like I could pass the torch." I knew she wanted to die. And if I hadn't come into the room at that moment, she probably *would have.* But as soon as she told me in that moment, (in a whisper) "I wish my husband was here."...

Interviewer: Did she die that night?

Nurse: She lived for 48 hours. And her husband was at her bedside when she did pass. It was as good as it could be. She was finally at peace, and he was there with her, which is what she really needed and what he needed too, I believe. It was pretty amazing, experience.

Interviewer: Were you scared?

Nurse: I was scared that her husband wouldn't make it in time. I was scared that she wouldn't be able to get that peace and comfort that she needed at that time....She wanted her husband there. So it was almost a responsibility to make sure that he was there.

Interviewer: So when she said to you, all I want to do is die, what did you say?

Nurse: I think I—I don't know if I really said anything. Or If I just sat with her and held her hand. I don't really know. I know I said to her, "I know this is hard." I think I was more focused on what I could do to make her more comfortable. And she, was ready to die and I respected that. I didn't feel like I needed to say, "you'll make it..." Just kind of, be okay with that. And it was, and she was okay with it. And we were doing the right thing. It definitely was. But, that's what we do. We try and, put our stuff aside, and say, "Alright. What is it that you need? And, how can I help you get there?" The team even came the next morning. I was taking care of her the next day and they came to me and they said that they knew that I had stayed after my shift. I felt a little confused especially learning this new protocol—that allows you to give narcan for someone who's gotten too much medicine. They said, "by you sitting there with her and stimulating her, you made the protocol work, because if you went in there and she couldn't respond, you would have had to give the medicine, the narcan." So they validated that my decision was best for the patient's comfort.

Interviewer: It's interesting because the protocol, for the protocol to work well it requires someone with really good judgment and presence.

Nurse: Absolutely. And had there not been presence...

Nurse 2: She would have had to have the narcan.

Nurse: Exactly! And you have to be there, "I'm waking you up." "Okay, but I don't want the medicine." And they go back to sleep for a minute. And, "Hey, you need another breath! Come on!" And watching the time, watching the clock tick. Seconds and seconds and seconds... feels like an eternity (murmurs of agreement.)

Nurse 2: It must have been nice though to get the acknowledgement from the team. That they respected....

Nurse: Yes. It really was.

This example provides a thick description (Geertz, 1970) of the meanings and qualitative distinctions encountered while trying to provide comfort. Multiple strategies were tried, and the nurse offered presence, and gentle stimulation in order to avoid giving complete reversal of the pain medication that would have catapulted the patient back into pain. The nurse recognizes the importance for the husband and wife to have the husband present at the bedside, and ensures that this happen. Presence and accompanying a person during a time of suffering is a profound comfort measure. The nurse has the courage to respond to what is at stake for the patient and her husband in the situation and takes definitive action. Human presence and solace augment the judicious use of pain medication, and make the decision not to reverse the pain medication with narcan, but rather sit with and coach the patient to breathe safe and ethical.

LIMITING THE IMPACT OF PAINFUL PROCEDURES AND THE USE OF RELAXATION, VISUALIZATION, DISTRACTION AND FUN

A pervasive understanding of nurses is that they bring comfort, nurturance, and foster independence and recovery. It is a practice that cannot be understood without understanding patient concerns and without making qualitative distinctions (Dreyfus, 1991a; Taylor, 1985a; Taylor, 1985b). To comfort others, one must be able to make qualitative distinctions between patient concerns and context, between connection and separation, and between coping and caring (Benner & Wrubel, 1989). Daily, nurses do procedures that inflict pain, such as giving injections, changing dressings, assisting the patient with coughing, deep breathing, and difficult mobility after surgery, retraining weak muscles, and many others. Inflicting pain conflicts with the nurse's self-understanding as one who provides comfort and nurturance. Nurses justify interventions that inflict pain by their greater good as life-sustaining measures that promote recovery. This justification is difficult for new nurses who have not had sufficient experience with the efficacy of treatments to be convinced or be convincing that the painful procedure is essential to recovery and in the patient's long term interest. For example, one new graduate nurse had to give large doses of antibiotics with noxious gastrointestinal side effects to a child with a bone marrow transplant. She found it difficult to carry off a convincing story of the importance of the medications because she had not yet seen a successful bone marrow transplant patient recover. However, seeing the child respond to various antibiotic therapies, and move from being withdrawn and listless gave her a first hand appreciation of the efficacy in the therapies (Benner, Tanner & Chesla, 2009). This first person witness to successful treatment is far more powerful in enabling one to cope with the pain infliction than scientific reports of efficacy.

Medical personnel, including nurses are at risk for focusing on what seems immediately therapeutic. However noxious procedures such as feeding a premature infant before they are ready to suck and swallow can have long term negative consequences. Nurse Mary-Anne Bennett describes learning from returning children and adults who were once in the neonatal intensive care.

Nurse: We wanted to address feeding because babies get what's called oral aversion because there are so many bad things, noxious things done around their mouth. We found that we are very good at feeding. We could feed a baby, even if baby wasn't sucking, we could get the food in, but the parents couldn't, so we show the parents: do this, do this, do this. Then we researched things, and found out that was really bad because the more you, not force food down the baby's throat, but encourage them in ways to swallow when they were not ready, that when they were 3 months old, that's when they could <u>refuse</u> to eat. That's around the time that it happens. Before that, feeding is reflexive...the suck and swallow, you put something in and they [swallow]. But at 3 months, they can refuse to eat. We were seeing that. We were seeing that babies come back who failed to thrived. I had one baby came back who was a year old and she was only 12 pounds. She JUST wouldn't eat. So, we formed a task group. We went to a lot of conferences and tried to find out what the newest information was. With these twin girls, we just come back from conference and they were at the point about to start eating. So I explained to mother what the issues were with feeding, because everybody wants to feed the baby, because we say, "as soon as they eat and maintain their temperature, they can go home." So that's the focus and parents get right into it, right away. In a bad way, sometimes. So, I explained to mother and father, this is what we are going to do to try to prevent problems down the road. It might take longer for the girls to EAT but it would be better for them in the long run. I told them how we were going to reach the goal of successful feeding.

Interviewer: How was that?

Nurse: What we were going to do was not give them a bottle, right off the bat, which is normally what we do. Then we can see if they can swallow without having an apnea spell. So I said, "we're not doing bottles at all. We're going to put the babies to breast, not for nutrition, but just to get them used to being at your breast, the smell of the milk. They may taste it. They do a lot of that mouthing so they lick, but they don't really suck and swallow. But, that's a very positive experience because they're skin to skin with the mother and they're getting a taste of milk and it's all good! There's nothing bad about that. Nobody is shoving something into their mouth and expecting them to swallow when they can't do it without distress. So I explained this to the Mother and she got on board right away, 'cause she understood and she knew I had the experience, also, to say, "I've seen this down the road. I don't want to....I want these girls to succeed in a different way." So, we set up plan, we wrote up a little care plan, and asked people to follow it. That was the problem...is that staff, and not only staff, but physicians didn't want to do it. Because their goal is to <u>get the baby out</u>. As long as baby living and eating, everybody's happy. They aren't seeing results of this. Months and years later, many kids don't eat at 7, 8, 9 years old. They have trouble swallowing because of that oral aversion. So we had to get the staff on board.

Interviewer: How did you do that?

Nurse 2: Both parents were on board and the mother came twice a day to hold the infants to her breast. One physician cared for these infants, and was able to <u>see</u> what we were saying. And the bottom line is, it makes it sound like the babies stayed in the hospital longer, but they actually went home before their due dates. We just didn't have them choking and having BAD experiences before they were mature enough to have a normal feeding. The problem was because people thought that they are big and growing nicely so people said they should be taking bottles. We'd be like, "well, every time you open the door to the isolette, the baby's color turns. They become mottled and their saturation level would go down. They can't even maintain themselves in an awake state, so why would you think that they could suck and swallow "she has no ability to.... she has no motor stability to be able to <u>barely</u> be <u>held</u> outside of her isolette. Why would you think that she could do the task of bottling?" When you said that to someone, to other staff members, then they mostly understood. They're like, "yeah, you're right." But it would be the junior staff that say (dogmatically), "she's 35 weeks! She <u>has</u> to take a bottle today, because that's a number we picked out of the hat. And they'd say (reluctantly), "oookaaay." They would try this approach.

Interviewer: So you are putting the baby to the breast, just letting it taste. Some would ask, so, at what point ?...

Nurse 2: Eventually baby starts nursing

Interviewer: So the baby, <u>on its own</u>, just takes to the...

Nurse 1: Because it's reflexive. They are going to do it. You just have to wait, and that's what nobody wants to do.

Nurse 2: There are some babies that are mature at 35 weeks and are able to do that. But these girls took 38 weeks. They were born 14 weeks early, so they weren't probably going to go home much before... they were SO sick. I don't think it really delayed their process of going home. It let us, because we were their advocates and their parents were their advocates, we were able to see the babies mature every week and even though they might not have been where you wanted to start at 35 weeks, they weren't ready. But, at 37and a half, they were ready and they ate, like within 5 days. It was a quick process once they... but if your forced it before that, it wasn't going to work.

Nurse 3: It was proactive because down the line, they won't have feeding problems.

Interviewer: This is new knowledge, uncovered in practice, from very observant nurses theorizing about "What could be better?". Have you noticed what happens with these babies 3 months down the road?

Nurse 1: Well these girls are almost close to 2 [years]. They are big chunky monkeys. They love food and eat everything. They walk, they have words, they're very social, you'd be hard pressed to guess that one of them was born dead with an Apgar of 0.

This is a good example of following the baby's maturational lead and avoiding bad feeding outcomes with careful, well timed introduction of oral feeding. More research needs to be done is this area. It is also a powerful illustration of how important comfort is to well-being. Traumatic painful experiences can have a lasting impact in children and adults.

The following observation of Extra Corporeal Membrane Oxygenation [ECMO] illustrates a nurse's attempt to bring some comfort to an infant in the midst of this procedure:

Nurse: What I do, more so in that situation, is tend to the baby emotionally.

Interviewer: Can you give me an example of tending to that particular baby emotionally? What were some of the things that you did?

Nurse: Oh, stroke her head and talk to her. And comfort her.

Interviewer: Comfort her? How?

Nurse: Oh, I just...

Interviewer: An outsider would never imagine, how do you comfort a baby on ECMO?

Nurse: Oh, you hold their hands because they're not paralyzed or heavily sedated. You give her something to hold on to. They're sedated but not paralyzed, so they can still move. They open their eyes, they grope around. So you touch, especially if they are awake and looking—and this baby was at some point alert, and I just I looked into her eyes and I talked to her and sing to her, and, I don't know, stroke her face or kiss her ears. You know, like a little thing. Things that people do with babies.

Interviewer: All the comforting practices (Observational Interview).

This extraordinary human attempt to rescue is a heroic procedure—keeping a human context in the midst of the intrusive technical intervention sustains the nurse as well as the infant. The comfort flows in both directions.

Pain is a major diagnostic indicator and nurses learn to judge levels of suffering not only by the patients' expression but also by the context of the pain, the patient's physiological responses, and the level of pain medication being given. Nurses who guide and coach patients through painful procedures run the risk of asking too much or too little from the patient. In the following clinical observation the nurse is coaching a newly admitted burn patient with third degree burns on his hands to stretch the hand tissue by flexing his fingers:

Nurse: (To patient) Can you do me a really big favor, and it'll help you out too? Try and make a fist. Now, before you do it,

Patient: It's going to hurt.

Nurse: Yeah. But before you do it, just let me tell you how to do it correctly.

Patient: Okay (his eyes are closed because of heavy sedation to mitigate his pain).

Nurse: Lot of people... I want you to open your eyes, Jim. A lot of people do this (demonstrating flexing her fingers in toward her palm quickly and frequently but incompletely making a fist). Okay? Now, that will actually be harder for you. Just very slowly squeeze your hand. And when you feel like you can't squeeze it any more, stop for a minute and take a break. Don't open your hand, and then try and squeeze it down a little further. Okay, keep going. You have to stay awake for this, though.

Patient: All right (opening his eyes).

Nurse: Yeah, it's kind of a drag I know, but you have to Jim, so let me see you make a fist on this hand. Bring it down, now, you want to put all your fingers all the way down to your palm, okay?

Patient: It feels like it's going to split.

Nurse: Yeah, I know it feels that way, but it won't.

Patient: Mm.

Nurse: Just keep going, I promise.

Patient: As long as you promise.

Nurse: I promise (Observational Interview).

Courage is required by the patient and the nurse. The nurse coaches and guides while acknowledging the pain. In this situation, the patient received pain medication that made him sleepy and he was also naturally afraid of hurting his hand. Such a situation is fraught with difficulty. Astute judgment and skillfulness are required. The patient relies on the nurse's past experience with other patients and trusts the nurse's reassurance that his skin will not split. The nurse's confidence encourages the patient to try the painful stretching of his fingers.

Nurses come to associate certain levels of pain with certain procedures and conditions, and these expectations govern their coaching and eventually the permissibility of pain expression (Strauss, Fagerhaugh, Suczek & Wiener, 1982). While the experience of pain is private and individual, suffering is public and can be judged by context and patient expression and movement (Rubin,2009). It is an unfortunate fallout of coping with inflicting pain that nurses judge patients' ability to withstand suffering. Judging the "reality" of pain is also an outcome of parsing the world in subjective and objective terms. Pain, that is considered "subjective" or due to fear or "being weak" (in these judgmental terms), can be dismissed because it does not point to important "objective" injury or disease. While it is essential to judge the severity of pain for diagnostic purposes, the ethic embedded in preventing suffering and providing comfort requires attention to all pain expression. The skill of providing comfort measures often augments effect.

The skill of involvement aligned with expertise in assessing suffering allows the nurse to acknowledge and ameliorate pain to the extent possible while being supportive and comforting when it cannot be relieved or removed. The unavoidable infliction of pain must be done without the kind of distancing or coping that ignores the pain, so that whatever comfort measures can be used are. Denial of pain causes the denial of comfort. Too much sympathy or too much distance are equally problematic. Persons in pain needs an "other" who can help them get through painful procedures by coaching them and bearing respectful witness to their plight.

Sometimes holding the patient's attention through distracting talk that takes them out of the immediate threatening situation helps the patient get through a difficult and painful procedure when artfully and judiciously done. When it works well, it works because there is a strong connection between the nurse and patient. In the following interview, a nurse recounts such a situation with a patient who had been in an automobile accident and was at risk for stray metal particles from the accident:

Nurse: It could have gone into her chest or to her stomach. I mean the physics of it, I mean [the metal] could have gone anywhere. So then the next step is to take her to interventional radiology to see what vasculature damage was done. And that's where I got a lot of satisfaction out of it, because I had to stay up there with her and monitor her, and I was pretty generous with the morphine because she's had a big hole in her leg and I think that was pretty reasonable. And I was there with the pulse ox and everything, so I gave her a lot of morphine. So we had to sit around and wait for a long time while they're shooting dye, taking all these pictures. And so I decided just to chat her up. I'm like so, 'What do you do? What's your husband do? How many kids do you have?' And we just talked and talked and talked and she said, 'You know, I've got five kids,' and her husband was the co-founder of this very, very famous restaurant in San Francisco that just recently closed and they own five other restaurants, and she's talking about the restaurant business and her kids and cooking. We just—and chat,

chat, chat for two hours, I just totally chatted her up. And she was a very nice lady, and very interesting to talk to. And so she said, 'Where did you go to nursing school?' And like I said, we just chatted it up, and...

Interviewer: Did you have in mind some aim or particular...?

Nurse: I wanted to keep her distracted because they had to put a femoral line in her and give her dye, and the dye makes you uncomfortable. You get a hot flash and sometimes your bladder burns—it's uncomfortable. And I figured my goal was to keep her distracted from everything else that was going on and at this point...she was afraid she was going to lose her leg. I mean at one point when she was in there, she said, 'Don't take my leg off, please. And so I kept her appraised of what's going on. I said, 'You know, the vascular films look good,' and 'It's a bad cut, but, you know...' I kept her appraised of what was going on with her injury, but at the same time I wanted to keep her distracted so they could do what they needed to do. So that's what I did and it was really great! I got a card later...days like that are what make it worthwhile to be a nurse, and... She had a congenital anomaly in her leg so it missed all the main arteries... And she basically, she gave herself a fasciectomy. Because they just took her to the OR and just debrided the wound a little bit, and that's all they really did. And then I think a week later they did a skin graft. And I went up and saw her about a week later. I went up to the floor and saw her because like I say, she was such a nice lady..., every time I see her. She comes by the ER sometimes, or she'll send me a note and just say 'Again I want you to know how much I appreciated that.'

The nurse is aware that she is "chatting the patient up," using social connection and distracting talk to distract the patient during the frightening time of waiting and the discomforts of the diagnostic procedures. This distraction augments the effects of the liberal pain medication. Once again, the comfort flows in both directions. The nurse finds great satisfaction in being able to distract the patient and be with her during the ordeal. Both patient and nurse remember the connection. Much focus is placed on therapeutic communication in nursing school; however, the nurse is left to learn about informal, ordinary social talk as a way to stem the tide of fear and keep the person connected to their world during periods of high threat.

Pain management and the infliction of pain are made more difficult in a societal context that has strong sanctions against drug dependency. Patients who require frequent and large amounts of pain medication over time are sometimes suspected of liking the drug too much. Clinicians are not alone in this concern. Patients who have a past history of drug addiction share similar concerns. For instance, a burn patient who was a former crank (cocaine related drug) user repeatedly denied pain or the need for medication. The nurse's concerns grew and as she probed his history, the patient voiced his fear about becoming addicted again. This conflict has spawned unenlightened practices and discourses of control rather than care around pain management.

Increasingly we find that nurses are incorporating complementary therapies into their approaches to comforting patients. Nurses often use guided imagery or visualization exercises to help patients relax. Usually they draw on any relaxation or meditation practices the patient has used in the past. The following example demonstrates how Priscilla Stoddard, an expert nurse anesthetist, draws on clinical imagination to blend many comforting measures such as comfort through connection, the use of rituals and familiar objects and new discoveries for distraction. The example illustrates how these practices are integrated into the therapeutic and safety aspects of her work:

CRNA: Kaylee is holding her "dolly" who is to accompany her back for her nap and she's sitting in her mother's lap, head against her chest, eyeing me with a healthy degree of suspicion. I proceed by saying, " I will be there to meet you when you enter the room but I will have my mask up. (I lift my mask into place so she can visualize my appearance). Though I have my mask up, you'll probably know me by my voice. I'll be telling you a story about rainbows as you go off to sleep. Did you know that there are about 100 rainbows on the ceiling in this room?" Kaylee scans the ceiling for rainbows, seeing none of course. I continue, "as I am telling you a story, you'll be breathing through what looks like an airplane pilot's mask. Nothing I'm going to do is going to bother you and I will be with you the whole time. The mask may smell a little funny, like when you go to the gas station with your Mom or Dad. You know how that can have a strong smell. You and Dolly are the only ones in the room who will see the rainbows. Would you like that?" Now her interest is piqued and she sits up and nods her head affirmatively.

The rainbow glasses are an idea that I acquired somewhere around 1996 when my son did a science fair project on rainbows. I saw these in a science catalog and we used them for his science project display. It occurred to me when I saw rainbow glasses in a science catalogues that they had great possibilities for helping to ease the transition of children who are typically anxious and sometimes crying into relaxing while they undergo anesthesia. If a child is really traumatized by being in the hospital, it doesn't always work but for most children, it is a fanciful diversion. I've affixed them to a regular glasses frame, after removing the lenses, so they can be worn like glasses. The key is to use them in tandem with a hypnotic effect, which I employ through the telling of a story. In my first year of practice as a nurse anesthetist, I worked along side an anesthetist who believed in the value of hypnosis and swore that he once helped a woman through a C-section with only hypnosis as her anesthesia. Though I'm not so extreme, I have certainly seen the benefits of calming patients by having them key into my voice, having that single focus, while I simultaneously administer the anesthesia. I have instructed the staff in the room that I want to have the child key into my voice and only my voice as they go off to sleep.….

I apply the mask, first to dolly and then Kaylee, a combination of nitrous oxide and oxygen. (Nitrous Oxide facilitates the rapidity of induction. Once she's through the reactive period, prior to intubating, I switch to 100% oxygen. The functional residual capacity of children is much smaller than adults leaving less time before severe oxygen desaturation if the airway deteriorates. 100% oxygen allows the anesthetist more time.) She breathes in holding Dolly, both swaddled in warm blankets. "Now, here come the rainbows" and the circulating nurse places the rainbow glasses over her eyes. I say: "Do you see the rainbows? Kaylee nods affirmatively as she scans the ceiling. I continue, "There are about a hundred rainbows. It's going to start smelling kind of strong. If you don't like the smell, just blow it away. Breathe in and blow it away. Nothing's going to bother you. You're just watching the rainbows and they're getting more colorful as you breathe."

As I raise the electric bed up to my height, I continue in a calm but even voice "Kaylee, you're going to feel like you're rising up to the rainbows, like in a hot air balloon. You're feeling very sleepy. Imagine that you and Dolly and Mom have packed a picnic lunch and you're floating above [hometown] looking at all the colors. As you breathe deeper, you'll notice the colors getting brighter, orange, blue, red. They're all getting brighter...... Now, you're getting so sleepy, you can't even keep your eyes open. You're going to take a great nap now." I continue a bit longer until it's apparent she's no longer hearing me. Her airway remains good and she has reached stage II of anesthesia, as her eyes are deviated and her breathing irregular. (I'm watching her chest for retractions and listening for upper airway occlusion as her tongue relaxes and falls back. At the slightest indication, I slip in an oral airway to displace the tongue forward and keep the airway patent) Her heart rate is still high around 150 and her vital signs are normal as I tape her right eye shut in preparation for intubating. (The tube and circuit come in from the right side and it's possible to give the patient a corneal abrasion when distracted intubating, not noticing what hits the right eye so I tape it shut.) I want to observe the left eye as another indicator of anesthetic depth so I tape it after intubation.

Protection, nurturing, connection and visualization are blended in the spirit of play and adventure, as Kaylee is prepared in advance for what she will experience in the O.R. The rainbow glasses do not work for everyone, but when they do, they provide a focusing point. The nurse's voice gathers up and guides Kaylee's attention so that she falls to sleep peacefully, which contributes to her calm post-operative emergence from anesthesia. This kind of comfort stands in stark contrast to the thrashing, crying, and fear that is too often observed. Comforting another human requires attunement, connection and imagination. In addition to the delight and comfort that Priscilla's novel invention as an intervention provides, as importantly, it enables much better physiological and pharmacological management of children during induction. Nurses have taught us how many comfort measures, like the rainbow glasses are born from clinical imagination and often present themselves when caring for a patient in distress. Whenever possible, fun can emerge as a form of distraction and way of coping with discomfort. Nurse Pat Ferencz reveals how ordinary, everyday interests like sports can open up one's imagination about how to make a demoralizing intervention a bit more fun and approachable:

Nurse: I admitted a 14-year-old boy, Jared, with a diagnosis of abdominal pain, r/o appendicitis. As I did his admission assessment, I wanted to make him comfortable. So, I told him I had two very important questions for him: One, was he a Red Sox or Yankees fan? And two, was he a Patriots fan? Jared laughed and said, "Red Sox, of course, and Patriots, but I like the Steelers, too." Finishing my assessment...I didn't feel he had appendicitis. Although his belly was softly distended and he had some pain with palpation, it was not centrally located or focused in the right lower quadrant. Jared had no difficulty climbing off the exam table or walking—two things that are usually difficult for a child with a true appendicitis. I felt he either had early gastroenteritis or constipation.

When the surgeon called back, he stated he wanted a barium enema done for Jared's CT and not PO contrast. "Great!" I thought. "Just what a 14 year old will want to hear." Most 14-year-olds, especially boys, get embarrassed when you ask about bodily functions or need to examine them, although they do like to joke about bodily functions. I went into Jared's room and explained the barium enema and CT, letting them know this would be able to give the surgeon a good picture of what was going on in Jared's abdomen and whether or not he would need to go to surgery. The look on Jared's face showed me he was mortified. He said, "That part of my body is for exit only." But he agreed to "do the test and get it over with.".... Jared said he wanted his dad to go with him but told his mom to wait upstairs. When Jared returned from CT, I asked how things went and he said, "Not bad. It was okay." But he wouldn't want to do it again. I explained to Jared that once his body was ready to get rid of the barium from the enema, it might be difficult to push out, as it is like clay. I also explained that he might have gas pains from the test as well, and the best way to make the pain go away is to "fart." Shortly afterwards, the surgeon called back and told me the CT was negative for appendicitis but that it showed Jared was constipated and ordered a Fleet enema. "Great," I thought to myself. Just what Jared is going to want to hear.

I went down to Jared's room and explained I had good news and bad news. The good news was his appendix was fine, but he was constipated, which was causing his abdominal pain. Jared and his parents both stated they were glad he wouldn't need surgery. I explained to Jared that to help him get rid of the "poop" inside of him, we would need to do an enema. "Not again," he said. I told him it wouldn't be the same as [the barium]. Jared responded with, "I think I need to go now." As he didn't need the enema right away, I told him he could go ahead and try to go on his own, but that I would need to see what he had done when he was finished. Again I got the look of "You've got to be kidding." I joked with Jared that there's nothing more a nurse likes than to see poop. I told him I would get him a "hat" for the stool to go in. "Not a baseball hat," I joked. It's a plastic container we call a hat. I went to the supply room and got a hat and a piece of tape on which I wrote "Yankees" and taped it to the front of the hat, as Jared does not like that team. When I brought it into the room, Jared and his parents all laughed. I told him he would get to "poop on the Yankees." ....He wasn't ready to do the enema, so I explained that we could wait and see [if he could go without the enema], it wasn't an emergency and he was spending the night in the hospital anyway.

After experiencing more abdominal pain, Jared did agree to have the enema, later exclaiming, "That was it?" Jared's pain resolved after the enema and its subsequent effects. What was memorable was Jared's and his parents' appreciation for getting him through an "uncomfortable, embarrassing experience", both physically and emotionally.

Despite his embarrassment, the nurse's skillfulness in creating fun and distraction in Jared's world of interests allows Jared to become comfortable with her, to the point that he prefers that she give him the enema over a male nurse. The nurse's connection with Jared enables him to accept what will be needed to relieve his pain and, in turn, guides her to patiently follow his timing. The use of humor and distraction require relational attunement and timing. The nurse and patient need to have sufficient common understandings for humor to work. This is why it is so difficult for humor to communicate and work across cultures. So the nurse must tread lightly in using humor, making sure that the situation is right for the patient, and that the humor is good natured and shared.

COMFORTING THROUGH FAMILIAR RITUALS AND ROUTINES

Routines and rituals are used to establish a sense of predictability, coherence, continuity, and comfort. Establishing the normal rhythms of day and night is a challenge in a brightly-lit, noisy critical care area. Therefore, establishing routines and rituals is an act of culture creation in an alien environment, as a pediatric critical care nurse points out:

> **Interviewer:** Are there any little tricks to the trade with that?
>
> **Nurse:** As far as getting them to sleep?
>
> **Interviewer:** And, weaning them?
>
> **Nurse:** Giving them a routine so that they know—that is more of a pediatric comfort measure. Like at home with kids, you give them dinner, a bath, you read them stories, or they watch television for an hour and they go to bed at 8:30. So, we create a schedule that's this way, so that they don't sleep all day. They get up in the morning and they have breakfast and they have their play therapy or whatever they do and they have lunch, they watch TV for an hour, they take a nap for two hours, then they get up and do whatever is appropriate for that kid. We designate sleep periods like in the afternoon. Because sometimes these guys will sleep all day and be up all night. Then if they're having trouble, like if they're still up at 1:00 in the morning...then the mother comes to visit the baby in the morning and he's sleeping all day long. If that happens we'll put him on chloral hydrate to see if we can get him more on a day/night schedule. Then we do not give him sedation except for maintenance during the day.

Cycles of rest and recreation are created in a crowded schedule of vital signs and therapies providing small islands of normal non-painful events and predictability. The above discussion led to further discussion about weaning patients from sedatives, in ways that did not create withdrawal problems and that fostered a more normal day and night cycle:

> **Nurse 1:** Back into day/night and getting them off of mega doses of barbiturates and some of our Neurosurgical patients are in barb coma and they need to be weaned. I've heard that barb withdrawal is very unpleasant and that you need to be a little bit nice about taking them off the drugs.
>
> **Interviewer:** Do you do similar things in ICN?
>
> **Nurse 2:** We don't have so much routine. I think the kids just end up getting their times stretched out. Some kids need a routine.
>
> **Nurse 3:** Well, the round the clock kids, the ones with the primaries get very hyper about it usually. They're either kids who are maybe failure-to-thrives where they just really don't want them to cry and be agitated for long periods because they're already not gaining weight. Or, sometimes really twitty preemies who tend to go into bronchospasm if you don't give them their sedation fairly regularly. They agitate themselves into ending up on higher ventilatory settings at being hand-ventilated, and all this. And, they make themselves sicker, literally.
>
> **Nurse 1:** We also use very small doses.
>
> **Nurse 2:** We're on the low side of therapeutic.

Cycles of comfort and rest are recognized as crucial to the "failure to thrive" infants, but they are probably no less important to any ill infant, child, or adult. These normal restorative measures are increasingly being researched (Bruyna, 1981; Daiss et al., 1986). However, the experiential and scientific wisdom about the importance of sleep and rest is seldom sufficient to overcome the press for and imbalance in the technical care that many units are designed to deliver.

Adults too need cycles of rest and comfort, and the maintenance of their circadian rhythms of day and night, as was discussed earlier. Adults who have rituals and spiritual practices can experience these as a familiar anchor. This expert nurse enriches our clinical and moral imagination to see how one may follow a specific patient's lead to provide spiritual comfort in the midst of everyday physical care:

Nurse: We had a patient who was having unstable angina. He had multiple MIs [myocardial infarctions] and a poor ejection fraction, and he came in with chest pain and unstable angina. He was totally mentally alert and coherent for two days. And he was being tended to by a loving family, very giving. On Sunday night he had deteriorated and required a lot of lasix for flash pulmonary edema. He got an arterial line; he is on nitro[glycerin], and doing fair. I came in on Monday morning and there was a new nurse who was on and I was asked to back her up. So I went in with her after I had done the assessment of my patient, I'd gone in with her and was helping her get organized for the day. And she was busy calculating her drips and looking at her arterial line and pressure tubing and everything. And I attended to the patient. And I brushed his teeth and his dentures, and washed his glasses and he asked me for some toast and tea, and I went and got that. And by the time I came back he said, 'Before I have this, will you get my shaving kit?' And I got his shaving kit, and he had a prayer in there that he said every day, and he said, 'I want to say my prayer.' I knew the prayer and I said it with him. And he thanked me and said: 'I have been saying this prayer every day for a long time and I've been saying it even more frequently now that I know that I'm very sick.' And he was sharing that he was not really afraid of death and he felt strong even though he was very sick. Well, I was off for a couple days and by the time—or, excuse me, that day he went into flash pulmonary edema and required intubation and so he was not doing very well. He was very agitated with his endotracheal tube and required fentanyl and he wasn't pavulonized [paralyzed], but he did require a lot of fentanyl and ativan. Two days later I came on. The same nurse was taking care of him and I was asked again to back her up. And he was still intubated but by this time he was made a DNR. I guess his family and he had extensive talks [about death] prior to this admission, but didn't really realize how imminent it was. And so he was a DNR and that day I helped the other nurse in the morning. And she was doing all her drips and everything. And I pulled out his shaving kit and I got his prayer and I said his prayer to him. And he was lucid enough to know that I was saying it. He held my hand and he obviously couldn't say it with me because he was still intubated, but he held my hand and nodded his head when I was finished. And that day he died. And it was just very moving to know that on his last day I prayed with him.

Birth, illness, injury, loss, recovery, suffering, and dying are human events whose meanings and practices exceed technical reductions of medical disorders to be fixed or cured. Even if comfort measures such as rituals, religious practices, and routines did not have a scientific medical legitimacy of providing a sense of well-being and calming the stress response (and they do have this scientific rationale based upon empirical research) (Benner & Wrubel, 1989), they would still have human legitimacy related to human goods—a life worth living and the very acts of creating culture, human connections, and traditions.

SUMMARY

In nursing and medicine we live out the tensions of objectifying the body, treating it as a collection of physical structures and mechanical functions so that we can overcome the aversion and human taboos of inflicting pain, doing surgery, and distancing blame and shame from the vulnerabilities associated with embodiment. (Benner, Janson-Bjerklie, Ferkelich & Becker, 1994e; Young, 1997) The scientific objectification of the body is necessary for the therapies of medicine, but therapies are absolutely dependent on larger human goods such as decreasing suffering, preserving human concerns, prolonging quality life, and recovery. Objectification and distancing are useful for coping with the terror of inflicting pain and facing the risk of death, but they are only useful for circumscribed periods and always run the risk of usurping human concerns. Comfort measures can appear ordinary and relatively ineffective when compared to repairing heart defects surgically, yet these very heroic procedures are dependent on comfort measures and cannot be sustained without them (Benner & Wrubel, 1989). The challenge is to create organizational and unit cultures that can accommodate both the science and human goods associated with confronting the human realities of risk, suffering, loss, and death and offering whatever comfort measures can be offered.

REFERENCES

Affonso, D., Bosque, E., Wahlberg, V., & Brady, J. P. (1993). Reconciliation and healing for mothers through skin-to-skin contact provided in an American tertiary level intensive care nursery. *Neonatal Network, 12*(3), 25–32.

Bell, R. P., & McGrath, J. M. (1996). Implementing a research-based kangaroo care program in the NICU. *Nursing Clinics of North America, 31*(2), 387–403.

Benner, P., Janson-Bjerklie, S., Ferkelich, S., & Becker, G. (1994). Moral dimensions of living with a chronic illness, autonomy, responsibility and the limits of control. In P. Benner (Ed.), *Interpretive phenomenology, Embodiment, caring and ethics* (pp. 225–254). Thousand Paks, CA: Sage.

Benner, P., Tanner, C. A., & Chesla, C. A. (2009). *Expertise in nursing practice: Caring, clinical judgment, and ethics.* New York, NY: Springer Publishing Company.

Benner, P., & Wrubel, J. (1989). *The primacy of caring: Stress and coping in health and illness.* Menlo Park, CA: Addison-Wesley.

Bosque, E. M., Brady, J. P., Affonso, D. D., & Wahlberg, V.(1995). Physiological measures of kangaroo versus incubator care in a tertiary-level nursery. *Journal of Obstetric, Gynecologic, and Neonatal Nursing, 24*(3), 219–226.

Bruyna, M. A. (1981). Planned periods of rest in the intensive care unit: Nursing care activities and intracranial pressure. *Journal of Neurosurgical Nursing, 13*, 184–194.

Chesla, C. A. (1996). Reconciling technologic and family care in critical-care nursing. *Image: Journal of Nursing Scholarship, 28*(3), 199–203.

Daiss, S. R., Bertelson, A. D., & Benjamin, L. T. J. (1986). Napping versus resting: Effects on performance and mood. *Psychophysiology, 23*, 82–88.

Dreyfus, H. L. (1991). *Being-in-the-world: A commentary on Heidegger's Being and Time, division I.* Cambridge, MA: MIT Press.

Foucault, M. (1973). *The birth of the clinic: An archeology of medical perception*. New York, NY: Vintage.

Goffman, E. (1961). *Asylums*. Garden City, NY: Anchor.

Habermas, J. (1984/1987). Lifeworld and system: A critique of functionalist reason. *The theory of communicative action* (Vol. II). Boston, MA: Beacon.

Henneman, E. (1986). Brain resuscitation. *Heart & Lung, 15*(1), 3–11.

Holden, T. (1992). Dialogues with excellence: Seeing Joan through. *American Journal of Nursing, 92*, 26–30.

Ihde, D. (1990). *Technology and the lifeworld: From garden to earth*. Bloomington, IN: Indiana University Press.

Koenig, B. (1988). The technological imperative in medical practice: The social creation of "routine" treatement. In M. Lock & D. Gordon (Eds.), *Biomedicine Examined* (pp. 465–496). Dordrecht, The Netherlands: Kluwer.

Logstrup, K. (1995). *Metaphysics*. (Vol. 1). Milwaukee, WI: Marquette Uinversity.

Logstrup, K. E. (1971). *The ethical demand* (T. I. Jensen, Trans.). Philadelphia, PA: Fortress Press.

Madjar, I. (1991). *Pain as embodied experience: A phenomenological study of clinically inflicted pain in adult patients*. Palmerston North, New Zealand: Massey University Press.

Mitchell, P. (1986). Intracranial hypertension: Influence of nursing care activities. *Nursing Clinics of North America, 21*, 563–576.

Rubin, J. (2009). Impediments to the development of clinical knowledge and ethical judgment in critical care nursing. In P. Benner, C. A. Tanner, & C. A. Chesla (Eds.), *Expertise in nursing practice: Caring, clinical judgment, and ethics* (pp. 171–198). New York, NY: Springer Publishing Company.

Stannard, D. (1997). *Reclaiming the house: An interpretive study of nurse-family interactions and activities in critical care*. (Unpublished doctoral dissertation, University of California, San Francisco, San Francisco, CA.)

Strauss, A., Fagerhaugh, S., Suczek, B., & Wiener, C. (1982). Sentimental work in the technologized hospital. *Sociology of Health and Illness, 4*(3), 254–278.

Stretkowicz, V. (1996). *Florence Nightingale's notes on nursing*. (Revised ed.). Philadelphia, PA: Curtis Center.

Taylor, C. (1985a). *Human agency and language: Philosophical papers 1*. (Vol. I). Cambridge, England: Cambridge University Press.

Taylor, C. (1985b). *Philosophy and the human sciences: Philosophical papers II*. (Vol. II). Cambridge, England: Cambridge University Press.

Taylor, C. (1989). *Sources of the self*. Cambridge, MA: Harvard University Press.

Taylor, C. (1991). *The ethics of authenticity*. Cambridge, MA: Harvard University Press.

Thollaug, S. (1991). *Domesticating the environment of critical care units*. Paper presented at the American Nurses' Association.

Vitello, J. (1984). Recalled perceptions of patients administered pancuronium bromide. *Focus on Critical Care, 11*(1), 28–35.

Young, K. (1997). *Presence in the flesh: The body in medicine*. Cambridge, MA: Harvard University Press.

7

Caring for Patients' Families

*F*or human beings, who are social beings prior to being individualized within a culture or family, the family is the basic unit of care. The family creates and constitutes the social context within which most illness occurs and is resolved (Litman, 1974). Human responses to illness are shaped by the family to a greater or lesser extent. We are defining family as any significant other who participates in the care and well-being of the patient. Caring for patients' families recognizes patient's particular familial social context, as well as the reciprocal relationship that exists between patients and their families. It is difficult, if not impossible, to map patient/family onto a strictly Cartesian model of medicine. Thus, nurses use multiple frames of reference, medical, social, care concerns and the mutual interactional and constitutive roles between patient and family. A PACU nurse spoke of that when she said:

> **Nurse:** You have to care about the patient, but you also have to care about the members of the family, too. Because, essentially, they are an extension of the patient. They also need the information, the reassurance, and the guidance.

Acute and critical care nurses with expert family care skills care for the family as an extension of the patient (Stannard, 1997). However, providing this level of patient and family attentiveness can be challenging, especially given the high demands of healthcare today. Acute and critical care areas are highly medicalized, and clinicians focus their immediate attention on patients' life-threatening and/or altered pathophysiological states and on stabilizing interventions. Feelings of anxiety and sorrow for the patient are initially put aside so that the nurse can focus on the immediate interventions at hand. Even family members want the focus of attention to be on the critically ill or injured family member. Caring for distressed family members, by convention, has not been the traditional style of coping with time sensitive and high demand interventions. Although patients may express the grief and terror associated with catastrophic illness or injury, they are often sedated, emotionally dampened, or even unconscious. Death anxiety, fear, and sorrow are palpably present and located in all their immediacy in the family. Thus, caring for the family invites acknowledgment of the patient and family's plight and, at the same time, creates emotional labor for nurses and other healthcare providers. For all of these reasons, it takes astute clinical judgment, wisdom, skill, and coming to terms with the human significance of illness and injury to care for family members of the acute and critically ill.

The purpose of this chapter is to describe nurses' care of acute and critically ill patients' families, highlighting the clinical judgment and skill required for this important

TABLE 7.1
Caring for Patients' Families

▓ Ensuring that the family can be with the patient
▓ Providing the family with information and support
▓ Encouraging family involvement in caregiving activities

relational work. Although family interventions and activities are bounded by the particulars in any given situation, nurses with expert family care skills care for patients' families in three primary ways, as shown in Table 7.1.

The nature and intent of family care can vary based on the situation and the nurse's and family's stance. Stance toward the family can be defined as the habits, practices, concerns, and skills the nurse brings to the situation (Stannard, 1997). Situational conditions, such as the patient-family care environment and the patient's clinical status, make some family-oriented interventions and activities possible while prohibiting others. The environment in a busy ED on a Friday night, for instance, will not allow for the comparable level of attentiveness and quality of family care that can be provided in that same ED on a quiet afternoon.

Other situational conditions that have been identified as important factors in nurses' ability to provide family care include the unit culture and the patient and family's length of stay (Benner, Tanner & Chesla, 2009; Chesla & Stannard, 1997; Darbyshire, 1994; Moore et al., 2003; Stannard, 1997). The tempo, mood, climate, and culture of any nursing unit make certain kinds of caring practices possible while discouraging others. These factors, as well as the patient population and unit staff, influence how nurses interact with patients and their families. A "family-friendly" unit culture, for example, is a unit culture with a socially embedded ethic of family care. This kind of unit culture has been shown to greatly influence nurses' openness to sharing and learning from one another in developing and extending their family care practices (Stannard, 1997). However, the opposite is also true. Less than optimal family care or breakdown between nurses and families has been shown to occur frequently in ICUs with a "family-restraint" culture (Chesla & Stannard, 1997). Family care can also take on a different character based on how clinicians and family members understand the patient situation. Family-oriented activities and interventions often become even more prominent when the focus shifts from providing heroic, life-saving or life-sustaining measures to ensuring that the patient has a comfortable, dignified death. For example, Tracy Davis, a pediatric ICU nurse, describes a drowning tragedy involving a toddler who had gotten out of the truck and wandered off while his family was unloading their boat. The critically ill toddler was doing poorly after a prolonged resuscitation:

Nurse: Gabriel was a 2-year-old, blonde-haired, blue-eyed boy…whose pH on arrival to [our unit] was 6.91, his temp was 84 degrees, and his pupils were fixed and dilated. He was already showing signs of cardiovascular instability and we were barely maintaining his blood pressure with [pressors]…When I met his parents, their devastation was apparent. At a time like that, it is a challenge to find any words of comfort that do not sound hollow and meaningless, but I had to try. I introduced myself and told them how beautiful I thought their son was. I then gently told them about Gabriel's condition. I knew they would not be able to fully process a lot of technical terms, so I tried to be as direct as possible. This is so hard when all of the things you are saying are the most awful words any parent can hear…Gabriel's condition continued to worsen throughout the day. We had to get him warmed to a normal temperature so that we could do some neurological testing. I noticed that his dad was especially quiet and had isolated himself from other family members…I walked over to him and sat down next to him. As I told him how very sorry I was about Gabriel, he began to cry. He then explained how it was his job to make sure the kids were in their lifejackets before they got out of the truck. He had forgotten to do this on this trip. His guilt was beyond measurement. A few quiet moments passed while he cried and I put my arm around his shoulder. There were really no words I could say to make this man feel better or less guilty at that moment… After a while, I asked him to tell me about his son. He started telling me about a lively, happy, joyful child. His love for Gabriel was immense…His wife was very close to their 4 year old daughter and he was very close to Gabriel. One of their favorite rituals was bedtime. He told me of their routine. Gabriel would get in his Barney pajamas and slippers and his dad would rock him and read him a Barney bedtime story before bed. It was their special time together at the end of the day. As he told me this, he began to cry again, saying he could not believe that he would never be able to do this again… The next day, the neurologist put Gabriel through a series of tests. They told us what we already knew—this sweet boy was brain dead. Gabriel's aunt was a nurse. She had asked me if there was anything she could do to help his parents. I decided to take her up on her offer. Knowing what was coming, I asked her to have someone go to their home and get Gabriel's pajamas, slippers, and storybook. She probably thought I was nuts, but I had developed a good relationship with Gabriel's family and she trusted me enough to do what I asked. After telling Gabriel's family the news that their son was dead, we went through the agonizing tasks of discontinuing life support. All of his family had the opportunity to hold him…I told the parents that I was going to clean him up so they could hold him one last time and asked if they wanted to help me. His dad spoke right up and said yes. This is when I told him my idea. I showed him Gabriel's pajamas, slippers, and book and told him that Gabriel's aunt had brought them from home. I explained that I thought he might want one last opportunity to go through their bedtime ritual together. He cried very hard but nodded his head yes. Together with his parents, we got Gabriel dressed and carried him to the Quiet Room. I had already put a rocking chair in there and the dad sat down in it with Gabriel in his arms. I told them I would be in the hallway if they needed me. I could hear his dad reading to him. It was quite emotional. Both of his parents were very grateful to me for helping them…I know that the pain and guilt the dad felt will never go away. In an otherwise hopeless and tragic situation, I believe I gave this dad one last memory. I hope it was the start of the dad's recovery.

Although caring practices and interventions related to patient death are more fully described in Chapter 9, this story illustrates how the patient's clinical status influenced the care this family received. The nurse's empathy and skillful read of the parents in this situation guided her in the difficult task of truth-telling, emotional presence, and skillful involvement. When the nurse shifted her focus from saving the patient's life to helping the family confront their child's death, new ways of attending to and responding to the grieving parents were discovered. Recognizing this transition and re-directing her practical activities toward the dad's leave-taking rituals required the nurse to have a good grasp of the patient and family situation, and to stay open and remain flexible to the parents' shifting understandings. In response to the dad's concerns, the nurse compassionately staged the bedtime ritual so that the parents could hold their child in this very familiar and special way one last time.

Some family-oriented interventions and activities may also be more accessible than others depending on the nurse's and family's stance. It is possible for nurses to work in acute and critical care environments without attending meaningfully to patient or family concerns beyond the "guest relations" level of being courteous and polite—or what is commonly known in business circles as service excellence (Berry, 1999; Stannard, 1997). However, when one experiences first-hand the human side of acute and critical illness, it is seldom possible to return to previous levels of distance to the human concerns of illness. Many nurses described how being a patient or family member of a hospitalized loved one changed their patient and family care practices. This is illustrated in the following interview excerpt from a neuro ICU nurse:

> **Nurse:** We've had a lot of problems with families being upset because we didn't let them in and they had to wait so long to see the patient. We didn't want them to see their loved one all bloody or dirty, because we felt it made their anxiety worse... Before I was a patient, I would just let families wait. But <u>waiting</u> is <u>very</u> hard and I now know how that feels. So if I get a patient back from surgery and the family hasn't seen the patient for 12 hours, I'll go outside and say, 'So-and-so is kind of messy right now, but I just want you to come in and say hi, so excuse the mess.' And then they'll come in and say hi and then they'll leave. So, I guess, being a patient has changed the way I practice.

Experiencing hospitalization first-hand opened up for this nurse a new understanding of what waiting for something feels like, which has subsequently changed her family care practices. Having the family come in for a quick "look see" following a long surgical procedure can diminish patients' and families' initial anxieties by decreasing the time they are apart.

These kinds of transformative experiences on the part of critical care nurses have also been described by others (Chesla, 1996; Stannard, 1997). It is our belief that if nurses shared their stories with others, powerful clinical lessons learned could be transmitted and extended. For developing nurses, the above exemplar, for instance, stimulates clinical imagination, attentiveness, and skillful ways of being involved in helpful ways. Having a clearer understanding about what is possible during some of the hardest interactions with families can improve one's sensibilities and guide meaningful interventions. The practice of sharing stories, however, requires the creation of interpersonal and institutional space in which nurses can both present and actively listen to one another's narratives of clinical learning (Benner, Tanner, & Chesla, 2009).

Likewise, when a nurse "bonds" with a family, the nurse-family relationship itself becomes an intervention of sorts. Through mutual emotional availability, openness, and trust, other interventions and activities become possible. One's stance shapes how one experiences and understands a situation, and as such, influences the options and possibilities for emotional involvement and family care (Stannard, 1997). For example, a neonatal ICU nurse discusses how her relationship with patients' parents has changed from being distant and peripheral to a stance that is more open to family members:

> **Nurse:** I'm just starting to get into parents. For 20 years, I worked nights and never had any contact with the parents. I'd get attached to various babies, but I hardly ever knew the families. And I'm finding more and more that I'm getting to know not only the parents of whom I'm taking care of that day, but I keep following up with kids that I had last week or the week before. I actually stop and chat with the parents and check on their kids.

Interviewer: Why do you think it changed for you?

Nurse: A lot of my friends have young kids now and I'm just getting into kids in general… You know, it's not just a baby that leaves here and that's the end of the story. They continue to have a story even if I don't see them (Observational Interview).

This nurse's involvement with children and their parents in her personal relationships has influenced her professional relationships, particularly with regard to patients' parents. Recognizing her friends' ongoing stories has encouraged this nurse to rethink patients' and families' stories and her involvement with them. Simultaneously, working day shift rather than night shift has allowed this nurse to have greater interaction with patients' families. Shift work, thus, is another kind of situational condition which can influence family care. This nurse's level of emotional involvement has now made certain caring practices possible (such as "following up" on patients and families for whom she has cared), and has enlarged her notions of caring work.

Because these three central family care practices overlap, nurses with expert family care skills seamlessly tailor their interventions and activities to the patient and family situation as illustrated in the following example from the PACU:

Nurse: Children definitely want their parents there as they're waking [up from anesthesia], and the parents preoperatively are told that they can be with their child as he or she is waking up. Well, coming out of anesthesia, there's that period of emergence, which, in children, can be manifested by the child being out of sorts, a little combative, whiny, crying, not really being able to open their eyes and tell you what's going on. Yesterday, I was taking care of a 10-year-old boy who was just waking up and he was crying with his eyes closed as mom and dad walked into the unit. And I would think for a parent to hear their child carry on like that would be extremely disconcerting. So, it's quite the task for the bedside recovery nurse to figure out what it is that the patient needs, as well as calming mom and dad's anxieties. Sometimes it's not a matter of the child being in pain, even though they're saying they're having pain. Oftentimes, it's just sheer anxiety—they're scared. They know something is different; they're in a strange place. They may have some discomfort, but they're scared because they don't have a complete grasp of what is going on, no control… So yesterday, I instructed the mother, 'Tell him that you're here and that he's OK. Tell him that the surgery is finished.' So mom was right there, holding his hand and speaking softly into his ear, telling him over and over again, 'Mommy is here with you. Relax, it's fine.' In the meantime, I noticed that he was doing a lot of facial grimacing. Looking on his anesthesia record, I saw that he had only received a small amount of fentanyl—a narcotic—so I felt that it was best to give him some more narcotic. So his mother was repeatedly whispering into his ear and re-orienting him and I was giving him an analgesic. That combination worked really well. The mother had a job, something to do. It kept her occupied and the drug that I gave took effect… And I explained to the mother that the child was still waking up from the anesthesia. I said, 'As you can see, he is not opening his eyes and focusing right on us and speaking directly to us, so that makes me think that he is still coming out from the anesthesia. It's important to touch him and stand close and keep repeating to him that the surgery is over.' And I assured the mother that, with a little bit of time, he would calm down and hopefully go back to sleep and then wake up a little more satisfied.

This PACU nurse recognized how frightening it must be for a child to wake up feeling cold, confused, and uncomfortable in foreign surroundings. She also appreciated how unnerving it was for parents to see their child in that condition. The nurse understood the phenomenon of emergence from anesthesia and articulated multiple reasons why the child might be "combative, whiny, and crying." Grasping what was happening in the clinical situation required discrimination and reasoning-in-transition on the part of the nurse. The nurse's clinical judgment guided how she intervened to specifically interpret the situation to the family and then coach them in ways that assisted their child. Ensuring that the parents could be with their child was critical to their understanding of the child's discomfort, the reduction in their own anxieties, and their appreciation and trust in the nurse and her instructions. In fact, the parents' presence most likely potentiated the narcotic's effect. Although the research literature examining the effects of family visitation on the patient is still evolving, one published study found that family presence correlated with decreased procedural pain and midazolam use in burn patients (Byers et al., 2001) and another found that parental presence in the PACU decreases negative behavior change at 2 weeks postoperatively (Lardner, Dick, & Crawford, 2010). This story underscores how tremendously powerful familial presence can be.

Once the parents were at the patient's bedside, the nurse provided them with information and reassured them that their child's behavior was normal and expected. The nurse also encouraged and coached the mother to talk to and touch her frightened son. This level of parental involvement was beneficial for all of the involved parties, and would not have been possible if family access had not been ensured in the first instance. Although ensuring family access is not always thought of as an intervention, this nurse was able to provide better patient care through the mother than she herself could have provided. While family care practices generally overlap as they did in this clinical example, to best articulate distinctions and highlight how each is central in family care, the aspects will be discussed separately.

ENSURING THE FAMILY CAN BE WITH THE PATIENT.

A crucial aspect of family care is ensuring that a family can be with their ill loved one, as family access promotes family cohesion, connection, and closure; fosters patient well-being; and provides the family with information. Yet, historically, many acute and critical care settings have severely restricted family access, thereby limiting nurse-family interactions and, in some cases, nurses' development of family care practices (Chesla & Stannard, 1997). Commonly cited rationales to limit family access include: concerns regarding patient stability, infection, rest, and privacy; the effect of visitation on the family; space limitations; and healthcare providers' performance abilities. While some of these concerns have merit, numerous studies have investigated family visitation and found no adverse effects on patient stability and infection or any negative consequences on family members (Ballard et al., 1984; Bay et al., 1988; Bru et al., 1993; Burke et al., 2009; Fiorentini, 1993; Fuller & Foster, 1982; Fumagalli et al., 2006; Hendrickson, 1987; Hepworth, Hendrickson, & Lopez, 1994; Kleman et al., 1993; Kowba & Schwirian, 1985; Lazure & Baun, 1995; Lewis et al., 1991; Nicholson et al., 1993; Oehler & Vileisis, 1990; Paludetto et al., 1981; Prins, 1989; Schulte et al., 1993; Proctor, 1987; Schwab et al., 1983; Simpson & Shaver, 1990; Solheim & Spellacy, 1988; Umphenour, 1980; Wranesh, 1982; Yu, Jamieson & Astbury, 1981).

Traditionally, setting limits on family access has been done in the spirit of allowing for clinicians' exclusive attention to the ill patient's needs or most recently, to be HIPAA (Health

Insurance Portability and Accountability Act) compliant. These limits have probably also served clinicians by providing protection and distance from the human significance of facing death and loss. Regarding HIPAA, under the latest iteration of the privacy rules, healthcare providers are allowed to disclose protected health information at their discretion to persons assisting in an individual's care, including family members and close friends (Roberts, 2003). But some clinicians use HIPAA as the reason to limit access to nursing areas or even to develop family care skills. It is true that some families do better and worse than others in supporting their ill family members at their bedsides. A family member crying uncontrollably at the bedside, for instance, can upset the patient and disrupt care. This kind of interruption in care can cause staff dissatisfaction with family visitation (Garrouste-Orgeas et al., 2008). Another family member, though, may cope quite well, given the circumstances, and can provide the ill patient with solace and comfort. Likewise, some patients respond well to a family member's presence, while other patients may prefer to be alone. It is for this reason that we encourage nurses to think of family presence as an intervention. When titrating a vasoactive drip, for example, the ICU nurse will typically monitor the patient's physiologic responses. Likewise, it behooves the bedside nurse to monitor the patient and family member responses during visitation, especially in the early phase following admission to any nursing unit. Families may still make palpable their fear and sorrow, which can cause emotional labor for the nurse. Learning to cope with the anxiety and grief associated with critical illness or injury while remaining emotionally engaged and open to the patient and family is a human and social involvement skill that characterizes expert nursing practice (Benner, Tanner & Chesla, 2009,). Nurses caring for wounded warriors returning from Iraq and Afghanistan have had to learn to incorporate family care early in the acute and rehabilitative care since family care is so crucial in the patient's long term and complex recovery (Kelly, Benner, Benner, In Progress, 2010).

Although some nurses are more likely to promote family unity during socially sanctioned times—such as birth and death—many families want and expect to be together at other times as well. Families especially want to be with their ill loved ones when they take a turn for the worse (Stillwell, 1984). Yet, this is precisely the time when family-focused care presents the greatest challenge as clinicians attempt to save the patient's life. An ICU nurse told us:

> **Nurse:** I think it's hard, you know, because the sicker the patient, the less you want visitors. But at the same time, it's more important to have visitors... But you don't want a lot of people around the bedside because if you've got to get to that patient quickly, it's like, 'Out of my way!' So, family visitation in an intensive care unit really takes a lot of nursing judgment. I think it's really hard to set hours (Observational Interview).

As this nurse points out, ensuring family access requires judgment. Unit policies that limit family access and involvement as a strictly enforced rule do not take into account the variety of patient and family situations nurses face daily. We favor family care guidelines over rules, because guidelines offer nurses and other healthcare providers the flexibility to respond to the unique needs and strengths of patients and their families in particular situations. While this nurse admits "it's hard" to have "a lot of people around the bedside" when the patient is doing poorly, she also realizes the ethical import of ensuring family access at precisely those times.

Requiring the services of an acute or critical care nurse, by definition, means that a particular patient's condition warrants close observation by a highly trained professional.

Death is always possible. Because the family constitutes the patient's world, ensuring a family's access to their ill loved one is an ethical issue. An ICU nurse wrote about a clinical incident that highlights this very point:

> **Nurse:** A 44-year-old man walked into the ED at 1 a.m. after having complained of abdominal pain all afternoon... He was placed on a monitor and while the nurse was drawing his blood, the patient VFib arrested. He was resuscitated for about one hour and then sent to the ICU. On arrival to the unit, the patient was 'on his head' [in Trendelenburg] and his BP was 50/palp with wide open [vaso]pressors, an antidysrhythmic, and IV fluids. His heart rate was in the 60s with an 'unknown rhythm'—irregular with a very wide QRS. At the scene were three medical residents and one intern, one surgical resident and an intern, seven nurses, and a multitude of consults now waiting outside the room to see the patient. The patient's family was waiting directly outside the unit doors... As the arrest progressed, the patient continued to get worse, not better. The medical resident who originally saw the family in the ED continued to go out and inform the family of the patient's changing status. As yet, the family had not seen him since he walked into the ED... We did everything we could to save this young man, but he was pronounced dead at 2:30 a.m. After the arrest, none of us wanted to leave the room because we knew the patient's family was right outside the unit. Finally, the senior resident and the patient's nurse went out to speak with the family while the rest of us cleaned him up. This episode was very important to me because I felt as though we had deprived the family of their last chance to see their loved one alive. This man walked into the ED and now he was dead. This one episode has changed how I feel about having patients' families visit while the patient is critically ill.

This powerful clinical incident illustrates the ethical challenge of balancing heroic interventions with the human significance of illness, loss, and death. Because families, by convention, are frequently separated from their loved ones in a critical situation, few clinicians consider this to be an inhumane practice. Yet, research has repeatedly shown that family members want to be with their dying loved ones and be given the option to be present for resuscitation efforts and invasive procedures (Barratt & Wallis, 1998; Bauchner, Vinci, & Waring, 1989; Bauchner, Waring, & Vinci, 1991; Bauchner et al., 1996; Boie et al., 1999; Doyle et al., 1987; Duran et al., 2007; Eichhorn et al., 2001; Fraser & Atkins, 1990; Hampe, 1975; Mangurten et al., 2006; Mazer, Cox, & Capon, 2006; Meyers, Eichhorn, & Guzzetta, 1998; Meyers et al., 2000; Powers & Rubenstein, 2006). A patient's death can threaten the very identity and world of the family. Although physical death occurs in the dying patient, the social level death is felt in the patient's surviving family long after the physical death has occurred. Denying a family the opportunity to be with their dying loved one does not take into account the world-defining nature of the patient-family relationship.

Family member death is one of the most significant transitions a family will experience—along with birth—which is why so many family members have expressed the desire to have the option to be present while their loved one is undergoing resuscitation and invasive procedures. These sentiments are slowly beginning to spill into the popular press which will only increase the consumer pressure to allow for family presence (Harder, 2001). This moment in time is akin to the social pressures in the 1950s when obstetricians routinely kept fathers out of the delivery room and were forced to change their practice due to changing public opinion. The nurse will still need to interview the family to ensure that their concerns and wishes are honored. Not all family members will want to bear witness to the patient's crisis care, and their wishes too must be met with appropriate care and information and without judgment or coercion to be present if this is not the family's preference.

Although family access recognizes and reinforces the family's preeminent position in the patient's world (Chesla, 1996), family presence during a patient crisis can bring forth strong feelings of emotion which can interfere with clinicians' performance abilities. A flight nurse spoke of this when she said:

> **Nurse:** When the family's there, it puts a whole different light on [the situation]. It isn't just an airway anymore. [The family] makes it more real. You have to really <u>focus</u> and say, 'Okay, this is what I need to do,' and <u>try</u> to separate yourself from the emotion...You just have to sometimes put a wall there.

As discussed in Chapter 4, healthcare providers commonly engage in a temporary objectification of the critically ill patient when performing life-saving measures. This protective practice often becomes more difficult when the family is present, because the "airway" can suddenly transform into a person who is an integral part of a loving family. If nurses dwell in these emotions, they may be unable to provide the necessary life-sustaining therapies. As a way of coping with the intense emotional pressures, nurses focus their attentions on prioritizing and performing their actions and on separating themselves from the emotion-filled situation. Stannard (1997) also found that nurses with expert family care skills typically distanced themselves from patients' families during times of crisis. It is important to note, however, that these nurses became fully engaged again with a family once the patient's condition stabilized.

We believe that with appropriate resources (such as adequate preparation of the family, support personnel to help the family through the resuscitation, and debriefing sessions and supportive work with staff), the option of having families stay with their loved ones during a resuscitation and invasive procedures should be extended to all families in all areas. However, the flight nurse's observations point to the necessity of having adequate staffing so that the family is supported by other team members who are not engaged in the immediate life-saving efforts. Additionally, this excerpt underscores the additional emotional load associated with a family's presence during a crisis situation. On-going supportive sessions and debriefing with staff are necessary to assist them in coping with emotion-filled situations.

Even in more routine circumstances, separating a critically ill patient from the family requires a great deal of trust on the part of the family. An OR nurse points to the social and emotional work of this separation:

> **Nurse:** Parents want to know that they're handing their child over to a decent, kind human being. So it's very important to make eye contact, sit down, use touch—all those non-verbal communications.

Attentiveness and connection at these junctures when a family hands their loved one over to be cared for by strangers can decrease familial anxiety and fear. Hasty or poorly orchestrated transfers can increase the family's anxiety. Time is helpful in building trust and ensuring a smooth transition, however, nurses with expert family care skills who work in areas with rapid turnover rates (such as procedural areas), have learned to use powerful non-verbal communication, such as that which was described by the OR nurse above, to make a connection and foster trust in a very short timeframe. Ensuring family access, no matter how short the duration, serves to maximize the time patients and family members can spend together. This is illustrated in the interview excerpt by a flight nurse who was preparing to transport a traumatically injured child:

> **Nurse:** It's really important to have the family come in if you can... If it's not that busy, we try to have the family come in the whole time we're there so that we can interact with them a little bit more and because you're taking their child away—especially if you're flying. The family may have to drive three hours to get there (Observational Interview).

Realizing that anything can happen with a critically ill patient in 3 hours, this flight team typically ensures family access to their loved one prior to transport. This patient and family-centered ethic promotes the integrity of the family unit and enables family members to touch, hug, kiss, and say goodbye to their loved one.

In another situation, an ICU nurse ensures that a newly admitted patient and his family have some time together before the patient is intubated:

> **Nurse:** Mr. D was a 31-year-old man who...had flu-like symptoms for a few days...got increasingly lethargic and ended up in our ICU. On admission, his speech was barely audible and he could hardly move. His wife and mother accompanied him and they were extremely upset and scared. I asked the family to wait in the waiting room until we had him settled. After assessing Mr. D, we decided he needed to be intubated to protect his airway. While we were preparing for the intubation, I let his family in for a short visit.

What is covered over in this nurse's account is the flurry of activity that inevitably occurs when a critically ill patient is newly admitted to an ICU, particularly in the midst of preparing for an invasive, life-sustaining procedure. Not only did the nurse and the other healthcare providers need to get the patient "settled," but they also needed to fully assess and treat his worsening condition. The nurse's clinical judgment and skill in grasping the patient's physiological condition enabled her to weigh the risk of having precious pre-intubation time elapse with the benefit of ensuring that the patient and family could be together, if only for a short time. Because the nurse understood the family as an extension of the patient, she skillfully folded her care of the family in with her care of the patient. By ensuring family access prior to his intubation, the nurse enabled the family members to verbally communicate with one another—something that would not occur again in this case for several weeks.

While patient access is important and valued by families, family presence is significant and favored by patients (Duran et al., 2007; Eichhorn et al., 2001). Because critically ill patients are often heavily sedated with multiple pharmacological agents or are unconscious, many clinicians assume that family access benefits only the patient's family. Yet, a family's presence can provide the ill family member with love and support, which have significant healing powers in their own right. An ICU nurse speaks to that by recalling a patient and family for whom she had once cared:

> **Nurse:** I used to work in a trauma center in the Midwest. I cared for this 23-year-old patient with a severe closed head injury, fractured femur, and chest and abdominal injuries... The physicians told his family that he wasn't going to live. Well, <u>every</u> single day, his mother came in and read him the local newspaper. Because he came from such a tiny town, this was a little one-sheet paper. You know, like, 'Mr. Smith sold his hardware store today.' She did that every single day. But on Sundays, she wore this

God-awful red dress that <u>he</u> [the patient] bought for her for her 50th anniversary or something. And it was just the ugliest dress. We used to say, 'What is she wearing that for?' But she'd come in and take his hand and say, 'It's Sunday. I'm wearing your favorite red dress.' We had him for three months. He was transferred to rehab and a year later he came back to see us. Do you know what he said, what he remembered? Feeling that red dress. When he woke up, it was a Sunday, and he said to his mom, 'It's Sunday. Where's your red dress?' She hadn't worn it that day. But he <u>heard</u> her. He heard that Mr. Smith sold his hardware store.

This powerful story points to the under-determined nature of this and many other clinical situations where the critically ill patient is expected to die but survives nonetheless. While the multiple therapies and interventions used in this case undoubtedly helped the patient's chances for survival, the mother's continued and supportive presence was certainly central in his healing and eventual recovery. This story also highlights the healing power associated with meaningful and significant caring rituals. Because the mother was ensured access to her comatose son, she was able to read the town newspaper to him on a daily basis. In a familiar voice, the mother relayed comforting news about people and places of significance to him. By wearing his "favorite red dress" on Sundays, the mother provided her son with a supportive and orienting presence which he remembered when he woke up from his coma. Finally, this story underscores the importance of family access to both the family and the patient. Although many critical care nurses continue to think of families as "visitors", healthcare providers are, in fact, the visitors in the patient-family relationship. Ensuring family access recognizes and respects the life-long and world-sustaining relationship between patients and their families.

Using a broader notion of "family", nurses can help coordinate pet visitation, which can be a powerful intervention that helps to pull the patient back into the familiar world that may be lost in an acute or critical care environment. Susan Foy, an ICU nurse, described a clinical incident in which a young woman was brought into the ICU following her second suicide attempt in less than 2 weeks. Following the tricyclic antidepressant overdose, the patient was unresponsive, on a ventilator, and decompensating:

Nurse: While the [nursing] supervisor and I were at [the patient's] bedside, her parents were telling us that her golden retriever was lost without her at home and [they] were thinking what a good idea it would be if she could only see her dog—maybe it would lift her spirits and help her fight to live. At first, I thought that would be out of the question since it was a breach of hospital policy, but I looked at the supervisor and asked whether this was possible. While looking at the patient lying there in bed hooked up to everything for life support, [the supervisor] said, 'Let's do it!'…A few hours later, the nursing supervisor and the parents had "sneaked" the dog up the back elevator when it was quiet. Before the dog entered the room with the parents, I had weaned off the paralytics and lightened her sedation so that [the patient] could open her eyes to see the dog and touch him…The dog cautiously approached the bedside and sniffed [the patient's] hand as her dad lifted her hand to touch the dog's face. [The patient] reached out her fingertips to touch her dog and her dad lifted the dog to lay beside her on the bed. I was watching [the patient] to ensure that her heart and respiratory rates weren't compromised. Her vital signs were fine and she was calm for about 30 minutes and the dog was very still during this time. It was then that I realized that this moment was 'meant to be'. Tears rolled down [the patient's] cheeks when she recognized her dog's presence.

Unfortunately, in this case, the patient's clinical condition continued to deteriorate and she died 2 days later. However, this bold intervention no doubt brought peace and even joy to the dying patient and certainly inspired in the parents strong feelings of doing *something* for their daughter in an otherwise powerless and tragic situation. With the advent of service dogs, therapy dogs, and pet visitation dogs, many facilities now have extensive policies and procedures in place (DiSalvo et al., 2005). But in this incident, the nursing supervisor and bedside nurse knew that the cost of breaking away from hospital policy was worth the therapeutic benefit to the patient and family. In addition to ensuring a family's physical access to the critically ill patient, nurses are pivotal in ensuring a family's emotional access to their ill loved one (Chesla, 1996). For example, a neonatal advanced practice nurse described a worrisome case which required intervention on the part of the nurse and the social worker:

Advanced Practice Nurse: One case that I look back on and feel good about was a newborn baby that I took care of who was born with hypoplastic left heart syndrome—one of the most complex kinds of congenital heart diseases you can have. There is a lot of mortality and morbidity associated with the disease and it requires a lifetime of surgeries... Anyway, this baby survived the first surgery, was weaned from the ventilator and extubated, and was doing well. But after several days, it became apparent to us that the mother wasn't coming to visit... So [the social worker and I] made contact with the mom and asked her to come and visit the baby... One day while I was holding the baby, the mother walked in and I was like, 'You're here, this is great! I'm so excited!' So I said, 'Let me put this baby down and get you a big comfortable chair and then you can sit down and be with him.' She wasn't making any eye contact with me and I could tell she was really scared. So I put the baby in her arms and told her that I'd leave her alone for a little bit. I came back and she was crying. And from that day on, she had bonded with the baby, she became so engaged. He's probably a year and a half old now and he's a wonderful, thriving, happy child. Every time she sees us, she expresses the role that we played in making her the mother that she is. And it didn't really take much, you know, obviously a lot of it came from within her. But we worked with her very closely during the entire hospitalization and taught her how to care for her baby. We tried to make him as normal as we could in terms of her being able to bathe him and hold him.

The disturbing and unusual lack of parental involvement in this case prompted the advanced practice nurse to contact the mother and encourage her to come and visit her baby. Because the baby required such an extreme level of medical interventions and was constantly at risk for dying, it was nearly impossible for the mother to bond with her child. Yet mother-infant bonding was essential, and without parental involvement and support, the baby would probably not have survived the multiple surgeries involved. When the mother arrived on the unit, she was warmly welcomed and was left alone for a few moments to "be" with her baby. Although many of the maternal feelings came "from within," several of the nurse's actions were central in creating new possibilities for the mother in terms of interacting and emotionally connecting to her baby. Ensuring physical access was obviously necessary before the nurse could encourage mother-infant bonding. By involving the mother in her infant's care, the nurse skillfully facilitated emotional connection, and simultaneously taught and coached the new mother important mothering skills.

When emotional connection already exists, nurses with family care skills help shore up patient-family bonds that may be weakened by prolonged illness or institutionalization. A PACU nurse discusses some of the approaches she finds helpful when working with patients and their families during the immediate postoperative period:

> **Nurse:** I've noticed that families are often afraid to get close to the person that's had surgery because they might hurt something, disconnect something, or they're afraid to be there. Oftentimes I find it necessary to give them permission to get close... Sometimes I'll put the side rail down, so that the mom or dad can touch their child and hug them. Because if the side rail's up, there's a barrier. But if you move the side rail down, they can get closer [to the patient]; it's a very helpful maneuver... I'll also often tell families that they can kiss and hug the patient... But you almost have to give them <u>permission</u> to love the patient and touch them the way they would like to, and I think a lot of people respond to that and need that guidance.

Many families do not have experience with acute care institutions and often have no idea what healthcare providers expect from them or what is safe in terms of interacting with their ill family member. In addition to their uncertainty, family members are usually very anxious about their ill loved ones. This excerpt points to the nurse's skillful coaching of families, which requires openness, judgment, and attunement. The nurse provides families with information and guidance, but also offers them possibilities for re-establishing connection. By eliminating obvious barriers and guiding families on how to "be" with their loved one in a foreign and frightening environment, the nurse assists families in emotionally re-connecting with recovering family members.

Most acute and critical care areas are designed to support multiple technologies for patient cure rather than care. By altering and managing the care environment and making it more conducive for quiet, undisturbed family time, nurses help facilitate sustained emotional connection between patients and their families, as illustrated in the following excerpt by an ICU nurse:

> **Nurse:** I took care of this one patient, a heart/lung transplant recipient who had a little bout of rejection and needed to stay in the ICU for four weeks. Just being in the ICU for 4 weeks was really a drag. So we pulled the curtain a lot so that the patient and his wife could be alone, because it's such a fishbowl atmosphere in here. That gave them some privacy so they could hold hands or just talk without somebody else right there (Observational Interview).

The nurse in this situation realized that the "fishbowl atmosphere" was not conducive to family privacy or spousal intimacy. The nurse's clinical judgment and grasp of the situation were essential to the success of this intervention. By reading the patient and family and recognizing the significance issues at stake for them, the nurse instantly grasped that quiet, undisturbed time was necessary to ensure sustained emotional connection between the patient and his wife. A nurse who is skilled at reading patient-family interactions and dynamics may recognize, for instance, that, in some cases, encouraging sustained emotional connection may exacerbate the patient's or family's discomfort. In cases such as these, a skilled nurse would be less likely to intervene in this fashion. However, in this situation, pulling the curtains and ensuring that the patient and his wife had private time together was crucial for them to tend to their relationship during this prolonged family crisis.

Although family access in critical care settings is frequently controversial, nurses are often concerned about the integrity of the family unit when family members are not physically present. For example, an ICU nurse intervened by encouraging the husband of a critically ill patient to more actively involve his grown children in his wife's care during her last few weeks of life. The 45-year-old woman was emergently hospitalized for sepsis and respiratory failure:

> **Nurse:** When [the patient] was first admitted, the family lived here for two or three days. But then the father sent [the children] home and would not let them come back to see her. And the patient wasn't really doing too well. So I said to the husband, 'You know, your wife isn't doing very well and if she dies and your kids don't see her, they might resent you for not allowing them to come [and be with her]. Your wife may not make it. Maybe you should rethink your decision.' So, that weekend, the kids came in to see her and...she looked terrible. Her kids are young, 18, 20, 21—they're in college. But they seemed to be very supportive of one another. It seemed like they were coping and doing all right (Observational Interview).

As the situation became clearer to the nurse, she assisted the husband in coming to terms with his wife's clinical deterioration and encouraged him to reconsider his children's lack of involvement in their mother's care. Looking ahead, the nurse recognized that the husband's coping strategy of protecting his children might actually cause his grown children additional grief if they were not allowed to see their mother or engage in any leave-taking rituals. By telling hard truths, the nurse re-framed the situation for the husband and helped him to consider the possible ill effects of his decision. This risky intervention on the part of the nurse required a good grasp of the clinical situation and an astute read of the family based on her relationship with them.

Most people appreciate from experience that a picture is worth a thousand words. One of the most important pieces of information a nurse can provide the family is the patient. Ensuring family access initiates the vital and multi-directional flow of information among ill patients, their family members, and the healthcare providers. A PACU nurse describes the essential role families play in informing healthcare providers about their ill family members:

> **Nurse:** There are so many little vital secrets families have that can help us in the care of the patient—things that we can never get from the medical record. You know, the whole gestalt of who that person is—that can only come from a significant other.

The stakes are even higher with critically ill "silent" patients or patients who are unable to meaningfully interact with the environment. In these cases, nurses and other healthcare providers often "know" the critically ill patient through the patient's family (Benner, Tanner & Chesla, 2009, 1996; Stannard, 1997; Tanner, Benner, Chesla & Gordon, 1993). Several nurses, for instance, described looking at family photos and listening to family stories as approaches that enable them to meet and know the "silent" critically ill patient. In another example, an OR nurse recalled a pediatric patient for whom she had cared that required special home care following the surgical procedure. The nurse informed the patient's surgeon of the unusual family circumstances, to which he asked, "How do you know that?" She replied, "Because I talked to the family, that's how." The OR nurse then told us, "It cannot be stressed enough how much information we can find out from families in a very short amount of time." Gleaning this information, especially in a compressed time frame, requires on the part of the nurse skillful questioning, an unrushed demeanor, and an openness to learning about the patient from the family.

On occasion, though, families are not able to travel extensive distances, get away from work commitments, or access certain restricted areas within hospitals, such as the OR. Those families must often rely on the information provided to them via technology—phone reports, web/email updates, and text pages. Many nurses described "virtual visiting" or the practice of providing families with detailed information through some technologic platform that paints a picture of the patient for the family. Virtual visiting enables a family to receive enough information so that they can imagine their family member's plight and feel connected. Nurses provide concrete connections so that the separation anxiety is diminished. For example, an OR nurse reviews some of the information she might pass on to parents when they are virtually visiting from the surgical waiting area while their child is undergoing a craniotomy:

> **Nurse:** For example, I'll say, 'John went to sleep without any problems. He didn't cry, he held his mask, and he just drifted off to sleep.' Or if he cried, then I would say, 'He cried a little bit, but he probably won't remember it because of the anesthetics.' I usually try to tell the family something specific, rather than 'He's fine.' I don't think that's enough. And each time I call them I give them a little bit of information. 'Well, we just moved the microscope again, so now we're working under the monitor.' Or if we have finished, I'll say, 'We finished the bone work and now we're down to the dura'—because most families know what's going on with their kids. And if they don't know, then I tell them... But the information lets the family know what's happening and what still has yet to be done (Observational Interview).

By receiving frequent and detailed telephone reports from the nurse, the family is able to stay informed and be partially involved, in spite of their physical distance from the patient. As in this situation, expert nurses further recognize that a family's experience of waiting time can be excruciating when minutes feel like hours. Keeping the family informed is a moral judgment and act to alleviate unnecessary distress and fear whenever possible.

In another incident, Luigina Maniscalco, a nurse working in a Special Care Nursery, described a situation in which a mother delivered a 34-week baby by emergency C-section but suffered complications following her delivery, necessitating maternal admission to the medical ICU. The parents had not had the opportunity to see or hold their son yet. After Luigina did her assessment, her empathy for the mother was exhibited in a unique way.... from the baby:

> **Nurse:** To me this was a tragic situation: Mother and Baby had to be separated... Watching Bryan on the warmer, I remembered Mom had not been able to see him. I took Polaroid photos of Bryan, so Mom could feel that she was part of his care. I wrote a letter to Mom with a crayon, from Bryan.
>
> **Dear Mom,**
>
> **I am doing OK. I am on a warmer with a heat lamp on to keep me warm. I have tape on my chest that attaches me to a monitor. My nurse Gina had to give me a boo-boo in my right hand to start an IV—she said I needed this**

because I cannot eat right now. Gina said you wanted to breastfeed me and she did not have any of your milk now, so the IV is my food. Gina also had to give me another boo-boo and take blood and send it to the lab. She told me you had to have blood sent to the lab too and she told me I would be just fine. I love you and miss you and cannot wait until you can hold me. Gina took pictures—she said I am beautiful and she said you would think so too.

Love, Bryan

I went to the MICU and asked Mom's nurse if I could see her for a few moments... I was told by Mom's nurse that she was uncomfortable and kept asking about the baby. I wanted Mom to see/know who was taking care of her baby.

When I introduced myself to Mom and told her I had photos and a letter from Bryan, she began to cry and asked if I would read the letter to her... As I was reading the letter to Mom, Dad arrived; I now read the letter to both of them. As I read, both Mom and Dad gazed at the photos of Bryan. I handed the letter to Dad when I was finished reading it to them. I promised Mom I would return at 11 pm ONLY if she wanted me too. Mom said "yes" for me to return. I left the MICU. Bryan was very stable for the rest of my shift.

I returned to the MICU at 11pm to talk to Mom. The nurse reported that Mom settled down after my initial visit... I again gave Mom a new Polaroid (because baby's change so quickly. I did not want Mom to miss-out on her baby) and gave her a good-night letter to read from Bryan.

Dear Mom,

I am tired now and going to sleep. You need your rest too.

I love you,

Bryan

I told Mom Bryan had a comfortable night and that he would most likely transition nicely. I said good night and told Mom I would be back tomorrow....I got to see Mom the next evening. [She was now on the Post-Partum unit.] When she came to the SCN, she remembered my name and thanked me for "letting her be with her son" when she was so sick....She stated "because of the pictures I was able to rest comfortably through the night". As Mom approached the bedside, I helped her sit at his isolette and saw the anxious look in her eyes as I was getting Bryan ready to be held by Mom. I will never forget the look of peace and serenity in Mom's eyes when I handed Bryan to her. She was where she needed to be. She embraced him and kissed him and cried and told him she "loved him forever"....

[At] Christmas, Mom and Dad sent me a card stating they love to read Bryan's letters to them. "Thank you for his letters."

This is an example of creating visitation opportunities when none exist and the significance it holds to feel close to a loved one. The imagination and caring on the part of the Nursery Nurse made this creative intervention possible and enabled the parents to be part of their child's care—even when separated in different nursing units. Virtual visiting will never replace physical presence or the need for family access, but facilitating this form of visiting is another way that nurses can extend their care to include patients' families. In this situation, the expert nurse provided the needed connection at the moment but also a life-long cherished memory.

PROVIDING THE FAMILY WITH INFORMATION AND SUPPORT

Another central aspect of family care is nurses' provision of information and support to patients' families. Information has been identified as a crucial component in coping and family satisfaction (Doerr & Jones, 1979; Nyamathi, 1988; Zawatski, Katz & Krekeler, 1979), while support, in the form of nurses' caring behaviors and interactions, is enormously influential in shaping the care experience for both patients and families (Benner, Tanner & Chesla, 2009, 1996; Burfitt, Greiner, Miers, Kinney & Branyon, 1993; Chesla, 1996; Holland, Cason & Prater, 1997; Stannard, 1997; Warren, 1994). Taken together, these two nursing interventions are highly valued by families and are even more meaningful when family access is ensured.

Nurses provide families with orienting information, help families grasp changing clinical relevance, and impart discharge instructions and information. Orienting information quite literally orients and familiarizes the family with the situation at hand, and includes interpreting for the family the surrounding equipment, the patient's condition, and the anticipated trajectory or big picture. Several nurses described formal orienting activities for families, such as tours of the ICU before their loved one's surgery. The practice of preparing families for their initial visit is another kind of orienting activity, as illustrated in the following excerpt from a PACU nurse:

> **Nurse:** So we always make sure, 'Do you know what it's going to be like?', because I've had families come to me and say, 'I had no idea he was going to look like that' or 'I didn't know she was going to behave that way.' So we usually brief the family on what to expect before they're at the bedside. Sometimes it's <u>scary</u> to see your loved one in that bed all pale and white.

Briefing a family beforehand by painting a picture of what they can expect to see and hear in terms of their loved one, of the immediate bedside environment with its supporting technology, and of the pace and activity of the unit is an orienting activity that prepares and assists the family in coping with the change in their loved one's condition. This familial coping through change can also be thought of as family transition work. In an elective surgical case, for instance, the patient's family may not have confronted illness and the possibility of death until they see their recovering loved one "all pale and white." Nurses' preparatory work can dampen the initial shock and help a family with their important transition work.

In another example, a pediatric ICU nurse describes her involvement with the parents of an 8-year-old boy with Respiratory Syncytial Virus (RSV):

> **Nurse:** I tried to keep the parents informed so they would know what was going on. I tried to keep it simple and gauge the mother's reactions, but I was getting the feeling that she didn't understand what I was talking about. Just the look on her face, it didn't look like she was understanding me (Observational Interview).

Relaying clinical information to patients' families in language they understand is often quite difficult, especially when one considers the various language barriers and the complex concepts, such as antibiotic resistant strains, that nurses are required to translate to families as part of their daily practice. The nurse in this situation "tried to keep it simple", while other nurses spoke of using analogies and drawing pictures to convey the orienting information they were attempting to impart.

The nurse in the case above realized from the mother's facial expressions that she did not understand what the nurse was telling her. Reading a family member's response to the information presented requires keen perceptual awareness, and in some cases, cross cultural skills. Rephrasing, reframing, and repeating are helpful strategies when there is a lack of comprehension on the part of patients or family members. Listening to the patient's and family's interpretation of the situation can best inform nurses about gaps in understanding.

Anxiety can also make the comprehension of complex or detailed material even more difficult. A neonatal ICU nurse points out:

> **Nurse:** When a baby is that ill, usually the family is fairly stressed out. A lot of times they don't retain what you tell them. You have to explain things several times before it actually sinks in. So you have to be really patient with them sometimes when they ask the same questions over and over (Observational Interview).

Assuring that the family is ready to absorb information is a form of judgment and timing which is crucial for effective delivery. Patience comes more easily when the nurse remembers the family's plight. Just as nurses can read family members, so too, can family members read nurses (Stannard, 1997). Families often recognize when the nurse is simply informing them as part of her or his job and when the nurse is informing them to provide understanding. A nurse's rushed and unwelcoming behavior will often escalate family anxiety. Understanding, and therefore patience, can be expressed by setting the tone, slowing the pace, and listening and responding to a family's concerns.

Nurses set the tone in their interactions with patients and families, as illustrated in the following nurse-family interaction, which occurred in the PACU:

> **Nurse:** Recently I cared for a 20-year-old cerebral palsy patient, who also had a developmental delay. He was coming in to have a pelvic tendon bilateral release done, and he was in his wheelchair. He was highly anxious and his parents were very, very anxious too... I'm sure they felt rushed and also just the impending anxiety of having this procedure done made them nervous. I could tell that the mother was extremely anxious about getting her son from the wheelchair into the bed and getting his clothing changed. And I conveyed to the mother, 'It's fine. He's here. Let's let him just sit in the chair for a while; let him get accustomed to his surroundings. You have done great Mom and Dad. He's doing fine. You're doing fine. Just let him sit here and maybe in a few minutes, ten minutes or so, he'll feel more comfortable and we can help him get his gown on. And, in fact, I don't even have to be here, <u>you</u> can be the one to put the gown on him...' So, I'm reassuring the mother and the child, 'We will take our time; there's no rush, you can be here with him.' And as I am carrying on in that manner, the curtain is whipped open and in comes the anesthesiologist saying, 'Oh, hello. My name is So and So and we're going to do the IV now! Are we ready to go?' It was <u>totally</u> disruptive. So I calmly told the anesthesiologist, 'The patient has just arrived. We need a little bit of time. Mom is here with the patient. We're going to get dressed, and so we need a few minutes before you come in. This isn't the average case. The child needs a lot of support. So a few more minutes alone would be helpful.' Meaning, it will help you in your endeavor also.

By listening to the family's concerns and calmly reassuring them, the nurse successfully set the tone by dampening the emotional energy in this situation. She read the anxiety on the parents' faces and slowed the pace by suggesting that they wait a few minutes to let the patient get acclimated to his new environment. By encouraging the mother to get involved in helping her son change into the hospital gown, the nurse gave control back to the parents who were, up to that point, feeling helpless and out of control. Once the nurse created this emotional climate and space for the patient and family, she did not allow it to be disrupted by the anesthesiologist who was unaware of the situation. Assuring patient and family readiness, as this nurse pointed out, serves the healthcare team in their endeavor of an on-time start to the surgical procedure as well. In situations such as these, tone of voice and pacing are as important as the words spoken, since the goal is to dampen anxiety and create a sense of possibility.

Nurses also help families grasp patients' changing clinical conditions, which can be thought of as assisting the family to come to terms with whatever clinical turn has transpired. Although a clinical turn can indicate patient improvement, because of the nature of acute and critical care, many of the clinical turns that nurses remember helping families grasp were turns for the worse. Whether the patient's condition is improving or deteriorating, in order for the nurse to assist the family, he or she must first recognize the changing clinical relevance as described in Chapter 2.

For example, an OR nurse discusses an incident involving the family of a young child who is scheduled for surgery to correct a heart defect:

Nurse: This was a young, really educated couple and this was their only child... It was discovered in the preop area that the patient's peripheral IV [with an infusing vasopressor] had infiltrated, which basically increased the risk of her surgery. Her hand was really, really big. It was a terrible infiltration. And she could have some horrible complications postoperatively because they were going to put [the child] on the [cardiac-bypass] pump. So the surgeon, the anesthesiologist, an anesthesia resident, a surgical resident, and the preop nurse ganged up on this couple and said, 'Worst case scenario: your child could lose her hand if we do the surgery. But if we wait, she could get sicker and she really needs to have this surgery done. What do you want to do?' I stood back and watched the whole situation and I finally just piped up and said [to the parents], 'Would the two of you like some time to discuss this alone before we go into the OR?' And they said, 'Oh yeah, we really would.' I said, 'Give me your little girl, I'll hold her. She's doing fine. Let me take you to a conference room where the two of you can just sit down and discuss this.' Because everybody was so focused on getting the child into the OR and getting the show on the road, they didn't realize that the parents were just totally overwhelmed, I mean, they were speechless. [The parents] did go and sit down and they decided to proceed with the surgery. Unfortunately, I didn't have the opportunity to check on the child postoperatively because I left town for the week. But if the child had lost her hand—and they did say that it was almost a sure thing that she would need some skin grafting on that hand—I think the family wouldn't be as angry because they weren't forced into making a rapid decision.

Interviewer: As a result of your intervention?

Nurse: My strong bearing, yeah. But I think that they (referring to the healthcare team) just didn't have any concept of what it must have been like for that couple... The parents were just emotionally paralyzed, and I thought, 'If they say yes now and something

> happens to her hand, they're never going to forgive themselves.' They're always going to say, 'We didn't have the time to make the right decision...' It didn't take the parents long, it was just 15 minutes or so, but I'm glad for them that I did that, because regardless of the outcome, I think they were more ready to accept it and they wouldn't go around for the rest of their lives saying, 'Why didn't we ask for more time to make this decision?'

Recognizing the tremendous weight <u>any</u> parent would feel by having to make this particular decision rapidly, the nurse acted as a moral agent by giving the parents the opportunity to discuss their options in private and away from the rushed atmosphere of the preoperative holding area. Because the other members of the healthcare team were focused on getting the sick child into the OR as quickly as possible, their collective understandings and bodily responses created a crisis-like atmosphere, which only served to escalate the parents' anxieties. The nurse's skillful intervention created time for the parents, which not only transformed the high energy, high-stakes "crisis" into a less emotionally charged situation, but also afforded the family the possibility of coming to terms with the clinical turn in their child's condition.

As in the case above, helping families to recognize changing clinical relevance also assists family members in preparing themselves emotionally. This can range from preparing families to see yet another mechanical device attached to their ill loved one to facing the imminent death of their family member. For example, an ICU nurse told us of an interaction she had with a patient's concerned husband:

> **Nurse:** He knew me and when he was getting ready to say goodnight, he said, 'Now, you're going to call me if anything happens, aren't you?' I said, 'Yes, I always call you if something happens.' He said, 'Well, this bad thing happened and no one told me.' I said, 'I'll tell you anything. I'll wake you up to tell you we're going to X-ray or anything else you want to know.'

While phoning family members at home with changes in their loved one's condition meets a highly ranked family need (Hickey, 1990), it also informs and prepares the family for what they can expect the next time they arrive at the hospital. In the example above, a breach of trust occurred when a "bad thing" happened on a previous occasion and no one had informed the patient's husband. The loss of trust that occurred illustrates the social and emotional work required for all patient and family transitions. In response, the nurse promised the husband that she would tell him "anything" he wanted to know about his wife's changing condition. While this may take more effort on the part of the nurse, in the long run, it is required to keep interpersonal trust intact so that the help offered is experienced as helpful by family members. These ethical and relational skills are unfortunately often compromised or overlooked altogether in the rapid fire pace of acute and critical care settings.

In another example, a neuro ICU nurse describes how she worked with the family of a patient for whom she had cared who sustained major neurological trauma:

> **Nurse:** Well, when you work with a patient for so many days, you see the changes. Like with this one patient, he started flexing the day before, and he was a 3 on the Glasgow Coma Scale [which ranges from 3-15], and he had a pneumonia... It was just like all these things adding up. So I tried to tell the family that, you know, maybe it's time to step back a little and ask yourself what you want... You try to paint that picture that some of the families can't see, namely, that their loved one may be in a coma for a long, long, time.

This nurse not only gives the family the big picture (Benner, Tanner & Chesla, 2009, 1996), but also assists them in understanding the patient's serious condition by pointing to the worrisome clinical indicators that are "adding up." Ensuring that the family can be with the patient can ease this transition for the family, as the family members can witness many of the indicators that the nurse points out.

Clinicians usually recognize deterioration in a patient's condition, and thus, experience a shift in understanding, well in advance of the patient's family (Stannard, 1997). This occurs for primarily two reasons. First, clinicians' physiologic and scientific background and skilled clinical knowledge enables them to grasp the relevance of a patient's worsening clinical status. If clinicians have worked in a high acuity environment for a moderate amount of time, they are accustomed to making this transition, and, depending on the patient's illness or injury, they often anticipate this clinical eventuality. Many families, on the other hand, have never faced acute or critical illness before, and as such, can only hope and not predict. Second, while many clinicians may have developed emotional attachments to the patient and/or family, the deteriorating patient is still not their loved one. For a nurse, this shift is one of many in a career or profession, but to the family, this acute or critical illness on this day may transform their life as they have known it. Confronting the mounting evidence that suggests a downward trend is more accessible for clinicians than it is for the patient's family. These two reasons alone position clinicians and the patient's family to diverge in their understandings of the shared clinical situation, for they usually live in two very different experiential and emotional worlds. Nurses who help families grasp changing clinical relevance, thus, help to bridge the gap that often exists between clinicians and the patient's family (Chan, 2005).

Families of acute or critically ill patients appreciate honest information that is sensitively delivered. Compassionate truth-telling requires dialogue and relationship (see Chapter 9). Yet, nurses and other healthcare providers often struggle to provide a family with honest and concrete information when there are many clinical uncertainties. A neonatal ICU nurse speaks to that when she describes a severely neurologically impaired infant:

Interviewer: How frank and honest are you with the parents about your concerns?

Nurse: Well, I tend to say I don't know because...we don't know yet how this child is going to turn out—whether she's going to get better or worse. But I do try to be realistic with them. If they were to come in and feed her and see how she is, I might say, 'This might be as good as it will get and we just need to work out ways to deal with her as she is and to love her as she is.' It's really hard with neurological involvement—it's not about how <u>honest</u> you want to be, it's just that there are too many unknowns (Observational Interview).

Because of the under-determined nature of the infant's clinical trajectory, the nurse is reluctant to speak to the family in concrete terms. The information the nurse provides the family, thus, is guided by the patient's clinical condition. If the nurse continues to remain open to the patient's unfolding clinical course, as the patient's condition becomes more certain, so too will the information the nurse provides the family.

Expert nurses have learned from experience to stay open to the clinical situation, as critically ill patients' clinical conditions can fluctuate dramatically. Nurses described "miracle" patients that survived despite all odds, and stable, recovering patients that suddenly died. Overstating family information with absolute certainty or avoiding risk by denying a family vital information can cause unnecessary grief and distrust on the part of the family. These kinds of learning experiences have taught nurses with expert family care skills to impart family information in a realistic—yet hopeful—fashion that reflects the ambiguity inherent in the clinical situation.

Nurses also provide families with discharge instructions and information. This process is often delayed in critical care areas, because nurses want to ensure patient survival before launching into extensive discharge teaching which can build the family's hopes. Two neonatal ICU nurses discuss this issue below:

Nurse 1: Supposedly, discharge teaching starts the day of admission—that's what we tell ourselves...

Nurse 2: That's the theory, but what's the reality?

Nurse 1: Well, it's not really until the kids are extubated and start tolerating a lot of hands on intervention so that the parents can really get comfortable with them. It's teaching them what they need to know, how to feed their babies, and how to interact with them.

Delaying discharge teaching until a critically ill infant is less critical, can be extubated, and can tolerate parental interaction and activity also makes the discharge instructions more relevant to parents, as they can more readily imagine their child at home without the encumbrance of life-supporting devices. Also, the child's improved condition helps the parents to recognize that learning is essential.

While delaying the discharge planning process in critical care areas may seem logical, it also means that there is more information giving and teaching to be done in a shorter period of time. With shorter lengths of stay, nurses are often hard-pressed to provide all of the information families need to know. Another neonatal ICU nurse describes this tension:

Nurse: Babies are getting ready to go home, so the parents need volumes of teaching. Either it is their first baby or their first pre-term, so the parents are scared—and that requires a lot of teaching! We have to teach them to give baths, take their temperatures, give any med the baby will go home on, give them monitor teaching if the baby is going home on one, teach them CPR. It is quite a lengthy process and it takes time, which is challenging when you have four of these babies to care for (Observational Interview).

Teaching anxious family members requires patience, understanding, and good communication skills on the part of the nurse, which includes active listening as well as a firm grasp of the content so that it can be simplified and re-stated in multiple ways to ensure family comprehension. While the teaching process can be abbreviated or compressed, these "shortcuts" are often at the learner's expense. When patients are "healthy enough" for families to receive discharge instructions, staffing requirements are usually adjusted to reflect the lower patient acuity. But in the case of discharge planning and teaching, lower acuity does not mean that less time is required. The transition from the acute care institution to home is an important one and often requires intensive one-on-one nurse-family interactions. Given the amount of vital information nurses provide families so that they may safely and competently care for their recovering loved ones, staffing systems based solely on patient acuity and not on patient complexity or care needs are woefully inadequate.

In addition to information, nurses also provide support to families of critically ill patients through reassurance and by establishing trust and rapport. Illness or injury creates a crisis within any family. Reassuring a patient's family that a particular patient event or transition is common and expected can ease family members' fears and allay anxieties. For example, two PACU nurses discuss ways in which they reassure anxious family members in the immediate postoperative period:

> **Nurse 1:** You know, you've got to reassure them with something physical: 'Look! Oh, oxygenation is good, the heart's doing well, look there's no bleeding. Look at her appearance. She's doing wonderfully!'
>
> **Nurse 2:** I oftentimes make it a point to show the family member the dressing... And I think it makes a difference, because I would want to see the area that was affected on someone I loved. I wouldn't have the nerve as a bystander to pull up the covers and look for myself, but I would sure welcome the nurse who showed me the dressing if I was the family member.
>
> **Nurse 1:** Parents usually want to see a dressing, but with friends and spouses, I let them take the initiative. If they start talking about it, then I say, 'Oh, it's doing fine. Do you want to see it?' But if they don't talk about it or the patient's a very private person and doesn't want to be exposed, then I just leave it alone... You kind of have to take your cues from whatever interaction is going on.

These nurses realize the importance of emphasizing positive patient responses or outcomes to worried family members after their loved ones have undergone something as invasive as surgery. The nurses' dialogue also highlights their response-based practice, as they inform and support the family based on their read of the patient and family situation. Because of their experiential knowledge in working with recovering patients, these nurses can see when a patient is "doing wonderfully," while the family may only see their loved one as tired and pale. Nurses help family members reappraise their family member's condition based upon the foreign context of critical illness. Reassurance provides families with realistic hope, which meets yet another family need (Hickey, 1990) and is a major family coping strategy.

In another example, an OR nurse describes how she carefully watches patient-family interactions and "follows their lead" (Benner, 1994c) when providing family information and support:

> **Nurse:** Some families are more affectionate and tender than others, and we just have to work around that... I took care of a patient last week and the father [of the patient] absolutely refused to let anyone make contact with his eleven-year-old child. He sat on the bed with his arm around her, and no matter who asked her a question or tried to talk to her, the father answered for her. Even if she tried to talk, he would interrupt her. Nobody was going to get to his little girl. And he was also very domineering with his wife. The wife didn't make any comments unless she looked at him first, and any questions that came up that were directed to her, the wife would ask him. So, we had to work with that.

Interviewer: So what did you do?

Nurse: Well, once we got into the OR, she [the patient] was very verbal and cooperative and told us what she did and did not want. But in the pre-op area, I just sat on the other side of the child's bed and when I asked her a question, I looked at Dad first and then at her. And then a couple of times, I took Mom off to the side a couple of steps and said some things to her. She was <u>very</u> worried, so I wanted to give her some comfort... So if you pay attention to what's happening with the family, you can find out a lot about their dynamics and figure out a way to get in there to work with them (Observational Interview).

In this case, the nurse's ability to notice family interaction patterns enabled her to tailor her interactions and interventions to match what was both desired and required by the patient and her parents. Because the family was under a great deal of stress in anticipation of their child's surgery, the nurse understood that it was neither the time nor the place to attempt to change what might be life-long familial coping styles and interactional patterns. By working within the family's world, the nurse was able to respect the father's boundaries, while at the same time, provide the patient's mother with much-needed support and comfort. Once the child was away from her parents and in the OR, the nurse remained open to interacting with the child on the child's own terms.

As was illustrated in the previous case, developing trust and rapport or connecting with a family is central to family support. This human connection provides families with reassurance and support, knowing that their ill and vulnerable family member is in capable and caring hands. In another example, the same OR nurse discusses how she typically works with young patients and their parents:

Nurse: Well, I find it easy to get along with families and their kids, but I came from a family with lots of kids. First I usually try to deal with the parents. 'Hi, I'm So and So.' And then I look at the chart and ask them if they have any questions. But before that even happens, I can sense if that's the right thing to say or not, just by what's happening in the room. I sort of like to work off of what's happening with the child and the parents. Are they playing with the child? Is the child asleep? Is the family hovering over the bed? You know, lots of nonverbal clues. And, with practice, it doesn't take very long to assess what's happening. Someone who doesn't have a lot of experience with kids maybe can't do that. But I look at the chart and start talking with the family right away—parents, mother, father, grandparents, foster parents—whoever they are. And I don't exclude them from looking at the chart. I'll say, 'Oh, I see here it says such and such has happened. Was that recent?' Just little comments, something to say, you know, connect, I'm here. I find that once I have gained the confidence of the parents, it's much easier to deal with the child, and the parents are more willing to let you deal with their child.

This excerpt is instructive because it illustrates practical approaches that can assist nurses in establishing trust and rapport with families. Additionally, the nurse points to the work of creating smooth transitions from one care setting to another. It also highlights the skills of being present in the situation. The nurse lets the family set the pace and carefully enters the situation in accord with the family's stance. Like other examples of managing care transitions in this chapter, this nurse has found ways of developing trust and rapport with patients and their families in a relatively brief period of time.

In another example, an ICU nurse describes the importance of establishing a trusting relationship with a patient's family:

> **Nurse:** And the fact that I'm it—I mean they can leave the room feeling like they can get a good night's sleep... I get good vibes when the family says, 'Oh, you're on tonight. I was asking if you were going to be here.' [This] is what keeps me at the bedside.

This excerpt illustrates the power of many nurse-family relationships and underscores how the relationship itself is an intervention of sorts. The nurse understands remarks such as these to mean that a family trusts her to stand in for them. Standing in for a family means that the nurse will care for the patient while incorporating and representing the family's concerns in their absence (Stannard, 1997). By virtue of their relationship, the patient's family "can get a good night's sleep," knowing that their critically ill loved one is being cared for by a nurse they trust.

A nurse-family connection may develop into a relationship if the two parties are emotionally available and have enough interactional time together. But with decreasing registered nurse staffing levels and increasing patient acuity, time is often limited for direct care. In a recent study investigating nurse-family interactions in ICUs, Stannard (1997) found that nurses who valued their interactions with patients' families attempted to consistently work with the same patient and family over several shifts or would "follow up" with them if they had another patient assignment. Following up was a way to sustain the developing nurse-family relationship and was experienced by the family as a source of continuity that enabled them to entrust the care of their loved one to the nurse.

Due to shortened patient stays, we found in this study that many nurses followed up with patients and their families by checking on them after they had been transferred to another unit within the hospital or contacting them once they were discharged home. Some nurses also followed up by attending patients' funerals and helping families locate important community resources. This meaningful relational work validates the significance of the human and social connections that were made and allows for all involved parties to experience closure on unresolved issues and concerns. Though not a formal bureaucratic structure, this relational work is crucial to the social fabric of acute and critical care areas, and should be promoted by ensuring that there is adequate staffing and time for nurse-family interactions.

ENCOURAGING FAMILY INVOLVEMENT IN CAREGIVING ACTIVITIES

Encouraging family involvement in caregiving activities is another essential aspect of family care, and can range from minor involvement (e.g., asking a family member to pass an alcohol wipe) to major involvement (e.g., inviting a family member to assist with the patient's bath). Although numerous obstacles for family participation exist (including hesitancy on the part of nurses, unit policies that prohibit family involvement, and inadequate staffing and lack of time), studies have shown that families both desire and value involvement in their loved ones' care (Chesla, 1996; Coulter, 1989; Glaser & Strauss, 1965; Hammond, 1995; Li et al., 2000; Mitchell et al., 2009; Stannard, 1997). Simple acts of helping can: facilitate patient-family bonding and togetherness; promote patient healing and comfort; decrease a family member's sense of helplessness and anxiety; and assist family members in grasping their loved one's condition.

Many of the family involvement stories came from pediatric and neonatal nurses, as family participation in those areas also serves to prepare family members for their caregiving roles once their child returns home. While the same could be said for adult acute and critical care areas, the societal expectation and ethic of involving parents in their child's care is much stronger than it is for family members of adult patients. Yet, family members of chronically ill adult patients are often accustomed to providing direct care to their ill loved one. Familiar grooming and caring rituals by family members can evoke a sense of continuity and comfort for adult patients. On the other hand, hospitalization may provide a needed respite for family members from these usual caregiving activities. Thus, opening up possibilities for comfort care and direct caregiving activities for adults requires exploration of patient and family preferences.

Determining the extent to which family participation is desired requires the nurse to have keen perceptual awareness and good communication skills. An ICU nurse, for instance, told us that she typically tells family members, "You can do as much as you want or as little as you want—just let me know." Once a family's desires are known, nurses with expert family care skills slowly involve families by acclimating them to their ill loved ones within the foreign context of acute or critical care. For example, two neonatal ICU nurses discuss a family's reaction to their premature newborn infant and describe how the nurses in the unit responded:

> **Nurse 1:** The parents would breeze in, look at the baby, and leave. They clearly wanted to love their baby, but they didn't get what they had bargained for. That's epidemic in our nursery. People have this idea in their pregnancy that they're going to have this wonderful, cute baby and then they get stuck with this little <u>scrawny</u> thing. So it took them a long time to adjust. But we wanted them to start touching their baby. So we asked, 'Will you take the baby's temperature?' That's usually where we start or else we'll ask them to help us diaper the baby.
>
> **Nurse 2:** But I think you do it step by step. Like you said, we start with the thermometer and diaper change, and once they get comfortable, they'll start initiating that care by themselves.
>
> **Nurse 1:** And we also start parents off with skin care. We have lotions and I'll say, 'Why don't you do some skin care on your baby?,' and get them used to sort of handling their baby a little bit... With that one family, they ended up being very happy, but it took a lot of support and nurturing.

The parents wanted to love their baby, but they were blocked from expressing that love because of their own feelings of shock, disappointment, and fear, and by the overwhelming amount of technology required to support their critically ill infant. Recognizing and understanding the parents' position, the nurses invited their involvement by encouraging them to initially participate in a low-tech and non-threatening activity. These nurses have learned experientially that once parents get accustomed to their baby and to the foreign environment of the ICU, they begin to "see" the baby as a person and involve themselves in their baby's caregiving activities. Taking it "step by step" assists families in their own transition work of adjusting to their baby's condition and to their new roles as parents of a critically ill infant.

In another example, an advanced practice nurse described a patient who was admitted to the ICU for an upper gastrointestinal obstruction. The patient had ALS (amyotrophic lateral sclerosis) and had been cared for by his wife at home:

> **Advanced Practice Nurse:** The patient was on a home ventilator and his wife had been doing everything for him for the past two years... [Because the wife wanted to continue to provide her husband's care], I advised the staff nurses to back off so that we could assess what she knew and what she was capable of doing. In fact, she knew how to do his cannula care and clean his stoma, so we got her supplies. The only bone of contention was suctioning because she was using clean technique. I told her that [clean technique] was very acceptable in the home setting, but in the hospital, we needed to use sterile [technique]. She was resistant to that, but I basically told her that there was too much risk for infection if we used anything other than sterile technique. So she warmed up to that... And I gave her positive strokes like, "You're doing such a great job. You really have this down pat... As long as you're interested and want to continue, we'll make sure that you have the equipment and supplies you need and be available to help." I think there is a tendency sometimes [on the part of nurses] to do everything [for patients] when they're initially admitted. Here I felt the appropriate intervention was to back off.

Determining whether direct caregiving was desired in this situation was imperative, since the act of helping could be perceived as a burden if involvement was unwanted by either the patient or his wife. By carefully and socially negotiating the wife's involvement in her husband's care, the advanced practice nurse ensured that the work of caregiving was not insensitively shifted from the healthcare providers to the family, but was instead based on the desires, abilities, and usual caregiving patterns of the particular patient and family.

By convention, nurses working with adult patients typically provide all patient care. It requires judgment to know when to step back and create the possibility for family involvement in providing direct care. In the above example, one can imagine that the wife's needs for caregiving and respite fluctuated during her husband's hospitalization. By working closely with the wife and taking her lead (Benner, 1994c), nurses presumably shifted back and forth from providing care to supporting the wife while she provided care. Providing respite for family members when the emotional and physical demands are too great requires judgment, flexibility, and openness to the patient and family situation.

While the above examples have dealt with neonatal and adult patients, incorporating family care into pediatrics is a front-line comfort and support for children who do not easily transfer their allegiance and trust to strangers. A parent's soothing and familiar voice and presence is the most powerful organizer and coach, as illustrated in the following example where a PACU nurse describes how the patient's mother assisted her in the care of the recovering child:

> **Nurse:** Yesterday, I had this patient whose O_2 saturation was low, and we had to keep asking the child to breathe deeply. So I got the mother to coach the child to breathe deeply every single time that happened.

By inviting the mother to remind her child to breathe deeply whenever the saturation monitor alarmed, the nurse provided the most effective prompting and coaching possible. She also enabled the mother to be a helper, rather than merely an observer. Helping not only enables family members to feel useful and active in their loved one's recovery, but it also makes the task of bearing witness to their loved one's suffering more bearable, since taking direct actions is a form of coping in its own right.

Coordinating certain patient activities to meet the family's schedule, such as delaying a bath until the patient's wife can assist, can also promote family involvement in their loved one's care. Since many patient-related schedules are arbitrary, rearranging activities to more fully involve the interested family member is yet another way of extending patient care to include the family. For example, a neonatal ICU nurse described planning an infant's feeding times around the mother's schedule:

> **Nurse:** The patient's diagnosis was intrauterine growth retardation. She's not our tiniest baby, but she's under 1000 grams. Her mom, I think, had high blood pressure. That restricts blood flow to the placenta which retards growth. That's probably why she's [the baby] so small. But these babies can be very sick... So, what we're doing is teaching her to bottle [feed] even though she gets gavaged at other times. For instance, if I knew her mom was coming at 5:00, I wouldn't gavage her this time, because I'd want her to be awake and ready for mom. So we try to plan it (Observational Interview).

Assuring that the baby's feeding times are coordinated with the mother's schedule requires additional time and attentiveness on the part of the nurse, but gives the mother the message that her presence and involvement in her baby's care is valued. The baby's alertness and eagerness to eat can also further engage the mother in her baby's care. Involving parents in the care of their premature and critically ill full-term infants is crucial for parent-infant bonding, and is as important as any medical intervention.

Family involvement in caregiving activities also assists families in grasping their loved ones' conditions. Since many acute and critically ill patients suffer from numerous setbacks and frequently have dramatic clinical turns, nurses are instrumental in helping families to see the big picture. While nurses also convey this information verbally, involvement in direct caregiving often makes the patient's clinical deterioration or improvement more tangible to the family. In the next example, a neonatal ICU nurse describes how she is currently working with the parents of a 1-week-old critically ill premature infant whose clinical status is slowly improving:

> **Nurse:** I think this baby will do very well, but there are always ups and downs. He may have some setbacks with feedings or something, but so far he is doing well. The other thing in his favor are his parents. They have been very actively involved and are very responsive to the baby. The mom is really sensitive to the baby and the baby's signals. I talked with her and showed her some of the baby's ways of communicating, like his way of saying, 'I have had enough.' Parents are so concerned about 'Is my baby going to live or not' that you need to work with them and show them what their baby is saying. This is important as we get past these really crucial days when you know that the baby is going to live and is going to be here awhile. You need to be thinking of what the baby needs developmentally. Sometimes you need to encourage the parents to hold their baby's hand. And other times you have to say, 'The baby is getting all worked up, let's draw back a little.' Also comfort measures—helping parents figure out what the baby likes. Can they find their hand? Do they like lying on their tummy or their side? (Observational Interview).

Because this nurse has a good grasp of the clinical situation, as well as expert coaching and communication skills, she is in the process of helping the parents move past their initial fears that their baby might die and is coaching them instead to be attentive to their baby's developmental needs. By sharing her understanding of the baby's anticipated trajectory, the nurse is preparing the family for future patient transitions. Working closely with an experienced nurse, thus, not only helps the parents prepare for possible clinical eventualities, but also enables them to learn general "tricks of the trade" and specific caring and comforting practices that are tailored to their infant's preferences and responses.

Learning and practicing patient comfort measures is highly valued by family members, but the family's involvement in providing the care can also promote patient healing and comfort. A less experienced neonatal ICU nurse wrote about a clinical case in which she learned how comforting family involvement can be, for both the patient and family:

> **Nurse:** It all started one morning after a very busy twelve-hour night shift. I was very tired and all I wanted to do was to hurry up and finish the night's work so that I could go home. The phone rang and it was the mother of the baby I was caring for—she wanted to come see her new baby. I reluctantly told her she could come up. When she arrived, she had numerous questions about how her daughter was doing. I didn't have very loving thoughts toward her daughter because one of the reasons I had been so busy all night was due to the fact that her daughter had cried inconsolably all night long. As I was speaking to this mom, her daughter (as usual) was crying, so I asked the mom if she wanted to hold her. Of course, she said yes, especially since she hadn't held her yet. As I handed the baby to her, the baby's IV disconnected and blood began leaking on the baby, the mother, and the floor. It was all I could do to keep from screaming. The mother, however, didn't seem bothered by the mess just created. She just began to rock and sing to her daughter, and for the first time that night, the baby quieted down and began looking at her mom. The mother had tears in her eyes and looked at me and said, 'You don't know how happy you've just made me. This is the happiest day in my life. I've waited so long to hold my baby.' (The mother had three previous miscarriages). The mom must have said this four or five times to me. All this took place in about fifteen minutes, and no I didn't get out on time that morning, but I surely learned an important lesson. Even though I may not feel like doing something for a parent because it is not in <u>my</u> best interest, it may be in <u>their</u> best interest or in the <u>baby's</u> best interest, and that is what really matters.

In this case, the baby finally stopped crying once she was held by her mother. This narrative highlights the tremendous healing power of mother-infant bonding, but can also be extended to point to the importance of facilitating patient-family functioning and relational closeness across the lifespan. While the nurse was trying to finish up her shift so that she could leave the hospital on time, the mother was experiencing the "happiest day" because she was holding a new life—her baby—which already had become a world-defining relationship for this new mother.

Preparing patients for discharge and helping families to safely care for and understand their loved ones' conditions and needs necessarily requires family involvement in transferring caregiving work from healthcare providers to patients' families. The transition from the hospital to the home requires planning and teaching, especially as patients, families, and healthcare providers face shorter hospital stays, increasing patient acuity, and decreased staffing. While discharge instructions and information are crucial for a smooth and safe transition, so too is the "hands-on" practice families need in order to provide care to their recovering loved ones. For example, a neonatal ICU nurse describes her unit's family involvement practices in relation to ensuring discharge readiness:

> **Nurse:** We have the parents do as much of the activities of daily living—taking the temperature, repositioning, range of motion—we encourage them to do as much as they can so that by the time they go home, they'll be perfectly comfortable handling their baby (Observational Interview).

By working closely with families throughout the entire hospitalization, this nurse and others in her unit maximize parental first-hand learning. Learning the skills entailed in infant care are compounded by the added technical procedures and anxiety over the baby's well-being. Anticipating the adaptations and contingencies of care at home require clinical forethought, coaching, and familial involvement in planning and caregiving. Risks and demands must be realistically assessed.

When patients are discharged from the hospital with more complex conditions requiring sophisticated technological support and corresponding levels of family vigilance, more intensive discharge planning and family involvement is necessary. An advanced practice nurse describes the work involved in assuring discharge readiness for adult patients who require mechanical ventilation at home:

> **Advanced Practice Nurse:** One area that I'm responsible for is the discharge planning for patients that are going home and require mechanical ventilation... It's becoming more and more of a burden to send people home, because what used to be thought as a less expensive alternative is actually a more expensive alternative... And those cases are always very challenging because there are so many different aspects of care that need coordinating... Even though a family may want to get [their loved one] home, we spend a lot of time in the beginning asking [family members], 'Do you really understand the burden that you're accepting, the 7-days-a-week, 24-hours-a-day accountability?' And, it amazes me how often physicians will say, 'Well, Sandy wants to take Fred home on the ventilator, and doggone it, it's a good idea. Let's just do it. We'll get this done in a couple of days and then we'll send them home.' And I'm like, 'Wait a minute. Time out. Have you talked to the patient about this? Have you talked to the family?' Because a lot of times, the family is agreeable and then when they get involved, the burden [is just too much]. And there's so much guilt associated with wanting to do the best thing for the patient. But [a family] never really knows what they're getting into until they're doing it. That's why it's so important to get them on a teaching schedule. Because the skills—whether it's tube feeding, suctioning, or skin and wound care—all those things they're going to need to know how to do when they get home. And teaching those skills is really nursing driven. The ventilator piece is really just a small part, because there's a limit as to how much you can really do in the hospital. You need to get the DME (durable medical equipment) company to go out to the house and do a safety assessment. You need to make sure the electrical systems are compatible. The family has to write letters to the fire and electrical companies so they're put on a priority list. [That means] that if there's an emergency or if they don't pay their electric bill, they don't get their power shut off. But all of those pieces have to be in place... So, I basically use a check list to help me coordinate all the activities that need to be taken care of. That's one piece. The second piece is the teaching tool we developed, which essentially lists the different caregivers that are going to be providing

different kinds of care... And one of the things we stress is that families can't just talk about it, they have to perform it—repeat demonstration. Because, to me, the issue of competency isn't necessarily what they tell you, but if they can perform the skill safely... But the key is really organizing and planning these things well. Otherwise, it's a disservice to the patient and family once they're discharged from the hospital.

This excerpt highlights some of the difficulties associated with shifting caregiving responsibilities from healthcare providers to family members who may be unable to see other options. Because this advanced practice nurse appreciates the emotional and physical burdens that constant caregiving can create for family members, he ensures that patients, family members, and other clinicians are sensitized and prepared as much as possible for the transfer of care and transition to home. By keeping the patient and family's best interests in mind, the nurse is able to deftly plan and coordinate complex and vital discharge activities and patient-family learning plans. Ensuring that families can safely and comfortably care for their recovering loved ones is a central nursing responsibility. Preparing for and ensuring a smooth and safe patient-family transition is another way that nurses can extend their care to include both the patient and the family (Mahrer Imhof, 2003).

SUMMARY

We have sought in this chapter to highlight important, yet often taken-for-granted, judgment and relational skills which nurses use daily in their interactions with patients and families. While nursing schools are beginning to introduce more relational and family content in their curricula, much work is still needed (Benner, Sutphen, Leonard & Day, 2010). As such, nurses continue to learn and refine their skills through trial and error learning in specific situations and by exposure to the role-modeling of others. By presenting nursing narratives that point to three central aspects of family care—ensuring that the family can be with the patient, providing the family with information and support, and encouraging family involvement in caregiving activities—we hope to transmit and extend acute and critical care nurses' family care practices.

REFERENCES

Ballard, J. L., Maloney, M., Shank, M., & Hollister, L. (1984). Sibling visits to a newborn intensive care unit: Implications for siblings, parents, and infants. *Child Psychiatry and Human Development, 14*(4), 203–214.

Ballard, K. S. (1981). Identification of environmental stressors for patients in a surgical intensive care unit. *Issues in Mental Health Nursing, 3,* 89–108.

Barratt, F. & Wallis, D. N. (1998). Relatives in the resuscitation room: Their point of view. *Journal of Accident & Emergency Medicine, 15*(2), 109–111.

Bauchner, H., Vinci, R., Waring, C. (1989). Experience and reason: Briefly recorded. *Pediatrics, 84,* 907–909.

Bauchner, H., Waring, C. & Vinci, R. (1991). Parental presence during procedures in an emergency room: Results from 50 observations. *Pediatrics, 87,* 544–548.

Bauchner, H., Vinci, R., Bak, S., Pearson, C., Corwin, M. J. (1996). Parents and procedures: A randomized controlled trial. *Pediatrics, 98,* 861–886.

Bay, E. J., Kupferschmidt, B., Opperwall, B. J., & Speer, J. (1988). Effect of the family visit on the patient's mental status. *Focus on Critical Care, 15*(1), 10–16.

Benner, P. (1994). The role of articulation in understanding practice and experience as sources of knowledge in clinical nursing. In J. Tully (Ed.), *Philosophy in an age of pluralism: The philosophy of Charles Taylor in question* (pp. 136–155). New York, NY: Cambridge University Press.

Benner, P., Tanner, C. A., & Chesla, C. A. (2009). *Expertise in nursing practice: Caring, clinical judgment, and ethics* (2nd Ed.). New York, NY: Springer Publishing Company.

Benner, P., Sutphen, M., Leonard, V., & Day, L. (2010). *Educating nurses: A call for radical transformation.* San Francisco, CA: Jossey-Bass.

Berry, L. L. (1999). *Discovering the soul of service: The nine drivers of sustainable business success.* New York, NY: Free Press.

Boie, E. T., Moore, G. P., Brurmett, C., & Nelson, D.R. (1999). Do parents want to be present during invasive procedures performed on their children in the emergency department? A survey of 400 parents. *Annals of Emergency Medicine, 34,* 70–74.

Bru, G., Carmody, S., Donohue-Sword, B., & Bookbinder, M. (1993). Parental visitation in the postanesthesia care unit: A means to lessen anxiety. *Child Health Care, 22*(3), 217–226.

Burfitt, S. N., Greiner, D. S., Miers, L. J., Kinney, M. R., & Branyon, M. E. (1993). Professional nurse caring as perceived by critically ill patients: A phenomenologic study. *American Journal of Critical Care, 2,* 489–499.

Burke, C. N., Voepel-Lewis, T., Hadden, S., DeGrandis, M., Skotcher, S., D'Agostino, R., Walton, S., & Malviya, S. (2009). Parental presence on emergence: Effect on postanesthesia agitation and parent satisfaction. *Journal of Perianesthesia Nursing, 24*(4), 216–221.

Byers, J. F., Bridges, S., Kijek, J., & LaBorde, P. (2001). Burn patients' pain and anxiety experiences. *Journal of Burn Care and Rehabilitation, 22,* 144–149.

Chan, G. (2005). Understanding end-of-life caring practices in the emergency department: Developing Merleau-Ponty's notions of intentional arc and maximum grip through praxis and phronesis. *Nursing Philosophy 6,* 19–32.

Chesla, C. A. (1996). Reconciling technologic and family care in critical-care nursing. *Image, 28*(3), 199–203.

Chesla, C. A., & Stannard, D. (1997). Breakdown in the nursing care of families in the ICU. *American Journal of Critical Care, 6*(1), 64–71.

Coulter, M. A. (1989). The needs of family members of patients in intensive care units. *Intensive Care Nursing, 5,* 4–10.

Darbyshire, P. (1994). *Living with a sick child in hospital: The experiences of parents and nurses.* London, England: Chapman & Hall.

DiSalvo, H., Haiduven, D., Johnson, N, Reyes, V. V., Hench, C. P., Shaw, R. & Stevens, D. A. (2005). Who let the dogs out? Infection control did: Utility of dogs in health care settings and infection control aspects. *American Journal of Infection Control, 34*(5), 301–307.

Doerr, B. C., & Jones, J. W. (1979). Effect of family preparation on the state anxiety level of the CCU patient. *Nursing Research, 28*(5), 315–316.

Doyle, C. J., Post, H., Burney, R. E., Maino, J., Keefe, M., & Rhee, K. J. (1987). Family participation during resuscitation: An option. *Annals of Emergency Medicine, 16*(6), 673–675.

Duran, C. R., Oman, K. S., Abel, J. J., Koziel, V. M., & Szymanski, D. (2007). Attitudes toward and beliefs about family presence: A survey of healthcare providers, patients' families, and patients. *American Journal of Critical Care, 16*(3), 270–282.

Eichhorn, D., Meyers, T., Guzzetta, C., Clark, A., Klein, J., & Calvin, A. (2001). Family presence during invasive procedures and resuscitation: Hearing the voice of the patient. *American Journal of Nursing, 101,* 48–55.

Fiorentini, S. E. (1993). Evaluation of a new program: Pediatric parental visitation in the postanesthesia care unit. *Journal of Perianesthesia Nursing, 8*(4), 249–256.

Fraser, S., & Atkins, J. (1990). Survivors' recollections of helpful and unhelpful emergency nurse activities surrounding sudden death of a loved one. *Journal of Emergency Nursing, 16*(1), 13–16.

Fuller, B. F. & Foster, G. M. (1982). The effects of family/friend visits vs. staff interaction on stress/arousal of surgical intensive care patients. *Heart & Lung, 11*(5), 457–463.

Fumagalli, S., Bonicinelli, L., Lo Nostro, A., Valdoti, P., Baldereschi, G., Di Bari, M., Ungar, A., Baldasseroni, S., Geppetti, P., Massetti, G., Pini, R., & Marchionni, N. (2006). Reduced cardiocirculatory complications with unrestrictive visiting policy in an intensive care unit: Results from a pilot, randomized trial. *Circulation, 113,* 946–952.

Garrouste-Orgeas, M., Philippart, F., Timsit, J. F., Diaw, F., Willems, V., Tabah, A., Bretteville, G., Verdavainne, A., Misset, B., & Carlet, J. (2008). Perceptions of a 24-hour visiting policy in the intensive care unit. *Critical Care Medicine, 36*(1), 30–35.

Glaser, B. G., & Strauss, A. L. (1965). *Awareness of dying.* Chicago: Aldine.

Hammond, F. (1995). Involving families in care within the intensive care environment: A descriptive survey. *Intensive and Critical Care Nursing, 1,* 256–264.

Hampe, S. (1975). Needs of the grieving spouse in the hospital setting. *Nursing Research, 2,* 113–119.

Hanson, C., & Strawser, D. (1992). Family presence during cardiopulmonary resuscitation: Foote hospital emergency department's nine-year perspective. *Journal of Emergency Nursing, 18*(2), 104–106.

Harder, B. (2001). Opening the curtain. *U.S. News & World Report, 131*(9), 64.

Hendrickson, S. L. (1987). Intracranial pressure changes and family presence. *Journal of Neuroscience Nursing, 19*(1), 14–17.

Hepworth, J. T., Hendrickson, S. G., & Lopez, J. (1994). Time series analysis of physiological response during ICU visitation. *Western Journal of Nursing Research, 16*(6), 704–717.

Hickey, M. (1990). What are the needs of families of critically ill patients? A review of the literature since 1976. *Heart & Lung, 19*(401–415).

Holland, C., Cason, C. L., & Prater, L. R. (1997). Patients' recollections of critical care. *Dimensions of Critical Care Nursing, 16*(3), 132–141.

Kelly, P., Benner, P., Benner, R., Kenny, D. J. (2010). Nursing clinical knowledge development: an approach for continuity of care for war injured service members. "Analysis of Family Participation in Care" Federal Tri-Service Research Grant. In Progress.

Kleman, M., Bickert, A., Karpinski, A., Wantz, D., Jacobsen, B., Lowery, B., & Menapace, F. (1993). Physiologic responses of coronary care patients to visiting. *Journal of Cardiovascular Nursing, 7*(3), 52–62.

Kowba, M. D., & Schwirian, P. M. (1985). Direct sibling contact and bacterial colonization in newborns. *Journal of Obstetric, Gynecologic, and Neonatal Nursing, 14*(5), 412–417.

Lardner, D. R., Dick, B. D., & Crawford, S. (2010). The effects of parental presence in the postanesthetic care unit on children's postoperative behavior: A prospective, randomized, controlled study. *Anesthesia-Analgesia, 110,* 1102–1108.

Lazure, L. L. & Baun, M. M. (1995). Increasing patient control of family visiting in the coronary care unit. *American Journal of Critical Care, 4*(2), 157–164.

Lewis, M., Bendersky, M., Koons, A., Hegyi, T., Hiatt, I. M., Ostfeld, B., & Rosenfeld, D. (1991). Visitation to a neonatal intensive care unit. *Pediatrics, 88*(4), 795–800.

Li, H., Stewart, B. J., Imle, M. A., Archbold, P. G., & Felver, L. (2000). Families and hospitalized elders: A typology of family care actions. *Research in Nursing & Health, 23,* 3–16.

Litman, T. J. (1974). The family as a basic unit in health and medical care: A social-behavioral overview. *Social Science in Medicine, 8,* 495–519.

Mangurten, J., Scott, S. H., Guzzetta, C. E., Clark, A. P., Vinson, L., Sperry, J., Hicks, B., & Voelmeck, W. (2006). Effects of family presence during resuscitation and invasive procedures in a pediatric emergency department. *Journal of Emergency Nursing, 32*(3), 225–233.

Mahrer Imhof, R. (2003). Couples' experience of living with cardiac disease: An interpretive phenomenological study. (Unpublished Doctoral Dissertation, University of California, San Francisco.)

Mazer, M. A., Cox, L. A., & Capon, J. A. (2006). The public's attitude and perception concerning witnessed cardiopulmonary resuscitation. *Critical Care Medicine, 34*(12), 1–4.

Meyers, T. A., Eichhorn, D. J., & Guzzetta, C. E. (1998). Do families want to be present during CPR? A retrospective survey. *Journal of Emergency Nursing, 24*(5), 400–405.

Meyers, T., A., Eichhorn, D. J., Guzzetta, C. E., Clark, A. P., Klein, J. D., Taliaferro, E., & Calvin, A. (2000). Family presence during invasive procedures and resuscitation: The experience of family members, nurses, and physicians. *American Journal of Nursing, 100*(2), 32–43.

Mitchell, M., Chaboyer, W., Burmeister, E., & Foster, M. (2009). Positive effects of a nursing intervention on family-centered care in adult critical care. *American Journal of Critical Care, 18*(6), 543-552.

Moore, K. A., Coker, K., DuBuisson, A. B., Swett, B., & Edwards, W. H. (2003). Implementing potentially better practices for improving family-centered care in neonatal intensive care units: Successes and challenges. *Pediatrics, 111* (4 pt 2), e450-460.

Nicholson, A. C., Titler, M., Montgomery, L. A., Kleiber, C., Craft, M. J., Halm, M., Buckwalter, K., & Johnson, S. (1993). Effects of child visitation in adult critical care units: A pilot study. *Heart & Lung, 22*(1), 36-45.

Nyamathi, A. M. (1988). Perceptions of factors influencing the coping of wives of myocardial infarction patients. *Journal of Cardiovascular Nursing, 2*(4), 65-76.

Oehler, J. M., & Vileisis, R. A. (1990). Effect of early sibling visitation in an intensive care nursery. *Developmental and Behavioral Pediatrics, 11*(1), 7-12.

Paludetto, R., Faggiano-Perfetto, M., Asprea, A. M., Curtis, M. D., & Margara-Paludetto, P. (1981). Reactions of sixty parents allowed unrestricted contact with infants in a neonatal intensive care unit. *Early Human Development, 5,* 401-409.

Powers, K. S. & Rubenstein, J. S. (2006). Family presence during invasive procedures in the pediatric intensive care unit: A prospective study. *Archives of Pediatric & Adolescent Medicine, 153,* 955-958.

Prins, M. M. (1989). The effect of family visits on intracranial pressure. *Western Journal of Nursing Research, 11*(3), 281-297.

Proctor, D. L. (1987). Relationship between visitation policy in a pediatric intensive unit and parental anxiety. *Child Health Care, 16*(1), 13-17.

Roberts, D. W. (2003). Privacy and confidentiality: The Health Insurance Portability and Accountability Act in critical care nursing. *AACN Clinical Issues: Advanced Practice and Acute Care, 14*(3), 302-309.

Schulte, D. A., Burrell, L. O., Gueldner, S. H., Bramlett, M. H., Fuszard, B, Stone, S. K., & Dudley, W. N. (1993). Pilot study of the relationship between heart rate and ectopy and unrestricted vs. restricted visiting hours in the coronary care unit. *American Journal of Critical Care, 2*(2), 134-136.

Schwab, F., Tolbert, B., Bagnato, S., & Maisels, M. J. (1983). Sibling visitation in a neonatal intensive care unit. *Pediatrics, 71*(5), 835-838.

Simpson, T. & Shaver, J. (1990). Cardiovascular responses to family visits in coronary care patients. *Heart & Lung, 19*(4), 344-351.

Solheim, K., & Spellacy, C. (1988). Sibling visitation: Effects on newborn infection rates. *Journal of Obstetric, Gynecologic, and Neonatal Nursing, 17*(1), 43-48.

Stannard, D. (1997). *Reclaiming the house: An interpretive study of nurse-family interactions and activities in critical care.* (Unpublished doctoral dissertation, University of California, San Francisco.)

Stillwell, S. B. (1984). Importance of visiting needs as perceived by family members of patients in the intensive care unit. *Heart & Lung, 13*(3), 238-242.

Tanner, C. A., Benner, P., Chesla, C., & Gordon, D. R. (1993). The phenomenology of knowing a patient. *Image, 25*(4), 273-280.

Umphenour, J. H. (1980). Bacterial colonization in neonates with sibling visitation. *Journal of Obstetric, Gynecologic, and Neonatal Nursing, 9*(2), 73-75.

Warren, N. A. (1994). The phenomena of nurses' caring behaviors as perceived by the critical care family. *Critical Care Nursing Quarterly, 17*(3), 67-72.

Wranesh, B. L. (1982). The effect of sibling visitation on bacterial colonization rate in neonates. *Journal of Obstetric, Gynecologic, and Neonatal Nursing, 11*(4), 211-213.

Yu, Y. H., Jamieson, J., & Astbury, J. (1981). Parents' reactions to unrestricted parental contact with infants in the intensive care nursery. *Medical Journal of Australia, 1,* 294-296.

Zawatski, E., Katz, B., & Krekeler, K. (1979). Perceived needs and satisfaction with nursing care by spouses of patients in the coronary care unit. *Perceptual and Motor Skills, 49,* 170.

8

Preventing Hazards in a Technological Environment

Nearly 100 years ago, the first ICU opened its doors to care for critically ill patients (Hilberman,1975). Since then, critical care areas have evolved into the most intricately designed and technologically complicated settings in inpatient facilities (O'Donnell, 1990). Concurrently, acute care areas, which were originally designed to be technologically sparse, have taken on an increasingly medicalized, specialized, and technologically sophisticated character. Technology, thus, is a taken-for-granted backdrop in healthcare today, ranging from the commonly used (e.g., automated supply and medication cabinets) to the esoteric (e.g., automated anesthesia system named McSleepy [McGill University, 2008]) and includes everything in between. Scientific and technologic advances have enabled clinicians to cure, in many cases, what was once incurable.

As technology proliferates, the nurse, who is the front line user of the technology, must be in active dialogue with engineers and technicians about the impact of technology on the nurse's overall vigilance and grasp of the patient's needs and clinical status. For example, now that a new standard of practice is to tightly monitor and control blood sugars, to what extent does this new monitoring and control interfere with other technical monitoring and interventions? Human-technology interface is always an issue. The technology must be designed so that it does not exceed the user's attention span and ability to respond, or show up as a distraction.

The classic often used example from the Movie "Top Gun" is that of the "top gun" pilots' cockpit that was designed to facilitate the pilots' expertise rather than inhibit it. Cockpit design included measurements and instrumentation readings that, at one time, exceeded the pilots' ability to use or even process the level of complex information while skillfully flying the plane. In the hospital, informatics automation goes too far when the computerized information management disrupts the nurse's use of paper and pencil as a strategy for remembering her or his patients, or provides too much information to be processed or made accessible in fast paced clinical practice arenas.

Technology is never without risk and/or possibility. As one of the nurses in our original study stated in relation to patient well-being and technology use, "If technology is not helping, it is usually hindering or even threatening the patient's progress." New technologies usually raise new clinical and ethical considerations. For example, some clinicians may continue to have the monitor screen and sounds on when a patient is actively dying and only palliative care is being given. The monitor serves as an intrusive disruption of a quiet and respectful

TABLE 8.1
Preventing Hazards in a Technological Environment

▨ Performing practical technology assessments

▨ Engaging in safety work

▨ Effective use and assessment of performance of technical devices

relational human space between family members' and patient's last moments because it unwittingly shifts their attention to the technology instead of towards the patient. A crucial orienting component of acute and critical care nursing practice is preventing both actual and potential hazards in the technological environment, since technology use is never without risk.

Technology is so pervasive in acute and critical care areas that it is often difficult to even recognize a therapy or device as a technological "thing" when it is commonly used in daily practice. Take, for instance, the stethoscope: before its invention, clinicians relied on basic patient assessment skills, such as inspection, palpation, percussion and listening directly to the chest for heart sounds. However, once developed, the stethoscope provided clinicians with a new assessment parameter, namely, auscultation. Few clinicians today, however, think of the stethoscope as a piece of technology. Thus, technology is on a continuum that ranges from time-tested "things" that have been extensively studied and judged to be safe (e.g., a nasal cannula for oxygen) to "things" that seem very hazardous with a great potential for causing patient/provider complications (e.g., an aerosolized experimental drug with carcinogenic and teratogenic warnings). We are defining technology broadly to include any drug, instrument, device, machine, or treatment that is used in the care or support of an acute or critically ill patient. Given the right set of circumstances, even safe technologies can present hazards or cause harm (Titler, 1993). The purpose of this chapter is to describe the nursing knowledge, judgment, and skilled know-how surrounding the use and management of technology, which includes three central patient safety requirements for nurses listed in Table 8.1.

Because these aspects of practice are all related to the safe and prudent use of technology, they frequently overlap, as illustrated in the following example from an experienced advanced practice nurse who works as a clinical nurse specialist (CNS) in a medical ICU. As background to the story, the CNS became aware of esophageal manometry, which was a new technology that measured mechanically ventilated patients' work of breathing. After a thorough review of the scientific literature and extensive discussions with the manufacturer and end-users at other facilities, the CNS wrote a proposal to purchase the monitoring device for use with select patients:

Advanced Practice Nurse: We had a patient who failed every weaning attempt, despite the fact that we were using a weaning protocol that we had developed and researched several years ago. There are a lot of theories about the best weaning approach, but I think the consensus at this time is that it isn't always the specific strategy as much as whether one uses a consistent approach... But this patient had failed multiple weaning attempts and the medical team continued to use the same strategy, thinking that somehow the patient was going to turn around and get off the ventilator.

One of the things that I noticed when I went into the patient's room is that she was very tachypneic. She has been on the ventilator for well over a month and was clearly dependent to the point that a tracheostomy had already been performed. She had very high resting ventilation requirements. Her minute ventilation was somewhere around 15 to 20/liters a minute—and that's a high ventilation requirement by <u>anyone's</u> standard. They were using a weaning strategy for her that works in the majority of our patients, where we gradually reduce the rate of ventilatory support in a stepwise fashion over a period of time. And then there's the clinical assessment that is done on a daily basis and in between the step changes to make sure that the patient is tolerating the wean. One of our terminating criteria for these weaning trials is an increased and sustained respiratory rate.

This lady was breathing around 35 times a minute. And I remembered that she had a high resting minute ventilation. My first thought was, 'She's not going to come off the ventilator if she's requiring that kind of support.' So I asked to have her respiratory mechanics repeated, where we measure spontaneous tidal volume off the ventilator completely. Her vital capacity, negative inspiratory force, and other parameters—with the exception of her high respiratory rate and the high minute ventilation—were within the normal range...

So I suggested using the respiratory mechanics monitor, which actually involves placing a nasogastric tube (NG) with an esophageal balloon in the patient, so that we could quantify her work of breathing. And I'm not a really strong proponent of technology just because it's available. Its availability shouldn't dictate its need or use. The clinical assessment is really the most important. But when you're sitting on the fence and you've tried what you normally do and that doesn't work, it isn't <u>unreasonable</u> to think of other approaches... I didn't want to put something in her nose if she really didn't need it. On the other hand, I thought these measurements might give us some information that we were missing in order to wean this patient from the ventilator. So, everyone was agreeable to try to quantify her work of breathing... We placed the NG and the patient's <u>resting</u> work of breathing, as I recall, was much higher than a usual workload. So we abandoned the standardized weaning strategy and we put the patient on a pressure support mode only. We increased the level of pressure support so that her work of breathing was within a normal range. And the medical team, more or less, went with whatever parameters I gave them because they didn't understand this device. So rather than titrating her ventilatory support to her respiratory rate and minute ventilation, we titrated the level of pressure support based on what we considered to be a 'tolerable workload' for the patient. Now the problem with that is that the normal physiologic range for work of breathing is based on normals. And this patient's workload may be higher than normal, but it still may be tolerable. So, we used a visual analog scale to get feedback from the patient as to what work of breathing was tolerable for her. This was a 100 millimeter visual analog scale, and 100 was the worst or least tolerable and 0 was the best or most tolerable... So we titrated the level of pressure support down in slow increments based on her monitored work of breathing and her feedback from the visual analog scales...

We also used other strategies. We made sure the nursing staff understood the importance of getting her out of bed every day, and we were more aggressive with her physical therapy. Because physical therapy is a consult service, if they think a patient isn't 'stable,' they sometimes sort of back off. So patients can fall through the cracks unless people call them and get them back onto the case. In any event, the patient wound up weaning off the ventilator over the course of about a week and a half.

I'm not certain that it was the respiratory mechanics monitor that we used, because her work of breathing never really got within a normal range... But as we backed off on the pressure support, her work of breathing seemed to plateau and her level of dyspnea didn't worsen... I'm also not certain that if I <u>wasn't</u> there, this <u>wouldn't</u> have occurred... But I don't think her work of breathing would have been monitored, and it's hard to know whether physical therapy would have gotten more actively involved independently or if somebody else would have stepped in and recommended it. By intervening, I think I played a part in accelerating this patient's [recovery].

This exemplar highlights many aspects of expert nursing practice and, in particular, illustrates safe and tailored use of technology. Because the patient had a high respiratory rate and minute ventilation, the CNS grasped that the standardized weaning protocol was not going to work with this particular patient. The nurse's in-depth knowledge of respiratory physiology and pulmonary pathophysiology, together with his knowledge about the new technology, enabled him to suggest and implement an alternative weaning approach. Abandoning the standard weaning protocol was not without risk and required clinical judgment, communication skills, innovation, and a firm grasp of the clinical situation.

Since the CNS had more familiarity with the new device than the rest of the healthcare team, he guided clinicians in titrating the amount of pressure support to the patient's monitored responses. This required the nurse to impart his skilled know-how to others in terms of safely managing the monitoring device and interpreting its data in relation to the patient's experience. By eliciting patient feedback using a visual analog scale, clinicians could ascertain whether or not the increased work of breathing was tolerable to the patient.

The patient's successful wean from mechanical ventilation after a month of ventilator dependency is testimony to the balance of both high-tech and low-tech interventions. Although this patient was an excellent candidate for the new monitoring device, the nurse carefully evaluated using yet another piece of technology. The nurse's maxim "the availability [of technology] shouldn't dictate its need or use" guided his practical technology assessment. The human costs and risks to placing a NG tube with an esophageal balloon for monitoring purposes were weighed against the benefit of more information. Low-tech interventions, such as getting the patient out of bed daily and instituting an aggressive program of physical therapy, were as important as the high-tech monitoring device and ultimately assisted the patient in weaning from the ventilator. While the safety practices related to technology use generally overlap in expert practice as they did in this example, to best articulate distinctions and highlight how each is central to protecting patients from technological hazards, the aspects will be discussed separately.

PERFORMING PRACTICAL TECHNOLOGY ASSESSMENTS

A practical technology assessment can be defined as weighing the risks and benefits of a given technological intervention with a particular patient by assessing the actual and potential side effects and possible sequelae, as well as the ongoing critical evaluation to determine if a technological intervention is appropriate or useful for a particular patient. Technological interventions must be critically evaluated in order to prevent technological proliferation (Stannard, 1995). A practical (or informal) technology assessment differs from a formal evaluation, in that, a formal technology assessment is the "process of designing and conducting investigations which enable reasoned judgment regarding efficacious, effective, and efficient patient care" (Sibbald, Eberhard, Inman & Sprung, 1993, p. 1778).

Healthcare spending in 2008 rose to $2.4 trillion or 17% of the gross domestic product and it is expected to rise to 20% of the gross national product by 2017 (Pennington & DeRienzo, 2010). The sheer cost of our current system, coupled with unacceptable patient outcomes in some areas/patient populations, underscores the importance of rigorous and systematic formal technology assessments and outcomes research to help guide clinicians' purchasing decisions and technology utilization (Stannard, 2011). At the federal level, the Agency for Healthcare Research and Quality (AHRQ) devotes a large amount of funding to support research projects that assess the clinical utility of medical technologies and interventions. On a more local level, many healthcare facilities utilize third party services, such as the ECRI Institute, to assist with value and efficacy analysis. Additionally, more clinicians are routinely turning to databases such as Cochrane Collaboration, Campbell Collaboration, and the Joanna Briggs Institute for evidence-based guidance.

While formal and rigorous scientific evaluation of technology is essential, as are comprehensive systematic reviews that guide evidence-based practice, so too are the continual practical technology assessments nurses conduct directly with patients. Practical technology assessments ensure tailored and reasoned use of appropriate technology for particular patients so that patient needs and the goals of therapy shape technology use rather than vice versa. This is distinguished from formal technology assessments which are based on large cohorts of patients and comprehensive systematic reviews which are syntheses of many research trials. We believe that practical technology assessments assist clinicians' in their ability to meet the commonsensical—yet oftentimes hard to attain—goal from the Centers for Medicare and Medicaid Services (CMS), namely, to make sure patients get the right care at the right time. We describe everyday technology assessments in order to improve thinking-in-action related to technology use and to link these informal assessments to more formal technology assessments and outcomes research.

A common practical technology assessment is limiting unnecessary and unwarranted intervention. In an excerpt cited in Benner, Tanner, and Chesla (2009, p. 164), a nurse describes caring for a patient who required mechanical ventilation for an acute exacerbation of chronic obstructive pulmonary disease (COPD):

> **Nurse:** She was trached and we were actively weaning her. We put her on a mask for about 10 hours during the day and then put her back on the vent at night. They had an A-line [arterial line] in her for about 50 days and were planning to put in a new one. I said, 'Why are you putting an A-line in her? She doesn't need one.' 'Well, she's vented—she needs to have one.' I said, 'No, one machine does not give you the criteria to put in a line. We know what her gases are. We know when she's going to get into trouble. She tells us by other parameters'.

Because this nurse had worked with the patient before, she knew the patient's responses and understood when the patient was "going to get into trouble." By convincing the medical team to follow the patient's embodied parameters or physiologic and behavioral indicators of impending respiratory failure (e.g., rapid, shallow breathing, fatigue, and anxiety), the nurse was able to prevent an invasive and uncomfortable procedure that was no longer needed to monitor or manage the patient's condition. The nurse's clinical and ethical grasp of the patient situation prevented possible patient complications stemming from the placement of an indwelling arterial line, such as infection, thrombosis, limited mobility, discomfort, unnecessary daily blood loss, and further trauma to the patient's radial arteries. Limiting unwarranted intervention in this case also helped to control costs, although the nurse's actions were, first and foremost, driven by the needs and demands of this particular patient. By increasing the reliability and appropriateness of technology use, practical technology assessments may secondarily reduce costs.

As with the previous example, more technology is not always better, nor is it the solution to every problem. Each new monitoring device provides clinicians with more data, some of which is interesting or redundant but oftentimes not essential. East (1992), for instance, found over 235 different categories of information at a critically ill patient's bedside one morning on rounds. A breaking point is quickly reached when there is simply too much patient data for clinicians to interpret and manage. Information technology should be designed to increase clinicians' grasp of the situation and attentiveness to and engagement with the patient. An overabundance of patient data can overwhelm the clinician or demand too much attention away from the patient's concerns and clinical signs and symptoms. A maxim that can guide intelligent and wise utilization of technology is to use technology when the data provided will likely change or direct the course of treatment.

In another example, an experienced neonatal ICU nurse recalls an incident in which her knowledge of predictable infant transitions guided her judgment in limiting several unnecessary interventions:

Nurse: This case involved 36-week-old twins who were both admitted to the ICN. One of the medical residents mentioned that one of the babies' lungs 'sounded really junky' and that his 'color wasn't right.' About that time I had walked up to the bedside and was helping the nurse do a few things. So I asked the resident if the baby had been deep suctioned over in the delivery room. He said, 'Well, no.' Meanwhile, he was asking for a tray to put in an [umbilical arterial] line and he wanted to put the baby under a 30% hood. I just kept looking at the baby. His respiratory effort was really minimal and I was thinking, 'This kid is not sick.' So I hesitated and the resident looked at me like, 'You know, you need to hurry up.' Well, I didn't hurry because I didn't feel like I needed to hurry. So I deep suctioned the baby and I asked the resident to listen. I said, 'Why don't you listen and see if he sounds any better?' So he listened and said, 'Do you really think you suctioned the lungs?' And I said, 'No, I know I didn't suction his lungs. I suctioned behind the trachea and down his stomach.' And I said, 'One thing I've learned over the years is that sound sometimes radiates to the lungs, so that you think they sound junky when they're not. So if you deep suction a C-section baby, all of a sudden they sound clear and they don't need chest percussion and things like that.' He looked at me and said something about, 'Well, I guess you're right.' But the nice thing about that case was that there were three nursing students standing at the bedside, taking it all in. I think had it been somebody who had been right out of school or had been a nursery nurse for only a few years, they might have immediately gotten the hood and put the line in the baby. But the baby would have weaned to room air in a matter of minutes... So I felt really good about that because the baby didn't need oxygen, didn't need a line, and proceeded to do quite well.

Knowing certain clinical facts (e.g., that the baby was a C-section baby who had not been deep suctioned) and using expert assessment skills enabled this nurse to understand that the baby was not in acute respiratory distress. Although the nurse intervened by suctioning the baby's esophagus, her single intervention successfully averted more traumatic interventions, such as the placement of an umbilical arterial line, the initiation of oxygen therapy, and aggressive pulmonary toilet. By clearly articulating her rationale and concerns, the nurse shared her experiential wisdom with the physician and modeled a practical technology assessment for the student nurses.

Another maxim nurses taught us is: if a technological device is not helping, it is probably hurting (Benner, Tanner & Chesla, 2009). In the next example, an ICU nurse describes a chronic critically ill patient for whom a technological device was no longer useful:

> **Nurse:** We had a patient in our unit for exactly six months, and we were trying to gear him, not so much to be discharged, but to at least be transferred to a facility closer to his home. He was on a low flow air bed for five out of the six months, and I was trying to get him to achieve some more normalcy in his life. Even though nurses often make the decision to put patients on those beds, they forget to take them off those beds. It took a lot of red tape just to get him off of this bed. I find that when the patients are really sick, those beds don't bother them. But when patients start feeling better, they don't really like those beds. So I got him off of that bed, and I saw a big change in him over the next week. He became a lot more independent because he was more able to control his environment. That was my intention from the beginning. He could push a button and move himself about, and he could get in and out of the bed more easily... I could see him more reality oriented because he had sheets under him, and he started to participate more in his care... We all assume that low flow air beds are a wonderful thing because they're great for the skin, but there is a point where I think they are not therapeutic. Patients can't hear well while they are on them, it's hard for them to move around, and it's not a natural environment.

While low flow air beds can help in preventing skin breakdown, like any other technological intervention, they are not without risk to the patient. Recognizing that the patient was no longer benefiting from the specialty bed, the nurse transferred him into a regular patient bed and saw a dramatic improvement. For this patient, the high-tech bed represented critical illness and dependence. Technology dependency has great symbolic power to make the patient feel helpless and estranged from her or his everyday world. The feel, taste, and touch of everyday life beckons the patient into the familiar world, thereby diminishing institutionalization and dependency. Being in a regular bed increased the patient's activity level and engagement with the world, and helped the patient to realize that he was, in fact, getting better. By eliminating an intervention that had outlived its usefulness, the nurse assisted the patient in moving one step closer to wellness, both physically and mentally.

It is becoming more common to have dedicated rounds in acute and critical care areas to assess the usefulness and appropriateness for select technological interventions, such as central lines and urinary catheters. As this nurse so astutely observed, "nurses often make the decision to put patients on those beds, [but] they forget to take them off those beds." The same holds true for many types of technological devices commonly used in inpatient areas. Ensuring that clinicians round with purpose and assess the utility of technological interventions for each patient is an excellent way to remove unnecessary technology, prevent technology-associated complications, and reduce cost.

Weighing the costs and benefits of any given technological intervention with a particular patient is a critical aspect of a practical technology assessment and informs its appropriate and ethical use. A number of nurses working in maternity areas described early maternal struggles with breastfeeding and the inevitable discussions regarding bottle vs. breast. In each expert example, the maternity nurses made suggestions based on what would work best for that particular mother and baby in that situation. Kathy Giannelli, describes a new mother who also wanted to breastfeed her new baby, but was having difficulties:

> **Nurse:** When I got into the patient's room for the first time that day, the mom was already trying to nurse the baby again. I asked her if she had gotten any sleep even though I already knew the answer. She had that bleary eyed look that a lot of sleep deprived moms have. She said, 'Not really, the baby was breastfeeding almost every two hours and he cries all the time. I can't be doing it right. I don't think he's getting enough. I think he's starving!' Her eyes started to fill up at this point and she started to cry. I said, 'That's not true. It takes three days for your breast milk to come in and until that happens, the little bit of colostrum or first milk that the baby gets is all he needs...But, I will have a lactation consultant come in to help you.' She said, 'Someone was in yesterday and when I asked her if it would be alright to give [my baby] a little formula, the lactation consultant said, 'Absolutely not! You should only breastfeed him. A bottle will cause nipple confusion and it isn't good for the baby.' Then [the mom] said, 'I feel like I'm such a bad mother. I'm so tired and my nipples are cracked and sore...I don't know what to do. I don't think I can do this.' By this time, she was really crying and trying to feed the baby at the same time. I sat down on the bed, hugged her, and said, 'You know, some of the lactation consultants can be very rigid and unbending on what is right and wrong in breastfeeding. Others are very flexible. This is your baby. You can do what you want to do. Usually, we tell moms that if they want to breastfeed, it is very important to try to have the baby nurse to stimulate milk production but then you can supplement the feeding with a half ounce of formula if the baby doesn't seem satisfied. I can get you something to help with the soreness and we can also help get the baby latched on right so that your nipples don't get worse... Most of the time, there is really no right or wrong way to do things...You have to do what is right for you, your husband, and your baby...If you really want to breastfeed, stick with it. You can give the baby bottles occasionally—it won't hurt him. But, breastfeeding isn't for everybody, so don't ever let anyone make you feel like you're a bad mother if you choose not to breastfeed. Try not to worry too much about what is right or wrong—just love him.'

This incident shows response-based practice at its best. Kathy shows incredible compassion and reassures and empowers the frightened and tired mother. But instead of pushing the mother toward one method of feeding, the nurse skillfully reminds the new mother that it is her baby and, ultimately, her decision. Over the years, a massive amount of research evidence has been compiled showing that breastfeeding is by far the preferred method of feeding for a multitude of reasons. Yet, not all mothers are able to breastfeed. This mother, like others, is filled with angst and guilt about being a bad mother based on the pedantic stance of the lactation nurse to breastfeed only. Kathy plants the seed that this might be the case in this situation and tries to assuage the maternal guilt. Happily, the new mother was discharged to home with her baby the next day and, while she was still working on her breastfeeding, the baby was crying less and sleeping in between feedings longer. Weighing the costs and benefits in this situation required the nurse to teach, support, and monitor the new mother's progress with breastfeeding, all the while knowing that another intervention might be needed.

Because of the calm, smooth performance of expert nurses like Kathy, it is easy to miss that weighing the costs and benefits involves knowing the research, knowing the patient's situation, and seeing what's possible. Here, evidenced-based practice weighs in favor of breastfeeding. Mindless application of the best knowledge or cutting edge research findings leaves this patient distraught. The expert nurse astutely grasps that a new mother cannot breastfeed well when very anxious and attempting to live up to other's expectations. So, Kathy's most skillful intervention is allaying mother's concerns, empowering her as the mother, and creating a calmer climate where successful breastfeeding is possible. Comfort and compassionate interaction replaces the need and costs of a technological intervention. Further, the intimacy between mother and baby is preserved.

Another maternity nurse, Nancy McClorey, describes a complex patient situation involving a mother who wanted to breastfeed her new baby. Given the intrusion of technology in this new mother's care and the distress experienced as a result, Nancy skillfully tames the environment for all affected while weighing the costs of introducing yet another potentially helpful apparatus. Here, the expert nurse points to her notion of good in guiding her judicious use of technology:

Nurse: Lori was a 30-year-old, G1P1, in her first post-op day following a cesarean section, necessitated by her tachycardia, borderline high BP and elevated thyroid hormone. She had a 5 a.m. consult with Dr. K, an endocrinologist, who ordered blood work, ultrasounds, EKG and a cardiac consult. I met Lori at 8:30, as she had left the floor early for ultrasound. When I first saw her, I recognized an anxious woman who was in pain. Lori was stooped over, guarding her abdomen and grimacing. I first offered Lori pain medication, which she received gratefully, assisted her to the bathroom and then back to bed. While assessing Lori, I asked her about Dr. K's visit. Lori told me she wasn't happy about being woken at 5 a.m. and then told me it left her anxious. "Was she that sick that the doctor needed to come at 5 a.m.?" I explained that, although extremely inconvenient, 5 a.m. was Dr. K's routine time for consults. I reviewed with Lori the tests Dr. K had ordered as I'm sure she was groggy upon just waking at the time of consult. She had already placed a call to her mom who was on the way to the hospital. While I was with her, Lori called her husband. She tried to tell him about the consult, the tests, and what the doctor was looking for. She became a little frustrated and emotional with her husband's questions. Upon her request, I spoke to him to explain Dr. K's "routine" 5 a.m. consult time, the tests ordered and assured him that Lori was very stable.

The transport team arrived to take Lori for a cardiac echo and an EKG before her mom arrived. Lori said her mom would be worried when she arrived, especially if she was not in her room. I promised her I would watch for her mom, introduce myself and reassure her. Lori's mom arrived shortly after Lori had left the floor. I could tell who she was by the worried look on her face. I introduced myself and showed her to Lori's room. She was teary, worried and obviously concerned. She told me "nothing ever seems easy for Lori. Lori had a hard time getting pregnant and now this." I told Lori's mom the timing of the consult was routine for this particular doctor. I assured her Lori was comfortable, very stable, and would return to the floor within the hour. I asked if she would like to see her grandson. She did, so I brought the baby and stayed while she visited with him. I wasn't able to leave the infant with her, I explained, per hospital policy. [After taking] the baby back to the nursery, I took Lori's mom a cup of tea to sip while she awaited her daughter's return.

While Lori was off the floor, I needed to educate myself, as one of the tests ordered for Lori was an adrenal challenge. I was to give Lori an injection of a medication I wasn't familiar with and have her blood drawn pre and a timed post draw. I started with the hospital pharmacy. I read the medication insert the pharmacy sent as requested. I spoke with the pharmacist concerning the likelihood of a reaction and how well the medication was usually received by a patient. I spoke with the med/surg nurse educator. I needed to know if the test was common practice on the med/surg floors and was there anything specific to the test I should be aware of. I also placed a call and spoke to Dr. K. to know in her words what she was looking for with all this testing so I was better able to explain the testing and reason for it to Lori. I was also concerned about breastfeeding after the administering the medication as this was a priority for Lori and the baby would need to be nursed upon Lori's return. The medication was not in Dr. Hale's drug reference book and the manufacturer stated, "transfer unknown. Use with caution." I engaged our lactation consultant at that time. She in fact emailed Dr. Hale, who upon review of the medication offered explanation as to why the med and breastfeeding were not contraindicated. After a phone call to the Pediatrician with this information, I was able to assure Lori on her return that breastfeeding need not be interrupted.

Upon Lori's return, I immediately brought the baby to her, as she had not yet seen him. I gave Lori and her mom some time with their new son/grandson. The blood work still needed to be drawn. I offered explanation of the lab tests as told to me by Dr. K, which educated Lori and her mom and answered their questions so they were more at ease. By noon that day, Lori had all the testing done and could concentrate on her recovery and the infant. Before I left for the day, I made sure Lori knew of her pain management plan that we had discussed earlier. I reviewed her breastfeeding plan for the next 16 hours. I reminded her that Dr. W, a cardiologist would visit her in the early evening as requested by Dr. K. After a bumpy start to the day, Lori was comfortable and more at ease.

During report the next morning, I learned Dr. W had ordered a Holter monitor to be started. So far, all tests were negative, except the continued elevated thyroid hormone. I also learned the infant had "nursed all night" and continued to be "fussy".

Upon greeting Lori this morning, I recognized a tired mom whose priority was to shower. I explained the order for the Holter and let her know I would call the technician to time the start after her shower. After breakfast and her shower, pain in control, Lori was able to focus on breastfeeding, which she continued to say was a priority. When I observed the infant's latch, I noted he was unable to maintain suction for more than a few sucks at a time. I again engaged the lactation consultant, who with Lori's permission set her up with a supplemental nursing system (SNS) as the infant was 48hr+ and was in need of more calories/fluids than provided by his unsustained latch. This intervention proved to be successful, as the infant was able to rest a few hours so was Lori. I also gave Lori an electric breast pump with instructions, to assist her milk production. Before I left for the day, Lori demonstrated both the SNS feeding system and the breast pump. I am careful to introduce this "technology" with breastfeeding as not to overwhelm the mom, but Lori was very receptive and appreciative as her goal was to breastfeed for 6months.

Lori went on to stay 2 more days at the hospital. Her medical condition proved very stable. She was in need of thyroid replacement hormone and encouraged to follow up with her PCP within the first week or two after discharge as this could potentially affect her milk supply…[I inquired and found that] Lori and her new baby were happy, healthy and thriving when they were discharged.

In her exhausted state following birth and a C-section without relief of pain, this new mother was unexpectedly awakened and was faced with a barrage of technology. Not only was the need for technological testing frightening, but it impeded mother's ability to attend to her priority—her newborn son and breastfeeding him. Nancy understands that the benefits of the diagnostic technologies in this instance far outweigh the costs as there could be a significant underlying disease. She responds to the multiple layers of distress by easing mother's pain and then skillfully comforts and educates Lori and her husband about their concerns. Notice that Nancy, like other expert nurses, invests significant effort to reduce the intimidation induced by using multiple needed technologies. She balances the human emotional costs of technology use with exquisite caring practices which include the calming, comforting, and respectful effect of serving tea to grandmother. This expert reveals in her attentiveness and responses that she understands the human costs, even when technology is used in the best of ways. Further, Nancy incredibly responds unreflectively to the feelings of alienation and helplessness that technology can elicit by bringing the newborn grandson which connects grandmother in a strong, practical, and human way. Countering the negative effects of technology with human connection is truly nursing at its very best.

We easily imagine how critical care nurses are constantly faced with taming the technologic environment, but the everyday care of patients throughout other specialties also presents nurses with challenges, as seen above. In the course of a 4-hour morning, Nancy astutely perceived another technology (a medication) that could foil mother's hopes of breastfeeding. She engaged in clinical inquiry about the problems of safe medication administration and its transfer into breast milk as she thoughtfully gained the scientific knowledge needed to ensure safe breastfeeding.

In the midst of the numerous technological and frightening assessments that the mother was experiencing, Nancy remained attuned and noticed the infant was unable to latch on for more than a few seconds at a time, which meant that he did not get the calories and fluids he needed in a 24 hour period. Nancy worked with the Lactation Specialist and also gave the new mother an electric breast pump to assist with milk production. As Nancy told us, "I am careful to introduce this 'technology' with breastfeeding [because] I don't want to overwhelm the mom, but [this patient] was very receptive and appreciative as her goal was to breastfeed for 6 months." Because Nancy had tamed the technological environment and created a realistic comfort with it, the introduction of another technology was well received.

Technology use can also bring about unintended effects that can eclipse any benefits derived from the technological fix. In this next clinical incident, a radiation oncology nurse, Brenda Silvia, was working with a patient and her husband in an outpatient oncology clinic:

> **Nurse:** Beth has metastatic ovarian cancer which is quite evident by the wound on her abdomen. She and her husband presented to my clinic for a consultation regarding how to best manage her pain and copious amounts of drainage. She appeared very well groomed and beautifully dressed. When speaking with her, I felt she kept a distance, both in a physical and emotional sense. It wasn't until the physical exam by the physician that I could see the reason behind Beth's 'distance'. The wound on her abdomen was extremely large and had lots of yellow/green drainage and a <u>horrible</u> odor. I could see the embarrassment on Beth's face when the dressing was removed. She spoke of the great difficulty she had in keeping a dressing in place, the odor under control, and her clothes clean. During the exam, her husband sat quietly in the chair against the wall and appeared totally impassive. After the physical exam by the doctor,

Beth was given time to clean up and then she and her husband would be relocated across the hall to our consultation room to discuss the treatment plan. I moved Beth's husband first. When I was alone with Beth, I asked her if her husband was always this quiet and her response bothered me. She said that he hasn't really been talking much since her disease progressed through her skin. The drainage and the odor issues had become such a problem that they no longer sleep in the same room.

The remainder of the consultation visit progressed as they usually do...I provided Beth and her husband instructions on how to better control her pain, then spoke with them as a couple regarding cancer diagnosis in general and what it can do to families and relationships. I addressed the issue of odor and advised them on several ways to help contain the odor after consulting with our enterostomal therapist on the subject. I was recommending the use of charcoal dressings when the physician came into the room with research articles on the use of honey in controlling wound odor. The patient and her husband seemed skeptical, but agreed to try it as this seemed to be a cheaper alternative to the charcoal dressings. Beth's husband seemed to 'come alive' with the realization that, in addition to the radiation helping to reduce the wound itself, there were other measures that could help with the drainage and odor problems.

Beth's radiation started one week later and on the first day I could tell by the look on her face that something was wrong. I took her into an exam room and she started to cry. The honey was creating a mess for her. It was mixing with the drainage and running down into her clothing, then becoming more sticky as it dried. She didn't know how to tell us that she didn't want to continue with the physician's suggestion. I reassured her that the physician would not be offended and that since we weren't sure how it would work for her, it was ok for her to not continue it. I reminded her that she has the right to refuse any and all treatments suggested to her. I spoke again with the enterostomal therapist regarding any other solutions to the odor problem and the use of P.O. Flagyl was made. This time, it was the physician who was skeptical, but after a little coaxing and a quick review of the literature, he agreed to write the prescription.

About two weeks after the initiation of radiation treatment and being on the Flagyl, Beth's eyes took on a sparkle. She was wearing more fitted clothes and her make-up was just so. I mentioned my observations to her and she confided that she was no longer sleeping alone.

By being open to the patient and family, this nurse was able to hear their concerns and to tailor the healthcare team's interventions to meet those needs. The nurse worked collaboratively with her colleagues to secure what was considered to be the most affordable and effective intervention to deal with the wound drainage and odor. But, the honey was causing other, bigger problems for the patient to manage. This can be thought of as a revenge effect of the technology (Tenner, 1997). Revenge effects are not side effects, but instead can be thought of as unintended effects that detract from or even negate the intended benefits of the technological intervention itself.

When the patient returned to the clinic, the nurse deftly assessed that "something was wrong". Because of the inherent power gradient between patient and provider, the patient did not want to "offend" the physician and risk any repercussions in her life-saving treatments. With her strong ethical bearing and exquisite clinical grasp, the nurse reassured the patient that it was "ok to not continue" while simultaneously performing a practical technology assessment. Through renewed collaborative efforts, the nurse secured a new technological intervention in the form of an oral antibiotic, which not only treated the wound drainage and odor problem, but brought the patient and husband together again with renewed feelings of intimacy and a possibility for health and life.

Because acute and critical care areas are so laden with technology, clinicians can easily succumb to technological faddism. The routine use of pulmonary artery catheters is an example of a technology that was once considered standard treatment for critically ill patients and that has only recently come under formal scrutiny (Shah, Hasselblad, Stevenson, Binanay, O'Connor, Sopko & Califf, 2005). An interview with two OR nurses illustrates the lure of new technology for many of the surgeons with whom they work:

Nurse 1: The surgeons get all these dandy new instruments...and then they want to have them every time. And the more stuff you show them, the more they want. They get kind of megalomaniacal and they want five of these and 10 of those, and, they're like $1200.00 a piece.

Interviewer: So who gets them? And who decides who gets them?

Nurse 2: Well, sometimes what we do is we'll see how often they actually use it before we spend the money.

Nurse 1: And it depends on whether it's expensive.

Nurse 2: The Clinical Nurse IV of the service sits down with the surgeons and asks them what they need for the next year. She then prioritizes by asking them 'How much do you really need it? It would be nice, but can you do cases without it?'

Nurse 1: It all depends on how much it is and what it is.

Nurse 2: And how often they're really going to use it.

Determining whether a new technology will advance patient care is a critical evaluation that, in this particular institution, a clinical nurse with administrative duties helps the surgeons to make. As illustrated above, clinical and ethical issues must be considered when purchasing any new technology, such as its ability to improve or enhance patient care. Other considerations include the immediate and long-term impact the technology will have on the patient, family, and healthcare providers, as well as any down-stream effects, such as the necessity for additional training and changes in staffing that may be required to accommodate the new technology. Thus, pressing into the future and anticipating the technological trajectory when performing a practical technology assessment requires knowledge, clinical judgment, and moral imagination.

While the above example deals with surgeons and the appeal new technologies holds for them, all clinicians in acute and critical care are at risk for getting "swept away" by technology (Tisdale, 1986). By way of example, an ICU nurse told us:

Nurse: You know, technology's great. But I find all the new nurses and orientees are <u>so</u> excited about the equipment. They see an 'exciting' patient as one who is connected to an LVAD (a left ventricular assist device), a balloon pump, and jet ventilation. I tell them, 'This patient is <u>sick</u>. And yes, technology is worthwhile, but, I've seen patients connected to all that [equipment] and they still die.'

Learning to temper unbridled enthusiasm for new gadgets and devices can be achieved by focusing steadfastly on the patient and family rather than the technology. Technology is never an end in itself; therefore, its design and use must be subordinated to patients' and families' needs and concerns. In the above example, the nurse is trying to demythologize technology. As she said, "I've seen patients connected to all that [equipment] and they still die." Overuse and over reliance on technology are more likely if technology is given excessive unexamined, magical powers. Reflectively and carefully assessing each technological intervention in relation to the needs and demands of the particular patient fosters appropriate and ethical use of technology.

When no good solution to a problem exists, a practical approach is to limit the technological interventions to those that are absolutely necessary (Benner, 1994). An example of this follows in which a PACU nurse discusses the use of physical restraints on a recovering patient for whom she had recently cared:

> **Nurse:** I was taking care of an elderly woman, she was about 85, close to 90 [years old], and she had a femoral popliteal bypass. When she came out to me [from the OR] she was intubated. At the time we needed to restrain her because she was very active, and the possibility of extubation was threatening. We then extubated her and she remained restrained, but she was clearly very uncomfortable. I gave her pain medicine, and that helped for a little while, but she really seemed like she wanted to be in a fetal position and the restraints disallowed that. So, I just said, 'I'm going to take the restraints off and see what happens.' I took them off, she tried to get out of bed, I calmed her and petted her back into bed. I told her the rules: she had to stay in bed and if she stayed, I wouldn't have to put any restraints on her. And she was a little lady and not really thrashing that badly, so I just elected to leave the restraints off. Even though it was a little more difficult for me to manage her with them off, I just felt that, for her, the freedom to move her extremities was more important than restraining her. And all I needed to do was every five minutes put her down in the bed. And then her son came, and he was very kind and gentle and loving towards his mother. So I asked him to stay and help me.

The nurse weighed the risks and benefits of using physical restraints, a form of technology, on an elderly patient who was recovering from the effects of general anesthesia. Initially, when the patient was at risk for self-extubation and the nurse's attentions were focused on patient stability, she felt restraints were warranted. However, once the patient was successfully extubated, had received pain medication, and was still uncomfortable, the nurse could no longer justify physical restraints. The nurse admitted that the unrestrained patient was a "little more difficult" to manage, but her ethical and clinical judgment could not justify patient restraints for the sake of nursing convenience. In some situations, there is a fine line between warranted use of physical restraints for the safety of the patient and inappropriate or abusive use. Good judgment is needed to distinguish between the two. Thus, electing to leave the patient unrestrained was both an ethical and clinical decision.

All technological interventions must be weighed judiciously because many interventions can begin a devastating technological cascade, which can be thought of as a self-perpetuating trajectory, usually beginning with a single technological intervention that unleashes a multitude of other problems which need to be treated with still other interventions. One can imagine, for instance, that if left restrained, this patient in the example above might have become more anxious, confused, and combative. To cope with her in that state, the nurse might have had to pharmacologically restrain her, which would have altered the patient's hemodynamics and interfered with the patient's recovery from anesthesia. In this case, the son's presence provided comfort and prevented the use of unnecessary technological interventions.

An example of a technological cascade is described below:

Nurse: Shortly after completing the wound, ostomy, and continence certification process, I began evaluating patients on the inpatient units. I distinctly remember being asked by a nurse on the [medical] unit to come and evaluate a 'leaky G-tube'. After reviewing the patient's chart, I remember thinking, 'This is going to be a straightforward consult.' The patient was admitted to the hospital following a cerebral vascular accident (CVA). She was initially stabilized in the ICU and later transferred to [the medical] unit. The CVA had left the patient with right sided paralysis, expressive aphagia, and failure to thrive, which required the insertion of a G-tube for nutritional support. The primary nurse assigned to care for this patient was becoming overwhelmed with the amount of care the patient required…The patient's G-tube was draining gastric juices onto her skin which required dressing changes every hour. The patient had become agitated with each interaction which was upsetting for the nurse.

Upon entering the room, I introduced myself as the 'skin care nurse' who was going to help with the leaking tube. The patient began to become agitated with rapid leg movements and moaning…I began my assessment by exposing her abdomen and G-tube site. I was immediately taken aback by the 'raw meat' that had taken over her abdomen. The caustic gastric drainage had started to macerate her entire abdomen… My first priority was to medicate the patient and provide the care she so rightly needed.

In this clinical incident, the skin specialist, Susan Gagne Rego, went into the patient's room expecting a "straightforward consult" and instead confronted an entirely different technological trajectory—a cascade of sorts. The technology that was utilized to treat failure to thrive ended up causing another series or a cascade of related problems, including a major wound on the abdomen necessitating frequent dressing changes and pain and agitation issues. Fortunately, for this patient, the skin specialist promptly mobilized resources and got the patient placed on a low flow air mattress. Additionally, the patient was placed on pain medications on a round-the-clock basis and a treatment plan was developed and implemented to heal the excoriated abdomen.

Unfortunately, not all technological cascades can be contained or halted. Some spiral out of control and consume all physiologic reserve, as is the case in this clinical incident:

Nurse: I was caring for an elderly lady who came from a nursing home and who was septic from her gall bladder. They gave her a bunch of fluids in the OR—she was pretty sick. She was 93 years old and not waking up after her surgery. She had her surgery at 1:00 p.m., and by 6:00 a.m. she really wasn't doing much more than opening her eyes once in awhile. One of the residents decided that she needed some narcan [a narcotic reversal agent], but I thought that since she was old and had gotten a lot of narcotic, it just probably hadn't cleared her liver yet—I wasn't too concerned that she wasn't waking up yet… After the third year resident ordered the narcan, I can remember standing there with it in my hand thinking that I shouldn't give it—that I should wait until the rest of the team came by—because she was stable and doing okay. She had a good blood pressure and a good heart rate, she just wasn't awake. Well, I gave it and the lady's blood pressure went up to 210/120 and she moved into full pulmonary edema because of the acute vasoconstrictive effects narcan can have on the lungs. She was blowing pink, frothy sputum across the room. She had to go on a vasodilator drip to control her blood pressure and her blood gases were terrible... Ultimately this lady had a two-week postoperative course in the unit and died. She was just too old to survive such an insult.

While this particular narcotic reversal agent is commonly given and time-tested, that does not mean that it is a benign agent or without side effects. The drug's action in this particular patient, who was elderly and already compromised, initiated a technological cascade of interventions. This tragic case underscores the need for on-going practical technology assessments that critically evaluate the reasoned use of technology with specific patients.

Although most technologies carry risks, many are crucial—if not life-saving—in supporting and treating critically ill patients' life-threatening physiological conditions. For that reason, acute and critical care nurses do not always limit interventions based on their practical technology assessments. For example, an ICU nurse who was caring for a leukemic patient on neutropenic precautions and who had frequent diarrhea told us:

We were in there changing the bed every one to two hours, and he was getting psychotic because he couldn't sleep. So finally we just told the doctors, 'Look, we have to put in a rectal tube. We've got to weigh the risk of his [lack of] sleep against the risk of putting in a rectal tube in somebody with such a low platelet count.'

This intervention was subsequently safely carried out. The nurses in this case clearly grasped that the rest and comfort this particular patient would receive secondary to their intervention far outweighed the more general risk of possible bleeding associated with the insertion of a rectal tube. This decision cannot be generalized to other neutropenic patients. Judgment implies both risk and uncertainty. Adding, withholding, or withdrawing technological interventions requires astute reasoning-in-transition about the particular patient. In this case, the technological intervention provided the patient with much needed rest and comfort.

The challenge is to design and use technology in ways that augment good clinical judgment. Skillful use of technology and clinical judgment is illustrated in the following observational interview of a neonatal ICU nurse while she cared for a critically ill 12-hour-old premature neonate. Because the baby's lungs were not fully developed, in order to properly ventilate him, the baby had to be intubated, paralyzed, and sedated. An excerpt of the observation begins after the nurse had suctioned the baby:

Nurse: The baby actually seems to do well with hand ventilation, which is a useful thing to know. Some babies saturate better when you hand ventilate them and other babies don't like it at all. He doesn't really seem to care one way or another. It actually looks like the skin on the down side of his head looks very good—he's got a little bit of redness...

Interviewer: What should it look like?

Nurse: Well, I mean you're looking for skin breakdown, although he's not really old enough and hasn't been laying on one side long enough to get any. But that's the point of turning his head from side to side is maintaining the muscle tone of the neck and also to give us the chance to not have pressure on it. And I'm also going to turn him just a bit—good boy—turn him just a bit on his side to get him off his back. Babies do not really like to be flat on their backs anyway. It's better for them developmentally to be kept on their side and try to keep their hands and feet flexed, which he naturally can't do since he's on versed.. But we try to position them as developmentally correct as possible.

Interviewer: What concerns you about his being on versed?

Nurse: Well, all of the side effects of immobility and the fact that you can't interpret by his activity what various things mean. Versed takes away a lot of information that you would normally have... I'm going to put his hands up to his face because that's a comforting thing for babies. Even though he can't really move, at least we can put his hands where he'd like them to be...

Interviewer: How will you make the decision that the baby no longer needs versed?

Nurse: We follow his sats and blood gases. Once the baby starts having arterial oxygenation of over 100 consistently, the doctor would probably, at that time, start to make tiny, tiny changes by coming down on the ventilation. Right now, the fact that the baby is on fairly high pressures on the ventilator and is so fragile, you don't want the baby moving at all and making his own respiratory efforts. But once he gets <u>down</u> somewhat on the ventilator pressures, he would be at less risk of having a pneumothorax caused by barotrauma. So at that time we would think about letting him wake up a little bit (Observational Interview).

The nurse adjusts her attentiveness and judgment based on the loss of information due to the baby's pharmacologically induced paralysis. This story also illustrates many of the clinical and ethical trade-offs clinicians must make when caring for critically ill patients. Using paralytic agents must always be carefully weighed. In this situation, because the baby is so fragile, sedation and paralysis are necessary in order to ventilate him adequately. Although these pharmacological interventions are used to mitigate the risks of ventilatory therapy, they also introduce new technological risks of their own, putting the baby at high risk for developing other secondary complications, such as skin breakdown and muscle wasting. While the medical treatments are aimed at saving the baby's life, the baby's comfort and development are central in the nurse's concerns. Subsequently, she provides comfort measures and positions the baby the way he would position himself if he were able. These caring practices are equally important to the baby's long-term well-being. Comfort measures that treat the infant like a normal baby preserve mobility and skin integrity but also accord the infant with human status and concerns. Because the clinical and ethical risks of using paralytics are so great, this particular technology will be discontinued as soon as it is safe for the baby. Initiating and limiting interventions in a clinically and ethically sound fashion, thus, requires ongoing judgment, knowledge, and attentiveness.

ENGAGING IN SAFETY WORK

There is a deeply rooted ethic in acute and critical care of protecting patients and humanizing the environment as the use of technology grows. This is a working out in practice of the ethical principles of beneficence and nonmaleficence (do the most positive good and do no harm, respectively). Engaging in safety work requires a constellation of skills and involves the practical activity of creating, maintaining, and repairing patient and family environments that are safe from actual and potential technological hazards. While expert nurses have always tended to safety issues, the Institute of Medicine's seminal works (2000, 2004), brought safety issues to the fore.

Ensuring a safe environment in the acute and critical care setting is no small achievement. Acute and critical care areas are intricately designed, technologically-laden, and staffed and supported by multiple and overlapping systems. Although the environment itself can be hazardous to patients, families, and staff (Rogers, 1997; Sommargren, 1995), actual and potential hazards can also be caused by a breakdown in established safety systems. Yet, many patients safely move through complex acute and critical care settings without complications or difficulty. Their safe passage is due, in part, to the skillful, but largely invisible, safety work routinely performed by nurses. An example follows in which an ICU nurse institutes isolation precautions to protect a vulnerable patient from developing an iatrogenic infection:

> **Nurse:** This weekend, I took care of a leukemia patient who was really septic, and he was a lot of work—not critical care work—but he was just busy. I think I made a difference in his care, because I went in and the first thing I noticed is that he had a zero white blood cell count and people were walking in and out of his room without any masks or gowning up or anything. So the first thing I did is I put him in isolation, strict contact isolation. He had a relapse of this before and the family knew exactly what contact isolation was and they said, 'Oh, we're so thankful you [put the patient in isolation]. We didn't want to say anything, but [isolation precautions] hadn't been done.' I think it was just overlooked, but they were really appreciative.

Even the family knew that the patient was at risk for added infection with such a low white cell count. This example illustrates that safety work involves sustaining standards of practice. Here, as in many situations, the problem is not lack of information or knowledge, but a lack of attentiveness and response to what needs to be done.

Daily, ongoing safety work is a taken-for-granted and invisible skill for two primary reasons. First, the skilled know-how of expert nurses in ensuring a safe patient environment often goes unrecognized until a breakdown occurs or the safety net they have created fails. Second, the practical ethic of protecting a person who cannot protect her or himself, historically is tied to women's work, such as preventing and protecting a child from harm (Ruddick, 1989). These gendered roots do not diminish the importance of safety work, but help to shed light on why this essential aspect of knowledge and skill has been largely unarticulated and uninvestigated.

The practical ethic of preventing patient harm often overlaps with clinical forethought (see Chapter 3) because anticipating possible patient complications and taking appropriate actions to prevent patient harm occur simultaneously in expert nursing practice. We want to call attention to daily safety work (which often relies on clinical forethought) as central to good nursing practice. It is a disciplined approach to ensuring that the environment is safe, and includes developing routinized safety practices such as checking the defibrillator on the code cart and ensuring that emergency bedside equipment is in working order at the start of each shift. Although policies and procedures mandate many aspects of safety work related to technology, they do not capture essential precautions in every situation. Therefore, noticing potential hazards and thinking-in-action must augment standard policies and procedures.

Simple activities, such as labeling IV lines, can prevent patient harm, as illustrated in the following example from a neonatal ICU nurse:

> **Nurse:** Because the baby's on [a pressor], we label the pump, the tubing, and the baby's wrist where it's going in. It's important whenever you have a continuous infusion of something like a vasoactive drug, that you label it clearly so somebody doesn't come along accidentally and use that IV to give a medication and give the baby a bolus—that would be extremely detrimental to the baby (Observational Interview).

Clearly labeling the infusion pump, the tubing, and the site to identify the infusing drug prevents others from inadvertently using the IV line for other purposes. Injecting another drug into an IV line that is dedicated for a continuous infusion will not only cause a bolus, but may also interact causing visible precipitation or invisible incompatibility in the IV line, making both drugs unusable and potentially harmful. Thus, while the activity of labeling lines itself is simple, the preventative necessity and power of this kind of safety work is large.

Other nurses spoke of securing and stabilizing equipment to prevent patient harm. Another neonatal ICU nurse describes some of the common safety practices in her unit:

Nurse: We keep the arterial line and the umbilical venous line, which we're transducing for a CVP, at heart level in order to get accurate readings. We usually clip them [to the side of the bed]... And also just the fact that the baby has a lot of wires and tubes, if you clipped them to the linen, they could get accidentally pulled. So this way, you won't dislodge something important. We keep the side rails up because, even on a baby who's [pharmacologically] paralyzed and can't move, you always assume that they can launch themselves off the bed somehow. His ventilator is also clipped to the [side of the bed]. It's important not to put any tension on the endotracheal tube because you don't have a lot of margin for error in a baby's trachea. The tube needs to be well below the bifurcation of the esophagus and well above the level of the carina, and that gives you about a centimeter of leeway on a kid this size (Observational Interview).

It is remarkable that nurses learn to live with such a demand for precision and high risk. Nurses' skilled know-how in securing and stabilizing extensive life-supporting equipment when there is very little room for error allows them to be respectful and vigilant without being unduly anxious. This example also points to the social embeddedness of nursing knowledge. While the nurse may develop her own style of securing equipment, she has also been socialized into her unit's shared understandings and ethic of preventing patient harm by routinized strategies for securing tubing. Safety work always involves local, specific knowledge. Environments and arrays of equipment must be rendered safe in particular settings and by particular staff. As the utilization of new technologies increases, the accumulated and shared clinical wisdom surrounding safe use of technology is further developed and passed on through the community of nurses (Benner, Tanner & Chesla, 2009).

In another example, a circulating nurse in the OR describes her concerns as she preps an incision site located on the patient's neck:

Nurse: What I think about in my prep is, number one, allergies, and number two, I don't want the betadine to pool under him so that he would get a burned neck. So, I think about safety when I'm doing the prep (Observational Interview).

This example illustrates the pervasive nature and ethos of safety work. The potential for harm from this relatively simple activity is notable. If the patient had iodine allergies, prepping with this particular solution would be contraindicated. But the solution itself can cause skin irritation, even in those not allergic to it. Knowing that, the nurse used the prep judiciously and therefore safely. If the prep solution had been allowed to pool near the cautery grounding pad, it could have resulted in a thermal injury. The nurse's activities protected the patient from harm and were oriented by her maxim, "Think about safety."

Later in the observation, the nurse engaged in multiple and simultaneous activities: she assisted others by tying their surgical gowns, helped the surgeon position the patient's head, counted surgical sponges with the scrub nurse, monitored the operating suite's temperature, and ensured that the requisite equipment and instruments were properly laid out and available. All of these well-orchestrated and routine activities are a form of safety work. In the background, a sterile field is maintained. Through careful patient positioning, the nurse can prevent nerve and muscle damage. Counting surgical sponges with the scrub nurse before and after the surgery is a form of surveillance which ensures that all patient-related items used during the operation are removed from the patient and accounted for. Because the circulating nurse is responsible for maintaining the temperature in the operating suite, she consults with the anesthesia provider as to the patient's temperature throughout the case to avoid either hypo- or hyperthermia. Finally, by thinking ahead and planning for patient contingencies, the nurse checks and double-checks necessary operating equipment and instruments. This kind of safety work requires an experienced clinician who knows the general trajectories of each kind of surgery and who can attend to details while keeping track of the whole situation.

Safety work—while invaluable in preventing patient complications—is often unnoticed unless it is missing, since its absence precludes smooth and safe patient care. Several OR nurses in a small group interview discussed how many of the surgeons with whom they work simply do not understand the essential work of the circulating nurse:

> **Nurse 1:** I was circulating one day for a particular surgeon. He said, 'You should be scrubbing.' After I tied his gown, he walked past me to the head of the table and said, 'Aren't you going to do any work today?' He said that because I was circulating, I wasn't the scrub nurse. And I said, 'Doctor, isn't it interesting that an RN is legally required to be in the room with a scrub nurse?' And he said, 'HUH!' and walked away.

> **Nurse 2:** Well, the surgeons I work with say, 'Anybody can circulate their cases.' Right! And we get so insulted, because we do very complex cases.

> **Nurse 3:** Very complex cases.

> **Nurse 4:** Circulating is much harder than scrubbing.

> **Nurse 2:** Circulating's hard. And yet, when they want to do a case and we don't have the staff, they'll say, 'Oh well, anybody can circulate.'

> **Nurse 1:** But that's because you <u>can</u> circulate—you're good at what you do!

The fact that thousands of patients undergo complex surgeries without complications on a daily basis is a cultural achievement and testimony to the pervasive safety work that expert OR nurses continuously perform. Ironically, their skills and expertise, in many ways, help to hide the value of their work. Because these nurses can simultaneously and deftly assess and monitor the patient's condition, coordinate the multiple activities associated with any surgery (such as anticipating resources needed for emergencies, ordering X-rays, arranging for specimens to be sent to pathology and/or the laboratory, checking blood products, and answering surgeons' pages), keep track and anticipate what each person will need, and provide documentation—all while ensuring a safe patient environment—the surgeons with whom they work do not "see" how vital their roles are. If one thinks of the surgical suite as a spaceship, the circulating nurse is mission control.

Yet, in spite of nurses' vigilant safety practices, system breakdowns resulting in patient complications still occur, as illustrated in the following story:

Nurse: We had a patient come back from the OR some time during the night and I took care of her the next day. She had an intra aortic balloon pump and when she initially came back from the OR, her foot was really mottled and it looked like they were going to have to take the balloon pump out because her circulation was being sacrificed. But it improved during the night, and by the time I took care of her, she had a good pulse. Her foot was cold, but they [the medical team] were happy with it because she had a pulse... Anyway, during the night after my shift was over, she lost her pulse. The nurse that was taking care of her kept telling the charge nurse who phoned the doctor repeatedly, but the doctor never responded. It turns out that the resident was really at fault for not coming to see the patient. But the next morning on rounds, the surgeon came in and right away whisked out the balloon pump and took her to the OR where she had an above the knee amputation of her right leg. After that, there was a big shakedown in the ICU trying to determine who was at fault. But it made me just so much more aware of everything that I'm doing and just making sure, double checking, that there really is a pulse.

When the human consequences are so grave, a safety net of responsible action on the part of all staff is required, regardless of title or position. This tragic story is instructive because it highlights the interdependence of the patient care teams. The nurse's attentive monitoring of the patient's pulse was not enough. She deferred responsibility and relied on action from the medical resident, which was not forthcoming. The informal nursing and medical expectation is that the nurse will go up the chain of command to get an appropriate medical response. Thus, safety practices can prevent patient harm, but only if appropriate action and intervention are taken when the situation demands it.

Another form of safety work is that of surveillance, which can be defined as the creation, implementation, and repair of specific safety systems that are designed to protect the patient from particular technological hazards. An example previously alluded to is the practice of counting surgical sponges at the beginning and end of each surgical case. Another kind of surveillance is checking blood products with another nurse or physician against the patient's blood type. These disciplined activities are considered standard practice and are aimed at preventing patient complications and injury. Surveillance differs from the more general skill of safety work, in that, safety systems are generally created and implemented with a particular error-reducing goal in mind. The chief objective of safety work is the broad goal of ensuring a safe patient environment.

As an example of surveillance, an OR nurse told us what she was watching for as we observed her at the start of a surgical case:

Nurse: Right now I'm just watching the surgeon's technique to see if he accidentally contaminates his gloves or anything... While draping's going on, people frequently contaminate their gloves and do not notice. So, the scrub nurse and I both watch (Observational Interview).

Both the circulating nurse and the scrub nurse vigilantly watch for inadvertent contamination. The nurses' attentiveness to keeping the sterile field intact is a form of surveillance aimed at preventing patient infection.

In another example, a neonatal ICU nurse described her unit's changing surveillance practices in response to admitting higher acuity infants:

> **Nurse:** We're working on developing a series of safety checks that each nurse will go through at the bedside. These checks aren't so critical in our unit now, but as we evolve into a more intensive care unit, there will just be more equipment and it'll be even more important to make sure that alarms are set properly or whatever.

Performing safety checks at patients' bedsides is a form of surveillance, as it enables the nurse to check, for example, the prescribed ventilator settings against what the ventilator is actually delivering to the patient. Checking waveforms, monitor alarm limits, IV infusion rates and solutions, and lines, sites, and dressings with the previous nurse during bedside report are invaluable activities, not only to catch and reduce errors, but also to convey practical monitoring and management information that is not captured on flowsheets, care plans, or kardexes. These safety checks also help nurses develop and extend their habits of attentiveness. As such, bedside reports with built-in safety checks are an excellent way to engage in surveillance work and to ensure patient protection from technological hazards.

Safety systems are also sometimes instituted to create a community of attentiveness around certain reoccurring hazards. Examples of this include "time-outs" to perform a multidisciplinary surgical safety checklist, recommended by the World Health Organization (WHO, 2009) to occur before anesthesia, before incision, and before the patient leaves the operating room, and independent double-checks by nurses for high-risk medications (Cohen, 2007). This front-line repair work often occurs at the unit level, and can result in the creation of new safety systems. For instance, in the OR, numerous healthcare providers question patients about their allergies and the nature of their surgery. While the frequent questioning may annoy patients and their families, the repeated questions serve as a built-in safety mechanism. This safety system only works, however, if multiple clinicians participate in the checking and double-checking of vital patient information.

Below, an OR nurse recalls an emergency pediatric surgical case in which she was asked to help. Because she was pulled from another case, she had no time to engage in some of her usual safety practices:

> **Nurse:** And so we're standing there putting the leads on the patient and I have to assume that anesthesia has done the patient interview. So I'm asking, 'How much does the child weigh? Does he have any allergies?' 'When was the last time he ate?'—all this kind of stuff. So, fine, I do the prep. But then I looked at the front of the chart, and there's a tag on it that said, 'Patient allergic to betadine.' And I had already prepped the patient with betadine. That's what happens when you take shortcuts. Things happen— just like doing the wrong knee—the patient gets something that he or she's allergic to. Everyone has to have the time to do the job they're supposed to do. And you can do it efficiently, but you still have to be given the time [to do it reliably]. And part of the problem that we face in being able to do our job is the first thing that people want to cut down on is nursing attention to the patient. They think that's <u>extra</u>.

Because the nurse in this situation had no opportunity to speak with the child's parents preoperatively, she relied on the information given to her by the anesthesiologist. Attentiveness and surveillance take time, commitment, and support, but the patient complications that are prevented by these safety practices far outweigh the cost of ensuring that nurses have sufficient time to engage in these practices in the first instance.

But as technology proliferates in healthcare and makes the work less transparent, the likelihood of new errors is increased (Reason, 1990). Consider the computer physician order entry (CPOE) systems that are beginning to evolve in healthcare systems across the country. These proprietary systems communicate to electronic pharmacy programs, which in turn, communicate with automated medication supply cabinets. While there is a push to have universal platforms, the current state in many healthcare systems is a complicated maze of different software programs with multiple third party patches in place to help the systems "talk" to one another. This disjointed series of systems does not even take the human factor into account (Benner, Malloch, & Weeks, 2010).

Recently, the Institute for Safe Medication Practices (ISMP, 2009) issued a bulletin describing different types of medication errors. Endogenous errors are caused by internal factors and arise within an individual who makes an error (such as a math error leading to a miscalculated medication dose) and exogenous errors arise from external conditions such as poor product labeling or unclear information. Independent double checks performed by nurses can help in eliminating both endogenous and exogenous errors, although, the ISMP admits that the double check systems will not catch all errors. System changes are necessary to reduce error frequency.

Yet, some system changes that are implemented are not always helpful and may even increase errors. Amanda Savage, an acute and critical care float nurse, speaks to this when she recounts a frustrating and ultimately tragic clinical incident:

Nurse: Prior to this [clinical incident], there had been numerous emails fired off about documentation. There was the addition of new 'process interventions' to document, despite the fact that nursing was already documenting these items. The new additions were [meant to be] 'more specific'. There was no removal of [items in] the present documentation, just additions upon additions. Everyone was gearing up for when Medicare would not pay for 'preventable' complications such as UTIs and decubitus ulcers. Additionally, at the beginning of the month before I took care of Mr. F, there were significant 'upgrades' to the present software, which required attendance at classes to learn about the changes.

This particular day, only 3 of the 7 laptops [on the unit] were working. The laptops are used for documentation of care, interventions, medications, and acknowledgement of orders. I was frustrated [already at the beginning of my shift] at not having the tools I needed. In the afternoon, I received report from the Emergency Department about an 80 year old man who fell at home and was found by his nephew. It was unclear how long the patient was [down], but physical findings were consistent with a stroke…Mr. F arrived to the unit with his nephew…Mr. F was able to talk, but his speech was slurred…When I examined him, he had left sided weakness in his arm, no movement of his left leg, and some right leg weakness. His pupils were equal and brisk. He was on some medication for his high blood pressure, but he could not recall [the name of the medication]. The nephew said he would bring the [medication] bottle when he returned. By this time, the laptops were all fixed so I grabbed one. It was now 5 p.m. and I completed the requisite assessment and 'process intervention' [documentation]. I took off his orders that included removing IV hydration. Between the assessment, process interventions, and physician orders, I spent a minimum of 40 minutes in front of a computer. I placed the patient on telemetry and he had a new onset of atrial fibrillation, so we had a cause for his stroke. I followed all the other orders and gave report to the night nurse at 7 p.m. I thought, 'Thank goodness this day is over!'. The patients were great, but it was the technology and pandering to the regulatory agencies which made my day too long. Anyway, I got home and did not feel good about something, but I could not put my finger on it. I just knew that I was missing something. I reviewed in my mind, 'Did I document this or that?' and remembered doing all that I was supposed to do. The problem was, I didn't do everything I was supposed to do, because I didn't use my brain—my thinking time in practice is now consumed by endless, redundant documentation.

While sleeping that night, I knew what I had missed. I actually dreamt about a CPK. Mr. F did not have a CPK done. He had been lying on the floor of his house for who knows how long and no one thought to draw a CPK and I had removed the IV hydration! I got up and called to ask [the nurse] to add a CPK to the morning labs.

I am a float nurse and I was lucky to be assigned to the same unit the next day. The first thing I did was make a beeline to check Mr. F's CPK result, but it was not there...I went to the lab tech and asked if she had drawn blood on Mr. F and she said 'yes'. I went in to see Mr. F and his mental status was diminished. I was [worried the patient had developed] rhabdomyolysis...I called the physician...When he called back, I explained that Mr. F had never had a CPK drawn, that I had asked the night nurse to add one, that the patient had a change in mental status and his weakness was more pronounced, and that I thought the patient should have IV hydration. The physician... was upset that a CPK had not been drawn in the ED and he OK'd the IV hydration...I called the lab and asked them what was taking so long and the person responded that there was no order for a CPK...The night nurse did not add a CPK because I do not have the authority to write or ask for labs. I put in the order and had the lab run stat. Sixty minutes later, a significantly elevated CPK came back...

I took care of Mr. F for the rest of the day. His mental status deteriorated, his kidneys were shutting down despite the hydration, and his weakness was profound. During the previous night, because the stroke was progressing, his nephew made Mr. F a DNR. The DNR was consistent with Mr. F's wishes. I spent the day ensuring that Mr. F was comfortable...

Normally, I am absolutely fierce about the appropriate care of patients with pancreatitis and rhabdomyolysis because they are routinely under-treated. But I hadn't been fierce with Mr. F. All the information I needed was there: elderly, lying on the floor, and differences in his lower extremities. The night before, I was so proud of myself for doing all the documentation and doing all the things expected of me. I did not use what I have always prided myself on—my thinking skills. I was so focused on finding working equipment and completing the mounting documentation in a cumbersome system that I missed what should have been second nature for me.

This chilling clinical incident resonates with most—if not all—clinicians who are currently involved with any clinical enterprise. The convergence of regulatory mandates (that frequently fall on nursing to monitor and manage), burdensome documentation systems and unreliable technological platforms, hasty and often ill conceived system-wide changes, and a continuing trend to limit and restrict nursing judgment at the state and national levels, all come together in this incident to create a perfect storm resulting in a tragic outcome for the patient and his surviving family. While the elements of this perfect storm are endemic in healthcare today, patient fatalities are, thankfully, rare. Unfortunately, more minor clinical incidents, with the same elements in play, are not uncommon. We believe that this incident (and others like it) should serve as a clarion call to bring the patient, family, and clinician judgment to the center of the healthcare delivery system again and to relegate documentation systems, technological "fixes", and regulatory mandates to their rightful place: in a supporting role.

EFFECTIVE USE AND ASSESSMENT OF PERFORMANCE OF TECHNICAL DEVICES

Another way that nurses protect patients from actual and potential hazards in technological environments is through their skillful and intelligent use of equipment, devices, treatments, and other technology. While many have criticized acute and critical care areas for their overabundance of technological "things" and have suggested that nurses spend more time nursing machines than they spend caring for patients, Hooper (1995) found that the equipment simply faded into the background for expert nurses. Instead, nurses saw "through" the equipment to focus on the information it provided about the patient's physiological condition. But in order for that to happen, a tremendous amount of skilled know-how, judgment, and knowledge are required.

Nurses usually learn how to safely manage equipment and interpret its performance "on the job" and through trial and error. Because there are always technological advances in acute and critical care areas, nurses must constantly learn and master new technologies, meaning they must not only know how to work with the equipment, but they must also know how it works. They must, as one nurse said, "Stay state-of-the-art." While formal inservices are scheduled to orient nurses to a new devices and greater emphasis is being placed on online computer modules to impart information and education across all shifts, little time is given for "hands on" demonstrations and simulations. Consequently, nurses usually become accustomed to and comfortable with a new device at a patient's bedside.

Having to learn a new device at a critically ill patient's bedside is challenging because of the multiple and competing demands on the learner. Learners do not learn well in stressful, high demand situations. Learning about new technologies under conditions that are far from ideal also puts the patient at risk. Patient complications can arise when a piece of equipment fails and the nurse is insufficiently oriented to the technology to properly troubleshoot and rectify the problem, as illustrated in the following example. Here, an ICU nurse recalls a harrowing experience in which she cared for a patient with a biventricular assist device who was waiting for a heart transplant:

Nurse: I think the most memorable equipment failure situation that ever occurred to me was the day when a patient's bi-ventricular assist device (VAD) failed. The patient was a bridge to transplant patient and he had been on the VAD for weeks... I hadn't been officially trained on the VAD, I was somewhat new here. I knew the patient because I was a traveling nurse who worked with him when he was in the coronary ICU. But once he was placed on this device, he was transferred to our cardiovascular ICU. Everyone who knew this patient had found him to be somewhat difficult, so they were like, 'You know him from upstairs, you take care of him.' And I'm like, 'Great! Cool! I'll learn about this new piece of equipment!' So I just kind of learned as I went and a few nurses gave me a quick inservice at the bedside. Anyway, the patient was stable enough that he could walk around, so nurses often went on walks with him. So we went downstairs for a walk. I'd been taking care of him for several weeks at this point, but I was still not an expert with the VAD. We just don't see them that often. So we went for a walk and the battery light came on. The patient assured me that, 'From the time that light comes on, we have half an hour.' But we decided to go back upstairs anyway... So we're wheeling it down the hallway and it stops. I just hear a very slow 'click...click...click...click,' whereas usually they go [faster], 'click-click-click-click,' you know, it's his heart. So I'm like, 'We've got to get you to an electrical outlet!

Interviewer: He's walking? There's no wheelchair?

Nurse: No, he's walking. He's pushing it! And it's a big piece of equipment, so now I'm pushing it and saying, 'We've got to get over to this outlet.' So we get over to a wall outlet and we plug it in and it's not speeding up. There was some way of switching it back and forth from AC to battery, but I was told, 'Whenever you take the machine out, flip it onto battery. And when you plug it back into the wall, it'll be fine. You don't need to flip it back.' That's what I had been told... So, I paged the perfusion team. They finally came and brought a battery pack—the OR's battery pack that you can use for transport—and we got him back up to the unit. Everything worked out fine, but, needless to say, a VAD class was quickly given!

This frightening clinical narrative points to the dangers of inadequate staff training and the necessity to have in place high-risk, low volume competencies. Without the proper knowledge and skills, this nurse was ill-equipped to think ahead, prepare for contingencies, and act rapidly in solving the problem associated with this crucial life-saving technology. Although the nurse paged the perfusion team and the patient was eventually transferred to the ICU without any adverse effects, the potential for cardiac arrest and patient death were great. This example underscores the necessity for on-going educational classes and demonstrations in an effort to prepare clinicians for safe technology use and to protect patients from technological hazards. Although organizations know that "trial and error" continue as a major source of experiential learning, situations where there is no margin for error call for a strong and safer administrative stance to safeguard patients and thoughtfully prepare clinicians.

In recent years, much has been made of the analogy between aviation and healthcare. Like aviation, acute and critical care nursing is increasingly dependent on advanced technology, but the systems in which nursing operates (including people and technology) are typically much more complex and variable than that of an aircraft and, as such, present greater challenges to maintaining high levels of safety (Webster, Stabile, & Merry, 2009). Charles Perrow (1999), a systems expert, has described the function of any technological or human system along two dimensions: interaction and coupling. The interaction between elements of a process or a device is considered complex if there are many sub-tasks necessary to implement at any point in its completion or implementation. The coupling dimension refers to the extent to which an action is related to its consequences. A system is said to be tightly coupled if consequences are closely linked to actions. Using Perrow's nomenclature, a nuclear power plant is complex and tightly coupled. What is less appreciated, however, is that the care of an acute or critically ill patient has similar system characteristics to the nuclear power plant and less similarity to the carefully controlled cockpit (Weick, 2009; Weick & Sutcliffe, 2007).

In the narrative above, the nurse had been assigned to care for the VAD patient even though she "hadn't been officially trained". We would argue that more healthcare facilities and schools of nursing should utilize high-fidelity simulation training, when possible, to capture the urgency and high-stakes nature of a decompensating patient situation without putting a patient or practitioner at real risk. Additionally, high-fidelity simulation can be used to explore failure modes of technology and human-machine interactions (Mudumbai et al., 2010). While there are many benefits to simulation, this approach cannot stand alone and should supplement situated coaching in real clinical situations, particularly on shifts where the least experienced nurses are assigned, and the use of narratives for learning in clinical arenas (Benner et al., 2010).

Safely managing equipment is only one aspect of managing technology. Nurses must also be able to rapidly and accurately interpret its performance. This requires clinical knowledge, skilled know-how, and respect for the device and the hazards it presents. Recognizing and discriminating between a potentially lethal dysrhythmia and motion artifact, for instance, requires clinical knowledge and judgment, and can make a critical difference in the patient's treatments and eventual outcome. This is illustrated in the next clinical incident, in which Debra Richards, an eICU nurse, works through technology to coach and mentor a new ICU nurse:

Nurse: It was a Monday morning at 8:00 a.m. when a new nurse in one of the ICUs pushed the call button in her patient's room that summons help from the [eICU] where I was working that day. I turned my camera on in the room and introduced myself. In a high, nervous voice, the new nurse said in rapid fire, 'Help! I'm just off orientation and I don't know what to do. The monitor says my patient is in VT—should I get a 12 lead? And honestly, I wonder if he's not seizing.' I pulled up the patient's ECG on my screen and all I saw was artifact, but his arterial line had a good waveform and read 100/70, his O2 saturation was in the mid 90's. I looked at the patient's [history]: Joe was a 75 year old male on a ventilator who was admitted for an acute MI a few days ago with no history of seizures. I looked at the patient with the camera: His face was calm, his color was good, his eyes were closed, and he didn't appear to be in any distress by his serene expression. I didn't see any myoclonic activity, but I saw tremors in his torso and limbs—he appeared to be shivering rather than seizing. [Using the camera], I looked around the patient's room to be sure that he was not being cooled by any device. I said, 'You've got a good artline waveform and his blood pressure is stable at 100/70. His O2 saturation is stable which leads me to think that it's not VT or seizure activity…It looks to me like he's shivering—does he have a fever?' The nurse said, 'I don't know. I just walked into the room and the monitor said he was in VT.' I told her that in between shivering, I could glimpse brief bits of normal sinus rhythm on the monitor. She threw up her hands and said, 'How do I know that he's not going in and out of VT? I think I'd better get a 12 lead.' Her voice was bordering on panic by this point. I reminded her that his B/P was stable so we had time to think this through. I told her that while protocols permitted a 12 lead ECG whenever a lethal arrhythmia was suspected, even a 12 lead would pick up the muscular artifact caused by shivering. She hesitated and then said, 'So, what do I do?' I had the impression that she wasn't going to believe me that the patient was in sinus rhythm until she could see it on the ECG herself. I looked at the patient's electronic orders. The patient had Ativan ordered prn. I suggested that she give the prn Ativan to see if we could decrease the shivering enough to get a clear ECG reading. She reluctantly agreed and left the room to get the Ativan. Her hands shook as she administered the Ativan and flush. The Ativan decreased the shivering to the point that it was only intermittent. I asked if she agreed that, when not shivering, the rhythm was a normal sinus rhythm. She smiled and agreed with my assessment. She was relieved that the patient wasn't in VT and on the verge of coding as she had at first feared. I asked what the patient's temperature was. She hadn't had time to take it yet and did so at my suggestion. Joe had a fever of 104... He had no order for Tylenol, so I offered to call the intern for her and ask for a Tylenol order. When I spoke to the intern, I updated him and obtained a telephone order for Tylenol. Back in Joe's room, I let the nurse know that the Tylenol was ordered and that the intern said he'd be by on rounds shortly. The nurse thanked me profusely...We made small talk for awhile...By this time, the shivering had stopped and the nurse had no doubt of the patient's stable heart rhythm and vital signs. When the intern arrived at the patient's room, I wished the new nurse a good day and turned my camera off.

The eICU at this facility serves as a resource and safety net for both patient and to nurses working in the ICUs. It is staffed 24 hours a day, 7 days a week, by expert ICU nurses. As is readily apparent in this clinical incident, the expert nurse calmly and skillfully coached the new nurse to systematically assess and "think through" the situation. The new nurse, fixated on the possibility that her patient was in ventricular tachycardia or VT, wanted desperately to obtain a 12 lead ECG for a definitive diagnosis. But, as the expert nurse wisely pointed out, the 12 lead ECG would only capture more of the motion artifact due to the patient's ongoing shivering. Helping the nurse to prioritize and stage the interventions, the expert nurse suggested the prn benzodiazepine to stop the shivering and reassessment of the ECG. Following that, the expert nurse suggested that the new nurse assess the patient's temperature. While the sequencing of these interventions may seem obvious to an experienced clinician, they can be overwhelming to a new practitioner—especially when the patient situation is perceived to be critical in nature. Through the extensive use of multiple technologies, the eICU nurse was able to mentor and guide the new ICU nurse through this learning incident.

Because the patient had cardiac-related problems, the new nurse expected cardiac complications and, as such, mistook the motion artifact for a serious dysrhythmia. If the expert nurse had not been available as a safety net and coached the new nurse to recognize that the supposed dysrhythmia was really only motion artifact, it is conceivable that unnecessary and unsuitable interventions would have been initiated. The new nurse learned a lesson that must be learned by every healthcare provider. Increasing perceptual acuity, however, requires experiential learning in clinical practice, openness to learning, reflection on practice, and an environment where teaching and learning are valued and supported with the goal of making practical clinical wisdom visible, intelligible, public, and cumulative (Benner, 2000).

Safely using equipment and interpreting its performance under high-stakes, high demand situations can be challenging, especially for practitioners who are less familiar, and therefore, less skilled with a given piece of equipment or interpretation of the data it produces. In order to safely care for acute and critically ill patients whose lives depend on the smooth and skillful management of various technologies, administrators and managers need to ensure that there are more experienced nurses on all shifts to assist less skilled practitioners. Practicing and learning alongside more experienced nurses (or virtually, as in the case of an eICU) not only improves the quality of the learning experience for the learner, but also ensures patient safety, as illustrated in the story below:

Nurse 1: I think a big part of our practice is that we work with a lot of equipment, and you have to really know that equipment and be able to troubleshoot it in the middle of a crisis when things aren't going the right way. One example I can think of...I participated in a code out on the floor recently... This patient arrested and by the time the nurses got there, [the patient's cardiac rhythm] had degenerated into a fine VF [ventricular fibrillation] as opposed to VT [ventricular tachycardia]. But when they put the quick look [defibrillator] paddles on the patient, they didn't see a rhythm. Because they didn't turn the [defibrillator] from 'monitor' to 'paddles,' they couldn't <u>see</u> the rhythm. It was a pure equipment problem.

Interviewer: And you were in what role?

Nurse 1: I was the charge nurse in the CCU and this happened at change of shift. Because the bed situation was really tight, I needed to know sooner than later if we needed to open up another bed [for this patient]. So I went out there to anticipate whether the patient was going to survive the code and be admitted to the CCU. So, the quick look dial on the defibrillator was key when they attempted to defibrillate the patient. Once they did get a quick look rhythm, the defibrillator didn't charge from the defibrillator itself. And what I suggested in the middle of the code was to charge from the paddles themselves and <u>that</u> worked, and we defibrillated the patient that way. Later, we checked the defibrillator and we couldn't reproduce what happened during the code. It's always that way! (laughs)... So, all in all, I felt like I impacted that situation in a positive way... And because of that, I'm teaching a class in the next couple weeks for these nurses in terms of responding to code situations and using the defibrillator.

Interviewer: Tell us more about how you came to this situation with the knowledge you had?

Nurse 1: We've always had defibrillators at the bedside in the CCU. We're <u>very</u> familiar with them. We check them every day, every shift. You always check your own defibrillator, that is the standard of practice that is set... That's probably why I know so much about defibrillators.

Interviewer: And the equipment they had for the code was not the equipment most of the staff were accustomed to?

Nurse 1: Well, they are [accustomed to it], but they don't have exposure to it like we [CCU nurses] do. They don't have patients that go into VT daily.

Nurse 2: They don't have to check that equipment every day.

Nurse 1: They don't even look at the defibrillator. When I was debriefing with them after the code, I asked, 'Do you <u>know</u> this defibrillator?' And a lot of the nurses admitted that they don't even look at it because it hangs out in the corner down the hallway and they rarely have to use it.

By virtue of the CCU nurse's experiential knowledge and skilled know-how in operating the defibrillator, she assisted the staff in troubleshooting the device and extended their clinical knowledge. Because the defibrillator was a commonly used piece of equipment in the CCU, this nurse developed an embodied skilled know-how in working with this machine. Without consciously focusing, the CCU nurse grasped instantly that the defibrillator was not set to "paddles" and later, was able to quickly suggest an alternate way to recharge the paddles when the machine temporarily malfunctioned. The nurse's embodied skilled know-how was reflected in her practiced, habitual, and context-sensitive response. However, as illustrated in this exemplar, habits of thought and action must not become mindless, lest they be overlooked or forgotten. A practiced attentiveness that stays mindful of inherent risks is required. What is in the foreground of the expert nurse's attention shifts with experiential learning (Benner, Tanner & Chesla, 2009)

Another essential aspect of preventing actual and potential technological hazards is ensuring that a given piece of equipment is accurate and precise. Some machines perform self-checks when turned on, whereas others require periodic manual zeroing and calibration. For example, while many technologic advances have been made with transducers (the component that is placed on an indwelling line that translates the vessel pressure into an electric signal that can be displayed on a monitor), pressure drift and waveform dampening can still occur. To ensure that patient treatments are based on reliable data, it is important to zero and calibrate any transducer if erroneous data are suspected. An ICU nurse spoke of that when she described her calibration practices:

> **Nurse:** I zero and calibrate my invasive lines at least every 4 hours. It's just something that I do. I realize there are theories out there that say you can zero less often. But I've come in and seen patients that are being treated for high wedges [pulmonary capillary wedge pressure or PCWP], low CVP's, or no blood pressure and the transducer is either 18 inches below the phlebostatic axis or 12 inches above their head (Observational Interview).

Because this nurse has witnessed inappropriate patient treatments based on inaccurate readings, she has heightened her routines of leveling and calibrating transducers. While this is a form of safety work, it is also essential to the safe management and accurate interpretation of a particular machine's performance.

Later, this same nurse cared for a critically ill and neurologically injured patient. She describes below some of her preliminary assessment findings:

> **Nurse:** The patient's really rhonchorous in her upper lobe, and she's wheezing in her lower lobes. Because she has very decreased breath sounds, I want to make sure that she has some pressure support and PEEP [positive end expiratory pressure delivered through the ventilator] to help her with her breathing. Her sats [oxygen saturation] are 100%, but I never really look at that very much unless it drops, because, in this case, her pulse oximeter is on her toe... So, even though it says 100%, it's not a good reading. The other thing is, if you notice, the pulse oximeter sensor is turned around so that it's measuring through the flesh pad instead of the nail. So I'll reposition the sensor. Her respiratory rate's a little elevated. She's on a rate of 12 [referring to the patient's ventilator setting] but she's breathing 22 to 26. So I'm going to suction her and see what I get (Observational Interview).

While the nurse skillfully assessed the patient, she also evaluated the way in which the technology was being used and therefore the accuracy of the data. She auscultated the patient's breath sounds and then checked the patient's current ventilator settings to see if adequate ventilatory support was being delivered. She has good reason to doubt the pulse oximeter. Incorrect sensor placement on a lower extremity can diminish the accuracy of pulse oximeter readings (Szaflarski & Cohen, 1989). By synthesizing patient assessment findings, prescribed therapies, nurse-initiated treatments, patient responses, and the supporting technology, the nurse assessed the critically ill patient's total picture. Grasping the total patient picture positions the nurse to think ahead and prevent complications before they occur, as well as to more fully understand unexpected patient responses and transitions.

In addition to ensuring accuracy and precision, nurses must also be able to discriminate between sensible and trustworthy patient data and spurious or aberrational data. Finely honed interpretive skills and seeing the unexpected are characteristic of expert nurses, as they commonly spot nonsensical laboratory results, suspicious hemodynamic values, and uncharacteristic assessment findings that are contrary to the patient's other physical findings. Catching the aberrational data and re-checking values before inappropriate treatments are initiated can prevent a host of serious patient complications.

For example, Kathy Giannelli, an maternity nurse, recalls a situation in which the patient's lab results did not correlate with her assessment of the patient and family:

Nurse: One day, at morning report, I learned that one of my patients, Nicole, was a recovering drug addict on methadone. She was a single 19 year old who had delivered her baby on the previous 3-11 shift by c-section…I was informed that Nicole's urine had come back positive for PCP or Angel Dust [that morning]. Policy at my hospital states that the patient has to have three consecutive 'clean' urines before [the patient] can breastfeed. I was also told that the father of the baby (Christopher) was 'involved' and had stayed overnight with Nicole. He was a recovering addict too, who had supposedly been clean for 2 years. On my unit, the nurse is responsible for the care of the baby as well as the mother, so now it was my job to inform Nicole that she couldn't breastfeed her baby. When I brought the baby into Nicole's room that morning, I had figured that I would be meeting just another addicted mother who didn't care enough for her unborn child to stay away from drugs. When I went into the room, Nicole was in the first bed by the door. She was a petite looking girl with dark shoulder length hair and big brown eyes. She had a tattoo on her shoulder and I made a bet with myself that it wasn't her only one…Christopher had more than a few tattoos on his arms and legs and had those oversized clothes on that look as though they were five sizes too big!… After introductions and checking the baby's ID band with the mother's, I put the baby in her arms. Then I said, 'Nicole, you aren't going to be able to breastfeed because your urine tested positive for PCP.' They both looked at each other and seemed confused. I went on to explain the hospital policy to both of them. Christopher asked what PCP was and as I told them, Nicole started to cry. 'I swear, I haven't taken anything except for my methadone. How could I? I've been on bedrest for the last month!' As tears rolled down her face, she looked down at the baby. I can't explain why, but at that moment, I believed Nicole. I have a daughter who is the same age and when I looked at Nicole, I was thinking, 'This could be [my daughter] lying there. Wouldn't I want someone to treat her kindly?' Christopher was getting angry, saying, 'Why would the clinic she goes to let her take her methadone home if they thought she was using? I've been with her the whole time.'…I told them, 'I will check into this and let you know what I find out. Until then, I will show you how to use the breast pump so that any breast milk you get, we can save until we get this straightened out. In the meantime, you will have to give your baby a bottle. They both thanked me as I left the room. When I looked at Nicole's prenatal record, I found that she had two other positive PCP urines at the end of her pregnancy. I felt so disappointed, because for some reason, I truly believed them. I went back into the room and told them what I had found. Again, looking confused, Nicole said, 'Dr. D never said anything to me—this is the first time

I'm hearing this.' Christopher added, 'I'm so mad at Dr. D for not saying anything—why wouldn't he say something to Nicole?' At this point, I really did not know what to think…I contacted Dr. D to tell him how upset Nicole and Christopher were and asked him about the positive urine results. He said, 'I didn't [tell them]—why should I? They were just going to do what they wanted to anyway.' To say the least, I was a little shocked at his response. I said to him, 'Wouldn't you want someone to say something if this was your daughter?' His response was, 'What am I supposed to do?' I wasn't sure what to do next, so I called our social worker. I explained everything to her and told her that I had a 'gut' feeling that Nicole and Christopher were being honest with me. She told me that she had problems in the past with the lab giving positive results, when in fact, the urine was negative. She said, 'I trust your judgment Kathy, so I'm going to call the lab and have them send her urine to another lab for re-testing.' I went back into the patient room and said, 'You could be trying to pull the wool over my eyes, but I really believe you and we're going to have your urine sent to another lab for re-testing.' Nicole started crying and said, 'Thank you for being so nice and for believing in us!' I was off the following day, so when I came back to work, the first thing I did was to ask about Nicole. I can't even begin to tell you how good I felt when I found out her urine had come back clean!

The outcome, in this case, would have been drastically different had the nurse not been able to push aside her initial judgments and be emotionally available after meeting the new mother and father. Kathy's perceptual acuity about the sincerity of the new mom flew in opposition of what could be a very likely problem of relapse. This expert nurse's intuition compelled her to pursue other possible reasons. By "trusting" them, new ways of attending to and responding to the parents were discovered. The technology, in this case, was the initial laboratory, which had failed by giving inaccurate results. By virtue of the nurse's openness and trust in the parents, she was able to question the validity of the lab findings and have another laboratory re-test the sample. This intervention had the happy consequence of allowing the new baby to bond through breastfeeding and created the possibility of a more confident and hopeful family that knew that someone trusted and believed in them. The technology in this clinical incident could have shut down this new family but, coupled with the nurse's ethical bearing, had it a transformative effect.

In combat zones, nurses frequently have to learn to simplify and go back to earlier technology (Richards, 2005). For example, complex I.V. pumps that calculate drug dosages and flow rates did not function well in the sand filled environments of the temporary "hospitals" in the sandy desert. Newly graduated nurses had to relearn to manage the I.V. drips without the aid of an I.V. pump for the infusions. Experienced nurses were able to reinstate the outmoded but workable strategy of indicating on the I.V. the amount to be infused per hour, and write the time intervals appropriate for the ordered flow rate on a strip of tape on the IV bag. Drops per minute had to be calculated and translated in to amount of I.V. fluid per hour by the nurses in order to ensure accurate flow rates.

Nurses in disaster settings and combat zones describe their many strategies, which they often called "jerry rigging," to alter technical equipment for use in the natural disaster or combat zone where supplies are limited. This points up the need for nurses to understand the purposes and functioning of technology that they use, in order to substitute, to adapt the technology for disasters, wars, or emergency situations where supplies may be limited or where the environment itself demands new design strategies for use of technology. In Iraq and Afghanistan care delivery has been streamlined and staged. Portable ICU's are embedded in the troops so that immediate emergency care can be delivered. Patients are then stabilized in the field hospital, before being transported from the field by air evacuation. Nurses have developed strategies for adapting technology and delivering critical care to wounded warriors in the cramped circumstances of air transport. For example, nurses have learned to carry the essential medications, sterile dressings, I.V. equipment, clamps, and instruments that they frequently needed because so little space was available to move to the "supply" location, once the flight was underway. The specialized circumstances of the airplane transport required that nurses adapt their care for completely new contingencies. They found that more pain medication was required, especially during plane take offs and landing, and scientific studies are currently being conducted to determine the physiological causes of this increased pain, drops in oxygen levels, vibrations due to acceleration and g-force, and other possible causes (Richards, 2005; Kelly, 2009; De Jong et al., 2010). The point of these examples is to underscore the importance of nurses learning about the purposes of technologies and imagine other means for accomplishing similar care goals when the technology breaks down or is unavailable. It is reasonable to expect that additional advanced preparation in technology design, management, and use may be added to nurses' studies in the future.

SUMMARY

We believe that technology should support the Institute of Medicine's (2001) six health quality goals: safety, effectiveness, patient-centered healthcare, timeliness, efficiency, and equitability. While the effects of healthcare reform are still unknown, it is likely that acute and critical care areas will only become more technologically complex in the future. Preventing both actual and potential hazards in the technological environment will remain a crucial component of nursing practice. This knowledge work requires well educated nurses who are well trained in the local and specific knowledge in their settings. Diminishing access and observation time with patients, diluting the skill mix with under-skilled technicians, and work overload all place great strain on safety work. Through practical technology assessments, nurses help to ensure that technology is used in a reasonable and ethical fashion. Nurses also engage in socially embedded safety work and surveillance practices that are aimed at preventing patient harm. Finally, by safely managing technology and interpreting its performance, nurses protect patients from actual and potential technological hazards. These safety skills require a strong sense of agency and attentiveness. In order to ensure patient protection in the technological environment, educational and clinical settings need to assure that these skills are taught and nurtured and that nurses have the adequate institutional structures (e.g., staffing and educational resources) to support these essential preventative patient care practices.

REFERENCES

Benner, P. (2000). *From novice to expert: Excellence and power in clinical nursing practice.* Menlo Park, CA: Addison-Wesley.

Benner, P. (1994). The role of articulation in understanding practice and experience as sources of knowledge in clinical nursing. In J. Tully (Ed.), *Philosophy in an age of pluralism: The philosophy of Charles Taylor in question* (pp. 136–155). New York, NY: Cambridge University Press.

Benner, P., Tanner, C. A., & Chesla, C. A. (2009). *Expertise in nursing practice: Caring, clinical judgment, and ethics* (2nd ed.). New York, NY: Springer Publishing Company.

Benner, P., Malloch, K., Weeks, V, (Eds.) (2010). *Nursing Pathways for Patient Safety.* Philadelphia, Pennsylvania: Elsevier International Press.

Cohen, M. (2007). *Medication errors* (2nd ed.). Washington, D. C.: American Pharmacists Association.

Connors Jr., A. F., Speroff, T., Dawson, N. V., Thomas, C., Harrell Jr., F. E., Wagner, D., … Knaus, W. A. (1996). The effectiveness of right heart catheterization in the initial care of critically ill patients. *Journal of the American Medical Association, 276,* 889–897.

De Jong, M., Benner, R., Benner, P., Richards, M. L. Kenny, D. J., Kelly, P., Bingham, M., Debisette, A. T. Mass casualty care in an epeditionary environment: Developing local knowledge and expertise in context. *Journal of Trauma Nursing* (17)1, 45–58

East, T. D. (1992). Computers in the ICU: Panacea or plague? *Respiratory Care, 37,* 170–180.

Foley, M., Arias, K., Rich, V., Saliba, G., Gallagher, S., & Stannard, D. (2011). Promoting patient safety: Ensuring the involvement of the frontline healthcare worker. *Perspectives: Recovery Strategies from the OR to the Home, 9*(1), 1–7.

Hilberman, M. (1975). The evolution of intensive care units. *Critical Care Medicine, 3*(4), 159–165.

Hooper, P. L. (1995). *Expert titration of multiple vasoactive drugs in post-cardiac surgical patients: An interpretive study of clinical judgment and perceptual acuity.* Doctoral dissertation, University of California at San Francisco, San Francisco, School of Nursing.

Institute of Medicine (2000). *To err is human.* Washington, D. C.: National Academy Press.

Institute of Medicine (2001). *Crossing the quality chasm: A new health system for the 21st century.* Washington, D. C.: National Academy Press.

Institute of Medicine (2004). *Keeping patients safe: Transforming the work environment of nurses.* Washington, D. C.: National Academies Press.

Institute for Safe Medication Practices. Independent double-checks are vital, not perfect. *Nurse Advise-ERR, 7*(2), 1, 3.

Kelly, P. (2009). *Nursing clinical knowledge development: An approach for continuity of care for war injured service members Tri-Service Nursing Research Award.* Unpublished manuscript.

McGill University. (2008, May 2). World first: Completely automated anesthesia system developed. *ScienceDaily.* Retrieved May 6, 2010, from http:www.sciencedaily.com/releases/2008/05/080501180308.htm

Mudumbai, S. C., Fanning, R., Howard, S. K., Davies, M. F., & Gaba, D. M. (2010). Use of medical simulation to explore equipment failures and human-machine interactions in anesthesia machine pipeline supply crossover. *Anesthesia & Analgesia, 110*(5), 1292–1296.

O'Donnell, J. (1990). The development of a climate for caring: A historical review of premature care in the United States from 1900 to 1979. *Neonatal Network, 8*(6), 7–17.

Pennington, C. & DeRienzo, N. R. (2010). An effective process for making decisions about major operating room purchases. *Association of periOperative Registered Nurses, 91*(3), 341–349.

Perrow, C. (1999). *Normal accidents: Living with high-risk technologies.* Princeton, NJ: Princeton University Press.

Reason, J. (1990). *Human error.* New York, NY: Cambridge University Press.

Richards, M. (2005). *Clinical knowledge development of nurses in an operational environment.* Tri-Service Nursing Research Division: MDA905-03-1-TS15 Study in progress.

Rogers, B. (1997). Health hazards in nursing and health care: An overview. *American Journal of Infection Control, 25,* 248–261.

Ruddick, S. (1989). *Maternal thinking: Toward a politic of peace.* New York, NY: Ballantine.

Shah, M. R., Hasselblad, V., Stevenson, L. W., Binanay, C., O'Connor, C. M., Sopko, G., Califf, R. M. (2005). Impact of the pulmonary artery catheter in critically ill patients: Meta-analysis of randomized controlled trials. *Journal of the American Medical Association, 294*(13), 1664–1670.

Sibbald, W. J., Eberhard, J. A., Inman, K. J., & Sprung, C. L. (1993). New technologies, critical care, and economic realities. *Critical Care Medicine, 21,* 1777–1780.

Sommargren, C. E. (1995). Environmental hazards in the technological age. *Critical Care Nursing Clinics of North America, 7*(2), 287–295.

Stannard, D. (1995). Preface: New technologies in critical care. *Critical Care Nursing Clinics of North America, 7*(2), xv–xvi.

Szaflarski, N. L., & Cohen, N. H. (1989). Use of pulse oximetry in critically ill adults. *Heart and Lung: The Journal of Critical Care, 18*(5), 444–453.

Tenner, E. (1997). *Why things bite back: Technology and the revenge of unintended consequences.* New York, NY: First Vintage.

Tisdale, S. (1986). Swept away by technology. *American Journal of Nursing, 86*(4), 429–430.

Titler, M. G. (1993). Technology dependency and iatrogenic injuries. *Nursing Clinics of North America, 28*(2), 459–473.

Webster, C. S., Stabile, M. & Merry, A. F. (2009). The challenges of technological intensification. *APSF Newsletter, 24*(3), 33, 35, 43.

Weick, K. E. (2009). *Making sense of the organization: Volume 2: The impermanent organization.* Chichester, West Sussex, Wiltshire, UK: John Wiley & Sons, Ltd.

Weick, K. E., & Sutcliffe, K. M., (2007). *Managing the unexpected: Resilient performance in an age of uncertainty.* San Francisco, CA: Jossey-Bass A Wiley.

World Health Organization (2009). *Implementation manual: WHO surgical safety checklist 2009.* Retrieved May 6, 2010, from http:www.who.int/patientsafety/safesurgery/en/

9

Facing Death: End-of-Life Care and Decision Making

Acute and, particularly, critical care settings symbolize a cultural commitment to hero-ically prevent death, even at great costs (Kaufman, 2005). Over 50% of patients die in hospitals in the United States and several European countries (World Health Organization [WHO], 2004). In this context of fighting to save lives, death appears as the enemy, and its naturalness is overlooked (McCue, 1995). Indeed what is considered "natural" in birth and death have been transformed by technological capacities to alter and sustain what is known as natural human life (Kaufman, 2005). It is little wonder that at the end of life, rhetorical questions and human issues get framed in confusing discourses of different moral and human sources such as medical, technical, biographical, religious, relational, and so on. Human aspects of hope, denial, grieving and letting go are in the shadows of a technical discussion of disease states, and treatment interventions (Spichiger, Wallhagen & Benner, 2005; Oakes-Greenspan, 2007; Sunvisson, et. al., 2009) Death disrupts North American cultural themes of constant progress and promises of technological breakthroughs that triumph over death. Death and dying may strain the cultural fabric of critical care settings if the work group has focused only on the work of saving lives and has not developed a culture that acknowledges and responds to the inevitability of death, and the resulting emo-tional labor of caring for the dying and their loved ones.

Lock (1996; Oakes-Greenspan, 2007) notes that the term, "end-of-life," bears connota-tions of a biomedical approach to death and recommend using the term "end of living" instead. In the last 15 years palliative care has grown and increasingly hospitals have devel-oped largely inpatient palliative care units (Meier, 2002). Practice guidelines have been developed (National Consensus Project, 2004) to assure quality palliative care. However the standards of palliative care are often not achieved in hospitals (McGrath, 2001; Meier, Morrison, & Cassel, 1997; Bruera, 2006). As a medical practice discipline, palliative care focuses managing symptoms and spiritual concerns of dying patients though typically focus on symptom management is dominant. Patients/families often describe problems with com-munication that blocked their experience of being well cared for at the end of life (Dunne & Sullivan, 2000; Keegan et al., 2001; McGrath, 2001; Rogers, Karlsen, & Addington-Hall, 2000; Teno et al., 2004). Spichiger (2010) studied 10 adult Swiss patients with advanced malignant disease and 10 close family members. The patients were 3 women and 7 men, with a mean age of 62.7 years (range = 38-85). The 10 patients were no longer treated cura-tively and expected to die during their current hospital stay or within a few months.

Spichiger's study (2010) confirms that despite efforts to focus on comfort and symptom management through balancing adverse and beneficial effects, this is not always achieved despite the best intents. She offers the following examples:

> ….For a patient diagnosed with vertebral metastases causing severe pain and paralysis, a disease-modifying intervention, radiation therapy, was suggested. The patient agreed and later stated that his pain completely disappeared after the first treatment, while he never mentioned any problems with side effects from radiotherapy. When another patient got diagnosed with a severely advanced esophageal cancer, neither surgery, nor radiotherapy, nor chemotherapy, nor the insertion of a stent was suggested, because, according to the specialists' judgment, none of these treatments would contribute anything to the patient's quality of life. This explanation was acceptable for the patient and his wife… The decision for or against diagnostic tests and medical treatments or the choice between available therapies, however, was not always easily made as the following example shows. This patient suffered from shortness of breath due to aspiration pneumonia and pleural effusions. Shortly after his admission, a tube was inserted to drain pleural effusions. This first drainage worked quite well and the patient's breathlessness was relieved to some extent, but only for a rather short time. Two weeks later, the physicians suggested a second drainage. At this time, the patient left decisions to his wife, and she only reluctantly agreed.,, The second drainage was problematic and hardly effective, because the effusions were encapsulated. The pain from the tube was well controlled; the patient did not suffer from the treatment. However, it did not alleviate his shortness of breath. The patient died a few days later. In retrospect, any positive effect of this second drainage seems questionable from a professional perspective, and this was clearly also the view of the family member. (Spichiger, 2010 p. 321).

Spichiger's thick description of patient and family experience with end-of-life care in the hospital, despite the best palliative care intentions cannot always be achieved. Predictions about patient's responses to intervention often are contradicted by the patient's experience. Symptoms cannot always be managed despite the best technology, medications, and clinical judgment. Spichiger (2004; 2010) concludes that what can be promised and achieved is not to abandon the patient/family, to offer compassionate communication, attentiveness and availability and presence to listen to patient/family concerns (see also Halpern, 2001).

Physicians experienced in hospital based palliative care learn to enrich their concerns and communication with patients. Oakes-Greenspan found that 6 of a sample of 14 physicians surveyed about their palliative care practice told a specific story about how working with a specific patient or family altered their understanding of their palliative care and improved their listening for meanings and concerns about dying from patients and families. For example, the following physician as a resident found it impossible to say good bye to a patient, and this altered his palliative care practice:

> … it wasn't that I was oblivious to the fact that there was a *person*, I was just way too scared to be able to *recognize* it. And I really had that very particular thought of not being able to be…the living person who said goodbye to the dying person. And…since then, I've often…I've often seen my role as that. As…as one of the representatives of the people who will continue on the planet for some time after, to be able to say goodbye and to thank the person, or to recognize their passing (INT1, 453-464, emphasis by participant) (Oakes-Greenspan, 2007. p. 58).

Nurses and physicians are taught over time by their patients/families that not every patient can be saved, and that staying within an interventionalist clinical stance and discourse is dehumanizing for the patient/family and the care provider (Oakes-Greenspan, 2007). Elisabeth Spichiger (2010) studied the lived experiences of families and their hospitalized family member. She defined end of life as "all the diagnostic and therapeutic interventions initiated and provided by the interdisciplinary team of health care professionals in the hospital within the context of their relationships to patients and family members with the goal to improve the patients' situation. Sometimes the critical care unit becomes the place where the last "heroic efforts" are made, "doing all that can be done" to save a life until the life support becomes clearly limited to the outcome of prolonging dying, then the patient/family, physicians, nurses and whole health care team must negotiate withdrawing therapies and enhancing palliative symptom management as therapies are withdrawn. It is at this juncture that death becomes orchestrated and managed in the ICU (Kaufman,2005). Bureaucratic and cost-savings concerns enter the dialogue about ending what has become dying prolonging futile care. This transition presents particular challenges to ICU staff who only recently have openly begun the discussion of end-of-life care in ICU.

Acute and critical care clinicians normally believe that patients who are dying should be admitted to palliative or hospice care. Despite this ideology, the transition from curative to palliative care and death often occurs in critical care areas. Mortality rates vary, but many patients die in critical care units often in the midst of heroic measures. It is often assumed that patients will be transferred out of the critical care unit once a DNAR (Do Not Attempt Resuscitation) order has been written. This assumption is rational enough and in keeping with the mission and understanding of critical care units to provide curative therapies; however, it overlooks the relationships that are developed among healthcare providers, patients, and their families:

> Maintaining DNR patients in an ICU environment raises ethical concerns, such as whether health care dollars should be spent to maintain these patients in such expensive settings. Couldn't these patients be cared for as well on a medical or surgical unit? Removing DNR patients from the ICU setting would free up beds for patients whose survival depends on the care provided in such a unit (Jezewski, et al.,1993, p. 308).

These authors overlook the human import of transferring patients out of critical care if the patient's death is imminent. Once life support therapies and/or a DNAR decision has been made, the patient <u>usually</u> dies within 1 or 2 days. Transferring a patient at that point is sometimes humanly and economically too costly, especially if there are no suitable private rooms for the patient and family, or no hospice-palliative care beds. Accounting procedures do not usually account for hidden costs, such as opening a new room and transferring a patient. If these hidden costs were accounted for, then it would seldom be considered cost-efficient to transfer a patient whose death is imminent. We found in our study that if death were imminent, patients were seldom transferred out of the unit to die. It was too jarring and disruptive to the care of the patient and family to transfer them to the care of staff they had not met. Such late transfers can be experienced as abandonment by patients and families and are avoided if possible. However if the space in ICU is crowded and noisy, some families prefer that their family member to be moved to a larger private room where the family can better attend to the patient with little disruption.

Recognizing and responding to the transition from curative therapies to DNAR status is a major area of ethical and clinical reasoning for nurses and physicians. This chapter will focus on the clinical and ethical discernment required for this transition, as well as common problems, nursing interventions, and caring practices for the dying patient and her or his family. Sometimes a death is thought to be imminent but does not occur. Predicting death is uncertain. And if a patient lingers, then it is usually more humane to transfer the patient and family to a quieter and more pleasant environment. Under these circumstances, attention must be given to helping the family members make this transition. While it is reasonable to systematically exclude palliative care patients from admission to critical care units, it should not be concluded that dying patients do not belong in critical care units, because this myth covers over the provision of safe, humane care of the dying and their families. Since patients frequently transition from potential recovery to dying, critical care clinicians must become skilled in recognizing and articulating this transition, as well as skillfully at providing palliative care once the transition has been recognized.

Attending more closely to the transition period from reasonable curative and palliative therapies to palliative care only when caring for the patient whose death is imminent can provide closure and development of skill in caring for the dying. In turn, a decrease in death avoidance should also increase the physicians' and nurses' ability to recognize and come to terms with patient transitions into end-of-life palliative care.

DECISION POINTS AND TRANSITIONS

Focusing on decision points and outcomes overlooks the critical patient transitions that lead up to decision points. Crucial decisions to forgo or withdraw therapies based upon at particular points in time does not capture reasoning-in-transition over time with clinicians, patients, and families. Throughout the process of approaching death, improvement in the patient's condition may signal a hoped for recovery (Lynn, et al, 1997). As Brody and colleagues (1997) observed:

> Forgoing life-sustaining treatment is not a single decision but it often occurs in a sequential manner over several days... For example, which treatments should be discontinued? What order should be followed or should all life-sustaining treatments be stopped simultaneously? What is the rationale at work in withdrawal of treatments, and what are the goals of medical care in this situation? ...There are few descriptions of what is actually done, much less what should be done... (Brody, et. al.,1997 p. 652).

Brody, et. al. (1997 found that decisions regarding resuscitation, endotracheal intubation, and dialysis occurred earliest, followed by decisions regarding vasopressors. Withdrawing or withholding transfusions, hemodynamic monitoring, fluid administration, antibiotics, and other medications occurred later. Forgoing enteral feeding and discontinuing ventilatory support were the last decisions. Whereas a decision to not intubate a patient was made early on for patients not already on ventilators, once patients were on ventilators, decisions to withdraw ventilatory support were late decisions and occurred after several other interventions were first forgone.

Patient and family narratives about a patient's concerns, fears, and hopes, along with a narrative account of the patient's clinical trajectory to date and a projection of the most plausible responses can improve both ethical and clinical reasoning as well as articulation and communication about the patient's possibilities for recovery. As an experiential critical care nurse interviewed by Sharon Kaufman (2005) points whether or not the ventilator, vasoactive drugs or even dialysis depends upon the patient's condition. Is the therapy a bridge to recovery, or is it merely sustaining a patient whose clinical condition continues to deteriorate. Kaufman asked if the ventilator should always be considered "life support" treatment:

> I think at some point in time the mechanical ventilator *can be* life support/ I don't believe that all the time it is. But let me clarify that a little bit. The patient with pneumonia comes in. And that is the only thing he's got, pneumonia. But he's not breathing well from it and it's really compromising his respiratory status, so we intubate him. Is that ventilator at that point in time life support? In my opinion, no, that's an adjunct to his therapy to get him well. If pneumonia is the only thing that he's got, then we can treat it and get him out. But the course of the disease can continue, ad he can end up on dopamine or any of the other vasoactive medications—again, depending on the course of the pneumonia. We may put him on that because we don't have his fluids up yet, or he's hypotensive and we just haven't gotten on top of the infection yet. Again my feeling is that that's an adjunct to therapy that's helping him bridge that point. It's a treatable problem…It is truly a very murky area, one that I don't think anybody has ever tried to capture, because my opinion of where life support sort of starts for that person may be very different than where life support starts for someone else (Kaufman, 2005, p. 238).

Speaking from a wealth of experience, evidence based practice goes on to point out that even dialysis may not be considered life support when it is used as a renal replacement therapy for kidney patients, whose kidney function returns. Currently renal replacement therapy is used in the care of severely burned patients early on to prevent kidney damage. As this nurse explains, the meaning of a life supporting therapy must always be seen contextually, depending upon the patient's condition. What may be an adjunct therapy can become life support if the patient's condition worsens. A decision at one point in time should anticipate future decision points based upon the patient's responses to therapies and transitions.

Glaser and Strauss (1965) pointed out the distinctions between 'quick' and 'slow' dying trajectories in terms of how care is organized and delivered. Even within critical care units, there are quick and slow dying trajectories. Some patients die quickly and with the expectation of survival intact on the part of the patient, family, and/or health team members. Slower dying trajectories, however, are much more laden with ambiguity. Despite the advanced knowledge and abilities to assess physiological responses in critically ill patients, nurses and physicians are unevenly aware when the clinical situation shifts from the expectation of possible recovery to an understanding that further efforts are futile. This awareness is socially constructed. No particular individual independently makes such a determination. Rather, participants in the situation are insulated by role delineations, habits and custom, and their respective levels of involvement with the patient. Only as the patient's transition progresses toward certain death is there clarity. Prior to that point there is a moral tension associated with the ambiguity about possibilities for recovery.

It is an ethical breach to either provide futile care or not offer patients the best standard of practice that will allow recovery—this can be thought of as justifiable heroics (Holden, 1992). Prognostic scoring systems such as APACHE II & III, developed by Knaus and associates (1991) can provide benchmarks and statistical guidelines, but they cannot substitute for ethical and clinical reasoning about particular patients. Prognostic scores can be brought into the individual and collective clinical thinking as points of reference for the healthcare team, the patients, and their families. An ongoing dialogue with patient and family/surrogates about concerns and the evolving evidence about the patient's trajectory are

TABLE 9.1

Facing Death: End-of-Life Care and Decision Making

▧ Assessing and organizing a reasonable level of care early in the treatment encounter.

▧ Recognizing and communicating the transition from primarily curative to palliative care.

▧ Planning and implementing attentive, palliative care for the dying patient and family, once the transition from curative to palliative care has been made.

▧ Facing death.

all required for the best possible clinical judgments and care. Initial assessments and developing a plan of treatment set up a basis for gaining a clinical grasp and ongoing clinical reasoning as the patient's condition changes. The understanding that death is a probable outcome typically occurs in incremental stages and is negotiated over time. The goal of this chapter is to model experiential learning from particular cases and encourage clinical leaders to design strategies for experiential learning at the unit level so that cumulative wisdom and effectiveness about reasoning-in-transition from curative to full palliative care can be enhanced in specific health care teams.

In our interview and observation data we found a great deal of consensus on humane end-of-life care, but nurses described multiple practical, ethical, relational, and communication ambiguities and blocks to such care. There was a high degree of consensus on creating deaths with dignity and possibility for closure, goodbyes, and healing of relationships. However, actualizing humane and appropriate care of the dying was impeded by inevitable and not so inevitable human and organizational limitations.

Areas of clinical judgment about critical care treatment decisions can be divided into four major practical clinical considerations as seen in Table 9.1.

ASSESSING AND ORGANIZING A REASONABLE LEVEL OF CARE

Assessing and organizing a reasonable level of care early in the treatment encounter requires good clinical and communication skills. Understanding the patient's story in relation to current illness and treatment goals is crucial, but is often disrupted due to fragmented care. For example, patients are frequently admitted with no information about advanced directives or current treatment goals. Finding out about the history may be delayed by emergency admissions in the middle of the night. However establishing, as soon as possible, guidelines for different trajectories and eventualities can help families and patients understand their situation and better participate in the planning, decision making, and facing transitions as they evolve. Assessing the patient and family understanding of the situation and their hopes, concerns, religious beliefs and expectations is the first step. This initial narrative understanding needs to be enriched and filled out as transitions are made. Keeping and revising a narrative understanding of an illness (including hopes, concerns, and past decisions) is critical to planning and implementing reasonable levels of care and critical to understanding patient and family transitions. This is the phase where relationships are established and difficult turning points can be outlined as a framework for understanding transitions as they occur. Facing the changes and redrawing boundaries occurs over time and requires stable relationships with nurses who have understood the patient/family hopes and plans from the beginning. The metaphor of snap-shot or one point in time decision making does not capture the relational work required for coming to terms with what is reasonable to offer. This is illustrated in the following exemplar, written by Patricia Nash in her Master's level class on theoretical and ethical perspectives in nursing. In this exemplar, the nurses bear witness and learn from a physician and mother who bravely faces her daughter's death and coaches her through it. Patricia Nash demonstrates the narrative history required to understand the ethical and clinical course that moves from high curative efforts to facing death:

Patricia Nash, R.N., M.S.N.: This episode took place about two months ago, and remains very vivid in my memory. It's about a patient named Gina. Gina was a 16-year-old diagnosed with leukemia. She had not gone into remission with chemo, and was admitted for a bone marrow transplant (BMT). She was in our unit for about two months. Through that period of time, I had been Gina's nurse only two times. I was aware of her condition and progress through general shift report. I often helped the bedside nurses caring for Gina when I was the charge nurse as well.

I remember once overhearing a change-of-shift bedside report about Gina. The night shift nurse was relating how Gina said, 'I just don't get a break; nothing about this has been easy.' Gina did indeed have a rocky course from the time she had been admitted. She was very nauseated with the chemo and she had dreadful mucositis after the transplant. She frequently spiked fevers and was on multiple antibiotics, including amphotericin which gave her rigors.

Just when Gina finally seemed to be coming around, she took a drastic turn for the worse, developing liver and renal failure. She became increasingly encephalopathic, and developed progressive respiratory distress due to fluid overload. At this point, the BMT team and the PICU team began discussing treatment options with the parents. The general consensus was that she would not recover from this insult. Gina would minimally require some form of acute dialysis to keep her alive. The risk of infection with the dialysis would potentially result in irreversible sepsis due to her compromised immune system. Gina was too confused to express her wishes for her care. The parents decided to try the dialysis and, if Gina did not show improvement within a week, they would consider withdrawing support.

Amazingly enough, Gina did improve after about four days. She was showing signs of bone marrow engraftment on her blood work. She appeared not to have suffered any neurologic insult from the encephalopathy. Gina's liver function test was normalizing and renal function was returning. She finally had gotten the break she so deserved.

But, tragically, Gina's good fortune did not hold out. A week or so into her recovery Gina started to feel short of breath, and required oxygen. A chest X-ray was done and diagnosed the worst. Gina had developed CMV pneumonitis, a frequently fatal infection for the BMT patient.

The BMT team approached Gina and her family as to their wishes for the extent of support Gina would receive if her condition worsened. I should say here that Gina was a remarkably mature 16 year old. She had been very proactive in the decisions around her medical treatment. Before undergoing treatment, Gina had decided to have her ova harvested for the future possibility that she may become infertile with treatment and would like children later. In making the decisions for her future medical support, she chose to be supported with drugs and volume administration, but to stop if intubation was required. In essence, she had designated advanced directives. The plan was to treat the CMV with antiviral medication, monitor her condition, and continue discharge teaching in the hope that she could at least go home for hospice care if she did not improve. The goal of going home had become intensely important to Gina since her CMV diagnosis. Though Gina didn't improve over the next week, she didn't worsen either, and a date was set to send her home.

I was in charge of the unit the night that Gina's condition deteriorated. It was a chaotic night in the unit and the staffing was tight. There were a number of unstable patients requiring me to help with bedside nursing in addition to my charge duties. Toward the beginning of the shift, I was aware that Gina was experiencing increasing respiratory distress, and that the PICU resident was spending a lot of time in that unit. I didn't 'internalize' how much she was deteriorating though, due to a number of other patients crashing at that time. At that point I had no understanding of the extent I'd be involved with Gina that night. I kept touching base with the bedside nurse, and she said that Gina was definitely worse, but that they were holding steady.

About half way through the shift, I finally went over to the BMT unit. All three of the nurses working that night were in Gina's room. I took one look at the patient and I knew she was on the downward slide. She was extremely restless, her body was limp, and she had a terribly anxious look in her face. She couldn't find a comfortable position in bed, and she kept asking for more oxygen. Gina's mom had been at the bedside most of the week. She had gone to the family house across the street early in the evening to try get some much needed rest, before Gina's condition had started to declined. Gina kept calling her on the phone to tell her how bad she felt. The relationship between Gina and her mom was incredibly close and supportive. Her mom was a very calm, almost serene person, and was able to relieve Gina's anxiety each time by talking with her. Since Gina seemed to calm with the intermittent phone calls, the team didn't feel it was necessary to ask her mom to come into the hospital at the time.

I pulled the bedside nurse aside to ask what was being done with Gina. She said the resident was frequently assessing Gina, but hadn't really done anything for her. She seemed very frustrated by this. She wanted some action by the resident to treat Gina's respiratory distress. This resident had not blended well with our team. From the first day in the unit, he had been labeled difficult, arrogant, a know-it-all that didn't know anything. I could feel that the tensions between the bedside nurse and the resident becoming increasingly hostile. I knew my role as mediator between the two would become more demanding as the night went on.

In order to resolve some of the treatment issues, I went and spoke with the resident about what he thought the plan would be with Gina for the rest of the night. He said that Gina's respiratory distress was definitely getting worse. Anything short of intubation was not going to make her feel more comfortable. I had asked if we could at least give some pain medication. The resident reluctantly consented to a very small dose. The bedside nurse also wanted to give some lasix in an attempt to decrease pulmonary edema, thus decreasing the respiratory distress. The resident agreed to try this as well, even though the diuretic was potentially contraindicated due to fluid balance issues. Gina was having enormous amounts of liquid stool output and was being fluid replaced at about a liter per hour.

Gina did respond well to the lasix and morphine. At least, she appeared more comfortable after the meds were given. The bedside nurse, resident, and I were somewhat surprised by our 'quick fix' of the situation. We hoped that we'd found a way to keep Gina comfortable for the rest of the night.

Of course that was not to be the case. At about 3:00 a.m. Gina's respiratory distress worsened. The nurses called me with an alarmed 'Come over quickly!' I dashed down the hall and entered the unit hearing Gina yelling, 'I want to be intubated, I can't breathe! I want to be intubated!' I remember feeling like time stopped, and a million thoughts were popping in my mind: 'She's 16 years old, if she wants to be intubated, we have to do that for her', 'I don't want her intubated, I don't want to see her go through that protracted death', 'Her mom should be here, why didn't I ask her to come in earlier when Gina first started having problems?' While thinking all of this, I could hear the resident and the bedside nurse having a heated exchange. The bedside nurse wanted to give more lasix. This was obviously a futile treatment, but it had helped before. The resident felt the end was near, and didn't want to intervene like 'that' anymore, but he didn't know what else to do to make Gina feel less 'air hunger'. I felt that all these critical issues had come to a head, and I needed to make decisions. As a charge nurse, I feel my role frequently requires me to be the team leader in the unit. Even though Gina was not my patient that shift, and I was certainly not her physician, I felt ultimately responsible for the decisions made. On one hand, the patient advocate in me wanted to be sure we were doing everything for Gina's best interest. On the other hand, I wanted to ensure that we wouldn't get carried away with the support we could provide for her, which I have seen happen in the past.

The bedside nurse had called the mother. Apparently, she had heard what Gina was asking for, abruptly dropped the phone, and rushed over to the unit. When she arrived, she was panicked. She came rushing in to Gina's room and hugged her, saying 'No honey, oh no, I'm so sorry.' I don't know if she was apologizing for not being there earlier or for what she was about to convince her daughter to accept, but it was a very power-ful moment. The mom just held her for awhile. Gina's anxiety diminished despite her still labored breathing. The mom started to talk with the resident and the bedside nurse about what they thought was happening, with Gina listening to their conversation. Gina then asked her mom 'Is this what its like to die? Am I dying?' Her mom tearfully said yes. Gina and her mom continued to talk quietly, and Gina decided not to be intubated. She became very peaceful then. Her breathing was increasingly agonal. She would occasion-ally talk with her mom, and denied feeling uncomfortable when asked. The resident frequently asked Gina and the bedside nurse if pain medication was needed, but Gina consistently declined the offer. Gina passed away about four hours later.

I realized an incredible respect for Gina's mother that night. She had taken all those issues I felt so burdened by, and made those decisions with Gina's input. More remarkably, she had realized that further intervention was futile, and she wasn't going to put Gina through that painful and undignified death. She had acted as Gina's most powerful advocate. I cannot imagine raising a daughter for 16 years, then having to tell her she is dying, and there is no alternative. Gina and her family had accepted very advanced medical treatment by undergoing the bone marrow transplant. My experi-ence has been that it's common for these families to want to continue to go to great lengths if there are complications, because they have invested so much up to that point. But Gina's mom had resisted that lure of the ICU's technology, the hope that if you can sustain life a little longer, the one-in-a-million chance of recovery will happen.

I also gained a new respect for the resident. The PICU nursing staff is largely composed of very experienced nurses with a strong belief in the team approach for decision making in patient care. I can see how that could be intimidating for a new resident. We tend to question everything and distrust all new residents until they are proven effective and safe in their treatment of 'our' patients. I think this resident prob-ably took the questioning of his orders personally, developing an attitude of defensive-ness toward the nurses. This, of course, made the nurses even more distrustful. In this situation though, he was very invested in Gina's care, and was truly trying to make decisions that were both safe for Gina and also in her best interest. He could have easily pushed for her intubation. Instead, he noted the futility of the situation, and tried to work toward making Gina more comfortable. He took the time to try to work that out with the bedside nurse, despite the mutual animosity.

I suppose, all in all, this experience led me to rethink my perception of patient advocacy. I have often felt that the nurse can end up as the only advocate for the patient, battling reactionary decisions that don't account for patient best interests and desires. It can be incredibly validating when others involved in the care of the patient—in this case the mother and the physician—are also in touch with those sensitive issues and act to uphold realistic and empathic outcomes for that patient.

This narrative illustrates the ambiguities and the cross over between biomedical reasoning and the human experience of facing death. Facing the death of a 16-year-old daughter is an unspeakable tragedy. Somehow Gina and her mother did this together. The narrative depicts the uncertainties, the wish dreams for an omnipotent rescue, and the struggle for wisdom in the heat of the situation. The clinical decisions for Gina were made in the context of an uncertain, rapidly changing situation and in the midst of suffering and fear. The outcome was probably the best to be gained in a tragic situation.

RECOGNIZING AND COMMUNICATING THE TRANSITION FROM CURATIVE TO PALLIATIVE CARE

Communicating to critically ill patients and families is a fragile process filtered through fears and hopes, and across levels of education and understanding. It is little wonder that patient questioning and listening for patient understanding is so fraught with misunderstandings and fragmentation. Often families do not understand the practical implications of the biomedical choices and treatments presented to them. The following is a dramatic example of translating and clarifying for the family the patient's daily experience of the current level of treatment that the nurses considered excessive. The communication with the family had not been clear because, from the nurses' perception, the cardiologist was giving this family false hope:

Nurse 1: They get around it because they'll be very vague.

Nurse 2: 'I have seen cases like this improve. You know we have one more thing that we want to try.'

Nurse 1: It's just kind of a vagueness and the family was reading into this vagueness what they wanted to hear.

Nurse 2: When somebody gives you not a black and white answer, the family, of course, is going to read into the more hopeful side... The nurses all got together and we said: 'We're not going to do this anymore.' So when the family came in, we sat them down and said, 'This is what's happening to your mom. This is what we do to your mom every day. Turning her, putting these tubes in, sticking needles. We do this to your mom every day and it hurts a lot. And she's not getting any better.' I said: 'No one here believes that your mom will improve. And I'm sorry you're being led to hope that. We believe that this is just pure torture for her.' The family thought their mom was just sitting there nicely and happy, and that her body was functioning. They had no idea that we were just shoving tubes and doing all these procedures.

Interviewer: Were there any repercussions or conversations you had later with the medical staff about different...?

Nurse 2: No. Actually the son came up to me and the daughter and talked to me later and thanked me. He said, 'Thank you for really letting us know what's going on.'

In the above situation, it was the general medical and nursing consensus that the treatment was futile and that the cardiologist was not being realistic with the family. The family did not understand the implications of the treatments for the patient's suffering, and they did not have a clear picture of the gravity of her clinical prognosis. The family was presented with the treatments that could be offered without being presented what the chances for recovery were. These transitions—communicating the human implications of treatment in terms of suffering and recovery of functional capacities—are left out of communications limited to only the precise medical language used to characterize the patient's disease progression and response to therapy. Nurses frequently felt morally compelled to clarify for the patient's family what the silent patient was experiencing by their daily interventions, and what the implications for daily life entailed in formally stated chances of survival. Care and communication were guided by the stated goals of care in the moment. Nurses who involve families in their loved one's care provide practical insights into their ill family member's conditions and daily experiences (see Chapter 7).

It is not unusual for treatment options to be presented in terms of what <u>can</u> be done without clearly presenting the probability of success for the options offered. In the past, the option of forgoing further therapies in situations of futility was not often provided. This traditional style of practice and language favored over-treatment to under-treatment. With the increase in for-profit managed health care, many institutions have inserted managerial strategies to curtail over-treatment. The new ethical temptation may now, in fact, be weighted in favor of under-treatment. Clearly the demand for sound clinical judgment and skilled reasoning about the particular patient in transition has never been greater. The following example illustrates the style of presenting what <u>can</u> be done rather than weighing carefully the option of not treating:

Nurse: This patient had originally come in for GI bleeding, but he was also end stage COPD. Well they start talking about 'Well, he could start bleeding and maybe we'd have to do surgery and he's got this breathing problem' and they don't directly say 'If his heart stops or if he goes into a rhythm that doesn't support life, do you want us to shock him? Do you want us to put him on the ventilator?' They don't go right into those questions—the questions you want them to ask—they sort of talk around it by saying the things that they could do instead of what they maybe should not do. They just present a bunch of 'coulds.'

Interviewer: And that's what they were doing with this man?

Nurse: Yeah.

We have a constricted language around facing death as a human passage and caring practices for the dying have been pushed to the margins of biomedical technological interventions. Medical interventions and curative therapies have become our symbolic language of caring about and valuing the patients. Not to do these interventions may be construed by the family and health care team members as "writing someone off."

It was evident in the interviews and observations that the discourse of prognostic scores—predicting death (knowledge about the disease and death as a biological event)—do not address the relational language and work of facing death as a human passage. These two distinct discourses, the biomedical-system discourse and the human lifeworld discourse, are often used symbolically and as proxies for each other. Telling the truth, by giving realistic predictions so that decisions can be made, does not adequately address the human processes of letting go, saying goodbye, and facing death. There are multiple levels of truth that nurses negotiate with patients and their families: truth in accord with objective facts about the disease, and truths about the uncertainties and facing the implications of death (including the cultural and religious truths about facing death). Nowhere is reasoning-in-transition more apparent than in end-of-life care, where making qualitative distinctions are central about whether the situation is one of genuine or false hope or of efficacious or futile heroic therapies.

Reducing this complex human event down to rational calculation about "what to do when" over-simplifies the demands of the situation by reducing them to decisions rather than finding a good path or being true to the possibilities in the situation as it unfolds. Decisional language is not rich enough to capture the relational issues, the understanding that unfolds over time, or the moral and relational import of the actual actions taken. And as Lynn (1997, p.179) points out, this was one of the problems with the SUPPORT study:

> Public language describes virtually all history in terms of choices and decisions. We say that 'It was decided to use a ventilator,' or 'My doctor chose to put me in the hospital because I was breathing so hard.' In medical ethics and law, virtually all actions are spoken of as decisions, and statements of optimum care systems focus heavily on optimum decision making. In a trivial sense, of course, such language is not inaccurate. For almost any action, another action was possible, and could have been 'chosen.' It is not at all clear, however, that the putative decision maker sees the options in this way... Intervention nurses spent a great deal of time explaining how a hospital works, the nature of the illness, and the resources available to help. Often, patients or family members would claim that he or she 'needs' to know what to do now. In a conceptual framework that assumes that decisions are what counts, they would have been understood to be seeking well-constructed decision trees and ways to elicit preferences [a rational biomedical discourse]. Taken at their word, however, they may really have simply been seeking 'a way to proceed.' (Lynn, 1997, p. 179).

Nurses are the ones who are present, who bear closest witness to the patient's and family's plight during the family's process of trying to understand how to proceed. The nurse's actions and orchestration of interventions depends on whether it is a situation of survival of death, or whether more aggressive curative therapies are warranted, and when or whether the focus should be on care, palliation, and facing death. Finding a way to proceed, reasoning-in-transition about the human experience of impending death (e.g., leaving loved ones, saying goodbye, and finishing one's life) may go at a different pace than reasoning-in-transition about the biomedical. The communication of the two separate truths requires distinct relational and communication skills. What one says about human death versus the biomedical event of death are different. Timing and dialogue about "what can be" as heard by loved ones are very different, as illustrated in the above interview.

By definition, all patients are admitted to critical care units in an attempt to save their lives. This intensive care context is radically different than that of hospice, and influences the reasoning-in-transition about what therapies, symptom management, and care are appropriate at different stages. Nevertheless, those who are in hospice care also constantly

undergo management transitions, so that appropriate interventions and symptom management strategies change in response to patient changes.

The following example illustrates the ambiguity and conflict that can occur when a patient is admitted to the ICU for treatment short of intubation. The transition of possible survival to dying in a painful state was rapid. The nurse describes the event complete with her moral anguish and learning from the situation. It is a situation of inadequate pain relief in the midst of limited but aggressive treatment. The nurse's honest appraisal of the breakdown and the excessive suffering demonstrate notions of the good, as well as practical moral reasoning during transitions:

Nurse: We had a transfer during the night and I was coming on to the day shift and this gentleman was transferred because of poor ABG's. He was, he had vasculitis and he was having hemoptysis, basically bleeding into his lungs. He was a Do Not Resuscitate by his wishes and his family's wishes. He came to us because they wanted to do everything they could up to intubation. So basically he'd been fairly stable over night, I mean it was pretty tenuous, but just before I came on at 6:00 a.m., his PO_2 dropped to 40. He was wearing a 100% non-rebreather at 6 liters and the nurse that was taking care of him during the night had tried to get a morphine order for him just for comfort sake because he was starting to get a little restless. The intern was very, very reluctant, uh, but he did finally agree to a subcutaneous morphine order, which the night nurse gave and it seemed to settle him down for a little bit. By the time I got into the room, he was starting to become more restless again, but we were also doing everything under the sun for him. It was a very busy time, hanging bloods and medicines. I watched this man just deteriorate before my eyes. He became so restless and tachypneic. He started to become incoherent and I found myself going out of the room three or four times to talk to the team about increasing his medication or putting him on an IV morphine drip, and they were very reluctant. They sort of agreed with me, but they were reluctant, they were waiting for his attending to come in to see him to make some decisions about him. They were waiting for the family to come in to see him. They wanted him to be awake for the family. They did increase the order for the subcutaneous morphine, which I gave him, but it didn't really make a bit of difference. So I sort of had to deal with each member of the team as they came on. It was early in the morning before rounds, and the resident came on, and she agreed, 'Yes, he should be on a morphine drip,' but they weren't ready to do that. And then, finally, our attending came in at the same time I'd drawn another gas which showed that he hadn't improved at all. Indeed, he was dying. He was a dying man and I was really torn because I knew that my priority was to make him comfortable. At the same time, I had all these orders that I had to do, hanging his meds and blood products and what have you. They finally wrote the IV morphine order and I already had it made up. I had one of the nurses make it up for me, and when I went to bolus the IV morphine, I looked up at the monitor and he started to brady down to about 30, and it was just, it was less than two hours from the time I started, but it felt like, it felt like 15 minutes, it just went by so fast, and it was just a very, very upsetting experience. I started to cry and I bolused it anyway. I hung the morphine, I knew it wasn't going to make a bit of difference, but I just felt very helpless and I felt as though I didn't do enough for him. I really, I wished—in retrospect—I was thinking about it afterwards, I wished that I had made the team come into the room with me and watch him, because I was watching him and I saw what he was going through. Bleeding continuously out of his mouth, and he was just so uncomfortable. And I wish that I had taken advantage of the people on our unit. They are wonderful and they come to your aid whenever you need a hand, and I wished I had brought someone in there...

Interviewer: Who do you mean?

Nurse 1: The other nurses.

Interviewer: The other staff, the staff nurse?

Nurse 1: Huh-huh. I wish I had had them in there to do the, kind of the medical tasks, while I dealt with this issue because I really felt like it was the priority, and unfortunately, I wasn't able to really make this man comfortable.

Interviewer: So what did you? Why do you think there was reluctance to give him morphine?

Nurse 1: Well, I think that, I don't know if they thought that the blood products, the platelets and the plasma, would help slow down this bleeding that he was having and—I don't know really what they were—I know they were kind of passing the buck in a way. They wanted to get a hold of this attending, and they wanted the family to be more involved, I think—he'd only been in the unit for a few hours. That's the whole problem with the ICU, the focus is on, you know, keeping someone alive, regardless. Especially when they first arrive. I mean after a few days and things aren't working out the way you think, they start to think, you know, perhaps this isn't what we should be doing for this person, but...

Interviewer: Was there a sense, did the house staff recognize that this man was dying or were they still getting to know him?

Nurse 1: Yes. Well, I think that they did. I mean I did get to them into the room at one point, and the resident in particular said, 'Oh, yes, this is, this isn't right.'

Interviewer: This isn't—what isn't right?

Nurse 1: The fact that this man can't breathe and he's suffocating. And I think that they knew that, but I think it took that second blood gas before they—I don't know if they thought he was going to miraculously have a better gas the second time around. There was nothing really that was done in between that would have made a difference.

Nurse 2: Was he at all lucid through any of this?

Nurse 1: He was when I first came on, but he did become incoherent. I mean, he was trying to climb out of bed, he was pulling his mask off, it was just awful, just awful.

Nurse 2: Was he expressing his uncomfortable...

Nurse 1: He wasn't saying anything, no, no.

Interviewer: Was he agitated?

Nurse 1: Very.

Interviewer: And were you inferring from his agitation, his...

Nurse 1: He was hypoxic and he was air hungry. He was just trying to breathe.

Nurse 3: And since they weren't going to intubate him, which would help him feel more comfortable breathing, you wanted to make him more comfortable the best way that you knew how.

Nurse 1: Right, right.

Interviewer: How long ago did this happen?

Nurse 1: Several weeks ago.

Interviewer: So just recently, relatively recently.

Nurse 1: Yes. It was terrible. It was probably one of the worst experiences I've had.

Interviewer: And what was, I mean, what was worst about it?

Nurse 1: Because he suffered so, and I feel as though we could have prevented that, we really could have. There was no need for it. And it's really my responsibility, you know, I mean sometimes the medical staff doesn't see that as their priority, but I think as nurses, we do and we should.

Interviewer: What did you, what did—go ahead...

Nurse 4: I was going to say, sometimes I don't think they understand just how bad things are just because they're a little bit more removed, you know what I mean? You're there all the time and you're seeing all the little fine changes, and all the little nuances that go on. If you can actually drag someone in the room and say, 'Look.'

Nurse 1: That's what I wished I had done. I mean they did that, I did get them in there once, but they—I think if I'd gotten them in there and kept them there...

Interviewer: Was it unusual that they wouldn't sedate him? I mean, did you find that to be unusual?

Nurse 5: It depends upon who's on it seems.

Nurse 1: Well, also, too because he was a new patient. And you don't send someone to an ICU, and then put them on a morphine drip and just let them die. You do that on the floor. They come to the unit to be cured...

Nurse 2: Sometimes they don't understand and they can't explain it well enough to the family.

Nurse 5: Yes and no. I mean, I've taken care of elderly, demented, 100-year-old people, whose sons are physicians or daughters are physicians, and they want their parents [to have a pulmonary line placed]—and what do you say to that? 'No, they're too old, I'm not going to Swan them?' You don't, you know, you Swan them. I'm not sure where—it was sort of one of those situations where you didn't have time. You questioned it, but you really didn't have time to get involved with it because there were so many other

Interviewer: Did the patient die some time after the morphine that you...

Nurse 1: Just as I was pushing it. I mean, he never even got it really. I mean, he bradyed down, as I was about to push the morphine, I looked up at the monitor and he was just beginning to...

Interviewer: You gave it anyway, though, huh?

Nurse 1: I hung the drip, too. And it was kind of silly, but...

Interviewer: I don't know if it was silly, but it certainly had some meaning for you. Sort of a need to do it. How did you recover? You said you cried.

Nurse 1: Well, I had, one of the other nurses was in the room with me and I talked to her about it. It's nice to have the support of your fellow workers. She was very supportive.

This narrative captures many of the contingencies and impediments to providing care of the dying in a rapidly moving trajectory. The culture and expectations of critical care push for rapid interventions. There is a humane and ethical concern that family members be with the patient and participate in decisions to withdraw therapies. The nurse experiences moral anguish because her patient suffers a needlessly horrendous death. She feels responsible for not being able to ensure that the physicians understood the patient's suffering. This is a narrative of ethical learning. One can imagine that this nurse will recognize a similar situation in the future and be able to act more effectively to get what is needed for the patient. This is also an example of a recurring ambiguity in clinical practice. The nurse does not defend her actions, though she understands how emergency treatment clouded her thinking-in-action. In retrospect, she wishes she had marshaled her colleagues more effectively and had insisted that the physicians directly observe the patient. The patient and family had agreed that intubation and extremely heroic measures were not in order, but treating with IV medications was acceptable. A transition occurred, and the patient's suffering increased, while the chances for his survival diminished. The moral situation changed, and the nurse was filled with frustration and regret over the patient's agonizing death.

The story illustrates the clinical variations in the decision not to resuscitate a patient. Patients, families, and healthcare providers have often agreed to stop short of intubation and chest compressions. This is sometimes called, in informal language, a "pharm code." But it is difficult in the actual situation to stop short of doing everything that one knows to be technically effective when the patient is dying and the agreed upon measures are not working. The following excerpt illustrates the practical ethos of pressing on to do everything technically possible once efforts at lifesaving have begun:

Nurse: We had a patient for a month at least, and he had gone from having an MI to becoming progressively worse and worse and worse. His situation was complicated by a lot of pulmonary problems. He ended up having lines put in and then eventually became intubated and just got progressively worse. I took care of him from when he had a small MI and was doing fairly well. And then I took care of him a lot during that time when he had lines in, and then I took care of him when he was intubated. Then the night he died, he was being taken care of by another nurse. That night he became progressively worse and the nurse needed a lot of help because she is new to our unit. And he was on dopamine and levophed and was maxed out, and couldn't hold his pressure and we ended up giving him plasmanate because we thought he was hypovolemic. The doctor called his family and they came in about 6:00 p.m. to see him—his two sons and his wife. Then at 7:00 p.m., right before report, he went asystolic and he had been modified to a pharm code. I was at the monitors and saw him go asystole, so I ran in there and [the other nurse] was in there and we ended up not calling a formal code because he was just a pharm code and the respiratory therapist was already in there. So we started bagging him and just pushed drugs. We had to ask the family to leave. During that kind of situation they don't have any rhythm and you're just pushing drugs and it's not doing anything because he's not being perfused and we couldn't do CPR. The nurse that was taking care of him one or two times before was upset. One of the nurses from the day shift that was in there helping stepped out and said: 'Are you sure you don't want us to do CPR? You know, the drugs that we are pushing are not working and we don't have a rhythm and we don't have a blood pressure?'

In the meantime we were paging cardiology stat and so by the time the cardiologist got there, probably ten minutes had gone by, but it seemed like an hour, because we just could push drugs and then wait and then push another epinephrine and then wait. I was just looking at him. He was by this time pale and dusky. The respiratory therapist kept bagging and you know we would watch the clock. Can we give another atropine or can we give another epinephrine? I just started crying because I had taken care of him so much and I had a really good rapport with him and his son. It took me a long time to get over that. I knew that he wasn't suffering, and I kind of wanted his death too, so he wouldn't have to go through the whole rigmarole of being coded. He was such a nice man and he had such a small MI. It was just so complicated that you think: 'Why does it have to be him?'

This narrative shows the anguish of losing a patient and illustrates the pragmatic distance between what seemed to be a rational decision to limit resuscitation to only medications and administering what turned out to be an inadequate treatment. In a cardiac arrest situation such as this, the administration of the resuscitative efforts were in vain. However, if the patient had not fully arrested, but instead had become very unstable while maintaining a cardiac rhythm with moderate hypotension, the drugs alone may have revived the patient. But this patient was dying and was not being cared for as a dying man. The nurse's sense of adequate resuscitation efforts and good care for the dying are violated. The limited, therapeutically invalid attempts to save his life continued to the very end. The nurse experiences moral anguish [Reich, 1984; Rushton, 1990] because she implemented ineffective interventions to save his life that were destined to fail, instead of facilitating a comfortable and peaceful death or administering a full resuscitation effort. Such irrational and dissatisfactory actions indicate lack of clarity about the nature of the patient's transition.

In rare instances, there is reason to decide on a pharmacological code which is in the patient's best interest. More typically, pharmacological or drug codes are a compromise between disagreeing parties' orders for resuscitative measures versus a DNAR order. In most instances, pharmacological codes are unsuccessful, cause the patient to suffer, and often needlessly separate the patient and family at the time of death. Nurses are then left with a situation of administering death through what is understood more as ineffectiveness and neglect than setting reasonable limits. Apparently this situation was clouded by a clinical understanding that this patient might survive. "Partial" extreme measures are fraught with ambiguity, and attentiveness to transitions into futility can prevent tragedies such as the one above.

We think it is helpful to name and characterize different commonly occurring transitions from heroic treatment to caring for the dying patient and family as they occur in critical care units. Transition into unacceptable levels of treatment and suffering too often goes un-named and un-discussed. Avoidance and "moving on" without confronting mistaken treatments is an ethical breach in team building and taking responsibility to learn from experience. Naming such transitions and clinical/ethical debriefing after such events can create a cumulative wisdom and improved clinical and ethical discernment by all members on the healthcare team. Setting limits is a reasonable strategy for keeping open to possibilities, but there are few worked out public understandings and language about what it is like to administer ineffective treatments in the name of saving a life, while watching someone die. The ethical violence to the patient/family is clear, but the nurse's moral anguish of administering ineffective treatments, and lack of attention to death as a human passage, becomes clear only with the nurse's first person account of her/his experience.

The nurse wants to be true to her responsibility to the patient and neither create unnecessary suffering or omit possible lifesaving treatment. There is little time for reflection in the situation and a 10-minute delay in the cardiologist's response heightens the moral conflict. Timing and progression of events are central to moral reasoning in practice. Timing and action are left out of ethical theories that focus only on justification of actions after the event (Beauchamp, 1994). Narratives such as the one above can enhance moral imagination (Murdoch, 1970/1991; Nussbaum, 1995), moral perception (Benner & Wrubel, 1982; Blum, 1994; 1980; Vetleson, 1994), and skillful ethical comportment (Benner, Tanner & Chesla, 2009), and breathe life into upholding ethical principles of fidelity, beneficence, and non-maleficence (Beauchamp, 1994).

PLANNING AND IMPLEMENTING ATTENTIVE, PALLIATIVE CARE

Once the decision is made to implement palliative care for a dying patient, how to plan and implement that care requires astute skills of involvement with the patient and family in order to ensure that death as a human passage and end of a particular life is attended to with respect and dignity. The Institute of Medicine [IOM] (Field & Cassel, 1997) notes that dignity is layered with cultural, social and person meanings and recommends that rather than trying to formalize the definition of what is "dignity" in ways that could cover all experiences, that those dying be treated in ways that convey respect for the person's inherent dignity:

> death dignified by care that honors and protects—indeed cherishes—those who are dying, that conveys by word and action that dignity resides in people, not physical attributes, and that helps people to preserve their integrity while coping with unavoidable physical insults and losses (p.25).

Anne Hughes (2001) did a study of what constitutes "dignity" in dying for the inner city poor and found that relational recognition practices that include respect and meeting the person as a person rather than "other" or a person who is dying. By contrast, Chochinov and his colleagues (2002) proposed an empirically derived model of dignity at the end of life. He interviewed 50 terminally ill Canadian cancer patients. Patients were asked how they defined dignity, and what particular experiences supported or undermined their sense of personal dignity. The respondents were asked for their opinions about what role "dignity" played in causing patients to request the hastening of an inevitable death. Chochinov and colleagues (Chocinov et al 2002) proposed a formal model that depicted the interrelationships of the three categories (illness related concerns, dignity conserving repertoire, and social dignity inventory). Dignity was identified as the outcome variable in their model. The five themes related to social dignity were: privacy boundaries, social support, care tenor, burden to others and aftermath concerns. The dignity conserving repertoire turned out to be a significant moderating variable in the model. The eight sub-themes of dignity-conserving perspectives were: continuity of self, role preservation, generativity/legacy, hopefulness, autonomy/control, acceptance, and resilience/fighting spirit. Three sub-themes were described for dignity-conserving practices: living in the moment, maintaining normalcy and seeking spiritual comfort. These "dignity conserving" repertoire for patients are related to existential skills of dwelling Weiss (1996; 2010; Sunvisson, Haberman, Weiss, Benner, 2009).

Sara Weiss (1996) describes the existential skills of dwelling as follows:

> . . . the following existential skills promote and sustain dwelling-in-the-world: (a) physical and cognitive capacities including memory and access to emotions which facilitate embodied participation in meaningful habits, rituals, and practices, (b) ways of being with people characterized by a self-in-relation-to-others based on practices of mutual recognition, and (c) caring or having current concerns or structures of meaning such that people and things matter; what is salient shows up in light of these concerns. (Weiss, 1996, p. 117)

Weiss notes Winnicott's (1953/1986, p. 256) observations of the links between the relational transitional objects established for children, religious meanings, and spirituality in adulthood:

> Winnicott (1953/1986, p. 256) talks about the "intermediate area of experiencing;" the part of the human being where the ability to recognize self and other and to accept reality develops. In infants, it is an area of illusory experience, where transitional object and transitional phenomena facilitate beginning object relationships. Winnicott asserts that this domain of illusion prevails in adulthood, because the tension between inner and outer reality can never be completely reconciled. It is in this region, outside the authority of any kind of reality testing, where artistic experience, religious feeling dreaming, and creativity exist and provide a bridge between inner self and world. (Weiss, 2010, p. 307).

Judith Wrubel and her colleagues (2009) found that living, dwelling in one's relationships and lifeworlds helps patients live their lives until dying, and contrasted those who experienced social death prior to physical death:

> Nineteen participants described living daily lives that embraced centrally self-defining concerns despite the spatial and temporal constrictions imposed by their illness. Of the 19, 12 died before the end of the study. Three types of central concerns embodied the participants' core values and personhood: (a) relational, (b) spiritual, (c) goal-oriented. These were not mutually exclusive categories. Most participants' narratives reflected more than one concern. Maintaining engagement with one or more of these central concerns was a source of positive feelings in the midst of the ups and downs of the illness, and recurring or ongoing pain and suffering. Thirteen participants (8 deceased, 5 nondeceased) did not share any of the central concerns held by the Maintained Lifeworld group. One or more of the following life aspects or disease conditions among these participants appeared to prevent the maintenance of a lifeworld: (a) relocation just before or during the study; (b) disease-caused cognitive impairment or preexisting psychiatric condition; (c) commitment to pre-illness goals that were no longer tenable; (d) ongoing substance abuse. (Wrubel, et al, 2008, pp. 1429-1430).

Wrubel and her colleague's work (2009) point to common concerns of nurses midwifing death in order to help patients to continue to live their lives until death, as evidenced by the exemplars presented in this chapter.

Weiss (2010) points out the importance of transitional objects helpful in developing object relationships in general. Her works points to the phenomena of holding open a horizon and a sense of possibility in old age and dying.

The nurses we interviewed reflected these concerns about lifeworld and relational ties being maintained at the end of living. It is here that one can notice a cross-professional overlap with the work of clergy in helping persons maintain their spirituality and lifeworlds in the midst of extreme illness:

> When concerned with recovery and coping with the human experience of illness, nurses focus on patients' life worlds-their families, communities, and the concerns that organize their lives. To do this, a broader view of rationality is needed. After all, giving birth, recovering from injury or acute illness, coping with chronic illnesses, and approaching death are all deeply embedded in people's life worlds and cannot be adequately addressed by a narrow, technical rationality (Benner & Sutphen, 2007, p. 108).

In our original study (Benner, Hooper-Kyriakidis, & Stannard, 1st edition 1999) and now in the last 10 years, we found that disagreements over the content and nature of comfort care are frequent. There was a distressing level of variation in the care of the dying patient, once it was decided that death was inevitable and there were no further viable life-sustaining treatment options. This is illustrated in the following interview:

> **Nurse 1:** There are like two camps. Some people say that just because they're a 'No Code' doesn't mean that if their blood pressure drops, we're not going to stand them on their heads and put them in Trendelenburg. Even though we're not going to start them on dopamine, we're still going to do other non-invasive treatments, anything we can to get that blood pressure back up. Give them a 100 cc's from their [IVs] instead of 50. Anything we can possibly do to get that pressure back up. And yet there's another group of people that feel like, 'Well, OK, their blood pressure's dropping, we'll just keep them comfortable and let nature take its course.'
>
> **Nurse 2:** Sometimes I find myself in either one of the camps.
>
> **Nurse 1:** Exactly!

These nurses express human conflict and uncertainty in facing and bearing witness to death. Staff development and ethics consultation can help clarify the conflicting goods of preventing prolonged suffering prior to death (i.e. extended or suspended dying) versus saving lives of patients who are not dying and may benefit from full resuscitation.

There were also examples of dying babies being given tactile stimulation to breathe, as is the usual practice for recovering premature infants. Nurses often failed to make the distinction between the ordinary life-saving measures for the infant who is not dying and appropriate care for the dying infant, and consequently prolonged the infant's dying by repeatedly interrupting apnea episodes through stimulation. This example illustrates the need to clarify and work through the practical ethics of caring for the dying when all treatment has been withdrawn. Suspending usually taken-for-granted practices such as stimulating infants during periods of apnea requires thoughtfulness and consensus on the need for palliative care.

The moral import of being the one who intervenes or withholds intervention closest to the dying person is not adequately accounted for in discussions of ethical decision making. We do not know how extensive the practice of manipulating the blood pressure of dying patients with DNAR orders is, and recommend research and quality assurance studies be done in order to understand this practice better. We speculate that the over-riding habits and concern for saving lives and the emotional and moral demands of being the one present at death cause nurses to intervene in ways that postpone death. The other temptation is to hasten death. We did not encounter instances of hastening death in this study. There has been insufficient discussion and clarification about what is meant by caring practices for those who are dying as Brody, Campbell, Faber-Langendoen, and Ogle (1997, p.547) point out:

> For 15 of the 52 patients, physicians specified that patients were to receive 'comfort care.' However, the subsequent care rendered to these patients varied substantially, from discontinuing all medical interventions except oxygen and morphine as needed, to continuing pressors and parenteral nutrition, initiating antibiotics, and drawing blood samples for serum creatinine determinations in a patient who declined dialysis... The main focus in the care of the dying patient has been on making the initial decision to forgo treatment; once physicians recognize that a patient is dying and further aggressive treatment is unwarranted, there is little guidance in deciding specifically which treatments to discontinue and what care to provide (Brody, et. al, 1997 p. 547)..

Our descriptive study corroborates this observation. There is much clinical wisdom and skilled know-how that could be imported from hospice care to critical care settings. Also, ethics consultation around differences in opinion and practices around palliative care are needed on a unit-by-unit basis to reduce variation in nursing care that is at cross purposes. In the following exemplar, Nurse Cindy Rogers recounts Marie's downward course of illness due to advanced stage breast cancer. She courageously advocates for the patient's transition into the hospice care at home that she and her family had requested.

Nurse: I first met Marie when I transferred to the inpatient oncology unit from the outpatient clinic. I had seen her a few times while working down there, so I was somewhat familiar with her history. She was only 44 years old and had been first diagnosed with breast cancer with advanced disease the year before. She had ignored a large breast mass for a year. She was the mother of two sons and one would be married soon. The other son was 16 years old. She had been separated from her husband, but he had reconciled with her to help her through her cancer. He seemed very loving and doted on her, staying overnight often.

This admission had been for a malignant pleural effusion and Marie had several thoracenteses and chest tube insertions, but the pleural effusion kept coming back. Another round of chemo was tried. She became neutropenic, and with a white cell count of only 100, she was a set up for a severe infection. She was transfused with several units of packed red blood cells. She was put on total parental nutrition and multiple intravenous antibiotics for a resistant pneumonia she had developed. She grew weaker, and her arms, legs, and abdomen ballooned with edema. Her skin was pale, translucent and shiny. Thankfully, her chest tube had been removed the week before, so her pain was well controlled on a small dose of Oxycontin.

Over the last few days Marie had developed a pulmonary embolus and was being treated with IV Heparin. Marie told me she was tired of these futile attempts to treat the ever-increasing problems caused by her cancer and the chemotherapy. She had not left that hospital room in a month and missed her home. Her husband had stayed almost every night, sleeping in a recliner. At night her husband asked about Marie's chances of survival, and I spoke in a low voice and said, "She will not survive this."

She asked me if she would ever get better. I told her what the doctor had already told her, gently, but honestly that the cancer had spread and was incurable. It had not responded well to the chemotherapy, and I told her more chemo at this point was probably too dangerous because she was so sick. She looked at her husband in shock and asked him if he knew she was that ill. She assumed all the suffering she had endured would resolve when her cancer was cured. Her husband told her, "You are in God's hands."

Marie, her husband, and I spoke of Marie's wishes should her condition decline further. She and her husband decided that if this was God's plan, then He knew best, even if His plan was to heal her by taking her to Heaven. I told her that I would stand by her decision.

I came in the next evening to find Marie had taken a turn for the worse and had been put on 100% oxygen. She and her family agreed that she was not to be resuscitated. They wanted her to go home with hospice. Unfortunately, her doctor was having trouble letting go, so while the doctor did write the DNR order, Marie was also started on continuous infusion morphine to help her breathing and was not referred to hospice. The doctor then was off duty for the rest of the day. I went to check her after report and found her comatose with agonal respirations. The oxygen mask looked so large on her small face, but she did look peaceful. Her husband asked me to explain what the PCA was. I told him it would deliver a continuous dose of morphine to Marie to keep her comfortable. He questioned why it was started, as Marie did not complain of pain, and she hadn't liked the way morphine made her feel previously. She was barely arousable. He told me he wanted to take Marie home. I knew the hospice consult had been cancelled, but I felt I needed to get this woman home in the morning to be around the things she loved. I knew her time was running out.

I shut the morphine pump off and told her husband that we would see if she woke up a little. If she was in pain, I could always medicate her. I paged the oncologist on call who came to the floor about 30 minutes later. I asked him to D/C the PCA and reinstate the hospice consult per the family's wish. I also asked for a Foley cath order for the patient's comfort. He agreed to the PCA and Foley but did not want to reinstate the hospice consult until the patient's own oncologist came in the morning. I had already called hospice prior to the doctor getting to the floor to try to catch the hospice nurse before she went home for the day. She had already told me she would come speak with the family on her way home. I told the doctor this, but he still wanted to wait and let the other doctor make the decision. He said, "It can wait until tomorrow."

I said, "Marie can't wait. She is so poor that she could even die tonight. Marie can't wait for her own doctor to come in. It would add days to her hospitalization. The hospice nurse assured me that if she met with the family tonight, she could arrange to have a hospital bed in her home in the morning." I wasn't letting the doctor leave the floor until I got the order. He relented and told me to write the order and he would sign it.

I went to Marie's room to insert the Foley and tell her the hospice nurse would be coming in. I saw that she was waking up out of the morphine-induced fog. After I inserted the Foley, Marie was really waking up. Her family came back in the room, and they were so happy to see her awake. They all had a good visit, and she was able to speak with the hospice nurse. After the consult, I could see Marie was getting restless. I asked her if she wanted something to help her sleep. "Not morphine!" she said, so I gave her a small dose of Ativan.

The next night I came into work and was told Marie was able to go home via ambulance that morning. Marie died three weeks later, and I'm sure she would not have lived that long if she had stayed in the hospital. Her family let us know that her death was peaceful, and she was surrounded by the things she loved. They thanked me for helping her to get home as was her wish.

Even today, with more emphasis on palliative care paired with curative care, some physicians think that an order for comfort care only or a DNAR order will cause patients' needs to be neglected. This is evident in the following nurse's written account describing a discussion between a nurse and physician, where the nurse is advocating for patient comfort and for a DNAR order:

Nurse: Tonight, I decided it would somehow be different. I sat down beside the physician and engaged him in a somewhat lopsided conversation (mine). I asked him about the patient's code status. His answer was 'Full code, of course', and 'why do you ask?' (I was thinking he really does not want to know, but I am going to tell him anyway. I must, I will, and here goes) I took a deep breath and with all the tact I could muster, I proceeded. I replied that given the insidious disease process and the terminal prognosis, the patient was not likely to survive this illness. At this point he countered with a garbled account of how some multiple myeloma patients are living longer now than just a few years ago. I decided to bring him back out of the research studies and to the reality of the situation facing us this night. I calmly explained to him as graphically as possible what a code would do the patient's already broken body. 'Do you realized that with the first downward thrust of CPR I would probably break at least half of his ribs and perhaps his sternum?' I asked. 'Should he survive a code, what quality of life would there possibly be?' I asked earnestly and sincerely. 'He is already in so much pain that when we turn him he frequently asks for it to be all over. How can we put this human being through anything more?'

The doctor didn't say anything for a few minutes. When I couldn't stand the silence any longer I asked him 'What are you thinking?' He replied, 'You won't like what I am thinking.' I replied, 'I really want to know.' (Inside I was saying, 'Come on, come on, talk to me'). He finally sat up very tall in his chair and stated 'No code patients do not receive the same care as other patients.' Quickly I went to the defense of the nursing staff. He then just as quickly said 'See, I told you that you wouldn't like it.' I took a deep breath and calmly said 'We both have a right to have opinions and to share them. We really don't have to agree. What it really important is what would really be in this patient's best interest.'

At this point, my other patient began ringing her light for the bedpan. I looked around for someone, anyone, to do the task for me. No one was available so I paused in my dialog saying 'just a minute' and meaning 'I am not through with this conversation as I have at least 2000 more words on the subject.' But to my dismay, when I returned to my still warm chair, the doctor was gone. I was distraught, but then there was the open chart. Lo and behold there were the words NO CODE BLUE written two inches high for all the world to see. I turned to one of my fellow nurses and asked 'What changed his mind?' She answered quietly, 'You did. While you were gone, he turned to me and said: She is right.' He then quickly wrote the order and left the unit.

Two days later, this patient died quietly and with dignity. No one fractured his already ravaged body. No one forced a tube into his airway. Instead his nurse and his wife stood at the bedside holding his hands and bid him farewell and a safe journey.

Why is this incident critical to me? I learned one quiet evening that one nurse can be a patient advocate. This incident has given me the courage to speak up many more times. I find that I now can easily approach doctors and discuss a patient's code status intelligently and compassionately.

The awareness of the living-to-dying transition is human, and the clinical knowledge surrounding this transition is negotiated with the patient, family, and the healthcare team. As noted above, this process is further complicated when dialogue about the human passage of death is couched only in rational biomedical decision making language. Sometimes doing "heroic measures," even if futile, are taken up as a symbolic way of saying that the person is worth every effort, and the worthiness is symbolically construed by extreme measures:

Nurse: Sometimes families want everything done and you don't think that there is a point to it. We had a patient, a young guy about twenty-six with AIDS. He was a nurse and his father was a physician. I mean clearly they should have understood the disease process and he had pneumosistis pneumonia and they wanted him transferred into the ICU. They wanted him intubated and put on the ventilator and full-speed support. He died within twenty-four hours of admission to the ICU. And that was what they all really strongly felt was important because they really didn't want anyone to write him off because he had AIDS. It was a real conflict. I know for the nurses taking care of him for that short span of time—they were why are we doing this? But it was really important for the family and they were certainly medical people. They knew this wasn't likely to turn around.

This situation is not unique to persons with AIDS. Despite the clinical efforts to determine which measures work, medical interventions can be used to signify commitment. The discourse of science is taken up as much as religion or art might be used to express hope, protest, or despair—a symbolically laden form of giving respect to the worth and value of life. The biomedical interventions become sacramental acts instead of rationally determined, effective measures. Despite all efforts to be as clear and rational as possible, death as a human passage is non-rationalizable. Acknowledging death as a human passage, and acknowledging the sorrow, fear, and anxiety of losing a loved one can help patients and families to shift the communication and attention to facing death and paying respect to the life that has been lived. Tact, clinical wisdom, and compassionate relationships are required.

We found many cultural practices associated with being with and comforting the dying and their family. For example, the person should not die alone. Religious practices should be honored. The person should be allowed to have last wishes and completion tasks done on her or his behalf. The person should know, if possible and in accord with cultural expectations, that death is imminent so that they can face death and effect any completion tasks, make amends, or say good bye (Gordon, 1997). The environment should be soothing and not intrusive and disruptive. The patient's wishes for comfort and alertness should be honored so that maximum comfort and level of alertness are facilitated within the limits of what is possible. "Death with dignity" is a mandate for keeping the person as intact with as much continuity with the person's life as possible. The mandate for dignity is laden with ethical content that calls for limiting depersonalizing technology while using its benefits wisely. Dignity and care also require setting limits to futile treatments and allowing for the person to be comforted in ways that are available for the patient and family.

In the business world, cultural and ethnic diversity increase the need for impersonal and generalized rules and procedures in order to smooth the business transactions between strangers who come from culturally diverse groups. It is tempting to think that we can import these impersonal bureaucratic and market practices into the sickness and health industry to reduce conflict, suffering, and to "solve" the problems of suffering and dying. But neither ethics nor medical care related to dying can be adequately dealt with by rules and procedures about the general or the typical situation. Strategic goal-oriented language is not rich enough to capture the significance of death as a human passage. Dying concludes the person's human story, and forever alters the lives of family and close others.

Human concerns related to dying are highly particular and culturally dependent as illustrated in the following small group interview discussion about a good death. Many nurses are clear about the notions of good and principles related to caring for the dying. Even so, the skillful ethical comportment for making this happen is not easy to actualize, in the midst of the uncertainty and emotionally charged atmosphere of death and in the face of culturally diverse understandings about dying:

Interviewer: Is there a conflict in the notion of good and the notion of how one ought to die that comes up in the unit around this? A conflict about how it ought to be done or how one ought to die? Or is there consensus on how it ought to be? That's what I'm wondering.

Nurse: I think there's pretty much consensus on how people feel like it ought to be, but you can't actually actualize that....

Interviewer: Is there any drive for creating as much consciousness before death as possible? I'm trying to think of the cultural practices around dying.

Nurse: With being able to allow their family member to die? Because they won't allow their family to die. And the doctors don't want to withdraw support against their will. You have a lot of discomfort and right up to the very end, a lot of times, the patient's actually dying right there in front of everybody. But even if they're frightened, they're afraid for you to do anything like take the [ventilator] off or stop an IV or give a drug or do anything that might influence the actual death. And you do have to sit back and do it their way if that's what they want. But, in general...

Interviewer: On the staff there seems to be a consensus.

Nurse: The staff isn't comfortable with that type of death. But they are comfortable with doing what the family... They try to get the families to see the light (laughs) you know. But if they're not going to see it, you can't go too much against their will. And sometimes doctors will be strong enough to do it whether the family wants it or not, withdraw some support measures, or not add anything. That's the other one. You're not going to... The patient's going to die, but they're not going to withdraw anything, leave them on 100% oxygen, but they won't add anything. They won't treat the bug that's growing that they know is growing, that's going to kill them. And that's really hard I think. That's really hard for the nurses in the ICU to deal with. They don't like that. And they don't like—they call it—not having any guts (laughs).

Interviewer: Can you just talk about the things that you think about when you walk in a room, or the things that, if they're not there, you would say, "This needs to be here."

Nurse: For a patient that's dying?

Interviewer: Yes...

Nurse: That's really a hard one to put on paper for me because it just sort of _is_. And some people... It's really cultural in certain ways too... But you sort of assess what that particular family needs. And when you come into a room, and if you're working with them for a long time, it just sort of is happening, what they need.

As intimated in the above discussion, the nurse follows the family's lead. Death is an individual and community event, laden with particularity. Individuals, families, and community members want to be attended to, with respect for their customs and their particular concerns. Such attentiveness to particularity and diversity requires knowing the patient (Tanner, Benner, & Chesla, 1993) and well developed recognition practices that allow for dialogue and understanding (Taylor, 1991; 1993). Strategic planning language focusing on prediction and control clashes with the storied human world of concerns, meanings, and relationships that come together at the end of life. The nurse's moral sense of preparing human space for dying is not the exception. Every time a death occurs without this ritual of setting aside time and preparing a place for death, it was experienced by nurses in this study as a nursing and human failure in care—a failure in having a death with human dignity. So while the heroic saving of lives robs many of leave-taking rituals, these rituals are there to be called up and recovered as illustrated in this and many other stories. The following story told by Nurse Clara Reagan demonstrates the hospice wisdom of allowing patients to complete unfinished business so that they can die in peace (Byock, 1997).

Nurse: Last year during the Christmas week was when I met Ben and Alice. Ben was in his seventies and had metastatic lung cancer. All his treatments had been on an outpatient basis and he had not been hospitalized until now. Ben had stopped treatment several weeks ago and had been home receiving hospice care. He had told his wife Alice that when he felt he was close (to death) he wanted her to bring him to the hospital to die. He told her he did not want her to remember him dying in their home. A few days earlier Ben told Alice it was time so Alice honored his wishes and brought him to our unit.

The first day I took care of Ben, he barely spoke. I asked him if he wasn't talking because he was too weak or because he was sad. He just shrugged his shoulders. I held his hand and told him we would take good care of him, that we would make sure he stayed comfortable and that we would also help support Alice as well. He smiled and squeezed my hand. I met Alice later that morning. It was then that she told me she had diabetes and had gone home to get enough insulin for a few days. She said she wasn't about to leave his side. I reminded Alice it would be important for her to take care of herself by eating and resting as much as possible. I set up a sleeping cart in Ben's room and showed her where our shower and patient kitchen was. Because Ben wasn't eating very much, I told her to fill out the menus anyway so she would have meals to eat.

Ben slept most of the day so I spent the time getting to know Alice and finding out as much as I could about them. It is always easier to be supportive in ways which are helpful and comforting to a patient and family when I have an established relationship over the course of several admissions and a long period of time. I wanted to gather as much information about Ben and Alice's life and get to know them so that they would not feel like I was a stranger to them. Since Ben had told Alice he didn't have much longer before he came in, I knew time was of the essence.

I asked a few basic leading questions but it only took one or two for me to realize that Alice just loved to tell their story and that all I had to do was listen. She told me that she had known Ben since they were small children. They lived a few houses apart and went to grade school together. She said, as they became teenagers she always thought Ben was the cutest boy in the neighborhood. Trouble was, so did all the other girls and at the time she thought Ben viewed her more like a sister so they never got together as a couple. Eventually they both moved out of the neighborhood and lost touch with each other. They both married and had families. Many years later, shortly after Alice's husband died she was at a bar and spotted Ben on one of the stools. She said she couldn't believe it. She said he was handsome as ever. Alice told me she noticed he wasn't wearing a wedding band so she casually went over and sat next to him and said," So, are you gonna just sit there or are you gonna buy me a drink?" She said Ben recognized her immediately and the two spent the evening catching up. Ben was also recently widowed and confessed to Alice that the only reason he hadn't asked her out when they were younger was because he wasn't sure she would have said yes.

She said she told him she wasn't letting him get away a second time and they were married a few weeks later and had been together ever since.

Over the next couple of days, Ben remained quiet but comfortable and I made sure Alice ate and kept her blood sugar under control. Alice spoke lovingly to and about Ben. She told him he was a good man who had showed her true happiness and love. She told him she would miss him but that she knew because of her faith that they would someday be together again forever.

At some point later that day, Alice called me into Ben's room. "Something's wrong with Ben." she said. When I got to the room, indeed Ben was having trouble. He was gasping for breath, drenched with perspiration and was profoundly cyanotic. He was sitting bolt upright in bed leaning forward in an attempt to catch his breath. He was mouthing the words help me. Looks like PE I thought to myself. "It's OK, Ben; I'm going to help you." I placed Ben in a non-rebreather mask and grabbed some IV Morphine from the Pyxis medication dispensing machine. As I pushed the morphine, a pastoral care chaplain happened to stop in. He took one look at Ben and immediately began saying prayers one would hear as a patient was taking his last breaths.

Alice must have recognized those prayers as well because she leaped into bed with Ben and embraced his upper body, cradling his head in her bosom. She began saying to Ben, "It's OK my darling, Go, Go to heaven. Spend Christmas with Jesus." Ben began to become very restless, his eyebrows frowned and he was shaking his head back and forth. I recognized that this was not restlessness associated with his PE; rather he was trying to tell us he was not ready to go at that moment.

I nudged the chaplain and motioned for him to stop the prayers. He caught on and started to say, "It's OK Ben, it's when you're ready." I gently told Alice I could be wrong but that I didn't feel like Ben was taking his last breaths, I think Ben heard me because he started to shake his head back and forth again as if to say, "No, I'm Not!"

I reassured Ben that the oxygen and morphine would help him breathe more comfortably and to trust me and try to relax and rest. Again I held his hand and he squeezed it.

A few minutes later, Alice had told me she called her kids to come in. I told her that was fine, that I was sure Ben would like to see them and although I felt Ben was not ready to go, he certainly had an acute, sudden change in his condition. The next thing I knew the room was filled to capacity. There must have been 12 or 14 people in the room. I got a quick introduction to Ben and Alice's family. I asked if Ben knew they were there and they said they hadn't tried to wake him. I gently stroked Ben's shoulder and told him he had a room full. He opened his eyes and they began to talk to him. I watched from the door and noticed Ben sat up in bed and literally scanned the room back and forth slowly and methodically as if he were looking for someone in particular. When he finished he plopped his head back on his pillow. Hmmm I thought. I wonder who's missing.

Eventually the room cleared out. Only Alice and two of her daughters remained. We chatted about the day and Alice said, "You know, I was pretty sure Ben was dying this morning. After all I know he's ready. He told me so at home before we left for the hospital." I told Alice I felt Ben might be holding on for some reason, maybe some one. I explained to her what I noticed when all the visitors were here and asked if perhaps there was someone that Ben might want or need to see. Maybe someone he hasn't seen in a while?

One of Alice's daughters said, "Well, it might be his son. He won't come. He hasn't seen his father in about a year and a half over something stupid. He's a jerk." Well I said I don't know for sure if that's it but I have seen this happen before when a family questions what a patient is waiting for when they feel he has accepted death yet appears to be holding himself back. Alice's daughter said, knowing Ben he probably was waiting for his son. Ben always hated that they weren't speaking but that he had tried to reconcile but that his son never returned his calls. I asked her if she knew how to reach him and she said she thought his business number was in the phonebook and would give it a try.

The next day, Christmas Eve, Ben was noticeably weaker. It had been several days without intake of any kind and his urine output was scant but still Ben was holding on. I asked Alice's daughter if she had heard from Ben's son and she said, "No I left a message. He probably doesn't believe me and thinks I'm trying to trick him into coming to see his father." I asked her if she really thought that was a possibility and she said yes. I asked Alice if she wanted me to try to call him and she said. 'Yes.' She knew it would bring Ben peace if he came.

I took the phone number and went to a vacant room and asked the operator to place the call. I too reached an answering machine. I explained who I was and why I was calling. I told him I knew he had received a message from Alice's daughter and that his father was indeed dying. I told him I knew nothing about the reasons he and his dad had not spoken in a while but that I hoped he would come. I told him I felt it would bring his father peace and that he may bring himself peace as well. I told him I had been caring for the dying for almost twenty years and know that guilt is something we inflict on ourselves. I told him I was reaching out to him and hoped he would be able to free himself and his father.

I told Alice I had left the message and would pray that he would come for Ben's sake. She said I should pray for a miracle because she thought it would be one if he came. I said, "Well then, maybe Ben will have a Christmas miracle."

I was off the next two days. When I returned, Ben's room was empty. I asked the staff when Ben had died and they said early the previous morning. I asked if his son had come but nobody knew.

Later that morning, one of the pastoral care chaplains stopped by. I asked her if she knew whether Ben's son had visited. She said he had. She said he came in quietly and asked to see his father. Only he and Alice were in the room and then Alice gave Ben and his son some private time. She said that Alice told her that because Ben was so close to death, that as much reconciliation that was possible under the circumstances happened. She also said she was certain Ben knew he was there.

She also said Ben died peacefully a few hours after his son's visit. Alice had said she was grateful for she knew Ben was truly at rest.

I said a silent prayer to thank God for Ben's Christmas miracle.

Clara Reagan has gained much experiential wisdom in caring for dying patients in her 20 years of nursing practice. She noticed Ben looking for the missing son as he surveyed the room full of his family. She remained curious and open and asked about why Ben was holding on, saying that he was not ready to die. She made the extra effort to phone the son, when she leared that he might not have believed his sister. She developed a bond with Alice and Ben by finding out about the story of their life together. Without this knowledge of them and their life together she would not have been as effective in midwifing Ben's death. Her practice demonstrates advanced skills of involvement and clinical imagination based upon staying open, attuned and curious.

In some cultures, it is inappropriate for the patient's well-being to tell them they are dying. It is enough for the family to know and they (in culturally sensitive ways) convey this to the patient and carry out leave-taking rituals. Although the North American way is to have a direct discussion with the patient, it does violence in some cultures and ethnic groups. We need to convey our understandings and notions of good but recognize that our notions are sometimes not cross-cultural. If we err, it is better to err on the side of taking the family's lead, even if one does not understand the background practices.

Leave-taking rituals require that the patient and family members have some awareness that death is near. The nurse's moral sense about a particular patient and family's right to know the patient is dying offers respect for the human passage of death and the person's right to know. It takes moral risk and courage to overcome the fear that such knowledge might create suffering for the dying person and her/his surviving family. For example, after all resuscitation attempts to rescue a man in acute liver failure, the decision was made by the patient, family and doctors to withdraw all therapies. The patient asked the nurse how soon he would die, and she answered, soon, probably within hours (Benner, Tanner & Chesla, 2009). The nurse was compelled to speak the truth by the man's direct question and desire to know. In this sense, the nurse's actions seem to be in the spirit of respect and dignity. It seemed wrong to her to hide the man's imminent death from him, robbing him and his family of the possibilities of doing the rituals of leave-taking that they needed to do. One is cut off from community by having the community/family awareness mixed in a cloud of secret keeping or mutual pretense (Glaser, & Strauss, 1965). Tolstoy writes in his story of the *Death of Ivan Ilyich* (Tolstoy, 1996):

> The worst torment was the lie, this lie that for some reason was accepted by everyone, that he was only sick and not dying, and that if he would only remain calm and take care of himself, everything would be fine...He suffered because they lied and forced him to take part in this deception...this lie that degraded the formidable and solemn act of his death (Tolstoy, p. 137).

Knowing that a patient's death may be soon allows the patient and family to face death. Having said that, however, each case is bounded by the particulars unique to each situation and cultural meanings, including the patient and family's desires, cultural practices, and their shared life histories.

FACING DEATH

The unevenness of facing death causes much moral confusion and anguish in critical care areas. Yet we do have multiple notions in various religious and cultural traditions about facing one's own death. Regardless of the religious or cultural tradition, those dying and those witnessing a death find uncertainty, mystery, wisdom, angst, anguish, and even hope in facing the actual time of death. As Gordon Stuart, a 33-year-old writer dying of cancer points out to his hospice physician, facing death is never an all or none thing, and thus, any sort of achievement or technique-oriented approach to care of the dying is bound to fall short in the face of death (Kleinman, 1988, p.147):

Gordon: I am dying now, aren't I?

Hadley: Yes, you are.

Gordon: I can look into my garden and see sunshine. I know that next week, maybe tomorrow it will be shining just as brightly, just as beautifully, but I won't be part of it. I will no longer be here. Do you know, can you imagine what it—it feels like to make that statement and know that it is true for you that you are dying?

Hadley: I think I can, but I'm not sure.

Gordon: All that nonsense that's written about stages of dying as if there were complete transitions—rooms that you enter, walk through, then leave behind for good. What rot. The anger, the shock, the unbelieveableness, the grief—they are part of each day. And in no particular order, either. Who says you work your way eventually to acceptance—I don't accept it! Today I can't accept it. Yesterday I did partly. Saturday I was there: kind of in a trance, waiting ready to die. But not now. Today it is the fear all over again. I don't want to die. I'm only 33; I've got my whole life to live. I can't be cut off now. It isn't just. Why me? Why now? You don't have to answer. I'm just in a lousy mood right now. You get maudlin and morally weak waiting for the end. I'm usually pretty good aren't I? Only sometimes something young and scared breaks out. Otherwise, I become like an old man, preparing myself—but over weeks, not years (Kleinman, 1988, p.147).

Facing death cannot be separated from living one's life and being in the world with one's own friends, family, expectations, and fears. Recognition, avoidance, denial, anger, and readiness can all go hand in hand for the patient, the family, and the professional staff alike. Often, no one is ready and death still comes. This is why one faces death rather than masters it. Facing death requires shared understandings among healthcare providers, the patient, and the family as illustrated in the following excerpt:

Nurse: We took care of a patient for months who was on the ventilator and she would get to the point that [her trache] would be buttoned. She would be off the ventilator and then she would tire out again at night and it was just so much work of breathing for her and she decided before everyone else that she was going to die. They had conferences with her husband, Bill, because Bill didn't want to let her go, and basically we waited for Bill. She waited for Bill to say O.K., you can go now, and if you tire out this time we won't put you back on the ventilator.

In this situation, it was difficult for nurses, physicians, and finally the husband, to accept that the woman was exhausted and had begun to experience the ventilator as a torturous device that was merely prolonging her death. The patient was still fully herself and alert. She was not clinically depressed, and when the nurse was able to see the extent of her debilitation and suffering, she was able to let go and accede to the patient's desires. It was a slow coming to terms with her reality instead of the preferences and illusions of those who did not want to let her go (including the nurses and doctors). This case is also noteworthy in that the doctors and nurses waited for Bill to come to the understanding that they had, namely, the patient's irreversible condition and clinical deterioration. Providing surviving family members the opportunity to discover and accept the understandings and transitions for themselves demonstrates an ethic of care that extends beyond the patient. Because the world-shattering experience of death occurs within the family, it is incumbent upon healthcare practitioners to include the patient's family when end-of-life issues are discussed (Stannard, 1997).

Family members' transition to facing the death of a child carries with it the sense of tragedy over the lost expectation and promise of a life not yet lived. Rituals of connection and letting go help people face the sorrow and inevitability of death. In the following excerpt, a nurse talks about the moral and human necessity of waiting until the father can come to terms with the death of his premature son:

Nurse: The morning before he [the infant] died, everybody except for the dad was ready to just extubate him and let him die. And the dad just couldn't make that decision, but by the end of the shift he was willing to agree to not restart the IV If it infiltrated, we wouldn't start it again. And if the ET tube clogged we shouldn't re-intubate. He could go that far but couldn't take that final step, which I thought was OK. So the way that the day progressed, we had the baby out of his bed and the mom, grandmother, and dad held him during the day and we just took care of him basically while they were holding him. And he had morphine every couple of hours. As the physicians came in they were getting these agreements [to set limits on treatment]... I had the attending physician be very explicit about the 'do not resuscitate' order. It was changed from just 'do not resuscitate' to stating 'do not resuscitate, no code drugs, no new IV starts, and no re-intubation' so that when I left and when the resident was in charge, if the person hadn't been around during the day and was not well apprised of the situation and what the conferences had been, it [the agreements to limit treatment] was right there in black and white. And, I could give all the information to the nurse coming on... It has to do with understanding how it is to come to terms with the fact that somebody you love is dying, and what kind of steps the parents needed to make. He (the father) has to be able to see, and it's really interesting to watch the process, because he was there all day long. He'd come and he'd be at the bedside for half hour and he'd be really teary and he'd leave for a few minutes and he'd come back. It was sort of just these gradual sessions of showing him more and more about how the baby was dying and the different things that weren't working anymore. And, giving him this extended period of time to come to terms with that. And then being able to accept the decision that he could make. I mean these parents are going to have to deal with the death. And they wouldn't have been [able to do that abstractly, from a distance]. Extubating the child, they have to live with that and that would have been a really difficult thing (Benner, Tanner, & Chesla, 2009).

This excerpt captures personal grieving of experientially moving through the sorrow of facing the death of a child. The decisions cannot be made outside the situation, nor understood without the parents and grandparents being <u>with</u> the child and feeling the changes in the child's condition. This process cannot be made more efficient without irreparably damaging the ones who are grieving—the community of care and memory. A measure of clarity must be achieved before the grief can be confronted and the death faced, not the least of which is that death is real and there are human limits in preventing it.

In a contrasting setting, hospice care at home, an advanced practice nurse points to a similar process of coming to terms with death at home:

Advanced Practice Nurse: I think that having the education in advance practice gives you a different perspective that you can look at the whole picture, which I think is really important in home care. I see children and you're never just treating the child, of course, it's the parents and the family, and it's really important to look at the whole situation. And I—listen and see where the individuals are coming from. And you know you're in there to follow doctors' orders, but you're also—In most cases I'm working with the family that has had a child with chronic illness, either a birth defect or an acquired illness, and there are a lot of issues around that dealing with mourning this perfect childhood they don't have anymore that they were expecting to get and didn't get. And with pediatric hospice, in my experience, parents never give up—they never give up. And they may give up one day but they don't really give up. They—they cannot give up. I don't think a stage theory works with parents at all. [She is referring to Kubler-Ross stages of facing death: denial, anger, rejection, and acceptance.] They go back and forth and they skip over some and they—they don't mourn in that way at all. They certainly start grieving before [the child dies] but they don't give up hope.

Very often when you're seeing a child at home, it's a child who has never been normal, whose quality of life has never been very good. And when they go into the hospital, the doctors see this child who has maybe very little cognitive ability and has been almost, you know, in a vegetative state since birth—and now this child is dying. They think, 'You know—well this is a good thing.' But when you go into the home, you see parents who <u>love</u> this child and they have taken this child and <u>loved</u> the child for what the child is, and what they have gotten from this child.

And we just had a little girl die this fall and she—and this was the case where the doctors were saying, 'Well, yes, she's dying and this is a good thing.' And the parents were not at all ready to let her go. And I think it was hard to see how much they loved her unless you went into the home and saw how the home was set up, and this was their first child and their only child, and she had never really ever been awake. She had never smiled except with gas, you know, and caring for her had been a tremendous burden. She had frequent seizures and she had a gastrostomy tube and would become very apneic with her seizures so she needed oxygen. She slept in the bed with them and she'd become a part of their lives. They loved her so much, so they were not at all at the point that the doctors and nurses were giving up and then she started having uncontrolled seizures. When we put her in the hospice program, and her parents were able to do that.

But in pediatrics, it's different because you don't—you don't sign a DNAR; we have modified DNARs. And—but I always talk to parents about calling 911 because often that will set up a chain of events that they really don't want and in this case they didn't want to do that but yet they were definitely not ready to let her go. And so in visiting them and in getting to know them over the period of months and, you know, being welcome in their home, I was at a good place to start talking to them about—I mean this child had never communicated in any way and she was close to two. She had never communicated like a normal baby would. But yet she did communicate with them. So this was a good—it occurred to me that this would be a good point because they loved her so much. I asked them—Jennifer's mother, 'What is <u>she</u> communicating to you now?' And this started a discussion that ended up with her mother looking at the idea that her child was telling her that she wanted to die, that she wanted them to let her go. And this was a different way for this mom and then the dad too, to look this. And the baby had the signs of impending death. You know, the urination had decreased and we talked about that somewhat and what Jennifer's body was sort of saying to us. And because they <u>loved</u> her, because they were very attuned to looking at how she could communicate and what she was telling them and what she needed—this meant a lot to them. And they could go with this and then they were able then to let her go. And they were able to start thinking about, you know, how it was going to be when she died and what they would need to do to let her go. And that was the point where they could turn that corner and do it. And they really—they did need to do it. It's not that they—I don't think they ever gave up hope, but they were able to face her death, and actually feel good about it in a way that the doctors and nurses had reached long ago.

I think that—I'm sure it is with adult patients, too, and with everyone who dies—but the person dies but the <u>parents</u> are left with those memories for the rest of their lives, and the siblings also. And I think it's really important because you're in there and you're more objective than the family and the parents, to remind—well to say to them that, 'You will live with this for a long time afterwards. The decisions you make have to be decisions that you can live with and that you can feel good about.' And that is one of your objectives; it affects how you deal with that family. I mean you can't force your—what you think is right on them. You have to really listen and try and understand what is important to them, what they need, and what is scary for them.

Dying alone and anonymously with no connections, rituals, or recognition practices is a bureaucratic nightmare created in our modern age. Having one's death precisely timed by oneself or others fits a strong North American tradition of <u>choosing</u> and <u>creating</u> one's own destiny. But choosing the timing and circumstances of death also collides with other cultural and religious meanings and practices to preserve life. In the following narrative, the nurse confronts the collision of the life and death of a particular person with death being considered as a biomedical mechanical failure:

Nurse: It's a pretty amazing story and I must say it has definitely changed not only my nursing practice but my whole life. It was this gentleman who was fifty-five years old. He was born on a farm, raised on the farm, and was a trucker. He was married and had two children. Somehow his wife had become blind. He was having problems with ventricular tachycardia. They had tried all of the different drugs and this was before we started putting in pacemakers for overdrive stimulation (close to eight or nine years ago). We had the old defibrillators and along with this, he was infarcting every time he had a prolonged period of ventricular tachycardia. He chipped away a little bit more myocardium each time, so he was into heart failure and was having chest pain and they put in a balloon pump. But he wasn't intubated. He was still breathing O.K. and was still alert and oriented.

He must have been shocked at least twenty times a shift or so over the course of a couple of days and it was just getting worse and worse, and his failure was getting worse and worse and his numbers were getting worse. He was deteriorating.

His wife was really involved in the whole situation. She would sit by the bedside. Then in the course of one evening, he started having a whole lot of ectopy but just was not responding to anything. And so we were coding him constantly and one time he went out and we started to code him and we shocked him and he came back and he woke up and he was just saying how he was angry at us. He said,... 'Don't do this anymore. I don't want you to be saving me.' He says: 'I just had a wonderful vision. I saw God and I am getting ready to go.' And we are all kind of looking at him thinking, well it's the lidocaine or something is wrong with this guy. And then he said, 'I need to talk to a Chaplain.' So it was early enough and luckily the priest was still in the hospital so we paged him and this gentleman came up and the patient wanted to be alone with the priest. And then he started quoting all the scriptures of verses in the Bible and things like that. His wife said, 'He doesn't know anything about the Bible. He has never even lifted a Bible in his life. He is a truck driver.' So he was talking to the priest and the priest came out and said, 'You know, he's really serious.' The priest felt that he was really serious about what he was saying and he had his last confession and told the priest some stories about his life that he didn't want anybody to know and things that he felt he let his family down with. The priest said, 'I really think this gentleman is serious. There is nothing wrong with him mentally or with the way he's mentating.'

So then he wanted his wife to be at his bedside and wanted to hold her hand. So she came in and she was holding his hand and maybe about an hour went on and he was doing just fine. Then all of a sudden he started going out again into ventricular tachycardia and started having all kinds of problems. So then we coded him again and this time he wasn't responding.

When we have codes ICU attendings or residents come up. And this resident comes running up from ICU and the first thing he says is 'Get the lady out of the room.' And we decided, let's leave her alone. And we just said, 'No, she is going to stay.' And the resident was really blown away.

We must have coded him for 45 minutes or so. And the wife sat there the entire time holding his hand, talking to him. All this craziness is going on all around her. When it was over, and she got up and thanked us all and just left. She said 'I know that is exactly what he wanted [to have his wife present at his death] and you let us do what we wanted to do at the very end.' And to her that was the most important thing.

It still makes me feel choked up inside that this is what happened [he was resuscitated against his wishes]. I very vividly remember the whole thing happening. That was definitely a situation where the nurses who had been there constantly day after day really got to know this guy, really got to understand that he was sincere [in wanting treatment stopped], and that maybe we should let him go or maybe we should let him make his decision on what he wanted and let the wife decide. And all the medical doctors and all the medical teams and all the wonderful medications we had and everything just were not what the man wanted. He needed time to be with his wife and to die the way he wanted to die. And it has always left a real impression that you have to understand the person, where they are coming from and maybe you do have to give in a little bit even though you want to push on. That it is a two-way street and if you can be convinced that somebody wants to die, it makes you start to wonder what medicine and nursing are all about sometimes. Maybe nursing is to give them that right, or to make sure that the doctors who just come running in to these codes and want everything run the way they are supposed to according to protocol, that you have to step in every once and a while.

Protecting the wife's wish to stay by the husband's bedside is central in the nurse's narrative. Also central was the pulling back the veil of the managed, secret, heroic death. One can only speculate how the wife would have experienced her grief if she had been forced to leave her husband's side. At least that ethical breach was not committed along with the unwanted resuscitation.

This is a narrative of working through a difficult passage. Though it happened eight or nine years ago, it is still fresh in the nurse's memory. The story is told as a form of moral instruction. The nurse is confronted with the problem of medicocentrism and paternalism—doing things for the patient's "own good" against her/his wishes. It is not easy to ascertain what the limits are, and certainly they were not determined in advance of this situation. Clearly the man and his wife initially wanted "everything" done. But the situation changed. The patient was ready to let go, and the medical staff weren't ready to change with him, to give him back the control over deciding when he had had enough treatment. It is unclear why the healthcare team did not listen to the priest, or why they did not have an ethics conference at the time of the patient's request. This is another example of how general ethical rules cannot replace judgment and praxis. Everyone must have known, ethically speaking, that the man had the right to say "Stop." But everyone was engaged in the life-saving process, or actually in the death-postponing process, and could not disengage from that. Ethical decisions made in the heat of the situation are often different than those made speculatively standing outside the situation (Taylor, 1993). What was good (death-postponing) became bad as the situation changed.

Advanced directives are helpful, but not a panacea for the confusion near the end of one's life because their explicitly stated desires and wishes often change in the heat of the moment. Discussions with prearranged surrogates can add flexibility and guidance to advanced directives. Advanced directives must be brought to the healthcare team's attention and discussed in relation to the particular illness experience. Writing up an advanced directive and living it out are distinct. For example, what may look like intolerable suffering to the outsider may be experienced quite differently to the patient. Likewise, the patient's own anticipations may be experienced quite differently than expected. The advanced directive provides a basis for discussing eventualities, and having prepared the directive is a basis for the discussion.

In another example (Benner, Tanner & Chesla, 2009), the wife of a man who had a heart transplant had not been able to face the death of her husband as long as talking about death was in terms of medical realities and treatments. After all, she and her husband had agreed upon heroic measures—after a heart transplant, at what point do you stop? The nurse introduced the ritual of reminiscing, which signaled to the wife the cultural practices of letting go and facing death. Entering this ritual space enabled the woman to reframe the situation from a heroic struggle against all odds and finally face the inevitability of her husband's death.

Allowing family members to say goodbye and confront the finality of death by seeing the loved one's body after death are common nursing practices. This is illustrated in the following interview of a nurse:

Nurse: Two or three months ago, I was working late at night; we were operating on an infant and the infant's parents were older parents. The mother was a nurse, but I didn't know it at the time. The child died in the operating room, and so I had called up to the unit to let them know that the child had died and asked them if the parents wanted to see the child. They said yes, the parents do want to see the child, and then, no they don't want to see the child. So I said, 'OK, I'm going to prepare the body for the morgue then.' So I did all of that. I prepared all the paper work, and I needed a signature from one of the physicians upstairs, so I went up stairs to the Pedi ICU.

As I walked into the unit, I saw the parents of the child there. And so I went up to the mom and dad, and I said, 'I'm really sorry for your loss.' The mother—I get all upset when I talk about it, because it's really upsetting (voice is quivering)—but, the mom said to me: 'Were you with her?" and I said, 'Yes, I took very good care of her, but unfortunately she didn't survive.' And she said, 'Well, you know, I don't feel like it's over.' I said, 'Well, would you like to see her?' and she said, 'Yes, I, I have to see her; it's not over for me if I don't see her.' So I said, 'OK, just give me a little while, and I'll go down and get her all ready and I'll call you and your husband so that you can come down.'

And so, I went back downstairs and I had checked to make sure that the child had been released by the coroner, and he said she had, so I took all the tubes out of her, and I took all of the IVs out of her. Then I washed her hair, and made sure there was no blood on her. I got her all fixed up really cute, and then wrapped her up in a blanket. I put her in a crib, and then I took her over to the Pedi wing of the operating room...

Then I called up the mom and dad, and they came down with a priest and all four of us went in there, and all four of us just kind of cried together, and it was pretty sad. But I felt better after the whole experience, and I think we all felt better about it. It was easier for the mother to have finalization after that. It made me feel good, and I think it made her feel good. And I know the husband felt better because the mother felt better.

Interviewer: What were you thinking about as this situation was unfolding?

Nurse: ...I saw her as a nurse. I put myself in her position, and thought, you know, what if this was my child? I'd want someone to be as caring and take as good care of her as I thought I did. I thought I did as good of a job as I could, as if she had been my own child. And I think that's what you do, when you meet people face to face, you become involved with them emotionally, even though you don't know them. Or you know them for such a short time, and then they become real to you, and when they do, it makes it that much harder.

This OR nurse captures an inside description of responding to another's suffering and doing what needed to be done. One can imagine that it was important to the mother to talk to someone who was present during her child's death. Seeing her child was essential to help the mother begin her difficult task of facing her child's death.

DISCUSSION: CURRENT ETHICAL DEBATES ABOUT END-OF-LIFE CARE AND DECISION MAKING

During data collection for this study reported in the first edition, and now 10 years later with the second edition, end-of-life care and public and policy debates around physician-assisted suicide and adequate pain relief for the dying are at the forefront of professional and societal debates. In the Obama Health Care Reform Debates, fear and political debates erupted about end-of-life care erupted. Daniel Callahan (1993) claims that we suffer from two biomedical illusions: first, that we have or will find a cure for human finitude, and second, that "the grandest expression of the respect we owe to life is to try to save life at all costs" (p.85). The dignity and worth of human life and the quest to save lives are both deeply held notions of good in the Greek and Judeo-Christian traditions. They become illusions when we imagine that we can ultimately prevent <u>all</u> death, that it is life-respecting to subject the dying person to futile treatments, and that biomedical interventions are the only means of expressing care.

The very real possibilities for cure and the real risks of subjecting patients to futile treatments that prolong dying in critical care create moral responsibilities among patients, families, nurses, and physicians. The human experience of facing death forms moral concerns and discussions about hope, suffering, and the possibility of death as the patient's condition changes. This is the dialogue about death as a human passage, the ending of a particular life and particular human relationships. The biomedical and scientific rational moral concerns create discussions about probabilities of success and failure of treatments and predictions of outcomes based on the best statistical data available. But these distinct moral concerns are seldom separated in human life. Sometimes nurses, physicians, and family members use biomedical and scientific probability language to convey concerns about death as a human passage. Indeed, it can seem that the language of biomedical science is the <u>only</u> appropriate or legitimate language for healthcare professionals since no definitive expertise can be offered about facing death. Talking about facing death as a human passage can seem to be the exclusive domain of nurses, chaplains, social workers, and psychologists. Biomedical language offers explanations and a sense of control and form central coping strategies in the Western world. Nurses often bridge the gap between the expression of the human significance of death and the discussion of biomedical probabilities and "rational decision-making" about end-of-life care.

Studies of end-of-life decision making and care tend to focus on rational calculations of benefits and burdens and statistical probabilities of survival and treatment outcomes, overlooking the ways that the process of facing death, of letting go of loved ones, influence the socially negotiated end-of-life care and biomedical decision making. The Robert Wood Johnson Foundation funded a large national study of end-of-life care and decision making. The SUPPORT Study (1995) was a two phase study that first conducted a 2-year prospective observational study with 4,301 patients, followed by a 2-year controlled clinical trial with 4,804 patients. This study has generated much public and professional concern. The descriptive phase of the study concluded that:

> Decision making was often far short of the ideal. Physicians did not know what
> patients wanted with regard to resuscitation, even though these patients were at
> high risk of cardiac arrest. Orders against resuscitation were written in the last few
> days of life. Most patients who died in the hospital spent most of their last days on
> ventilators in intensive care. We had not expected to find the high levels of pain that
> were being reported, especially in non-cancer illnesses. Except for the comatose,
> more than half of the patients with any one of the nine diseases[1] were reported (by

---

[1]The nine specific diagnoses in the SUPPORT Study were: acute respiratory failure, multiple organ system failure with sepsis, multiple organ system failure with malignancy, chronic obstructive pulmonary disease, congestive heart failure, chronic liver failure, non-traumatic coma, colon cancer and lung cancer.

the patient or family member) to have substantial pain, and we felt obliged to make pain a target of the intervention. The intervention phase of the study was based on this first phase descriptive study. Lynn (1997) describes the intervention:

...The intervention included frequent reports from the computer model for prognostication and reports from interviews with patients and their families. It was anchored, however, by specially trained and committed nurses who spent all their time counseling patients and families, convening meetings with physicians and others, eliciting preferences, making plans for future contingencies, and ensuring that the best possible information about prognosis and preferences was available for the care team. The nurses managed to carry out the intervention with grace, forcefulness, and timeliness. They had some communication with all of the intervention patients' physicians; prognoses were delivered for 94 percent of the cases, and, for patients who stayed at least a week in the hospital, the SUPPORT nurses averaged six visits... Once the data were unblinded, it was clear that the intervention had not improved outcomes in any of the five targeted problems:

1. The timing of a "do not resuscitate" (DNAR) order.
2. Accord between patient and physician about DNAR.
3. Time spent in an intensive care unit (ICU) in a coma or on a ventilator before death.
4. Pain.
5. Resource use (Lynn, Harrell, Cohn, Wagner, & Connors, 1997; see also, SUPPORT, 1995)

Except for pain management, the outcome measures were strategic and related to managing the disease process and timing of death. Patient and family preparation and support in facing death and the maintaining of openness and fidelity in relationships were not considered. Nor were grieving outcomes or family appraisals of care assessed Lynn, Teno,., Phillips, Wu, et al. 1997). Lynn (1997) concludes that the SUPPORT study placed too much emphasis on the rational decision making process and too little on the human aspects of facing suffering and death.

SUMMARY

The narratives in this chapter present the relational context for reasoning-in-transition that occurs as critical care nurses care for patients who move from hope for recovery to dying. Nowhere are the links between ethical and clinical reasoning more apparent. Facing death as a human passage, as these nursing narratives illustrate, cannot be reduced to issues of prediction and control without doing ethical violence. Developing cumulative wisdom about moving through possible treatment options to facing death can be enhanced in local units by sharing experiential learning such as the ones presented in this chapter. Keeping the patient and family story is part of bearing witness and forming caring relationships—both of which are necessary for safe passages in caring for the dying. Naming silences, mistaken transitions, and predictable errors between clinicians, patients, and families can create new possibilities in local healthcare teams. By retaining narrative memory about patients who have taught them lessons, clinicians can ensure that dignified and peaceful deaths are achieved more often in critical care areas.

REFERENCES

Beauchamp, T. L., & Childress, J. F. (1994). *Principles of biomedical ethics, 4th edition.* New York, NY: Oxford University Press.

Benner, P., & Wrubel, J. (1982) Clinical knowledge development: The value of perceptual awareness. *Nurse Educator*, 7, pp. 11–17.

Benner, P., Hooper-Kyriakidis, P. & Stannard, D. (1999). *Clinical wisdom and interventions in critical care: A thinking-in-action approach.* Philadelphia, PA: W. B. Saunders Company.

Benner, P., Stannard, D., & Hooper, P. L. (1996). A thinking-in-action approach to teaching clinical judgment: A classroom innovation for acute care advanced practice nurses. *Advanced Practice Nursing Quarterly, 1*(4), pp. 70–77.

Blum, L. (1980) Compassion. Berkeley, CA: University of California Press.

Blum, L. (1994). *Moral perception and particularity.* Cambridge, UK: Cambridge University Press.

Brody, H., Campbell, M., Faber-Langendoen, K. & Ogle, K. (1997) "Withdrawing intensive life-sustaining treatments: Recommendations for compassionate clinical management. *New England Jo. of Medicine, 336*(9), 652–657.

Bruera, E. (2006). Foreword. In H. Neuenschwander, R. Baumann, E. Bergsträsser, S. Eberhard, S. Eichmüller, H. Gudat, et al., *Palliativmedizin* [Palliative medicine] (p. 11). Bern, Switzerland: Krebsliga Schweiz.

Byock, I. (1997). *Dying well: The prospect of growth at the end of life.* New York, NY: Riverhead Books.

Callahan, D. (1993) *The role of emotion on ethical decision making.* New York, NY: Simon and Schuster.

Chochinov, H., Krisjanson, L., Hack, T., Hassard, T., McClement, S., & Harlos, M. (2006). Dignity in the terminally ill: Revisited. *Journal of Palliative Medicine, 9,* 666–672.

Chochinov, H. M., Hack, T., Hassard, T., Kristjanson, L. J., McClement, S., & Harlos, M. (2002). Dignity in the terminally ill: a cross-sectional, cohort study. *Lancet, 360*(9350), 2026–2030.

Doyle, D., Hanks, G. W. C., Cherny, N., Calman, K. (Eds.). (2005). *Oxford textbook of palliative medicine* (3rd ed.). Oxford, England: Oxford University Press.

Drought, T. S., & Koenig, B. A. (2002). "Choice" in end-of-life decision making: Researching fact or fiction?. *Gerontologist, 42 Spec No 3,* 114–128.

Dunne, K., & Sullivan, K. (2000). Family experiences of palliative care in the acute hospital setting. *International Journal of Palliative Nursing, 6,* 170–178.

Field, M. J., & Cassel, C. K. (1997). *Approaching Death Improving Care at the End of Life.* Washington, DC: National Academy Press.

Glaser, B. G., & Strauss, A. L. (1965). *Awareness of dying.* Chicago, IL. Aldine.

Gordon, S. (1997). *Life support: Three nurses on the front lines.* New York, NY: Little, Brown and Co.

Halpern, J. (2001). *From detached concern to empathy: Humanizing medical practice.* New York, NY: Oxford University Press.

Hawker, S., Kerr, C., Payne, S., Seamark, D., Davis, C., … Roberts, H. (2006). End-of-life care in community hospitals: The perceptions of bereaved family members. *Palliative Medicine, 20,* 541–547.

Heyland, D. K., Dodek, P., Rocker, G., Groll, D., Gafni, A., … Pichora, D. (2006). What matters most in end-of-life care: Perceptions of seriously ill patients and their family members. *Canadian Medical Association Journal, 174,* 627–633.

Holden, T., (1992). Dialogues with Excellence: Seeing Joan through. *American Journal of Nursing. 92,* 26–30.

Hughes, A. (2001). The Poor and underserved: Special patient population. In B. R. Ferrell & N. Coyle (Eds.), *Textbook of Palliative Nursing* (pp. 461–466). New York, NY: Oxford University Press

Jezewski, M. A., Scherer, Y., Miller, C., & Battista, E. (1993). Consenting to DNR: Critical care nurses' interactions with patients and family members. *American Journal of Critical Care, 2*(4), 302–309.

Keegan, O., McGee, H., Hogan, M., Kunin, H., O'Brien, S., & O'Siorain, L. (2001). Relatives´ views of health care in the last year of life. *International Journal of Palliative Nursing, 7,* 449–456.

Levenson, J. W., McCarthy, E. P., Lynn, J., Davis, R. B., & Phillips, R. S. (2000). The last six months of life for patients with congestive heart failure. *Journal of the American Geriatrics Society, 48,* S101–S109.

Lynn, J., Ely, E. W., Zhong, Z., McNiff, K. L., Dawson, N. V., … Connors, L. (2000). Living and dying with chronic obstructive pulmonary disease. *Journal of the American Geriatrics Society, 48,* S91–S100.

Jennings, B., Kaebnick, G. E., & Murray, T. H. (2005). Improving end of life care: Why has it been so difficult? *The Hastings Center Report* (Special Report, November-December), S1–S60.

Kaufman, S. (2005). *And a time to die: How American hospitals shape the end of life.* New York, NY: Scribner.

Knaus, W. A., Wagner, D., Draper E., Zimmerman, J., Bergner, M., Bastos, P., Sirio, C., A, Murphy, D., Lotring, T. & Damiano, A., et al. (1991). The APACHE III Prognostic system: Risk prediction of hospital mortality for critically ill hospitalized adults. *Chest 100*(6) 1619–1636.

Lock, M. (1996). Death in technological time: Locating the end of meaningful life. *Medical Anthropology Quarterly, 10*(4), 575–600.

Lynn, J. (1997) Unexpected returns: Insights from SUPPORT. In S. L. Isaacs & J. R. Knickman (Eds.), *To improve health and health care 1997: Robert Wood Johnson Anthology* (pp. 161–186). San Francisco, CA: Jossey-Bass.

Lynn, J., Harrell, F., Cohn, F., Wagner, D., & Connors, A. F. (1997) Prognoses of seriously ill hospitalized patients on the days before death: Implications for patient care and public policy. *New Horizons, 5*(1), 56–61.

Lynn, J., Teno, J. M., Phillips, R. S., Wu, A. W., Desbiens, N., Harold, J., Claessens, M. T., Wegner, N., Kreling B., & Connors, A. F., Jr. (1997b) Perceptions by family members of the dying experience of seriously ill patients. *Annals of Internal Medicine. 126*(2), 97–106.

Mc Cue, J. D. (1995). The naturalness of death. *Journal of the American Medical Association, 273,* 1039–1043.

McGrath, P. (2001). Caregivers' insights on the dying trajectory in hematology oncology. *Cancer Nursing, 24,* 413–421.

Meier, D. E. (2002). United States: Overview of Cancer Pain and Palliative Care. *Journal of Pain and Symptom Management, 24*(2), 265–269.

Meier, D. E., Morrison, R. S., & Cassel, C. K. (1997). Improving palliative care. *Annals of Internal Medicine, 127,* 225–230.

Murdoch, I. (1970/1991). *The sovereignty of the good.* London, England: Routledge.

National Consensus Project. (2004). *Clinical Practice Guidelines for Quality Palliative Care.* Retrieved September 10, 2006, from http://www.nationalconsensusproject.org/Guideline.pdf

Nussbaum, M. C. (1995) *Poetic justice: The literary imagination and public life.* Philadelphia, PA: J. B. Lippincott.

Oakes-Greenspan, M. (2007) *Running Toward: Reframing Possibility and Finitude Through Physicians' Stories at the End of Life.* Ph.D. Dissertation, University of California, San Francisco, Department of Physiological Nursing.

Rogers, A., Karlsen, S., & Addington-Hall, J. (2000). 'All the services were excellent. It is when the human element comes in that things go wrong': Dissatisfaction with hospital care in the last year of life. *Journal of Advanced Nursing, 31,* 768–774.

Sepulveda, C., Marlin, A., Yoshida, T., & Ullrich, A. (2002). Palliative care: The World Health Organization's global perspective. *Journal of Pain and Symptom Management, 24,* 91–96.

Spichiger, E. (2004). *Leading a life with a terminal illness: An interpretive phenomenological study of patients' and family members' experiences of hospital end-of-life care.* Doctoral dissertation, University of California San Francisco, San Francisco, Department of Social and Behaviorial Sciences.

Spichiger, E. (2010). Patients' and Family Members' Experiences of Hospital End-of-Life Care. In Chan, G., Brykczynski, K. A., Malone, R. E., Benner, P. (Eds.), *Interpretive phenomenology in health care research: studying social practice, lifeworlds, and embodiment* (pp. 313–336). Indiannapolis, IN: Sigma Theta Tau.

Spichiger, E., Wallhagen, M., & Benner, P. (2005). Nursing as a caring practice from a phenomenological perspective. *Scandinavian Journal of Caring Sciences.* Dec;19(4):.303-09

Stannard, D. (1997) *Reclaiming the house: An interpretive study of nurse-family interactions and activities in critical care.* Doctoral Dissertation, University of California, San Francisco School of Nursing.

Sunvisson, H., Habermann, B, Weiss, S. & Benner P., (2009). Augmenting the Cartesian medical discourse with an understanding of the person's lifeworld, lived body, life story and social identity. *Nursing Philosophy* (2009), 10, pp. 241-252.

SUPPORT Principal Investigators (1995) "A controlled trial to improve care for seriously ill hospitalized patients: The study to understand prognoses and preferences for outcomes and risk of treatments (SUPPORT) *Journal of the American Medical Association, 274,* 1591-1598.

Tanner, C., Benner, P. Chesla, C., & Gordon, D. R. (1993) The phenomenology of knowing a patient. *Image, 25*(4), 273-280.

Taylor, C. (1991). *The ethics of authenticity.* Cambridge, MA: Harvard University Press.

Taylor, C. (1993). *Explanation and practical reason.* In M. C. Nussbaum & A. Sen (Eds.), The quality of life. Oxford, England: Clarendon Press.

Teno, J. M., Clarridge, B. R., Casey, V., Welch, L. C., Wetle, T., Shield, R. et al. (2004). Family perspectives on end-of-life care at the last place of care. *Journal of the American Medical Association, 291,* 88-93.

Tolle, S. W., Tilden, V. P., Hickman, S. E., & Rosenfeld, A. G. (2000). Family reports of pain in dying hospitalized patients: A structured telephone survey. *Western Journal of Medicine, 172,* 374-377.

Tolle, S. W., Tilden, V. P., Rosenfeld, A. G., & Hickman, S. E. (2000). Family reports of barriers to optimal care of the dying. *Nursing Research, 49,* 310-317.

Vetleson, A. J. (1994). *Perception, empathy, and judgment: An inquiry in to the preconditions of moral performance.* University Park, PA: Pennsylvania State University Press.

Weiss S. (1996). *Possibility or despair: Biographies of aging.* Doctoral dissertation, University of California, San Francisco, CA.

Weiss, S. (2010). Dwelling-in-the-world: Realms of meaningful involvement in late life. In Chan, G., Brykczynski, K. A., Malone, R. E., Benner, P. (Eds.) *Interpretive phenomenology in health care research: Studying social practice, lifeworlds, and embodiment* (pp. 287–312). Indianapolis, IN: Sigma Theta Tau.

Winnicott, D. W. (1986). Transitional objects and transitional phenomena: A study of the first not-me possession. In P. Buckley (Ed.) *Essential papers in object relations.* (pp.254–271) New York, NY: New York University Press. (Original work published in 1953).

World Health Organization (2004). *Palliative care: The solid facts.* Retrieved 02/28, 2009, from http://www.euro.who.int/InformationSources/Publications/Catalogue/20050118_2

Wrubel J., Acree M., Goodman S. & Folkman S. (2009). End of living: maintaining a lifeworld during terminal illness. *Psychology and Health.* 1476-8321. Vol. 24 (10) Pp. 1229-1243. Doi: 10.1080/08870440802320463. Reprinted in Chan, G., Brykczynski, K. A., Malone, R. E., Benner, P. (Eds.) *Interpretive phenomenology in health care research: Studying social practice, lifeworlds, and embodiment* (pp. 337-358) Indianapolis, IN: Sigma Theta Tau.

10

Making a Case: Communicating Clinical Assessments and Improving Teamwork

A science-based clinical practice requires skillful communication of ambiguous clinical understandings and of practical and ethical concerns as they evolve so that sound clinical decisions can be made. Scientific findings and treatment rationales are sometimes divergent and can be sources of disagreement and misunderstanding.

The goal of this chapter is to describe the work of creating a communicative context for everyday clinical problem solving and teamwork and to point out areas of clinical judgment that are inherently ambiguous and therefore difficult to communicate to others.

Clinicians are being encouraged to use a more standardized communication, such as SBAR which stands for: (1) **S**ituation: after communicating the name of reporter and patient, a brief statement of the patient's problem is given; (2) **B**ackground: information relevant for the situation at hand; (3) **A**ssessment: a summary of what the clinician believes is the underlying cause and its severity; (4) **R**ecommendation: what is needed to resolve the situation (Pope, Rodzen & Gross, 2008). In the Carnegie National Study of Nursing Education (Benner, Sutphen, Leonard & Day, 2010), it was found that student nurses receive little training or practice in making a case to other team members or in interpreting what they think is most relevant about the patient's current situation. Part of the problem is that student nurses cannot legally take telephone orders unless they are on the phone with their clinical instructor as well as the health care provider. In fast-paced clinical settings this is difficult to coordinate, so often the student talks to the staff nurse, who makes the telephone call. Benner, Sutphen, Leonard & Day recommended that students and inexperienced nurses get practice in simulation labs in making a case (2010).

The following five clinical aspects are particularly challenging because they rely on clinical interpretations and assessments. Each of these five aspects would provide an excellent basis for developing simulations and inter-professional seminars around reporting ambiguous clinical situations. While the communication of SBAR is extremely useful, it focuses on the point when the clinical problems and definitive actions are clearer and definitive. Leading up to that clarity is the need to articulate and compare subtle, less definitive patient trends to other clinicians. Students and nurses alike need to be taught to bring early warnings about ambiguous patient changes to more experienced clinicians and provide narrative examples of observed changes and trends and then take steps toward confirmation and disconfirmation of competing possible causes and physiological states. This is

TABLE 10.1

Making a Case: Communicating Clinical Assessments and Improving Teamwork

- Communicating about clinical transitions
- Communicating missed time tables and unexpected changes in clinical trajectories
- Changing practices and developing new clinical knowledge
- Developing clinical knowledge about experimental interventions
- Team building: Developing a community of attentiveness, skill, and collaboration.

the most difficult stage of clinical reasoning and communication about that reasoning. It is much easier to communicate about clear cut well-documented patient trends and responses The five clinical aspects shown in Table 10.1 are examples of transitions that are predictably difficult to identify and communicate, yet crucial to timely assessments and needed interventions for patients.

Multiple concerns are usually at stake in communicating clinical knowledge and clinical reasoning. Becoming clearer about the skill of presenting ambiguous patient changes, patient concerns, and practical and ethical issues can improve communication and the reliability of clinical decisions. The first step is to better articulate the issues so that this vital area of communication and practice can better be included in the education of clinicians. As one nurse points out:

> **Nurse:** I had a teacher who would let the nursing student practice speaking with the physician...because when you get out of nursing school you don't really know how to communicate with the physician because you [don't usually do it]. You speak with your instructor or you speak with the nurse who's seen the patient and they take care of the physician part, but you never really learn how to communicate with the physician.

Gathering, interpreting, and communicating an ongoing and unfolding grasp of the patient's situation is not well taught in linear and rational-technical models (e.g., the nursing process) of clinical problem solving. Usually, little focus on interpreting particular clinical situations, and even less attention is given to communicating these interpretations in clinical teaching. Experience with many clinical trajectories and practice at articulating these clinical understandings are essential to the development of expert clinical judgment in order to move those judgements into effective action.

No clinician is infallible. Errors are reduced and clinical judgment is improved by clear communication, and by comparing and pooling experiential clinical wisdom. The style of clinical judgments varies depending on the kinds of evidence that are available to substantiate patient changes, and whether the understanding is primarily clinical or primarily about scientific understandings, standard practice, or critical pathways. Clearly marshaled evidence and explicit statements about clinical reasoning are best, but early communication of subtle signs and ambiguous changes can trigger the necessary vigilance for further data collection, clarification and problem solving. Overstating or understating the case for a clinical judgment create problems. However, when changes in the patient status are ambiguous, then it is best to acknowledge the ambiguity but call for additional watchfulness and confirmatory testing as indicated by the concerns. Much of this communication occurs verbally and informally since most external situations are unstable and unclear. Most clinical interpretations are necessarily tentative, as illustrated in the next example:

> **Nurse:** This gentleman is doing great. He had a liver transplant a few days back. His kidneys had shut down, so he was on CVVH (Continuous Veno-Venous Hemofiltration) intraoperatively and perioperatively. He's done very well. We're just worried—his hematocrit hasn't stabilized completely for us, so they're still discussing the plan... If you read a chart and know a patient you know that they don't always reflect—the charts do not always reflect the <u>whole</u> picture and what the plan is sometimes. Because we're still talking about what the plan is and there are a few options and people don't want to write that down yet (Observational Interview).

There is almost always a gap between what is being considered or speculated about and what is written on the chart. Clinicians make a case for a particular understanding of a patient's clinical condition and that interpretation is then subjected to validation, questioning, and counter interpretations. In this way, clinical understanding is enhanced by multiple perspectives. It is not sufficient to know what is going on clinically with patients; this knowledge has to also be communicated to and validated by other clinicians in order to generate timely responses. Gathering, ordering, and presenting the clinical data all require judgment and skill. The communication process involved in presenting a case, itself, requires judgment and skill.

Communication across disciplinary lines can be difficult, especially when there are status and power inequities. A cynic might conclude that exchanges among respiratory therapists, nurses, and assistive personnel or between nurses and physicians are over-determined by status and power. But if the exchange were <u>only</u> about power, then concerns for the patient's well being would be lost and all clinicians would experience cynicism and doubt about their clinical knowledge. Returning to the content and stakes for the patient/family and clearly stating clinical judgments and understandings often prevent issues from deteriorating into power struggles. Winning one's point at the expense of accuracy and fidelity to the patient's best interests is unethical and leads to confusion and loss of clinical grasp for the clinician, creating danger for the patient. Returning to "the good of the patient/family" is a form of ethical and clinical discernment that can be practiced and mastered when addressed at the individual, professional, and institutional levels.

Power issues are most evident when the clinical situation is changing and the available data needed to make decisions are not yet definitive. Yet, it is this ambiguous time of change that gives the necessary lead time to intervene regarding an emerging complication. Open communication and dialogue are crucial to the patient's well-being. This is illustrated in the following situation in which a patient with a thoracic abdominal aneurysm (TAA) repair returned from the operating room and developed cardiac tamponade:

> **Nurse:** The surgery was long. He had a huge blood loss. They brought him back to the unit very unstable... So there were basically four of us in the room managing the patient, the CT resident, the ICU resident, the charge nurse, and myself. [The first year] resident in the room could do everything... And the fellow [who was not in the room] finally gave us an order over the phone. He didn't know what was going on in the room, hadn't even seen the patient postoperatively, and he gave an order that we all refused to do.

Interviewer: What was the order?

Nurse: To start a drip that was inappropriate for what was going on with the patient. The patient was basically tamponading; he was bleeding into the space around his heart... The fellow wanted us to start dobutamine, but that was only going to vasodilate him further, increase the squeeze on his heart to—where? More blood into his chest?... I questioned the order. I brought it to the attention of the charge nurse and she agreed with me. The two doctors in the room were like: 'Start what?'

Interviewer: Had you been the one to have the conversation on the phone and take this verbal order?

Nurse: No, the resident in the room [went to the desk to telephone the fellow]. He took the order for dobutamine and gave it to me and I said, 'No.' He got back on the phone. I never left the patient. He got back on the phone and said: 'They don't want to start it.' And then the charge nurse who was there, said to him: 'Tell him we will start it when he gets here. We will have it all ready to go. He needs to come and look at the patient.' We made that deal with him. So he, of course, came up furious, and just as he got there the patient arrested. He basically turned to leave the room to go tell the family that that was it, when the other [house] officer, the surgeon said: 'Wait a minute. We haven't even opened up his chest yet. We don't know... If you would like me to, I would do it.' So the surgical resident, never having opened a chest, had the chest open within a minute and fully resuscitated the patient. We eventually got him back down to the operating room and this man survived. It was a long haul for him. He ended up on the ventilator for quite some time and was sick for awhile. He stayed in the unit for about another month to six weeks before leaving. But he did get better and left the hospital... And the interesting outcome on all that was that this fellow felt like we were blocking the care of the patient and went to his attending saying, 'Well, I wanted to start a dobutamine drip.' The attending was not all that familiar with the bedside management of the patient. So he basically called the other surgeons there 'clowns' and wanted to speak to somebody about the two nurses who wouldn't carry out the order until the ICU team and attending came around the next day and said, 'Congratulations on what a great job you did last night! The surgeon who stepped in and just opened the chest, that was phenomenal! And the dobutamine, who thought to start dobutamine?' All the other physicians around really questioned the order as well... Not so much as an outright apology was made to the surgeons who were there and helping out, but it was known that what they did was really appreciated in the end...

Interviewer: Did the resident have any rationale when he gave you the verbal dobutamine order?

Nurse: He was just kind of a middle man. He really didn't know what to do. He was new and he'd never been on this service before. I don't think he'd ever been in a situation quite like this before. While he was in the room, he basically looked to the other two surgeons who were in the room, even though they weren't part of that service. They had a lot more knowledge and experience, so he turned to them for help when he wasn't getting any from his [senior] fellow. The resident making the phone calls was asking for advice from his fellow. He wasn't quite sure. He kind of had to say, 'What do I need to tell him?' He couldn't look at the patient, the flow sheet, the picture, and put it all together well enough to relay what was going on. You had to spoon feed it to him, 'Now when you call, you want to tell him about the blood pressure, what's coming out of the chest tubes, et cetera...'

Interviewer: And were you saying that to him?

Nurse: Oh, everybody was. It was a group. Just one of those nights where everybody was in the room and nobody was leaving. But it was a group that worked well together. So it wasn't just my patient that night, it was everybody's. Even the ICU resident was going to the blood bank. Everybody was just doing...everybody acted as a nurse that night...

This exemplar illustrates many of the points to be made in this chapter: reasoning-in-transition, starting with a transition that was difficult to recognize because the patient's baseline condition was so unstable and because he continued to have chest tube drainage. Even though there are some power struggles in the situation, it is clearly more important to save the patient's life than "obeying orders" or maintaining traditional lines of authority. The role of the nurse in framing the clinical problem is evident in the example of coaching the ICU resident on how to make a case to the fellow on the phone (Benner, Tanner & Chesla, 2009). This example also illustrates the importance of team building and collaboration among the nurses, resident, and surgeons for good clinical problem solving. This example also highlights how actually seeing the patient's condition plays a role in achieving a good clinical grasp of the situation, especially in this particular presentation where chest drainage continued. The charge nurse backed up the physicians and nurses who were present, attending to the patient by insisting that the fellow look at the patient before giving an order that she also knew was inappropriate. It illustrates why it is best for the person who has the best grasp of the patient's clinical situation to phone the physician, if possible, so that the direct first-hand understanding of the clinical situation can be conveyed, and why it is preferable to have the person writing the order see the patient if possible (Benner, Tanner & Chesla, 2009).

Physicians become accustomed to having nurses make a clinical case and present the clinical data in a way that shapes and narrows the possible range of plausible interpretations (Benner, Tanner & Chesla, 2009). Presenting a clinical interpretation depends upon keeping track of the patient's condition and responses to therapies—synthesizing the ongoing reasoning-in-transition. This process is disrupted when care is fragmented, patients move to different units and settings, or when there is little continuity among the professionals who care for the patient. The patient's transitions should be conveyed along with the history of the changes in the patient's condition. Building in narratives about patients' transitions in patient records could prevent repeated episodes of deterioration due to a lack of understanding of the patient's history, trajectory, and responses to therapy. Clinical understanding is directional and temporal. In the situation above, the evidence for cardiac tamponade had to be marshaled in the context of the patient's unstable condition and unfortunately the case was not effectively made until the patient had a cardiac arrest.

In the National Carnegie Study of Nursing Education (Benner, Sutphen, Leonard & Day, 2010) it was found that clinical teachers struggled to teach students how to keep track of transitions or changes in patients' condition across time in response to their disease or treatment. While students are carefully taught to assess the patient's response to therapies, they do not often get the opportunity to work with their instructors to titrate intravenous medications in relation to the patient's responses to medications, particularly vasopressor medications. Also the time sequencing on a unit may not allow students to observe critical transitions in the patients. Simulation of patient transitions and in patient responses to vaso-pressors and other titrated medications are required to adequately prepare students for this central role in nursing care and has been identified as a major practice-education gap in nursing education (Benner, Sutphen, Leonard & Day, 2010).

Nurses typically present clinical data to physicians in pre-interpreted forms that dem-onstrate a narrative understanding of patients' trajectories and current conditions. Common clinical conditions come to be recognized as calling for common clinical interventions, and this routinizing of expectations creates problems when new science and technologies emerge. In the following excerpt from Benner, Tanner, and Chesla, (2009) a nurse presents a meaningful story of the patient's therapies and responses by linking certain therapies to changes in the vital sign record on the flow sheet (p. 99). Her account illustrates practical and impromptu clinical teaching and learning, interpreting, and presenting clinical judgments:

> **Nurse:** Our 24 hour flow sheets on the heart patients, that record the pulmonary artery pressures and other patient data, provides an area [of teaching] where I say, 'See how this affected urine output and this affected that and the heart rate affected this and going down on the dobutamine affected this?' So I'm always including the whole spectrum so they can see it on the paper and that's how I usually [teach] it. And then I also give little scenarios, 'Okay, so you see this and this and this, what do you think is going on?' Because they don't always cue in that cardiac output increased. They may be thinking of drugs or more concrete things rather than, 'Oh the heart rate went up just a little bit,' so I use the whole spectrum.

Patients' stories, as told by the flow sheet, are ways of teaching this storied under-standing about the interactions between vasoactive drugs, fluid, temperature, urine output, and the patient's hemodynamics. Yet student nurses and beginning staff nurses have to be taught to read and interpret the flow sheets. They have to learn how to identify and follow trends and changes. Going over the flow sheets with new nurses and physicians allows for common understandings and expectations to develop around treatment options. If new nurses fail to follow the local conventions for presenting the clinical "data," their message may be misinterpreted or missed. For example, a new graduate phoned two different physi-cians about a patient's deteriorating status. She gave all the appropriate laboratory data but did not emphasize the significance of the patient's changing blood gases. The patient was in metabolic acidosis and needed hemodialysis. The physician, accustomed to a meaningful ordering and interpretation of the data, failed to notice the blood gas changes (Benner, Tan-ner & Chesla, 2009). This points to the disparity between formal and informal expecta-tions. In the tradition of the Doctor-Nurse game (Stein, 1967; Stein, Watts & Howell, 1990), the nurse is only supposed to present the clinical data and allow the physician to make judg-ments about the data. However, such a complete separation is impossible and belies the fact that the nurse would not even call the physician unless he or she had made a judgment about the patient's clinical data and/or condition (Benner, Tanner & Chesla, 2009).

Open acknowledgment of ambiguity and reflection on the clinical judgment involved in communicating changes in the patient's condition invites criticism and improvement which can enhance experiential learning. We have ample evidence in this study that nurses continue to use indirect patterns of communication and deference to physicians in order to avoid conflict and get the interventions they deem necessary from the physician. How-ever, enlightened and liberated practice for both professional groups requires that these patterns of communication be abandoned for forthright communication about clinical understandings and judgments. There was also evidence, however, that this pattern is changing. For example, nurses from an intensive care nursery (ICN) told of the commonly heard joke about ICN nurses at their medical center:

Nurse 1: The ICN nurses used to have an awful reputation with the new medical staff. They would say: 'Oh, we've heard.'...With the rotation plan—

Nurse 2: Not being long enough, only a month.

Nurse 1: So its important I think that—and I think it is well deserved that we have a reputation of being assertive...

Nurse 2: There's a saying out there that: 'What three things you never have to say to an ICN nurse: What do you think?'

Nurse 3: 'Am I in your way?'

Nurse 1: Yes, 'Am I in your way?' or 'Here let me write you an order.' (Group laughs)

Nurse 2: 'Is there an order you would like me to sign?' (Group laughs)

That this is an "oft told joke" is evident in the joint telling of the sayings. It also reflects the common practice of assertiveness by these ICN nurses and that their assertiveness causes role conflict with physicians. It is encouraging that there are well established examples of a successful refusal of an order, of going up the chain of command, and of insistent warnings that were warranted and saved infant's lives. Telling these success stories and keeping them in the institutional memory reinforces the legitimacy and significance of the nurses' patient advocacy for improving patient outcomes.

Although physicians were not included in this study, we would be remiss to discount their expertise and judgment. In many cases of physician-nurse disagreement, the problem is unclear and complicated by incomplete communication or understanding. Thus, insistence, assertiveness, and going up the chain of command are no substitute for good listening and collaborative skills. Physicians anecdotally report that, in some cases, the nurse fails to listen, repeatedly calls to insist upon a treatment, and eventually persuades the physicians into writing an unnecessary order. For example, a nurse insisted on infusing albumin in an ICU patient with low serum albumin levels. When the physician repeatedly discussed why it was not indicated and shared current scientific findings, the nurse reported the physician to the chief of medicine, faulting his clinical knowledge and judgment because all the other physicians routinely treated similar patients with albumin. The chief, who agreed with the physician but had submitted to the repeated pressure to treat, took the opportunity to inservice the nurses and physicians about the inappropriateness of that particular treatment. This example illustrates how openness and listening to understand are essential skills in negotiating multiple clinical perspectives that focus on the patient's best interest. It also reflects how good and current science must inform experienced-based learning and updating and supplanting old practices.

COMMUNICATING ABOUT CLINICAL TRANSITIONS

Once a clinical situation has been redefined, for example, "This is heart failure rather than hypovolemia," then the relevance of certain signs and symptoms change as well as the indicated interventions. Before the clinical situation is redefined and while the evidence is mounting that the patient's clinical situation is changing or does not match clinical expectations, the change in patient status is experienced as a time of ambiguity, disturbance, or active problem solving (see Chapter 2). Gathering and presenting evidence and communicating about a sense of impending change requires clinical judgment. But fluctuation and changes in the patient's condition are the norm rather than the exception in most critically ill patients, as reflected by the following interview:

> **Nurse:** I would have to change the [patient care] plan in that sort of circumstance also. I mean, that's what primary nursing is all about. The fact that you respect your peers and your associates, and that the person who's at the bedside at the time is making the assessment and they have to do what's correct in their own nursing judgment for that particular time. And plans are subject to change over hours, not even days in our unit. Just because you were on yesterday doesn't mean that when you come on in the morning things haven't changed, and that's the real issue. Just because you make a plan and someone changes it, it doesn't mean they thought it was a bad plan. It just means that the situation changed.

Learning to effectively communicate clinical interpretations (especially early underdetermined interpretations) to others requires thinking-in-action and the ability to name subtle changes that point to transitions in the patient's condition. Clinical reasoning calls for reasoning-in-transition based on perceptual acuity about particular manifestations of the disease and on knowing the particular patient, all of which are interpretive. Interpretation is necessarily social. Multiple sources of ambiguity can disrupt communication because clinicians act in terms of a current and unfolding clinical grasp of the situation. If clinicians only focused on ambiguities or were locked into rigid plans and expectations, they would be incapable of thinking or acting in particular situations. Clinicians would lose their grasp and their ways to act. Instead clinicians tell coherent and plausible stories in order to communicate to others about how cardiac functioning is influencing renal and brain function and how these may be related to hemodynamics, body temperature, patient activity and so on, depending on the patient's particular clinical condition and trajectory.

In the following written exemplar, the nurse recalls the changing patient course where the patient was once conscious. The nurse had a very different appraisal of the patient's respiratory condition that was evidenced by her lung function tests. The situation is ambiguous before and after it is resolved:

> **Nurse:** The patient is a 40-year-old female who came to the MICU with a diagnosis of possible pneumonia, CHF (congestive heart failure), and CA (cancer). She was admitted with very poor ABG's (arterial blood gases) and history of idiopathic pulmonary fibrosis since 1981. The patient was told on admission that if need be, they would like to intubate her to treat her pneumonia and then extubate her in a few days. The patient agreed. Mrs. S. was intubated within 12 hours of admission after her CO_2 rose into the 90s and she became confused. Her ABG's began to deteriorate rapidly requiring maximum ventilatory [support] and drugs to sedate and paralyze her.
>
> Mrs. S. was an extremely ill women who was sedated and paralyzed for approximately three weeks. Since the patient was very anxious, she remained sedated for a few weeks in order to ventilate her effectively. During this time, Mrs. S. had multiple

procedures done to her (i.e., trache[ostomy], surgery for gall stones, many [invasive] lines and a few chest tubes). We had attempted on multiple occasions to try and wean her from the ventilator. However, her pulmonary mechanics were terrible and every time we tried, she seemed to get sicker and require more drugs to keep her comfortable and higher ventilatory settings to keep her ABGs adequate. During this time, the patient had no idea how sick she was or what we were doing to keep her alive.

Mrs. S. had a large extended family who were all very involved with her. Her entire family came to this country from Italy. She met and married an Italian man in this country and had two children—a son, 11 years old and a daughter, seven years old. Her role in the family was wife and mother. She was responsible for taking care of the children, looking after the house, and preparing the meals. Her family was well informed of the patient's status. They had grieved on many occasions because often times we thought that she was going to die. As the patient began getting better the family became extremely happy that Mrs. S. was alive and they felt she looked 100% better than the past few weeks.

Unfortunately, Mrs. S. was not happy with the way things were when she finally woke up from the drugs. She was alert and oriented—with no residual affects from the drugs. She made it perfectly clear that she did not want the ventilator or the trache[ostomy]. 'Take this (the ventilator) off!' 'When it pops off, I do fine on my own, so why do I need it (the ventilator) to breathe?' 'Can you take this out (tracheostomy tube)?' 'How can I go home [with a ventilator] and take care of my family?' The patient was weeping, crying, requesting that the ventilator be removed. She denied she needed it.

My concern was that Mrs. S. was not only appropriately depressed but also that she was denying the fact that she needed the ventilator. I was also worried about her inability to maintain her role in the home. All of her caregivers had come to the conclusion that Mrs. S. was now a chronic patient and while Social Services was looking for placement at an appropriate facility, she would remain in the MICU. Weekly meetings were being set up with the family to prepare them for this move.

While taking care of the patient, I was struck by her insistence that she did not need the ventilator. I wanted to try to attempt to wean the patient from the ventilator. I felt that we (the team) could at least try to decrease her ventilator settings enough so that a home ventilatory program could evaluate her. I also wanted to see if this was a possibility before I brought the issue up with the patient and/or her family. Therefore, my goals were to use this opportunity to attempt to decrease the patient's vent settings and to help the patient come to terms with the fact that she physically needed mechanical ventilation to live. I never expected the patient to be able to wean completely from the ventilator.

My rationale for this was that the patient came to the unit with a very poor lung status. Her mechanics were very poor but we never knew what they were at home prior to admission. Maybe they're still the same? Slightly worse? The patient also had a great desire to get off the ventilator and was willing to work hard at it. Why not try?

At rounds the next morning the following were present: two residents, two interns, attending of the month, private physicians, the nurse manager, and myself-associate nurse. A brief presentation was given by the on-call intern. No change was planned from custodial care; they were awaiting placement. All entered the room to assess the patient and talk with her. The patient was telling them how she felt she did not need the ventilator. The team did not respond.

The nurse manager was aware that I wanted to attempt to wean the patient if she would tolerate it. The patient's private physician left the room to write his note. The nurse manager and I left the room to approach him. Since the team had placed the patient in the mode of custodial care, I felt that I might need the assistance of her private physician to sway the team's decision. The physician was about to write his note out in front of the room. We approached him to bring up the issue with him. 'We've been talking about Mrs. S. and about how she's been saying that she doesn't want the ventilator. We would like to try and wean her from the ventilator again.'

The private physician said: 'We've tried that many times before and it hasn't worked.' I explained: 'I understand that, but the patient is now healthier than she's ever been. She really doesn't believe that she needs the ventilator, and I think we need to show her that, in fact, she really does need it. Also, if we can decrease her ventilator settings, she might be eligible for a home vent program. I was aware that the physician had been very concerned about discharge planning and I thought this might help my case.'

The private physician responded: 'Well, I'd be willing to try if Mrs. S. is.'

'I was going to bring up the issue with the team at rounds today. Maybe you'd like to talk with Mrs. S. before then?'

The private physician re-entered the room and approached the patient as the team was beginning to leave. At this point I was glad that the physician agreed to try. I didn't expect her to come out and say she'll try and work with us to get off the vent, but I was hoping that her private physician would hear what she had been saying to us for days ('I want this vent off !'). As the team discussed her plan for the day—no major change—I brought up the issue of weaning: 'I was wondering if we could try again to wean Mrs. S.?' The resident responded, 'I don't think that's such a good idea. We've tried it before and we ended up in worse trouble than we started.' (I knew it was going to be difficult to change the overall plan!) and I said: 'I realize that and I agree with you, but right now the patient is healthier than she's ever been. Now would be the ideal time to try. She's willing to help us and she wants off the ventilator. It's the best opportunity thus far.'

The resident responded: 'But nothing has changed.' I explained: 'She's changed. She's been asleep for over a month and has had no time to deal with the fact that she'll need a vent to live for the rest of her life. I'd like to try and decrease her [respiratory rate] if only to show her that she truly needs the machine to live. She doesn't know yet what it's like to breathe without the machine.' The intern interjected: 'That seems like a reasonable idea to me. If you told me I'd need a vent for the rest of my life after being asleep for one month, I'd think you were crazy.' At this point, everyone became quiet. I was glad that the intern felt that it was at least reasonable and I was happy that he tried to relate how the patient must be feeling to how he would feel. I was hoping that I could convince someone else that we should try. The attending then came out of the room and stood with the group.

The resident said: 'Well, do you want to just take her off the vent and put her on a T-piece? She won't last long.'

The attending of the month responded: 'No, I wouldn't do that; she's on maximum ventilatory [support] now. She'd do very poorly.'

The private physician said: 'I've talked with Mrs. S. and she'd like to try [getting off the vent]. Whatever you think would be the best way is fine with me, but I told her we'd be trying today.'

The resident said: 'You realize she's not going to do well.' I responded saying: 'I think we all agree on that point but the patient wants to try. Why not let her try? If we can decrease her ventilator settings maybe we can get her into a home ventilator program.'

The attending said: 'Her mechanics are terrible; she probably can't be decreased much more.' I explained: 'I know she has bad mechanics, but she may have been at home with mechanics just like this. She obviously had poor lungs before she got here. Why can't we just try?'

The attending responded: 'Well I guess we can. I'd like to get some numbers first. Do you think we could get numbers on her resting and exertional minute ventilation?' I said, "Sure."

The intern asked: 'So do you want to decrease her IMV?'

The attending responded: 'Let's wait for her numbers and then we'll decide how to proceed.'

The team moved on to the next patient and I called the respiratory therapist. He came right up and got the numbers. Mrs. S. was able to double her resting ventilation!!! This was definitely not expected. The respiratory therapist did the procedure two different ways just to make sure it was correct. I was stunned and very happy for Mrs. S. Maybe we would be able to decrease her ventilator settings after all.

Next, we called one of the chest physical therapists to work on inspiratory muscle training with Mrs. S. The therapist laughed at us when the respiratory therapist and I told her which patient we wanted her to see. However, she was pleasantly surprised to learn the Mrs. S. could double her minute ventilation. The therapist worked with Mrs. S. that morning and the patient was able to do inspiratory muscle training off the vent for 15 minutes!! We thought she would last about two to three minutes. I couldn't believe that Mrs. S. was able to do this. We continued to work with her to decrease her vent settings.

Mrs. S. was off the vent and discharged from the unit one week later. This exemplar was important to me because it helped to reinforce how much we, as health care providers, need to <u>listen</u> to what our patients are telling us and then act on that information as a patient advocate. I think the most important thing I did in this exemplar was to listen to my patient and pursue the issue with the team by using scientific rationale to back up what I wanted to do. The most unexpected thing that happened was that Mrs. S. was able to get off the ventilator. It was also good to relearn that a number (representing in this case her pulmonary mechanics) is really only a number. You need to look at the total picture for that number to mean anything.

The nurse and the patient's private physician advocated for weaning the patient from the ventilator, if at all possible, based on ethical considerations for the patient's right to refuse treatment. The nurse skillfully presented a case for weaning using the patient's ethical claims and advocating for the patient. The nurse, private physician, and the intern could imagine the patient's plight and argued for the patient's right to try to wean from ventilatory support. As this case illustrates, remaining open to changing situations and redefined trajectories and transitions requires clinical judgment and attunement. This is a vivid lesson about considering the patient's <u>particular</u> adaptation pattern and is a good example of the difficulty in arguing for a new understanding based on a changing situation. The situation had changed dramatically for the patient upon regaining consciousness, but the majority of the medical team continued to cling to an earlier understanding. After all, they had tried to reduce the ventilatory support before, unsuccessfully.

Focusing on achieving the best clinical understanding for the good of the patient requires respectful listening to the patient, the family, and the multiple health care team members involved. It is useful to rehearse direct styles of communication that will encourage respectful listening. For example, restating your understanding of the physician's clinical understanding and the rationale for treatment can open up the dialogue. Asking astute questions can also open up the dialogue. In some situations, it is helpful and clarifying to articulate one's clinical forethought and expected course of action, based on the physician's decision to treat or not. Similarly, asking the physician about her or his anticipated eventualities in the situation and then asking about treatment preferences for each eventuality can assist in understanding the physician's reasoning-in-transition. Backing off and acknowledging that the picture is not yet clear, but that the goal is to be prepared for the patient's sake and not for the sake of winning an argument, can reduce tension and encourage dialogue. The goal is to avoid locked positions that close down communication and understanding. Oppositional stances of winning or losing one's agenda prevent the <u>best</u> account of the patient's condition from being considered. After the immediacy and heat of solving a complex clinical problem, system improvement through debriefing and clarification of effective and ineffective communication patterns can improve communication processes and help the team to learn together.

COMMUNICATING MISSED TIME TABLES AND UNEXPECTED CHANGES IN CLINICAL TRAJECTORIES

Recovery from most surgeries has familiar patterns of progression and patient responses. With experience and expertise comes the ability to recognize the absence of usual responses (Benner, Tanner & Chesla, 2009). Absence of the usual can signal impending complications. When common expectations are missed, recognition and communication about the failed expectations are particularly difficult, since the number of plausible explanations for the missed time tables are usually numerous and inherently ambiguous. In the following example, the nurse notes that a patient was not waking up appropriately from his coronary bypass surgery. He was on a balloon pump and multiple vasopressors to maintain his blood pressure. The healthcare team was able to wean him off vasopressors, and his renal function returned, but he was slow to wake up:

> **Nurse:** Each day, I said, 'What do you think about having a CAT scan done on him?' to see if there was any other reason, because I hadn't given him sedation since surgery and [his response] is really unusual. Usually people start waking up, they move around, they shiver and shake, and you give them a little bit of morphine, but he had nothing... Anyway it just looked strange to me. It wasn't the usual course, even though he was so close to death when he came back—he had turned around in so many ways after [surgery] except for his neuro status. So we finally took him to CAT scan, and the report was that he had infarcted areas of his brain.

This is the usual kind of modus operandi thinking characteristic of clinical reasoning (see Chapter 2); however, communicating failed expectations is more ambiguous than communicating positive signs and symptoms. Becoming more articulate about specific expectations for typical patients, such as the ones spelled out in critical pathways, can assist in the increased ability to recognize deviations and communicate the variations noticed. As illustrated in the example above, the nurse interprets the patients' responses by stating the failed expectations.

We highlight the perception of missed time tables here because they are a crucial clinical problem solving tool and because they are subtle. They often begin with an uneasy feeling that things are not quite right (Benner, Tanner & Chesla,2009). The sense of being puzzled is not enough evidence for intervening, but it should stimulate a problem search and create a heightened level of vigilance. Alerting others that a patient does not seem to be responding as expected also signals the health care team to be observant and probe further as needed.

CHANGING PRACTICES AND DEVELOPING NEW CLINICAL KNOWLEDGE

Changing patient care management practices that alter patient responses and trajectories necessarily create the need for developing new clinical knowledge and judgment skills in new contexts. Increasingly, patients are having one-day surgeries and are discharged earlier. This increases the importance of making sound clinical judgments about when patients can be safely discharged from critical care areas, as illustrated in the following interview from PACU nurses:

Interviewer: So, it's a real judgment about when patients are ready to go.

Nurse 1: It's a collaborative decision. If I feel they're ready to go, and they (the anesthesiologists) feel that they're ready to go, then they go.

Interviewer: Where do physician's opinions fit in here? Or is that based primarily on a nursing opinion?

Nurse 2: We ask them before [we discharge them].

Nurse 3: We basically tell the physician when they're ready to go.

Interviewer: Because you're there and you know more about when they're ready to go more. But I was just curious about the politics of that...

Nurse 1: There are times where a physician says, 'I want this patient observed for "x" number of hours because of this.' I had a pediatric patient; I think she was from the Middle East somewhere... She had broken her arm and they set it somewhere else. The family went to Hospital X and got it reset. But it became all swollen. So this time, the physician wanted to be a little bit more careful. He wanted her here for six hours to make sure that there was no swelling before we sent that kid home. So there was nothing for us to do, you know; we watched television.

Nurse 3: Well, it's the nurse's responsibility to understand the simplicity or the complexity of the case, and then engage the physician when it's needed. For instance, in my previous example [regarding a woman with severe postoperative pain], I needed to engage the physician all evening because we were giving the patient very large amounts of opioids. It was his decision and mine that she go home but it was not a decision I could have made by myself, because of the extent to which I had given her these large volumes of drugs. But then there are the really simple cases where it's clear it's just going to be your decision. And you don't need to engage a physician. You just tell the physician it's time now. And then there are times where there are shades, one way or the other, where you need to engage your colleagues and say: 'What do you think? Come over here. I need a nurse consult. Tell me what you think about this situation. What would you do?' Often times it is helpful to have our colleagues' fresh perspective on a case that's become too difficult or complex for us, depending on what's going on that day.

Pooled clinical perspectives are often sought (Benner, Tanner & Chesla, 2009). Research is needed on the efficacy of informal consults for improving clinical judgment. While aggregate data and evidence-based medicine will be helpful for evaluating newer practices of early discharge and one-day surgeries, aggregate data will never replace the need for making clinical judgments about particular patients and particular situations. Institutional policies and ethics must support front line clinical decision making where ambiguity and risk can most reliably be recognized by clinical experts. Protocols and cost management strategies must not replace safety precautions where there is uncertainty or unpredictability about patient risk. Making an exception and delaying patient discharge based on concerns for patient safety should not require ethical heroics, but must be supported by institutional guidelines that give patient safety top priority.

The logic of limiting variability in practice through standardization works best for bringing sub-standard practice up to acceptable levels. However, reducing variability in the practice of expert clinicians reduces variability on the high end of performance. Reducing variability where innovation is needed impedes knowledge growth and the development of practice. The logic of evidence-based medicine works well for well-tested and high quality outcomes in stable situations, but aggregate data about health care outcomes does not inherently point to better practice, innovation, or the development of new clinical knowledge. The need for expert judgment in experimental versus well-tested therapies illustrates this.

DEVELOPING CLINICAL KNOWLEDGE ABOUT EXPERIMENTAL INTERVENTIONS

Critical care is a locus of the development of experimental interventions, such as minimally invasive surgeries, fast-tracking, new immunosuppression therapies in transplant recipients, and thrombolytic therapy after cerebral vascular accidents. Each major change in scientific understanding and therapeutic interventions call for clinical knowledge development.

The ethics of informing and teaching patients and families about changes in clinical situations where the disease or therapies are poorly understood or tested guides clinical judgment. The care of persons with AIDS provides a dramatic example:

Advanced Practice Nurse: Yes, this [caring for persons with AIDS] has been an experience where the health care providers and the patients have been in this together.

Interviewer: You've learned it together.

Advanced Practice Nurse: Yes, I worked here before the HIV test existed. And, when we didn't know—when number 1, I was a gay man, and number 2, we didn't know whether, as nurses, we would get it from the patients. And so, later we found who was infected and who wasn't on the staff. But in those early days, we didn't know.

It is hard to remember the kind of active clinical knowledge development that is required when confronting a newly encountered disease with unknown infectious qualities. Descriptions of the patients' illnesses and responses to therapies were crucial. In another example, after much more was learned about HIV and AIDS, the focus shifted to improved clinical assessments and therapies. The following interview and observation occurred in an outpatient setting for care of persons with Acquired Immuno-Deficiency Disease at a time when there were new Protease Inhibitors and a new viral load test available. Little was known about the meaning of the viral load tests or how the patient would interpret the information. This nurse practitioner discussed openly with clients whether or not they wanted or were ready for the new information the viral load test would give. The nurse also discussed with patients whether and when to start the Protease Inhibitors. Clinical judgment was involved in evaluating the impact and suitability of the new treatments for particular patients:

Advanced Practice Nurse: But the two people I saw this morning, first Frank and then James, we got into very different levels of discussion; that's partly a response to the kind of people they are, and the level of discussion they're interested in.

Interviewer: I could see the difference. One was a full collaborator.

Advanced Practice Nurse: Yes.

Interviewer: Frank was problem-solving every minute with you.

Advanced Practice Nurse: Yeah, you know, Frank is agonizing over whether the drug is the right one for him. And so he really benefits from hearing what my thought process was as I discussed the drug I was recommending. In fact, he's heard me state exactly that before, about why I picked which drug to recommend to him. He sort of needs to hear it again. The other guy is: 'Yeah, I'm fine, what you gave me is great. Thanks.' I certainly don't think it means one person is brighter or better, I don't mean to imply that at all. It's just the way they respond,... who they are and how they operate.

Interviewer: Yes and the way they understand the medication.

Advanced Practice Nurse: Yes.

Interviewer: I think good clinicians know a lot about that, but we don't articulate it very often.

Advanced Practice Nurse: But, when I have a patient who says, 'I don't know. You tell me what to do. I'll do whatever you say,'—that kind of thing. I don't do so well with those patients (laughs).

Interviewer: Yes.

Advanced Practice Nurse: I don't like that and I'm not comfortable with it. If it were insulin, I might be comfortable. But with these drugs, I'm much less comfortable.

Interviewer: Too much responsibility. That's a really good point, because it has to do with the clarity that you have about the risks of the treatment.

Advanced Practice Nurse: Mhum.

Interviewer: And with the insulin—you are pretty clear—it's really better for you to take it, so it's not so much of a weighty responsibility?

Advanced Practice Nurse: There are some people who will, initially, want you to decide for them. But there are people who you can bring along and engage them more, change their whole perception of health care, and they end up really enjoying the experience of doing well.

Interviewer: How do you coach them in changing that role? Can you think of a person that you've brought along in that way?

Advanced Practice Nurse: I can't think of anybody right now individually, but it's certainly happened.

And it just sort of starts with [instruction like]: 'Well, there's really no one best answer here. There are a few things we need to consider here. I think there's a general acknowledgment of the fact that we don't have all the answers. I think we need to have an appropriate awe [for the risks]. The clinical outcomes [of taking and not taking insulin] are so clear, compared to these drugs (Observational Interview).

The practical and relational skills of negotiating how and what treatment plan the patient can and will follow are not usually taught as a form of clinical judgment, yet these practical and interpersonal considerations play an enormous role in the clinical judgment of any practitioner. We recommend that students spend more time learning about and developing skills revolving around practical aspects of planning and patient education about treatments. The ethical demand for communicating and empowering the patient's decision making and self-care practices is a constant in good practice. The demand becomes even more urgent when the risks and benefits are not yet well-tested and the clinician has no certainty that the treatment benefits will outweigh the risks. This is a kind of practical technology assessment, which is further described in Chapter 8.

TEAM BUILDING: DEVELOPING A COMMUNITY OF ATTENTIVENESS, SKILL, AND COLLABORATION

Since the first edition of this book, increasing attention has been paid to the deleterious effects of extreme hierarchical structures and status inequities in hospitals. It is agreed that incivility is a major threat to good patient outcomes (Lower, 2008). In January, 2009, The American Hospital Association initiated a Standard for Accreditation (LD.03.01.01 JCAHO, 2009) that health care organizations define acceptable, unacceptable and disruptive behaviors of professionals and that they develop a process for managing those unacceptable and disruptive behaviors. Members of the health care team are expected to maintain professional relationships by demonstrating communication and interpersonal skills that show respect for patients, families and health care team members. They are expected to be sensitive to diversity among patients, families and staff as well. This impetus to "regulate" the improvement of workplace environments has come from evidence that civility, good communication, and collaborative improve patient outcomes (Baggs, 1989; Baggs, Schmitt, Mushlin, et al., 1999). Patterson and colleagues (2002) developed strategies for communicating when the stakes are high.

Team building is a central if relatively invisible role of nurses. Nursing and medicine are knowledge intensive and rely on other health care professionals whose work is also knowledge intensive. In order to develop sufficient practical know-how and common understandings about practice and roles, common expectations must be built. The daily work of communicating and negotiating similarities and differences in styles of practice and team building is all but hidden. Because nurses are the ones whose presence with patients in critical care settings is most constant, understanding and communicating about roles, relationships, and styles of practice are done primarily by nurses, as illustrated in the following example from the operating room. The language is replete with truncated examples and snippets of interactions as the nurses try to capture the variability and contingencies of the practice:

Nurse: I know some of the physicians' idiosyncrasies. They like things the same every time, generally, within the parameters of each individual patient. But, you know, if a surgeon is used to putting a stimulator on the right side and the patient wants it on the left, the patient wants to know why. If the anesthesiologist wants to give a certain medication and the doctor's used to another medicine, the surgeon wants to know why because if there's a good reason, I'll say, 'The surgeon doesn't want you to give that medicine because it interferes with the stimulation.'

Interviewer: So this is when you're in what role and you're helping out...?

Nurse 1: Well, my role is a little bit different. I'm not normally in a scrub or in a circulating position, although I perform in those roles as well. Today I performed as the stereotactic nurse, so my job is to coordinate the activities of the scrub and circulating nurse, as well as the room and the equipment, and make sure the cases go in the routine manner. So it's a little bit different.

Interviewer: But in any of these roles you are considering the information you have, based on your experience with these people, and you're jumping in to offer relevant information that perhaps one of the other nurses or surgeons or anesthesiologists don't have—the piece of information that...

Nurse 1: Perhaps. Or, maybe they do have. Or, maybe they feel uncomfortable saying anything. It just depends, you know. There may be certain situations where I wouldn't say anything.

Interviewer: Can you think of one?

Nurse 1: Not if the patient was going to suffer for it, no.

Interviewer: When you say, 'If the patient were to suffer from it,' what do you mean?

Nurse 1: Well, like if we're repairing an aneurysm and the patient's blood pressure is too low, and we have a young resident who doesn't happen to have a more senior resident in the room at the moment, and I look up and see that the blood pressure is 60—I'm going to say something. 'You know, our usual range is...' And if that goes nowhere, I'll say, 'Do you want to get your attending in?' I don't think the school of hard knocks is a good way for people to learn. It causes too much suffering.

Interviewer: I see what you mean.

Nurse 1: I think everybody agrees with that, even if their own dynamics are maybe a little bit different.

Nurse 2: Yes.

Nurse 1: Look at Linda. I'm sure she does it all the time, even though she works with surgery residents. 'Oh, you know, Doctor So and So likes this or that.' 'No problem.' 'Oh great.' 'Thanks.'

The filling in and pointing to the variability doesn't make for good prose, but it points to the integrative communication and team building skills characteristic of a complex socially embedded practice. Teams work in relation to the tasks at hand and the skills of the team members. The transition from the formal plan or outline of the work (e.g., a systems design) and a well-functioning social community makes the team work in real time, along with all the contingencies and relationships. It would be impossible to anticipate, predict, and control this teamwork because the collaborative interactions of the team are generative and synergistic (Benner, Tanner & Chesla, 2009, pp. 233-278).

While it may seem too idealistic to say that it is the "good of the patient" that governs team development, solidarity around working for the patient's best interests provides the necessary structure and content for coordinating and orchestrating the team's multiple perspectives, skills, and knowledge. What is actually "good for the patient" may be misunderstood or poorly worked out, but the work cannot even go forward without this guiding principle. Having this goal of working for the good of the patient creates the risk and vulnerability inherent in the work, because understanding the good is continually being worked out in less than ideal circumstances, fraught with contingencies, variability, and risks (Murdoch, 1970/1991). The fiduciary or covenant relationship with the patient and family (May, 1983; Pellegrino & Thomasma, 1988; Sharpe, 1997) guides good practice.

Pellegrino and Thomasma (1988) pointed out that the patient's vulnerability and the unequal power of physician (and nurse) and patient calls for a fiduciary relationship. Sharp (1997) summarized the meaning of a fiduciary relationship as one in which the fiduciary has expert knowledge and access to specialty resources. The fiduciary is "a person entrusted with power or property to be used for the benefit of another and legally held to the highest standards of conduct" (Rodwin, 1995). Sharpe went on to explain:

> Because the fiduciary relationship is based on dependence, reliance, discretionary authority and trust, the fiduciary's activity is regulated with regard to conflicts of interest and other potential threats to the welfare of the fiducie [The one who must trust the services of the fiduciary.]... (1997, p.204).

It is the peculiar vulnerability of the patient and the trust invited by the healthcare provider that together explain why healthcare providers, unlike shopkeepers, have <u>de facto</u> positive obligations of beneficence toward those whom they serve. As healthcare comes to be increasingly reinterpreted in the language of the marketplace—as "patients" become "customers," "subscribers," or "covered lives"—we risk losing sight of the fact that patients are not just the "consumers" of healthcare, they are its direct object (Sharpe, 1997, pp.204-213).

When this fiduciary relationship is breached, practice becomes confused and corrupted. Even what is best to do clinically becomes unclear if the clinician's relationship to the patient's best interests are lost. This is evident even in the extreme example of the operating room where the lines between patient and clinicians are purposefully veiled by the sterile drapes and the ritualized hiding of the patient as person (a necessary objectification) during intrusive surgical procedures:

Nurse 1: Sometimes the worst thing that I do all day is to give report and go home. You know, it depends on who your turning your case over to.

Interviewer: What do you mean 'the worst thing that you do?'

Nurse 1: The hardest thing to do.

Interviewer: Yeah.

Nurse 1: You've worked all day with this family and you've been calling the family and you've dealt with the patient—you've pretty much—You've made a contract with the family and the patient.

Interviewer: Yeah. You can have...

Nurse 1: When they saw—and they know you and you know them. And I often will go see family members on my way out. I will have my street clothes on and I'll say, 'No. We're just going to finish it tomorrow. We're all going home.' You know, with a smile. But sometimes you give reports to nurses that really haven't done a lot of your specialty and you just feel like a fool going over this, this, this, and this.

Nurse 3: You know they're going to take care of all the very basics things that are evident, that are easy to see. What you're troubled about is that there are so many variables that could happen. There is no way in a report that you can outline for them... 'Now if this happens you're going to need to take the following actions. [Lists many contingencies.] It sounds very vague but it's a reality. It's very difficult to leave your patient with someone you can't trust to do the basic things and even harder to know that they're going to take care of the rest of the things.

Nurse 5: Or make that extra effort.

Nurse 1: Mmm. Right.

Nurse 4: Who is going to make the entire outcome pleasant and smooth for every single person involved.

This interview conversation reveals the sense of responsibility that these nurses feel. They form a contract and bond with the family that they will be with and watch over the patient. Leaving before the surgery is over infringes on this informal contract, and comments are made about "work time" and leaving. The situation becomes morally difficult if the nurse has to leave the patient to a nurse who he or she feels is not as competent, so the conversation naturally flows into the coaching and direction the nurse provides for her replacement nurse. Weaving a tapestry of understanding and continuity as patients' conditions and settings change requires a narrative memory of the patient's story:

Advanced Practice Nurse: The new attending, Dr. C, understood the patient's poor prognosis, so she thought 'Well, what are we doing here?' Because we're doing this very, extreme CVVH—it isn't a chronic therapy—so why are we doing that if this is the [end of therapeutic options and the patient is dying], and I had to fill in. 'This is the plan, the patient <u>knows</u> what her prognosis is and she has accepted that—she's already planning what the funeral's going to be like, but this is what we need. We just want to get her home. She has a few more things to take care of and we just need to get the fluid off. And so having that information made a world of difference, rather than going to the attending and starting the conversation.

I'm here and as the doctors (residents) change, I provide the continuity of information... I have usually rounded already about an hour or so before the physicians round and have talked to the nurses about things, so hopefully they can participate in rounds. But a lot of times, the bedside nurse can't. So I will pass discussions about the plan on things to them when they miss rounds by asking, 'What's the plan from the ICU team?' I will pass that on to the nurses and sometimes with the respiratory therapists.

Even the style of telling about and piecing together the continuity and tapestry of care (Gordon, Benner & Noddings, 1996; Schindul-Rothschild, Berry & Long-Middleton, 1996) is characteristic of bridging, filling in, and coordinating the efforts of caregivers who work discrete shifts or who have only brief contacts with the patient. The nurse does not fill in all the relevant clinical detail in the example above, because she is pointing to the episodic and response-based nature of the work involved in completing the patient's story and of spelling off those who missed rounds. This integrative communication and team building function is vital to patient safety and well-being. One of the problems with a systems engineering approach (e.g., re-engineering and systems design) is that discrete functions, tasks, and goals are identified and designed into the system (Champy, 1995). However, the broad integrative functions and knowledge work required for reliability and solving problems on the spot are overlooked in a systems design approach, because the complexity of judgment, timing, and team work resist formalization (Bourdieu, 1980/1990; Dreyfus, 1992). Consequently, it is easier to focus on efficiency and recurring problems in a systems design, than it is to focus on the sequencing, particularities, contingencies, and reliability created by the front line problem solvers required to make any systems design work (Benner, Tanner & Chesla, 2009).

Calling attention to lapses in performance, for example, when a sterile breach is observed in the O.R. or sterile bedside procedure requires courage and clarity. The stakes are high for patient well-being and safety. The following example is common if you insert many possible other contraindications for continuing with a procedure that is already set up in a hospital. In this case, Carol Samuels, a cardiac cath lab nurse, tells the story of a child scheduled for cardiac catheterization until an ambiguous case of chicken pox is noticed:

Nurse: It was a normal morning this past winter in the cath lab. Michael came in with his mother for closure of his ASD (Atrial Septal Defect). The admission was the same as most others. Normal 6 year old, with normal vital signs, and a negative pediatric screen. No cough, no cold, no exposure to anyone with rash or infectious disease. Michael had not had the varicella vaccine. I told Michael's mother that we would get started shortly and he could change into his hospital gown. When I returned to give Michael his pre-op, I asked mom if she had any other question. She said no but there are 2 spots on his neck that he did not have last night when he went to bed.

I looked at the spots and wondered if chickenpox was a possibility. I really did not know but told mom that it would be best if Dr. Smith looked at the spots. Dr. Smith was the attending Cardiologist scheduled to close Michael's ASD.

Dr. Smith went in to talk to mom and look at Michael's spots. When he came out I was shocked when he told me, "Don't tell anybody" because no one can tell if it is chickenpox or just a bug bite. The implications of not telling anyone were too overwhelming to think about. I didn't say anything to Dr. Smith, however I know my eyes said enough. He told me we would change the order of the cases and Michael could be last.

I put Michael and his mother in a separate room and told mom not to let Michael leave the room. I explained the implications of chickenpox to other children in the Hospital and told her that many children could get seriously ill and possibly die if exposed to the disease. I told her that although Dr. Smith did not know if it was chickenpox, he was considering the possibility and since it was a possibility, we had to consider it real for now.

I guess I didn't really believe that not telling anybody was a good solution. I asked Dr. Smith if he would like to have an infectious disease consult to rule out chickenpox. "No, they wouldn't be able to tell yet either." I told the people who were scheduled to do the procedure that the order of the cases had been changed and reason that they had been changed. Of course, this set off a discussion on the best way to handle the case and what SHOULD be done. I told everyone that for now, we were isolating Michael and hopefully Dr. Smith would reconsider the infectious disease consult during the time it took to do the next procedure.

At the conclusion of the next case, Dr. Smith asked me to call infectious disease for a consult. The resident on call along with the attending Infectious Disease Physician came down with his flashlight and confirmed the diagnosis of chickenpox. We rescheduled Michael's procedure and sent him home to recover from his illness. When Michael returned 6 weeks later, I asked how he had done. Michael's case was not very bad, he only had about a dozen lesions on his body, however his brother came down with the worse case his mother had ever seen, with lesions all over his body, in his hair and in his mouth. I was happy to see them back and happy to know that in the end we had done the right thing for Michael and the other children in the Hospital.

In this particular situation, where the cardiologist and cath lab nurse have worked together closely for years, the nurse's intentional and blatant nonverbal "look" conveyed her shock about his questionable judgment. With few words, Carol clearly made her case when she suggested that an Infectious Disease consult was needed for a definitive diagnosis. Given the danger of potentially proceeding, despite the command not to tell anyone, Carol tells everyone and ensures that no nurse on the team will knowingly or mistakenly take this child to the cath lab and consequently expose a myriad of critically ill and immunosuppressed children to a disease that could be life-threatening. Although poised to do so, the team did not have to take a stand to ensure safety.

The work of team development and teaching are particularly evident in working with less experienced clinicians, such as interns and newly graduated nurses:

Advanced Practice Nurse: ...There are days when I educate the interns and am the person who has the expertise to make decisions about, you know, coumadin issues. Since we are the continuity, I think our attendings call on us to deal with some issues, maybe they get phone calls on outpatient issues and I think that they put it in our laps to deal with. So that's pretty common, but it just varies from day to day.

While all the allusions the advanced practice nurse has in mind are not spelled out in this interview, the flexible strategies necessary for teaching interns and new nurses while still getting the work done is a common nursing experience. Even in units where the support for continuity has eroded, many nurses still follow-up on patients and their families who are transferred to other units to ensure that patient/family needs are understood and met (Stannard, 1997). As the nurse stated, "We are the continuity." It is this continuity and stability in the team that can create institutional memory and cumulative learning over time.

The phrase "It varies from day to day," in the interview earlier, is worth taking seriously. It is difficult for the nurse to characterize the practice by one or two examples. Because of the variety of health care workers and the variability among patients, responding to that variability is part of the knowledge work of the nurse who has the most consistent presence in the system. Consultation between clinicians about a patient's condition often creates new clinical understandings because multiple clinical perspectives clarify and enrich clinical judgment (Benner, Tanner & Chesla, 2009, pp. 233-278). With increased use of advanced practice nurses in critical care areas, the boundaries between physician and nurse practice are even more blurred (Benner, Tanner & Chesla, 2009):

Nurse 1: I think that the difference between experienced nurses in our unit is that if you intuitively or empirically know something and the intern is your first line of defense, the more experienced nurses will go to the charge nurse or some other senior person and say, 'These are the things I'm seeing. What do you think?' And then we'll go up the chain of command. And I think that often you have to do that. Sue was telling me a story about this baby who was on peritoneal dialysis. She was born with very small kidneys. [The intern ordered lasix and the nurse refused to give it.]

Nurse 2: And the attending physician led the residents through—he kept saying to them, 'Now why wouldn't you want to give lasix?' And the residents would say something and he would say, 'I can't <u>hear</u> you.'

Nurse 1: Which attending was it, Joe?

Nurse 2: 'I can't <u>hear</u> you,' and so finally the residents got it—that they were going to put this baby at risk...

Keeping the patient's story is integral to the nurse's function as the practitioner who is most present. As in the above situation, collaboration with some team members comes only after learning from breakdown. In this case, the resident learned the value of the nurses' early warnings. The nurse moved up the chain of command and secured more appropriate medical interventions.

Nurses also commonly learn to make qualitative distinctions from physician colleagues who not only point out those distinctions in day to day practice during rounds, but also actively teach nurses at the bedside and in continuing education programs (See Chapter 2, Qualitative Distinctions). Further, it is often through clinical teaching relationships that collaborative relationships are born. In unit cultures where collaborative relationships are already established, active participation becomes expected:

Interviewer: With this particular baby is there anything—when the attendings come to the bedside—that concerns you? Are you a part of rounds or can you bring concerns to rounds—what's your role at this point?

Nurse: Generally when the doctors make rounds in the morning, it's an expectation that the nurse will be at the bedside, should listen to what's going on with the baby, and interject anything that is relevant or a new development that the doctors may not know about. We are to participate in rounds and be an active part of the team, not just follow orders blindly.

Interviewer: Is there anything about the management of this baby that you would like them to do differently or are you comfortable with the management?

Nurse: No, no, I'm totally comfortable with the management and it varies a lot from physician to physician.

Interviewer: How comfortable you are...?

Nurse: This baby is not really being managed by the residents. The level of his illness is so profound that he is managed at the fellow and attending level. They're keeping a very close eye on things. So a lot of times if you have a baby who's less sick, who's being managed by the residents who are less experienced, you tend to question things a lot more and to really follow up on things, going up the chain of command if there's something you're not certain about, but this is the 'top of the chain of command,' so, I don't really have any issues at all about how the baby's being managed.

Interviewer: It's interesting that you say this baby is so profoundly sick, because I look over there and I see what looks like a well nourished pink baby with sort of cute downy hair and...

Nurse: But an awful lot of equipment (Observational Interview).

The ease or dis-ease with which how a patient is managed, whether there seems to be a good clinical grasp and a good clinical response, is continually assessed by skilled clinicians, as illustrated above. The infant is very ill, but is being managed well so that he does not look distressed. This is distinct from the infant, as presented in Chapter 12, who is not as critically ill, but who appeared to be rapidly deteriorating because a new nurse was unclear about how to nest the neonate. The background for the appraisal of the patient's condition necessarily includes a sense of how well the patient is being managed and how well the patient's condition is understood and shared by all team members. In each local setting there are judgments made about who is available to provide the best clinical management and guidance. The following example from a neonatal ICU nurse is based upon the local situation of having a cadre of well-prepared advanced practice nurses (who, in this case, are nurse practitioners) available for consultation and immediate problem solving in ambiguous and transitional situations:

Interviewer: I want to explore for a moment how the nurses determine when to call you and when to call the intern. It sounds in this situation that the nurse first called the intern.

Advanced Practiced Nurse 1: Well, they might call the intern if they're around. But basically, if we [advanced practice nurses] are around, we will <u>always</u> be the contact person. Because the nurses know that we will go and <u>look</u> at the patient, and that even though the issue may seem really small, it's important to <u>them</u>. So, I think most of the time we will go in and look at the patient and attempt to problem solve.

Advanced Practiced Nurse 2: (very soft) I think they call us more than they do the residents.

Advanced Practiced Nurse 3: I think it depends on how responsive the interns have been. I've seen one of the nurses go to an intern and say, 'You know, I'm really concerned that this patient is bleeding from his G tube and from his trache[ostomy] and I'm really concerned about this.' And the intern is just like, 'Yeah, okay.' And then the nurses come directly to one of us (advanced practice nurses) and says, 'I'm really concerned. What are you going to do about it?' And we'll go in and look at the patient and take care of the problem. And so I think the nurses are under the stress and strain of having a lot of interns that <u>they're</u> not getting answers from, but they need answers. I think they've learned that, and I think [advanced practice nurse 2] is right, they <u>do</u> come to us for a lot of things.

Interviewer: Has this set up some friction... How does the team work?

Advanced Practiced Nurse 1: It's very dependent on who the interns are, but in general, I think that we work fairly well together. And they [the residents] realize that we do a whole lot of their work for them. So, it's like the nicer they are to us, the better it is for them...

Advanced Practiced Nurse 2: I think they know that they rely on us too.

Advanced Practiced Nurse 3: Yes, I think that...I also think that sometimes it's such a relief that we picked up on a patient who was really sick or dealt with something that was really big. Because it's such a relief that they didn't have to do it. And that is one thing on their list of a thousand things that they didn't have to do.

Advanced Practiced Nurse 1: And I think it's a result of the residents learning what we do and what we are capable of, the more they're around us. Knowing that we pick up issues on patients that are outpatients, and admit people from clinic because the interns don't go to clinic. It's us and the third year residents, and [they learn] that truly we're the consistent force, and that it's not unusual to admit somebody and find something that somebody else missed...maybe the patient had just been in the emergency room a couple days before, and so I think the nurses come to us, and say, 'Well, these questions aren't answered.' But instead of just saying, 'Okay, well, see you later,' we try to find the answers and if that means somebody has to be hospitalized, then that happens. That's fairly common.

Reflection on the patient's condition and communicating multiple clinical perspectives are needed in basic education programs for all health professionals, but are also needed in high intensity, high demand work settings. Debriefings among team members on cases where communication was effective and where there were breakdowns can help clarify misperceptions and improve interdisciplinary communication.

Getting to know the skills and talents of team members develops over time with experience, and use of this knowledge makes all the difference in enhancing the functioning of the team. This is illustrated by Lisa Mayer, an OB nurse, in the following example of a young woman admitted from the emergency room for acute abdominal pain:

Nurse: I helped her from the ER cart to her hospital bed. Her cold, clammy skin prompted me to check her pulse. Thready and fast. I immediately hooked her up to monitors and at the same time questioned her of her days activities. It was clear to me whatever was happening was serious. The patient was showing signs of hypovolemic shock. I called the doctors and made sure the I.V. was patent and turned the volume up sufficiently to maintain her blood pressure.

When the staff doctor arrived on the floor my heart sank. I hadn't had a chance to see who was on call. He was a very experienced OBGYN who took call very infrequently, and I had no confidence in his "high risk" abilities. After evaluating the patient he gave his orders. I agreed for the most part but asked for a couple of modifications. The patient had all the signs of gall bladder attack, but he needed a scan to confirm it. I was a little uneasy taking a patient to the basement for a scan, so I took the unit scrub tech, Penny, with me. The patient was sitting up talking and her pain had improved after I medicated her, but something told me to be prepared for anything.

The radiologist scanned my patient. The gall bladder looked great but there seemed to be fluid accumulating around the liver. "It clearly is not ascites" he said, "but there is definitely some fluid there." I asked him if he ever scanned a uterus and could he tell if there was blood coming from it? At the time I asked Penny to call the OB resident to come look at the scan and diagnose uterine rupture. The radiologist could not find the uterus. The OB resident arrived and after a debriefing with the radiologist he informed me that, a 22 week uterus does not rupture, besides there is no vaginal bleeding." I was not giving up, and I was not going to lose control of this situation.

By this time the patient was showing signs of confusion. I asked the resident to help me get her back to OB because we needed to move fast. She complained of shortness of breath on the way back to the unit. When we arrived the staff doctor took one look at her and called General Surgery and High Risk back up. We moved the patient to the OR so we could easily intubate.

Many doctors converged upon the OR. A surgeon began placing a CIV (central IV) for blood administration. Two anesthesiologists poked her simultaneously attempting art lines for her falling blood pressure. I was very worried, and I could see in her eyes she was scared. The doctors had taken over. High Risk OB arrived. The patient expressed she couldn't breathe, but everyone was ignoring her. Holding her hand and with the other on her shoulder, I reassured her she could do it and everything would be all right. She was losing control. I breathed with her, calming her down, constantly reassuring her she would make it until she was sedated and intubated.

Still unclear of the cause, the abdomen was opened. Her uterus had ruptured, and she was losing blood rapidly. A hysterectomy was performed. As doctors sewed her up, I bathed and dressed her dead fetus.

We transferred my patient to the ICU vented. After giving report to her new nurse I started to leave. I saw a middle-aged, very distinguished man sitting in the waiting room alone and horrified. I approached him with my hand extended. I introduced myself and told him I had been with his wife all day. I told him his wife was very lucky to come through this emergency, but would be okay. There was nothing he could have done to prevent this. I told him his son was bathed and in a safe place in OBICCU. He could see him anytime. He chose to wait for his wife to see him. I said goodnight and left him.

In this example, Lisa managed to get the medical expertise and experience that were needed for the patient, when she recognized that the attending physician was not very experienced with high risk cases. Without Lisa's clinical leadership and coordination of the team, the patient's care might have been delayed at great risk. Unfortunately the OB resident she summoned to C.T. scan to help make a diagnosis was convinced that a woman with a 22 week fetus would "never" have a ruptured uterus. The nurse's experience with high risk OB patients was greater than the resident's. Despite the ambiguity and confusion over the cause of the woman's acute abdomen, and various inter-professional disagreements, the patient was taken to the OR in time to save her life.

Team members who work together over time develop a standard set of expectations. For example, nurses learn to anticipate and prepare the kinds of information a physician will want before making a phone call. By knowing the physician, the nurse also knows the questions to ask before the end of the discussion that will focus attention on overlooked aspects of care. For instance, the nurse may know that the physician will want an X-ray after a particular change in the patient's condition. If the physician overlooks mentioning it, the nurse asks the question in order to ensure that the results are available during rounds the next morning. Physicians also learn to anticipate what nurses need in the care of patients. For instance, physicians commonly anticipate the nurse's request for comfort care measures, particularly late at night. This level of communication reflects areas of practice and perspectives that have already been negotiated and agreed upon, and thus, no longer require routine communication. In the following interview excerpt, it is evident that home care nurses are aware of their influence on medical decision making, and have learned ways of making their communication with physicians more efficient:

Advanced Practice Nurse: Basically what I always tell my patients is that I'm essentially acting as the eyes and ears of the physician and so I was on the phone continuously just doing the head to toes with what I was seeing, and what I was hearing with the stethoscope, and what his weight was, and the color, and—all those sorts of things. And most of it got turfed to the primary care physician so that, you know, I was interacting with him and with the pharmacist. But because it was all so new to everybody, we were all just hyper scrutinizing this particular patient.

Interviewer: Can you give me an example of when you were on the phone and can you remember when you were talking to the doctor and, reading the patient to the physician on the phone and...?

Advanced Practice Nurse: Well it's not one particular thing. We do an enormous amount of phone work. By definition, home care involves an enormous amount phone contact with the physician. So you're there on the phone and they're just firing questions at you, such as 'Do you know how much weight they've put on? What's the level of pitting edema? What are his breath sounds? What are the heart sounds?' 'What does the patient look like?' And hopefully you've got some lab values, but many times that can be a slow turn around thing. Sometimes you're patching through to a pharmacist at the same time. So it's really trying to just feed clinical information to the physician. It's at the time same concise [and] relevant. That was one of the things I had to learn: 'How do I just, well, collapse a very complicated patient down?' So that a physician in private practice who has had to see a patient every 15 minutes—because they have a managed care practice—and who doesn't have a lot of time to spend on the phone with you, when you're just very quickly trying to update them with 'what you really need to know to make a diagnostic differential.' So you weed out the stuff that they really don't want to hear—that's just going to waste time. So I can't give you a one-two-three...you just have to learn how to give the most relevant, succinct, and concise clinical information. If they really have confidence in what you're saying, and if their feedback is that they're going to be ordering very significant therapies based on what you're seeing, it can come back and slap them in the face if you don't know what you're doing. So it's really a clinical credibility thing. You know, the problem is like, 'How do you make yourself credible to someone who may not even know you,' when you have end-stage patients that you're dealing with.

This conversation points up the high stakes of inter-professional communication and the ways that medical decision making is situated by the nurses' clinical grasp and articulation of the situation in the absence of the physician. This interview also illustrates the costs of fragmentation of service, distance, and lack of collaborative relationships between health team members.

A specialized, local language usually develops to communicate commonly-understood clinical conditions, along with the indications for treatment. These common patterns can be taught to newcomers through case examples. Clinical knowledge may be guided or misguided by strong instances where nurses and physicians learned from a particular case. Shared clinical understandings develop around these shared experiences. For example, Hooper (1995) found that physicians and nurses referred back to memorable cases where they had learned new clinical possibilities or new clinical dangers. Establishing and communicating styles of practice are also illustrated in the following nurse practitioner interview. For example, an advanced practice nurses talks about understanding specific styles of physician practice. By this she means not only the common patterns of clinical diagnoses and treatments but also their relationships and communication patterns with patients:

Advanced Practice Nurse: I think what happens with the nurse practitioner is that, whoever your physician is that you work under their licensure, you take on their style, maybe not their style, but you take on their [patient care] management style. And that is helpful here because we have certain protocols that we work with. The protocols also really help us as far as creating a lot of continuity between us... I think that we all have a lot of similarities, but I think we also have a lot of little differences. And I think that's what makes it work really well. I might really clash within a family for one reason or another, but Jane might just do really well with them. And I think that what we've done, over time, is that we've learned each other's strengths and weaknesses, and we've used this to our advantage too, and I think it's made it an even a better group.

Protocols and critical pathways establish formal expectations and patterns of practice, but the description immediately moves to not only the similarities in practices but also the differences that make the team work well. The description slides into a discussion of the team, and the use of a different team member's particular style working with different patients/families with different personalities and needs.

SUMMARY

We have sought to highlight the work of building a social context for good clinical judgment based on clearly communicating clinical and ethical understandings between health care providers. Making these aspects of clinical inquiry and problem solving visible has many implications for clinical education (both in academic and service settings), as well as in practice and management. Too often, practical and ethical aspects of clinical decisions fall outside of the "legitimate" bases for making clinical judgments, yet decisions and actions depend on these aspects of clinical judgment. Science is necessary but not sufficient for becoming a wise clinician who communicates and works well with others to bring about the best outcomes for patients.

Systems engineering and organizational designs that overlook team building and the social fabric of clinical knowledge are doomed to failure because they are not sufficient for producing the necessary clinical knowledge, judgment, and relationships that can deliver safe, trustworthy care or teach the next generation of clinicians (Champy, 1995). The examples in this chapter present the fragility of the practice, as well as the vulnerability of the patient to trustworthy watchfulness and the concern of practitioners who collectively work for the good of the patient and family. Narrative accounts, such as the ones presented in this chapter, create a picture of the practical clinical reasoning and communication skills required for team building and orchestrating the care of patients. Perspectives of other healthcare team members and narratives from patients and families are needed to extend this dialogue. Interdisciplinary and collaborative practice experiences in basic and graduate education programs would facilitate learning the perspectives of other providers in making and communicating clinical judgments and ethical discernment.

Communicating clear, well-documented clinical evidence of patient transitions is relatively easy. But excellent practice requires that early tentative recognition of patient changes be communicated also. Communicating tentative judgments and early warnings requires more trust, respect, and willingness to listen. Clinical knowledge is negotiated (Benner, Tanner & Chesla, 2009). Conflicts also arise over the state of the scientific underpinnings for interventions, and mutual respect and listening are also required to come to the best decisions.

REFERENCES

Baggs, J. G. (1989). Intensive care unit use and collaboration between nurses and physicians. *Heart and Lung, 18,* 332–338.

Baggs J. G., Schmitt M. H., Mushlin A. I., Mitchell P. H., Eldredge D. H., Oakes D., & Hutson A. D. (1999). Association between nurse–physician collaboration and patient outcomes in three intensive care units. *Critical Care Medicine, 27,* 1991–1998.

Benner, P., Sutphen, M., Leonard, V., Day, L. (2010) *Educating nurses: A Call for radical transformation.* San Francisco: Jossey-Bass and Carnegie Foundation for the Advancement of Teaching

Benner, P., Tanner, C. A., & Chesla, C. A. (2009). *Expertise in nursing practice: Caring, clinical judgment, and ethics.* New York, NY: Springer Publishing Company.

Bourdieu, P. (1980/1990). *The logic of practice* (Richard Nice, Trans.). Stanford, CA: Stanford University Press.

Champy, J. (1995). *Reengineering management.* New York, NY: Harper Business.

Dreyfus, H. L. (1992). *What computers still can't do: A critique of artificial reason.* Cambridge, MA: MIT Press.

Gordon, S., Benner, P., & Noddings, N. (1996). *The care voice and beyond.* Philadelphia, PA: University of Pennsylvania Press.

Hooper, P. L. (1995). *Expert titration of multiple vasoactive drugs in post-cardiac surgical patients: An interpretive study of clinical judgment and perceptual acuity.* Doctoral dissertation, University of California at San Francisco, San Francisco.

Joint Commission 2009 Leadership Standards LD.03.01.01 http://www.jointcommission.org/SentinelEvents/SentinelEventAlert/sea_40.htm, accessed March 31, 2010.

Lower, J. S. (2008). Creating a culture of civility: Challenges and recommendations. *OR Nurse, 2*(5), pp. 10–12.

May, W. F. (1983). *The physician's covenant.* Louisville, KY: Westminister/John Knox.

Murdoch, I. (1970/1991). *The sovereignty of the good.* London, England: Routledge.

Patterson, K., Grenny, J., McMillan, R., Switzler, A., & Covey, S. R. (2002) *Crucial conversations: Tools for talking when stakes are high.* New York, NY: McGraw-Hill.

Pellegrino, E. D., & Thomasma, D. C. (1988). *For the patients good: The restoration of beneficence in health care.* New York, NY: Oxford University Press.

Rodwin, M. A. (1995). Strains in the fiduciary metaphor: Divided physician loyalties and obligations in a changing health care system. *American Journal of Law and Medicine, 21,* 241–242.

Schindul-Rothschild, J. A., Berry, D., & Long-Middleton, E. (1996). Final results of the AJN survey. *American Journal of Nursing, 96,* 23–28.

Sharpe, V. A. (1997). Why "do no harm". In D. C. Thomasma (Ed.), *The influence of Edmund Pellegrino's philosophy of medicine.* Dordrecht, Netherlands: Kluwer Academic.

Stannard, D. (1997). *Reclaiming the house: An interpretive study of nurse-family interactions and activities in critical care.* (Unpublished doctoral dissertation, University of California, San Francisco, San Francisco.)

Stein, L. I. (1967). The doctor-nurse game. *ArchGenPsychiatry, 16,* 278–284.

Stein, L. I., Watts, D. T., & Howell, T. (1990). The doctor-nurse game revisted. *The New England Journal of Medicine, 332*(8), 546–549.

11

Patient Safety: Monitoring Quality, Preventing and Managing Practice Breakdown

*P*reventing mishaps and mistakes, which we call practice breakdown, is central to the nursing role. Nurses are at the sharp end of patient care and are the patient's last defense against patient care error or unprevented hazards of hospitalization and immobility. It would be hard to assign a percentage of the nurse's work devoted to patient safety, because vigilance, monitoring and prevention and promotion of patient safety are so integral to nurses' work. This was evident in our original study of nurses caring for the critically ill (Benner, Hooper-Kyriakidis, Stannard, 1999) and two whole domains of practice were distinctly related to the nurse's focus on patient safety, a chapter devoted to safety issues related to technology use (see Chapter 8) and this chapter devoted to patient safety. The Joint Commission on Accreditation of Hospital Organizations (JCAHO) notes that almost 50% of their standards directly relate to patient safety including the 'right reason' for patient care interventions and medication administration. The following nursing taxonomy comes from an extensive study of nursing areas of practice standards and breakdown from the National Council of State Boards of Nursing (Benner, Malloch & Sheets, 2010):

> *Safe Medication Administration:* The nurse administers the right dose of the right medication via the right route to the right patient at the right time for the right reason.
>
> *Clearly Communicating Patient Data and Clinical Assessments; Documentation:* Provides relevant information about the patient and the measures implemented or needed in response to their needs.
>
> *Attentiveness and Surveillance:* The nurse monitors what is happening with the patient noting and responding to any changes over time.
>
> *Clinical Reasoning and Judgment:* Nurses interpret patient's signs, symptoms and responses to therapies, adjusting therapies by protocols or notification of Health Care Provider.
>
> *Timely, Accurate, and Skillful Interventions:* The nurse properly carries out nursing actions.

Interpretation of Authorized Provider Orders: The nurse interprets, and clarifies health care provider orders.

Professional Responsibility and Patient Advocacy: The nurse demonstrates professional responsibility and advocates for the concerns and needs of patients and families.

Criminal Behavior Mandating Reporting to the State Board of Nursing: Criminal behavior falls outside the sanctioned legal domains of nursing practice and must always be reported to State Boards of Nursing (pp. 12-15).

It is generally agreed that a narrow focus on discrete "errors" cannot sufficiently improve practice and prevent future similar practice breakdowns (IOM, 2004). Safety engineering and systems re-design can solve faulty structural, functional and processes that have been found to be sources of errors. However, "systems design" cannot solve all the situated thinking and actions in the moment required by health care providers and particularly nurses, delivering complex patient care. Where a broad, knowledge based situated thinking-in-action is required, the knowledge work, adaptability, and situated thinking-in-action of professional practitioners are required.

In clinical settings, the potential for breakdown in the care of patients is ever present. Here, breakdown refers to situations that unfold in undesirable ways as the result of team members' performance, the unavailability of essential resources, and/or system problems. Weick and Sutcliffe (2001) point out that mistakes don't start out as mistakes, but become so over time. In the best of circumstances, system design, staffing, and even the environment of critical care units are designed to manage crises and prevent breakdowns. Well educated, highly trained professional staff are able to recognize and intervene in dangerous situations as they occur and take actions to prevent reoccurrence. Monitoring and improving quality requires: 1) Clinical forethought (see Chapter 3), 2) system repair, 3) learning from mistakes, 4) identification of dangerous conditions, 5) averting accidents, 6) team building, and 7) the development of cumulative clinical wisdom (see Chapter 5).

By their nature, fast paced, highly charged, crisis situations are susceptible to breakdown. One might even define a critical or crisis situation as the repair of breakdown (see Chapter 5). The formal side of organizations focuses on developing structures, policies, and processes to prevent breakdown. The legitimization of these procedures, including the structures of risk management and quality monitoring, tend to cover over the import of informal front line quality development and risk management by nurses and other healthcare providers. Because nurses have continuous bedside presence, they play a key role in the daily repair of systems and team building (see also Chapter 10).

The goal is to highlight the daily clinical judgment and expertise required to prevent, intervene in, and correct system failures, since this is a large component of the nursing role even in the best of circumstances. Front line quality monitoring, development and managing breakdown may appear "obvious" to nurse readers, yet raising consciousness about this aspect of nursing work can provide better organizational and public language and improve formal organizational supports and sanctions. During the second phase of this study (1996–1999), at the time of writing the first edition of this book, nurses were even more occupied in correcting breakdowns due to rapidly changing healthcare systems.

Nurses' stories of everyday practice reveal that breakdown is not limited to the physical care of patients. It can include psychological, spiritual, cultural, and moral aspects of care. A team's inability to function collaboratively is a common source of breakdown, however blaming team members seldom improves the situation. Focusing on blame diverts attention from where it belongs—on the safety and well-being of the patient. Focusing on the patient requires that the team's energies be directed in achieving the best possible outcomes for the patient and family. Breakdown may be actual or imminent. An actual breakdown situation occurs when intervention fails to meet the patient's needs, either in a timely manner or at all. An imminent breakdown is a situation in which the actions that are taken are inappropriate or inadequate and will, therefore, predictably not serve the patient's best interests.

Depending on the nature and extent, breakdown situations may or may not compromise patient care or the patient's condition. Patient harm related to practice breakdown, and particularly related to formally filed critical incidents is now recorded (Benner, Malloch, & Sheets, 2010). The problem of patient safety and practice breakdown has received more attention since the publication of the IOM reports on patient safety (IOM, 2004; Institute of Medicine, 2001; Cooper, Gaba, Lianga, Woods, & Blum, 2000; Cronenwett, et al. 2007; Gawande,. 2007; IOM, 2003; IOM, 2000; Leape, Lawthers, Brennan, & Johnson, 1993). Patient complications and longer hospital stays due to breakdown are easily detected (Fridkin, Pear, Williamson, Galgiani, & Jarvis, 1996). Litigation is an all too familiar and highly visible result of breakdown. However, preventing breakdown or potential breakdown situations to reduce adverse outcomes for patients, for fellow team members, and for their institutions are not easily documented and typically shows up in outcome studies as fewer unfavorable outcomes rather than positive outcomes (American Nurses' Association, 1996a; 1996b).

Because patient care can not always be provided "perfectly," learning to manage breakdown is an essential domain of expert clinical nursing practice. This chapter will describe six pervasive aspects of expert nursing interventions when managing breakdown situations, as listed in Table 11.1.

Nurses commonly remember and describe breakdown situations when the patient's clinical condition was deteriorating. During these times, rapid problem identification and intervention are essential. This is illustrated in the following small group interview where an experienced nurse notices that a newer staff nurse needed assistance with a critically injured patient. The patient, who had been hit by a motorcycle, had multiple neurological,

TABLE 11.1
Managing Practice Breakdown

- The role of agency in managing practice breakdown
- Frontline quality improvement, monitoring, and risk management
- Shoring up imminent or actual practice breakdown
- Team building in the context of practice breakdown: Resolving sources of conflict and confusion
- Repairing and redesigning the system to prevent further practice breakdowns
- Contrast cases: Working against all odds and acceptance of practice breakdown—letting the system fail:
  - ☐ Minimizing health care system failures in destabilized work environments
  - ☐ Providing highly technical medical care without adequate nursing care and social services

orthopedic, and abdominal injuries. Additionally, there were communication problems with the family:

> **Nurse 1:** The new nurse caring for the patient had not thought of calling the trauma team. I think the new nurse was very stressed. The family was putting pressure on her. I think she was overwhelmed by the amount of care that this patient needed. So overwhelmed that I don't even think she knew where to go for help. Now I had a very busy assignment of my own that weekend, but I was just kind of checking things that you see out of peripheral vision that you end up 'butting in' [a slang American term for crossing boundaries, and intruding where assistance is not expected], intervening, whatever terminology you prefer. So I knew that the primary nurse was going to be gone for several more days. Although this beginning nurse and I worked the same shift over the weekend, I knew that at the beginning of the week we were going to be on opposite shifts. She was just beginning her day rotation and I was just going to my night rotation. So I really thought, well, now that you've kind of gotten involved, I really felt compelled to put myself up as an associate and become part of the team. And first of all making sure that this patient got the kind of care that he needed, and second of all, being on the team and being able to educate this nurse in how to create more of a collaborative team effort than this 'butting in' type of situation. So like I said, there are times when I feel very compelled, that 'you have to do something.'
>
> **Interviewer:** Why did you feel like you were 'butting in?'
>
> **Nurse 1:** Well, it really is intervening to me, to help the patient.
>
> **Nurse 2:** No, I would think she'd appreciate having that, someone there to tell her, you know, maybe what she should do, especially if she seems so lost.
>
> **Nurse 1:** Yeah, I really, I do think she appreciated it... I call it butting in, but I don't think they see me as butting in. I think a lot of times people appreciate the help that I give them.
>
> **Interviewer:** So was it effective when you went to your night rotation?
>
> **Nurse 1:** It was very effective. There were injuries on the patient that hadn't been picked up because of lack of experience, and even the trauma team had missed. One of the things that really bothered me was this patient wasn't moving his right arm, and I thought, 'Why isn't he moving his right arm?' He had some soft tissue injury but really no broken bones, he had a head injury but the location of the head injury shouldn't have affected the right arm. I said to the team the next morning when they came in, 'Gee, has anyone thought about a brachial plexus injury on this guy?' And they all went, 'Oh, gee, yeah—he's got a clavicle and a rib fracture.' The patient had been there for like 6 days already. So I was able to notice things like that that didn't get picked up...
>
> **Interviewer:** Were you right? Did he in fact have a brachial plexus injury?
>
> **Nurse 1:** Yes, it was a partial brachial plexus. As his neuro status improved, he did regain some function of his arm, but not completely, and when they did the EMG, he did have a brachial plexus injury.

The nurse moves from informal intervention to formal intervention by assigning herself as associate nurse. We get no more information about the family as the nurse's interview shifts to her efforts at identifying a missed injury (a brachial plexus injury), shoring up continuity, and attentiveness to this patient's injuries and recovery.

Preventing imminent breakdown and responding swiftly and definitively are highly valued in the immediate situation and are informally recognized. However, the skills required for such performance are rarely taught since the focus is usually on "doing things right" and achieving standards of practice. Monitoring and improving quality in front line practice renders complex medical care safe. When breakdown in the care of a patient occurs, an expert nurse often recognizes the problem and is compelled to intervene to correct the problem. Nurses often call this patient advocacy, since they are advocating for the best care of the patient in less-than-ideal circumstances.

Because managing breakdown is often a life-saving intervention, we recommend articulating the nursing skills and further developing strategies for ongoing system repair and team building as a part of systems/practice improvement. The most basic form of system re-design is ongoing re-design based upon discovering sources of breakdown. System design close to actual goals and functions augments a systems' engineering approaches where task analyses are done, work flow is charted, and new, externally created work designs are created (Champy, 1995). Such systems' engineering is necessarily skeletal, leaving out the many contingencies and practical knowledge embedded in the situation. Also one cannot "engineer" the human work of creating a culture of attentiveness, care, and self-correction. Team building and creating a community of attentiveness requires different skills and strategies than system design. Team building refers to developing the human and informal side of the organization, sometimes called organizational culture or "lifeworld" instead of system (Habermas, 1984/1987; Ihde, 1990). Developing the lifeworld involves developing a community of memory so that errors are not repeated and troublesome behaviors are changed rather than accommodated. Developing cumulative wisdom refers to local, specific knowledge about doing better as a result of learning from failures. Such experiential learning is essential to the complex knowledge work associated with the human and medical care required for the critically ill and injured. Developing a practice (e.g., a socially embedded form of knowledge) requires attending to the notions of good inherent in the practice (Benner, Tanner & Chesla, 2009). Practical wisdom is developed and based on experiential learning while pursuing and drawing on research about the clinical science related to practice.

THE ROLE OF AGENCY IN MANAGING PRACTICE BREAKDOWN

In the preceding story, the nurse acts as a moral agent by actively intervening to improve communication with the family and by detecting a predictable but unnoticed injury, thereby bringing needed medical attention to the problem. In order to appropriately intervene in a breakdown situation, the nurse needs to have a good understanding of the patient's condition, how it is likely to unfold, and what is needed to alter and improve the patient's care. For this, the nurse needs both formal and experiential knowledge and the courage and skill to act; that is, the agency to take a stand on issues of concern. As Benner, Tanner, and Chesla (2009) point out, expert agency requires:

> 1) excellent moral sensibilities (a vision and commitment to good clinical and caring practices); 2) perceptual acuity (the ability to identify salient moral issues in particular situations); 3) [skilled] know-how; 4) skillful engagement and respectful relationships with patients, families, and co-workers; and 5) the ability to respond in the situation in a timely fashion (p. 158).

The role of agency in managing breakdown can be crucial in making a difference in the patient's outcome because nurses are commonly working in situations of status and power inequities. Often formal and informal kinds of power clash. Although the development of agency is central to taking skillful action to manage breakdown, it does not assure that colleagues will respond appropriately. The collective vision of good practice and the struggle against poor practice depicted in these examples can be a source of empowerment. Overcoming system failures and social injustice requires action at the administrative, social and political levels.

One's ability to influence a social system depends upon social power and working relationships. For example, temporary, per-diem nurses' abilities to influence others may be hampered as illustrated in the following written exemplar where the per-diem nurse recognized early signs of the patient's changing neurological condition but had difficulty getting a timely response. Based on past experience, she could foresee the probability of rapid and life-threatening deterioration:

Nurse: First of all, I have been a critical care nurse for 17 years in intensive care. At the time this case occurred, I was working for a registry. I knew there was a reticence about having registry nurses work in critical care from my experience as an ICU staff and charge nurse.

I was called into work and arrived just in time to receive a very brief report from the unit head nurse, Sally, about a trauma patient, a 19-year-old, who had fallen off a truck. She told me he should be going to the telemetry unit, but since there was no bed available, he needed to come here for observation. She told me that this kid was alert and oriented, had a single peripheral IV, and his neuro status and vital signs should be checked every four hours. She asked if I was comfortable with this, and I said, 'Yes.' There was some question about his loss of consciousness. They didn't have time in the emergency department to really understand if there was a loss of consciousness. He had not been sedated, he had a negative CT scan, his labs all checked out. There was no evidence of neck, back, or abdominal injuries. Looked like he had good renal function. And evidently, his mom only spoke Spanish, but she was informed by a Spanish interpreter. By this time, the patient was getting ready to be wheeled into the ICU.

When the patient arrived, I noticed that all four of his extremities moved very strongly, and I remember seeing some fear in his eyes. He glanced around the room silently. I introduced myself, I asked what name I should call him, and he didn't say anything. He needed to get used to his surroundings before he was able to talk, I guess. In the meantime, I hooked up his nasal cannula to liters of oxygen. I noticed his IV was intact, his pupils were equal and reactive at about 2-3 mm; vitals signs looked pretty good. I explained everything, as I gently attached the blood pressure cuff, the pulse ox sensor, and the EKG leads. Everything looked stable including his cardiac rhythm.

At this point, I asked what his name was again and he said, 'Jose'. And I said, 'So what brings you here?' As he quietly studied my face—so he was tracking—he became very easily distracted by sounds and motions of the unit and he seemed restless. Perhaps this was anxiety. My instincts told me that this behavior was suspicious of an occult head injury. It was possibly, worse than what his clinical findings demonstrated. But then I had to ask myself how much of this was anxiety versus a cognitive deficiency. You have to be very careful when you look at a head injury. You have to remember that he is 19-years-old. I decided that he was probably a bit sensory overloaded.

I limited his visual field by using the curtains to cut the view off between the two beds, but I left the view between the window and the door open, so that he wouldn't feel too threatened. I asked again, 'What brings you here, today?' He shifted his focus to another nurse who walked by. So I asked a simpler question, 'Jose, can you hear me?' He turned his head and focused on the window behind me. I noticed no drainage from either ear, nor bruising underneath or behind the ears—no signs of a basilar skull fracture—probably a safe assumption. He said, 'Yeah, I can hear you.' I asked other questions to assess his level of orientation. He ended up telling me he knew where he was, but he did not seem to recall the date or the actual year. He knew that it was December, and he knew basically what day of the week it was, but he had difficulty with the year, first saying, '84, and I said to him, 'You know, I don't think it's 1984. Can you think a little bit more on this?' And he eventually said, 'I mean, it's 1987,' and then, following that, 'It's probably 1994.' I reiterated the question about why he was brought to the hospital. He yawned and said, 'I'm not sure; could I go home now?' I asked, 'Do you remember what happened this morning?' He swerved his head to see what was on my other side; I gently touched his arm to bring his focus back. He said, 'I can't stay here, you know. I don't have any insurance, no money to pay for this.' This indicated his ability to assimilate information which requires some higher level of orientation. He continued, 'I'm not bleeding, you know. If I'm not bleeding, why do I need to be here?' I explained, 'Sometimes we injure the inside of our bodies and can't see those injuries from the outside.' He came back with, 'Well, I don't hurt anywhere.' He didn't have any pain, that was good.

He continued to be a little bit restless. And I noticed that he was a little bit photophobic. I wondered if it was a neurologic symptom or if it had more to do with the sun beginning to glare in the window. So, at his request, I closed the drapes to the window. I asked him again if he remembered coming to the hospital, and his eyes stopped roaming at this point, and it was clear to me that that it was a good move to close the curtains. He stared into the space behind me and said, 'I woke up in the ambulance.' He had sustained a head injury severe enough to cause some degree of amnesia. Over the next few minutes he demonstrated some ability to engage in further conversation with me, but his restless movements concerned me. The bed wasn't comfortable, nor did he like the confinement of the side rails. Nevertheless he was able to tell me fragments of his memory, about how his hand lost control, he lost grip before he fell from the truck. He was concerned at one point about what his boss would think. In the next moment he told me he was unemployed. When I addressed his unemployment, he gave me various answers at different times. I found myself wondering how much of this was reality and how much of this was confusion.

I flipped through the chart, noticed that there were no orders for other drugs that I might need, such as cerebral diuretic therapy, in the event that he developed problems. I was a little bit concerned about that, but I didn't really have time to call. At this point Jose became very, very restless. He pulled himself up, almost as though he was going to leap out of bed and another nurse (Mary) in the room and I looked at Jose. I asked what he needed, and he didn't say anything. I ended up saying, 'Do you have to urinate,' he said, 'Yes.' I showed him how to use the urinal and then he threw it on the ground and said, 'I don't have to go now.' At one point after that Jose asked, 'Am I going to die?' Mary looked at him and offered a playful response, 'Die, no way, we don't allow patients to die.' Jose looked at me for, sort of like a validation of this, and I explained to him the need to stay in the bed for safety issues and that we would be getting him home soon. I was haunted by the nature of these vague symptoms. He seemed inattentive and as I'm thinking of all these things, I'm trying to come up with something I can call the physician about, to tell him about my uneasiness, about what I see in Jose. If you can't report something more specific than he looks anxious, you can't get help.

So, finally Jose closed his eyes; he looked relaxed. I asked the nurse (Claire) behind the curtain to help me determine if she would have called the neurosurgeon. We talked about what I saw and what I didn't see. She ended up not agreeing with me that what I saw was anything more than age appropriate anxiety. She also alluded at some point that I needed to be more concrete in my observations: 'You can't call a neurosurgeon to show him that you intuitively think that there's something here, You need more concrete evidence.' She explained that I couldn't access the neurosurgeon without going through this trauma physician, Dr. D. Jose began to arouse. He restlessly pulled himself up by the rails and then announced 'I'm going to barf.' I grabbed a plastic basin and shoved it under his chin. He gagged a few times and then flopped back to rest. At that point, I was ready to call Dr. D. when he walked in. I explained, 'Jose is nauseated, and just had some heaving.' My unfamiliar face left him with uncertainty about my observations.

Dr. D. looked at him, looked at his pupils. Jose remained silent as he tightly squinted his lids shut and thrashed his head side to side. Dr. D. said, 'You're going to do just great, Jose. You're going to do just great.' He asked a series of questions that ran together, didn't give Jose time to respond except to give an all inclusive answer of 'yes' to all of the multiple questions that Dr. D. asked. Dr. D. went to leave, but I asked, 'You've got to understand, I have this very uneasy sense about his restlessness.' He seemed to appreciate my sentiment and asked me very quickly, 'What do you think he needs?' He asked me if I thought he needed a sedative. I said 'No.'Jose at this point had drifted back to sleep, 'Not really. That isn't exactly what I had in mind. My sense is he needs another CT scan.' 'Well, we'll get one in the morning, in the meantime if you need anything, call me. And by the way, you should give him some compazine if he gets nauseated again.'

I went back to the bedside, and pushed the call light to talk to the charge nurse to ask somebody to get a hold of a neurosurgeon for me. Mary (head nurse) came over the intercom, I had no problems getting her to agree to call the neurosurgeon. The vital signs at this point looked great. Jose began to arouse. He shook and scooted to the foot of the bed. He was hanging his legs over the edge of the bed. I was urging him to sit up. He scooted back, he flopped over onto his abdomen, and now he is face down with both knees hugging the foot of the bed frame. He says, 'Leave me alone,' when I tried to get him to turn over and scoot him up in bed. I called Claire from behind the curtain, I pushed the call light again, and I pulled the ambu bag out of the plastic cover. I noticed that there was no mask there. Claire comes around and says, 'What's wrong,' and I said, 'I need a mask for the ambu bag.' She says, 'You know, his saturations look good.' I said, 'Yes,' but I motioned for her to look at Jose. Jose is still laying belly down, ah, stripped naked, not just physically, but of all sense of modesty now. This behavior seemed very, very peculiar to me. To Claire, this seemed as nothing more than age appropriate behavior. We attempted to get him pulled over, and pulled up in bed, and this was when Jose began to become restless. He combated our efforts against his 200 pounds of weight. Claire went to get Mary's help. He still had a normal sinus rhythm, his vitals were stable.

Before I had time to say anything, Jose started to seize—violent, tonic-clonic movements in all four extremities. I flipped the oxygen up, I pulled the pillow out from underneath his head, and I said to Sally, he is having a seizure right now, I need an intubation tray, I need a RT (respiratory therapist), get me some drugs, preferably some dilantin and valium, and get a doctor who can get this kid intubated. And down for another CT scan. She didn't hesitate. I hooked the ambu bag up, Mary walked in, we both pulled him over on to his back, pulled him up, I cranked the head up again. At this point I grabbed the ambu bag, attached the mask, and started bagging him. The RT came. I checked his pupils and saw a very large, fixed pupil, 6 or 7 mm, on the right side. I knew this was big trouble. I asked Claire to get some mannitol. He had a brain injury and his ICP was on the rise. His pressures were high enough to begin shifting his brain tissue to the other side, and that's why I asked for mannitol. I hung it to his IV, started a couple more IVs, pulled some blood out, handed it to Mary, told her to send it for a CBC and a type and cross match. I thought for sure he would be going to surgery. Sally at this point had come in to the room, handed me some drugs, valium and dilantin, and in my other hand, she put a telephone and she says, 'This is Dr. T., the neurosurgeon.'

I kept watching Jose and I said, 'Jose has just had a seizure, tonic-clonic in nature. His pupils, both of them now have blown and his vitals and sats are fine right now, and we're bagging him. He needs to be intubated, he needs something for seizures, I need to get him downstairs for a CT scan.' I was very direct with him, and he said without hesitation, 'Yeah, sure, get him down there, get the trauma physician up to intubate him, give him some valium, give him some dilantin, uh, get him down to CT. I'm on my way in to the hospital right now. I'll meet you down there.' Dr. D. walked in at that point, he says, 'What is going on? I was just in here.' I pushed the valium and the dilantin through two different IV sites. I had to be very careful with my calculation. As I was thinking about this, I was thinking about how helpful Dr. D. was going to be. It looked like he was losing it. So, I said, 'Yes, it's true, he didn't look this bad when you were here a few minutes ago, but right now we need to have him intubated so we can get him down for a CT scan.' He regained his composure, he checked his pupils, validated that his pupils were blown, and he ended up tubing this kid. And by about 10:38-10:40, we were going out the door. It seemed to be the longest distance I had ever traveled to any CT scan. Around 10:50, we were in the CT scanner. We were standing behind a glass partition and I spotted the crash cart over the corner. As I wondered if there would be dilantin, or mannitol, or valium on it when in walked Dr. T. He says, 'Wow, look at that, I can't believe this.' He pointed to the screen, there were two pictures. He points to one and said, 'That was taken this morning.' The dura was intact. It didn't look like there was any problem. On the other side, there was an opacity which represented blood and a severe shift of the brain tissue that needed urgent surgical intervention. He said, 'I hope it's not too late. How soon can you get him to OR?' 'I'll get him down there as soon as I can.' We got him down to the operating room by 11:05. I realized it had been just five minutes over an hour since the moment I had met Jose. My hope was that we got him into surgery in time since both pupils had blown.

As I returned to the unit, I remembered I took time out to call Jose's mom, I used a Spanish interpreter, we somehow found a way to tell her that Jose had developed a bleed in his head, and that we had to send him to surgery to take the clot out of his brain. We needed her to come urgently. She agreed that she would come as soon as possible, when she could find a ride.

Interviewer: And what happened with Jose?

Nurse: Well by the time I finished talking to the mom it was about 11:30. Two o'clock in the afternoon, I received a phone call from the OR, and Dr. T. said to me, 'I think you saved this kid.' I was overwhelmed. He continued, 'The surgery went well and this kid really has you to thank for it all.' Jose came back from surgery at 2:30, and he looked good. He did great, I did not expect him to do so well. Ah, I was told in the month to follow that he had swiftly recovered, without any neurologic deficit.

As the patient's deterioration became more evident with the seizure, the nurse was able to mobilize resources in order to respond to the patient's urgent need for intervention. As a registry nurse, she senses her own lack of recognition and marginalization in this work environment, but is nevertheless persistent on the patient's behalf. Moral agency entailed recognizing the clinical problem (even before quantifiable evidence was available); skill-fully intervening with appropriate therapies until medical support was available; and per-sistently working with, through, and around others until the patient's needs were addressed. Because of the nurse's agency <u>and</u> the responsiveness of the head nurse and the neurosur-geon, this patient narrowly escapes a devastating brain injury and death. It is still a break-down situation because an even earlier response to the patient's condition would have been possible if the nurse had been able to convince the physician and head nurse earlier. In the airline industry, this would be referred to as a "near miss" story.

Clinical understanding, based upon experience, creates authoritative (as opposed to controlling or authoritarian) knowledge. For example, a practitioner learns to trust his or her recognition of early changes in a patient's condition by experiencing or seeing a suc-cessful intervention or the negative consequences of <u>not</u> taking action with early warning signs. After such experiences, the nurse is more willing to risk taking earlier actions to intervene on the patient's behalf (Benner, 1994a). The avoidable injury or death of a patient creates a call to examine sources of the breakdown and preventing future such events. As noted in Chapter 10, all clinical understanding is ambiguous because is based upon inter-pretation. Therefore, communicating one's clinical interpretations requires good logical presentation and the ability to engage in thoughtful dialogue. Presenting clinical cases with phrases that invite dialogue instead of resistance can increase success. Practicing dialogical phrases that encourage listening, such as: "These are the changes I see (summarize them) and this could be related to other causes, but if it is increased intracranial pressure, we don't have much time to respond, and improve communication during high stress times."

Openness is crucial in the communication process. Coping strategies for dealing with a sense of failure, disappointment, and remorse can impede or enhance experiential learning about how to prevent the recurrence of such adverse events. Getting stuck in personal remorse and guilt, or getting stuck in assigning blame to others does not prevent reoccurrence. Blaming oneself or another instead of focusing on solving the sources of breakdown are forms of what Logstrup calls "moralism" (Benner, 1997; Logstrup, 1997). Instead of allowing the breakdown to direct action toward repair of one's own habits of communication, risk taking, assertiveness, or on system redesign, and team building to effect better outcomes in the future, attention is focused internally or externally on "moral failures." Excessive focus on negative emotions, such as guilt, distracts from problem focus. On the other hand, over-focusing on what others could or should have done, while ignoring one's own agency in the situation, may help assuage feelings of remorse, but secondarily, create feelings of powerlessness and victimization. Strategies of empowerment begin with acknowledging the sense of remorse or failure, seeking clarification or social support, and directing those feelings towards understanding the sources of the problem and taking concrete actions to prevent future breakdowns. Trying to work to create better outcomes for the patient rather than "win" arguments with other staff members usually creates new options for action.

FRONT LINE QUALITY IMPROVEMENT, MONITORING, AND RISK MANAGEMENT

We have many examples of nurses' constant monitoring practices. Vigilance, for instance, is required to render intravenous therapies safe. It is situation of breakdown when intravenous fluids infiltrate:

> **Nurse:** . . . And the baby kept kicking the night before. It's IV was in his foot, and he kept kicking it out. And Dad was really upset about that because his site was starting to get red from the baby trying to kick it out. So I stuck cotton over the top of it and he stopped kicking at it. It seemed like it helped. And I just made sure that every hour I picked up the cotton and checked the sites to make sure it was OK. And the next night I came on and they had switched the IV to the other side because they only last about 24 hours when they're in the peripheral. So I came in and it was a registered nurse and I was really concerned about the IV, because I remember how the baby kicked and kicked and if it came out with calcium we would have a big problem... So, I asked her at 11 o'clock when we changed shifts, 'How's the IV?' And she said, 'Oh, I just checked it and it's fine. It flushes great.' So, we got done reporting at 11:15 and the baby was really irritable and screaming, and I couldn't console and I thought, 'Something's not right.' So I lifted up the cotton and his little foot was so swollen. It swelled all the way back. He had a band on his foot. It was swollen all the way back to the band and the band was so tight that his foot was blanched. And all I could think was, 'I've got to get the band off, or he is going to lose his foot and his toes were white.' So I got my bandage scissors and I was able to kind of shimmy them back and forth underneath the band without hurting his skin and I clipped it off and I pulled the IV immediately and elevated his foot. When you pull the IV out, usually you get some blood back and I was getting all water from the infiltrate. It didn't slough. The calcium didn't stain it. Thank God! I was just so angry because I had asked her at eleven. And I thought, there is no way from eleven to 11:15 could he have—and he could have lost is foot! And if I had waited. You're supposed to check it every hour. If I had waited until 12:00 who knows what would have happened?

The consequences of infiltrated IV's with medication infusions can be grave, therefore constant vigilance is required. The attentiveness required for monitoring dangerous IV solutions makes a direct claim on the nurse and she experiences moral outrage over what she considers to be a less than vigilant response by her nurse colleague. Critical care units are replete with technology and interventions that require constant monitoring and surveillance (See Chapter 8). The nurse detecting the problem with the IV had cared for the same infant the night before and was aware of the risk of the peripheral IV. This example brings to light the professional code taught in nursing school, that attentiveness and responsibility for patients go beyond the patients assigned to the nurse's care. Nurses have a strong sense of the community of care (Benner, Tanner & Chesla,2009) required to provide safe care to all patients. There is a tradition of sharing expensive experiential lessons so that other patients and nurses will benefit from error reduction.

Working in familiar settings with familiar patient populations prepares the nurse to be alert to common problems and dangers. Moving from adult to neonatal or pediatric units is particularly problematic because equipment and dosages are so different as illustrated in the next interview:

> **Nurse:** I just think it's frustrating taking care of a child. When I was a traveler, I always got to take are of children, and I mean babies that had multiple problems. An intubated infant is, I think, very frustrating for a nurse that's not a pediatric specialist. You know, you, you look at that ET tube, you know it doesn't have a balloon on it, your bagging him thinking, 'Oh my God, my sats are going nowhere.' I think it's frustrating and I, I we either need to take courses in pediatrics or, and I don't even agree with that because you know, it's not my specialty.

Children are also sometimes placed on adult units at great risk to the child due to lack of knowledge about distinctions between adults and children. In the following example a medication error occurred when a child was given an inappropriate dosage of pain medication:

> **Nurse:** In was just as much my fault as anybody else's, he was supposed to be on 12.5 mcgs of fentanyl. The bag was empty when we came on and so I went to get the bag for the nurse, and I looked at the bag, and there was 50 cc in that bag, and I said 'Wow, you know this bag isn't gonna last very long at 12.5 cc', cause that's what the Pedipump was set at. So I hung it. And I went to orient. And it must have been one and one-half hours later, the nurse came up to me and he said, 'You know, why is your patient so obtunded?' and as soon as he said that, click, I went, 'Oh my God, 12.5 cc is 12.5 mcgs, not!', and I went in the room and he'd received that med all day long at that dose. So we turned it off.
>
> **Interviewer:** a normal dose for that patient would have been?
>
> **Nurse:** 12.5 mcgs, 1.2 cc on a Pedipump... And I don't know how the child ended up in the adult unit.' I said to the attending, you know, 'We're fighting a losing battle.' He agreed and said, 'Let's get him to Peds. They know how to handle this kid.' I probably should have said something to the resident earlier. But it wasn't my patient and I knew the nurse, and he knew the resident, and I thought maybe he would have questioned him, but he didn't....But 20/20 hindsight says I should've said, something [to the attending to get the child transferred to Pediatrics.] Usually I do.

Fortunately, the child survived the potentially dangerous medication error. The example points up the problem of shifting habits of thought and action from adults to children. The shift requires more vigilance because nurses accustomed to caring for adults have to reorient themselves and their practices of thought and action. As the physician acknowledged, they have to know how to "handle a child on pediatrics."

Another major area of front line quality improvement and monitoring is in patient/family education. Frequently patients and their families have not received adequate information to understand their treatment or to make wise decisions. In the following example, the patient was being worked up for cardiomyopathy and had not received enough information to sign an informed consent for a cardiac catheterization. The problem was compounded by communication difficulties with the physicians:

Nurse: She is a rule out MI, also post flu-like syndrome. She has been followed by an internist for several years and has been putting off any kind of cardiac work-up. He has not been very aggressive with her, actually rather conservative. She came in with full blown pulmonary edema, her extremities were actually purple and she was in very severe distress. But she did respond very nicely to diuretics and oxygen therapy. And now as you saw she is much more comfortable. Her second CPK enzymes are positive but only mildly so. The third set has been drawn so we should get more information.

...We are already starting the education with her and beginning to approach her about a heart cath for Tuesday or Wednesday of next week. Both doctors involved have mentioned it to her but not gone into great detail. They have told me she needs a lot of education. So I am gently doing that with her. She is doing well, she is asking a lot of very good questions. So that is really my priority with her, education. I have already taken her the cardiac booklets to look at and I am going to get the films set up for her. We have this VCR & film patients can watch so I will get her started on that. I think once she has the information and has some time to spend with it she will be in agreement to the cath. She doesn't want to be stampeded into anything and none of the docs have spent much time with her.

So right now again education seems to be the priority with her Diabetes. I guess the other thing is working with the two physicians. They have never even met yet. The cardiologist has not been able to spend a lot of time with her and he is just really pushed today. So she is dealing with a new doctor plus she has her own family doctor who has been her long-term physician but he seems to get very annoyed with her. He thinks she is just nervous. He doesn't really listen to her. He just goes into her room for a minute and then leaves. He goes on vacation as of noon today and he has just kind of dumped her on the cardiologist. So she is asking me a lot about the new doctor, the hospitals, the routines. So she needs trust and reassurance. I approach her in a very matter of fact way, I give her the information, and tell her we do a lot of heart caths and see a lot of heart patients.

The nurse is typically the one to discover when there have been communication problems causing a breach of trust, prompting her in this instance to step in and intervene on the patient's behalf. This is a front line interpretive and coaching function that picks up the loose ends, and smoothes communication and transitions between physicians and departments within the hospital.

SHORING UP IMMINENT OR ACTUAL PRACTICE BREAKDOWN

The second aspect of managing breakdown consistently found was "shoring up" breakdown. Shoring up is a way of intervening by offering support or assistance. In many situations, nurses shore up breakdown situations by stepping in, coaching, and augmenting healthcare team members to recognize actual or potential problems, to initiate appropriate therapy, and to alter interventions to improve the patient's care. It can mean coaching others into and through needed interventions or teaching them how to provide care in difficult situations. Shoring up also involves socializing and mentoring colleagues in ways that assist in their development of skilled clinical knowledge. At times, especially in a crisis, if the abilities of team members are limited, shoring up can mean stepping in and taking over until the situation is corrected or until appropriate resources are available to correct the breakdown. The following example from the operating room illustrates the ongoing attentiveness required to prevent mistakes:

Nurse 1: The students I have been working with have to write reports about their experience and they have to evaluate the person they were with. And so one of the students wrote, 'Well, not only does the nurse have to know everything about the surgeon and everything about the patient, but he/she has to be there to make certain—pretty sure that the surgeon does the right thing (laughter).

Nurse 2: She hit the nail right on the head!

Nurse 1: And the student's teacher told me that, and I said 'Well, that's pretty grandiose. But at least I impressed upon her the importance of our being there.'

Nurse 3: Well, you know, that kind of leads into... This incident didn't happen to me but it did happen to my sister who is an OR nurse, and she related it to me. It just happened to her recently and she was kind of devastated by this incident. They were rushing through a lot of 'come and stay' patients, and doing a whole bunch of knee surgery on these patients. And she had just taken her patient to the recovery room, and her second patient was being wheeled into the room by the surgeon and the anesthesiologist. And she didn't get a chance to look at the chart and she had a million things to do, and it was some young kid that was having his knee operated on. So, to make a long story short, they were about to make the incision in the leg when my sister said to the surgeon, 'You know, I didn't get a chance to look at the permit. I just want to check it because I haven't had a chance to.' So she went over, and sure enough the permit was for the left leg and they had prepped the right leg, and she said, 'Dr. So and So, the permit says 'left' and we've got the right checked out and I didn't get to ask the patient. Do you know? Is it the left or the right?' And the surgeon said, 'Oh my God! We've got the wrong leg prepped!' And so, she made a big difference. If she hadn't checked the permit, they may have finished the operation on the wrong leg before they realized, or maybe they would have realized it in the middle of the surgery, but it still would have been a huge mistake and everyone in the room would have been involved.

The routine checking and double checking of the informed consent by the nurse, along with interviewing patients and families, are surveillance functions necessary to prevent error when patients are at risk in a speeded up system of more surgeries in less time with fewer staff members (see Chapter 8). Nurses discussed trying to hold onto their practices of patient contact despite these market-driven pressures. Routine, built-in safety checks and patient/family contact are omitted only at the risk of grave errors. This system building and repair work of nurses is largely taken for granted and thus easily overlooked in a systems engineering approach. The nurses are amused at the student nurse's grandiose statement about nurses "knowing everything," but this is because this generalist knowledge of coordinating and orchestrating many specialists' work is seldom formally acknowledged as the crucial safety work that it is (Benner,2001). This overview knowledge is not the same as the surgeon's focused knowledge on particular surgical procedures, but it is the environment-creating knowledge of functions, goals, and competencies inherent in the work of surgery that enables surgeons to focus on surgery.

This is also evident in the emergency department where nurses frequently call in specialists when they see that the emergency department staff are out of their depth. For example, a nurse describes intervening in the inept, non-specialized care of a burn patient in a small hospital. The patient had been given lasix [a diuretic which is contraindicated] and was not being fluid resuscitated or appropriately covered to reduce heat loss. It was too much for the nurse to correct without finding a physician specializing in burn care to intervene:

> **Nurse:** The burn attending physician got on the phone and said, 'Do you know that Lasix is contraindicated?' ...[It was] frustrating for us because we had, hours and hours of catching up to do with the patient's fluid. I'm glad that burn nurses, like [one of the clinical nurse specialist in the Interview], are so knowledgeable and we can call and say: 'This is the screw up I have.' And they will respond: 'I'll be right down!' ...Okay, come!' Help us fix it.

The system of highly specialized medical practice depends not only on physicians requesting consultation, but also on nurses calling attention to clinical situations that require additional specialized knowledge. Because nurses are in the position to observe many different practitioners, they are also structured to prevent or intervene in breakdown by arranging for additional consultations.

Experienced nurses often coach newer nurses through unfamiliar situations. In these instances, particularly when help is requested, breakdown is smoothly managed. In the following story, the experienced nurse describes shoring up breakdown:

> **Nurse:** There was a severe COPD patient who a new nurse had been taking care of. He was just transferred out of the CCU and he all of a sudden became very agitated. He was on a 35% [O_2 face] mask at that point in time. I looked at his fingernails—you didn't need an O_2 SAT monitor to tell you that his O_2 SATs were dropping below 60. He probably had a P[a]O_2 at that point of about 50-56... I walked into the room and said, 'Put him on at least 70% now—we'll get the order later.' He was really getting anxious, his nailbeds were blue, he was getting mottled—he obviously needed more O_2... He was in VT, but a lot of people tolerate VT ...I knew this man from the CCU—he was not responsive to amiodarone... His IV was not as good as I wanted it to be—his return [blood return from the IV] wasn't good, so I started a new IV on him. The doctors then ordered pronestyl. The new nurse who was taking care of him had no idea how to load pronestyl. So I told her that we generally load this drug [precise dose and time given] and you watch the pressure. We're talking at the patient's bedside because I didn't have time to pull her out of the room. I told her how to do it... So we loaded him with pronestyl, and his heart arrhythmia responded.

This kind of instant in-the-moment coaching, what we refer to as situated coaching, and filling in are essential to prevent patient harm and to teach clinical wisdom to the next generation of practitioners who will then also be able to fill in and coach other new nurses. In all settings, administrators should plan for staffing patterns with some redundancy and back-up from more experienced nurses to allow for this on-the-spot clinical training and management of breakdown. When staff and working environments become highly destabilized, this ongoing staff development and patient protection is fragmented, if not lost, as illustrated in the following account of a critical incident that occurred during a nursing strike. The nurse who specialized in the care of cardiac surgical patients is a traveler doing orientation:

> **Nurse:** They wanted us to orient the staff. The hospital had just gone on strike. So there were a lot of <u>new</u> nurses, but there were some nurses who were in supervisory positions that started to do patient care and this one nurse who hadn't done bedside care in a long time said, 'Show me how to do this, work this IV pump.' So I went in to a fresh open heart patient's room and...all the patients, open heart patients there came back on nipride and nitro and milrinone. Automatically. And so I showed her how to use the pump, and I said, '...You can press 999 to open the IV pump door, but you <u>never</u> want to do that if you're giving fluid because you would just let the fluid run in.' I walked out of the room; I came back in and I looked at the monitor and everything was zero. <u>Absolutely everything.</u> And I looked at the patient, and I thought, 'Something's wrong here' and I remember, I just screamed, 'Bob!' [another nurse] and he came, you know, he came tearing in the room. We flattened the patient out, you know, I disconnected the pump, and I saw a 999. She had put 999 into the <u>Nipride</u> pump. (Horrified gasps from the background). And I just ripped it off of him and we gave him some fluid, and she was just standing there, and I thought, 'You're a supervisor... you're a supervisor!' And everybody had come running in the room, because I don't scream. You know, I try to handle a problem myself. You know, I assess as quickly as I can, but I thought, 'Oh my, she killed the guy. He was zero. This is just lovely.' But he came back, a lot of heart patients are so resilient.

> **Interviewer:** What did you do? You said you opened up the fluid?

> **Nurse:** I opened up the fluids and pulled all the drips off the IVS, and just gave him fluid and he came back right away.

The discussion continues, acknowledging the short action of this potent vasodilator. It is a cautionary tale about the risk to patients and nurses who are put in positions and settings where they are not knowledgeable. Sustaining attentiveness in such destabilized environments is impossible and shoring up "near miss" incidents becomes less likely.

TEAM BUILDING IN THE CONTEXT OF PRACTICE BREAKDOWN

O'Nora O'Neil, in her book, *Towards Justice and Virtue, A Constructive Account of Practical Reasoning* (1996) points out that team building and community development inherent in caring work require attentiveness and work, work which is so basic that it is the very fabric that holds together the possibility for acting in a social world:

> The fabric of feeling, culture and convention which sustains trust and communication is always fragile and vulnerable. It not only has to be preserved from damage and destruction, but to be shielded from mere indifference or neglect. It has constantly to

be created and sustained, recreated and renewed, to preserve 'the food of future generations'; and of the present generation. That 'food' will be reduced, and capacities and capabilities will fail at least for some, when nobody maintains and contributes to sustainable practices of communication, of toleration and confidence-building, of loyalty and engagement, of educating and encouraging, that will enable action, interaction and the development of human potential and culture. The social conditions for human life and interaction can be sustained and supported among connected agents only by attitudes and action that educate new generations, that develop individual characters and their capacities and capabilities and that foster and seek to improve civilizing institutions. To sustain and build confidence and trust, and with them the social fabric, we must not merely act justly, so refrain from destroying them, but help to breathe life both into current and into new practices and ways of life (p. 202).

Communicating and reaching consensus on clinical interventions are negotiated processes. It is a problem if clinicians cannot pass along their clinical understandings to their colleagues, because progress made under the care of one clinician will not be passed on to others which could cause the patient's condition to regress. This is illustrated in the following small group interview:

Nurse 1: This patient was in the hospital for three months. She was a 26-year-old girl that had 28 surgeries in her life for tracheal stenosis. She had a big family around her and she'd been in and out of the hospital so many times and she had just been married six months. The latest surgery was a colonic interposition and she had aspirated. She was intubated in an ICU on 100% oxygen with poor saturations. She was on high doses of multiple medications. Her pain management was not under control. She wasn't able to breathe when sedation was not adequate or no longer working. And over a course of time I got pain management service involved and an attending who very much agreed with me. And then multiple incidents happened where she almost died because of a problem with pain management where she'd lighten up too much and then desaturate and get really bad respiratory distress. Anyhow, we switched her to new drugs and she seemed to respond a little bit better. But we had her on so much medication and almost nothing seemed to be working... We had multiple meetings and three ICU rounds with the nurses. Always for the same thing, lack of communication between us. It's like I'd go home after being there for three days and come back and find everything undone, and everything switched, or the drugs given again that shouldn't have been given. Then I'd come back on and I'd start again and talk to pain management people. And we'd lower the amount of medication. I'd lower it just a little bit and see how she reacted to it and watch her heart rate. And usually within a few hours I had her heart rate back down and she would be relaxed and seem to be sleeping. The pain management people would make rounds and [comment]. 'Her heart rate's down, she looks good,' and then as soon as I'm off again you could see it go right back, even on the night shift a lot of times. I felt like I really made a difference the way I controlled her pain. It was hard to explain what I was doing to anybody. It was just my feeling for what she needed and it wasn't more medication. I felt like she needed less medication.

Nurse 2: You communicated it to us.

Nurse 1: Oh I know I did.

Nurse 2: Don't you guys change this!

Nurse 1: I did. I communicated it through meetings, through talking to all those services. The only service I felt like really paid attention, <u>really</u> paid attention, was the pain service. Everybody else reacted in their old patterns of how it's supposed to be.

This example points to the need to work on communicating successful clinical interventions so that gains made by one clinician are carried forward by the next practitioner. High use of temporary personnel and work overload without time for adequate communication make it impossible to sustain experiential learning and teamwork. As the nurse points out, such communication requires that clinicians pay attention and actively listen to accounts of successful interventions. Setting time aside specifically to focus on clinical understandings and successful interventions during "reports" to other clinicians raises the level of communication from what is written as the plan of treatment, to how the patient <u>responds to treatment</u>. The move toward more "efficient" reporting methods, such as taped shift reports, prohibit the dialogue between clinicians that is necessary for clear and complete communication about complex patients and their responses to interventions.

Informal patterns of communication and styles of practice are learned by nurses to facilitate teamwork and work flow. Status inequity between nurses and other team members is still an issue in nursing, so nurses weigh their interaction patterns with physicians centering on the patient. There is much left unsaid in the following interview excerpt, but it is evident that these advanced practice nurses have learned to create smooth interdisciplinary team communication:

Advanced Practice Nurse: And you get to the point where you know which service you're going to approach in which way. (Another nurse concurs.) You know, you deal with the neurologist differently than the neurosurgeons, you deal differently with the cardiologists, and you know, the intensivists, and everyone, and it's kind of, it's just really funny how you do that. But different services, you know, you can't get near their patients unless you play it the way that they want to play it. Which is fine. At first I used to buck that a lot, and do whatever I wanted to do and however I wanted to do it. But then again, it's not, it's not collegial, it's not helpful. So you have to figure out how to <u>do it</u>, without torturing anybody, including yourself... But you <u>learn</u> uhm, over the years, just as H. said, you have to look hard at yourself. And if you keep that patient as your centering point up front, you're going to get to where you need to be to make things happen for that patient. Then it becomes a win-win for everyone that's involved, but, I think, it takes constant reflection and constant correction.

REPAIRING AND REDESIGNING THE SYSTEM TO PREVENT FUTURE PRACTICE BREAKDOWNS

Experiential learning occurs when pre-understandings are altered, new issues are raised, and nuances are added to one's understanding. There is almost always something to learn experientially in clinical practice. The rapid response and the ad hoc nature of resuscitation teams creates a need for both thinking-in-action and reflection on what worked and what did not. When a resuscitation effort is poorly orchestrated, and perhaps even futile, there is much to learn and improve. An advanced practice nurse describes such a resuscitation:

> **Advanced Practice Nurse:** There was a code called. Usually in our institution when a code is called, a staff nurse from the ICU goes to the code, and it just so happened that things were kind of bogged down and no one could go to the code, so I was flipped the beeper and was asked: 'Can you go to the code?' And by the time I got to the code, this unit, that I had been working with before on mock codes, was in the process of doing this horrendous code on this baby that we had just transferred out the day before. So I knew the baby and knew the parents and everything. And so I was shocked to see that they were working on this baby, because this baby had HIV and was in multisystem organ failure and we had moved the baby out to essentially die on the floor that had sent us the baby. But—and so everybody was pretty upset, but there were eight nurses at the crash cart, stuff was flying everywhere. The baby had no access, and the fellows were running the code and screaming, and there were needles everywhere, so, the baby is in the middle on the board. No [IV] access. Respiratory [therapy] is there. There were probably three or four intensivists around the bedsides. There were lots of nurses there but they weren't doing what they were supposed to be doing. At that point of coming in, everybody was screaming, so I just started talking in a very soft voice and just saying, 'Calm down. You two, here; you there; you, stop; you know, you, over here, and more or less trying to get everybody to do what they had to do for this baby. And the baby was resuscitated. Throughout the entire process, it was fine, and it was obvious that what had happened was that somebody was looking for somebody to do something, to make a decision on this baby, but nobody was going to do that [a decision about whether or not to attempt resuscitation]. We were going from there to MRI (magnetic resonance imaging). Meanwhile, another nurse came up to take the patient to go to MRI. And I was going to go with the patient—it was obvious that the nurses weren't doing well, and they knew they weren't doing well. And my presence there, while they weren't doing well, made them feel more self-conscious. So I hung back, and after the baby left for the MRI, and all of them were standing there, I closed the door, turned around and said, 'How are you all doing, and what's going on here?' and they said:' We didn't know what to do.' I felt so badly for them. They really tried hard to do well for this baby,...so I started talking to them about some of the observations that perhaps in the future might be more helpful. I felt as though that wasn't working well either, and that was making them feel worse... So then I started picking up on what went well. 'Okay, so this is really what happened well. And this is what didn't happen well. But I hung back and we talked about it for a while, and I left when I thought that they would feel better.

This kind of on-the-spot debriefing and coaching is invaluable. The advanced practice nurse judiciously took the extra time that was needed to re-group and work through the feelings that such difficult resuscitations cause. Since she had been in a teaching role with this group of staff nurses, it was essential to spend time coaching on an actual code, complete with all its contingencies. We are left without knowing the outcome for the infant, and we are left without knowing whether an ethics consult was called.

New technology is frequently introduced in critical care units, post-anesthesia, emergency departments, and operating rooms. It is a problem when new technology is introduced with no preparation of the nursing staff (see Chapter 8), since the nurse's role in sustaining safe technical environments is crucial. In the following exemplar, an advanced practice nurse demonstrates her skill at system level repair in just such an instance:

Advanced Practice Nurse: This occurred in the neonatal ICU on a Saturday morning. One of our new anesthesiologists decided to put in an epidural catheter in a newborn infant during the night. Never been done before, no policy, no procedure, no anything. We're neonatal nurses, we haven't done epidurals in (laughs) if ever. It was very new and so I got a call that morning that they [the nurses] didn't know what to do. The catheter was already in, medication was already running and no one knew anything about it. The anesthesiologist came in and we had a large difference of—loud discussion. I explained that he was putting the patient at risk and the nurses at risk. That the nurses aren't inserviced [educated] on how to care for this and complications can arise and he also put the hospital at risk. We have no procedure for this and, even though it might have been right for the patient, it wasn't really right for the patient today. It might have been right in the middle of the week, but I wasn't right in the middle of the night. So we had a very lively discussion with the surgeons and everyone, and so I wrote up a plan for the day and actually the baby did well, but I think that was a negative situation where the nurses tried to call on their resource, being me, and knowing they were in over their heads, knowing that they were putting the patient at risk as a result of the physician putting something in place that no one knew how to care for. And that was kind of negative as a CNS. I found myself being very frustrated, that how can they do this to this patient

Interviewer: So, are things changed since then so that...

Advanced Practice Nurse: Yeah, I got actually an apology letter from the anesthesiologist and the attendings. They put them [epidural catheters] in now, but we've now prepared everyone to care for it. They apologized for doing it in such a manner.

This advanced practice nurse anticipates quality control problems with the introduction of new technology on the night shift, and moves to the system level to solve the problem. She is able to use formal lines of communication and change process.

While many of the examples about repairing and redesigning the system occurred at the unit level, we also found stories of breakdown at the administrative and executive levels that adversely affected the quality of patient care. In some situations, the multiple and rapid changes being approved at the executive level, without the benefit of a clinical perspective, altered the care delivery systems in ways that hindered or delayed patient care. In other situations, the restructuring of departments or the appointment of non-clinician managers over clinical areas created barriers in getting clinically relevant resources. However, there were also instances where power struggles between groups, particularly between physicians and nurses and between administrators and physicians, seriously compromised the care of patients.

CONTRAST CASES: WORKING AGAINST ALL ODDS AND ACCEPTANCE OF PRACTICE BREAKDOWN

While we found many examples of system repair, managing breakdown, and team building, we also found examples of clinical situations where the breakdown and destablization of the system was so great that the nurses could no longer sustain their practices of system repair and team building. We leave these examples from the highly destablilized health care systems because they serve as cautionary tales. Also with the sweeping reforms of the health care insurance industry and delivery system, the destabilization of the health care delivery during the transition to a more equitable health care system is predictable. Nursing shortages will continue, especially if more nurses do not enter graduate programs so that they are eligible to teach nurses (Benner, Sutphen, Leonard & Day, 2010). The need for more skillful nurses, particularly advanced practice nurses, will dramatically increase in the new health care reform that will provide access to health care for 32 million new persons. Never has it been more important for nurses to develop advanced practice roles, to meet the challenging improvements needed in the American Health Care System, to make it more accessible, more just and more focused on primary care and preventative health care. On March 23, 2010, President Barack Obama signed comprehensive health reform legislation, the *Patient Protection and Affordable Health Care Act* (also referred to as the "Senate Health Reform Bill"), into law, providing new coverage for millions of Americans. On March 30, 2010, President Obama signed into law a package of amendments (known as the "Reconciliation Act") to the new law. Now that the bills have been signed into law, the next steps toward implementation of this legislation begin. It is predicted that a much greater utilization of Advanced Practice Nurses will fill in wide gaps in primary health care and provide new services as are Nurse Practitioners and Clinical Nurse Specialists in acute and long term nursing care facilities. However, the sweeping new changes in health care delivery will, no doubt, cause a turbulent period of transition and system redesign as the system changes to accommodate more people.

The last major destabilization of the health care delivery system came in the wake of the failure to usher in health care reform during the Clinton presidency. The health care industry became even more profit-oriented (Weiss, Malone, Merighi, & Benner, 2002). Under the conditions of overwhelming and pervasive system problems, accommodating or making up for a failing system became the focus, or nurses resigned themselves to the moral failure of the system and their own complicity with that failure. The pervasive and anonymous forces of cost-cutting, down-sizing, and sense of threat became the foreground. Minimizing failure in destabilized work environments and providing highly technical medical care in the absence of basic nursing care and social work were two major contrast responses to ordinary management of breakdown.

The data collection for the second phase of this study occurred at the height of changes in the U.S. healthcare system to a more market-driven, managed care environment. Clinical narratives of front-line nurses (Benner, Tanner & Chesla,2009; Gordon, 1997; Schindul-Rothschild, Berry & Long-Middleton, 1996) reflect the strains and crises of this rapid change and the radical downsizing in hospitals. We would be untrue to the data if we did not call attention to the issue of repetitive system failure encountered in the highly unstable clinical environments we studied. Because of the destabilization of work environments, we found a heightening of the pervasive nursing work of system repair, redesign, and team building. Repairing or coping with breakdown was a prevalent theme in most of the interviews. We also found many expressions of moral outrage and anguish over patient suffering due to failures of the healthcare system. Two categories of repeated system failure stand out: 1) extreme downsizing and destabilization of work environments, and 2) the hazards of providing highly technical medical services in the absence of adequate supportive nursing care and social work.

MINIMIZING HEALTHCARE SYSTEM FAILURES IN
DESTABILIZED WORK ENVIRONMENTS

We encountered many examples of breakdown in meeting patients and families as human beings with dignity, in systems strained by cutbacks, rapid change, and no systematic planning for care of the uninsured. Christine Maslach introduced the term "burnout" as the loss of human caring (Benner & Wrubel, 1989; Maslach, 1982). Burnout may also be understood as a disengagement that interferes with one's sense of agency. While distancing can increase objectivity and problem focus, and can improve performance during times of crisis (see Chapter 2), complete detachment and disengagement make it impossible to see what needs to be done (Rubin,2009).

No doubt, work overload and chaos make it harder to meet others with kindness and respect. However, it is misleading to think that there was once a perfect system or a utopian time when meeting others who are different, suffering, and needy was "easy." Meeting those who are needy and suffering presents an ethical challenge regardless of the environment and circumstances, though of course, distressing conditions make this demanding emotional labor even harder. Logstrup (1997), a philosopher and theologian, points out that it is our most natural human response to try to alleviate the suffering of another; we have to have a reason not to respond to another human being's suffering (Martinsen, 2006). The "naturalness" of responding to the suffering of other human beings is a controversial and provocative philosophical stance, especially in a society that is riddled with violence or war. Complex bureaucracies, violent behavior, too many demands, and viewing "others" as wholly other (outside one's own community and even outside of humanity) are all sources of dehumanization that prevent healthcare workers from seeing another's suffering and trying to help. But what if we, as a society, stopped focusing on the "reasons" why we cannot respond to others' suffering and focused instead on alleviating suffering and violence in our society?

Taking individual responsibility in the absence of social action is self perpetuating and participates in oppressive structures. O'Neill (1996) points out that while care cannot thrive or compensate for unjust and neglectful systems, sometimes it is the only option available:

> The directly expressed social virtues are particularly important, and their neglect peculiarly undermining, when public institutions are bitterly unjust or destitution extreme. Although no amount of virtuous action can compensate for injuries of injustice, it can make some difference. Although nobody can care for and help others, so that any obligation to do so must be selective, and more selective still under the yoke of unjust or corrupt institutions, or in harsh poverty, the very fact that virtue can best be embodied in individual character, and hence exercised in dispersed forms, means that at times it survives when justice does not. Then, as in easier times, nobody can show concern or care for everybody, but some people may be able to show some care or concern for some others, and so forge and sustain forms of solidarity or friendship which ease the pain of poverty and injustice, even if neither can be mitigated. Sometimes dispersed acts of solidarity and support also have cumulative public effects: this is the power of the powerless even in hard times (p. 201).

The nurses in this study did not separate the issues of injustice, rapid change, and work overload from the ethical demands of meeting suffering, needy people. Work overload and de-valuing of workers by cutting daily staffing beyond reason, made it difficult, even impossible, for nurses to be open and attentive to patients and families who demanded too much of them.

In the following interview excerpt, the nurse reflects on her loss of the ability to listen to and seriously consider a patient's distress. A co-worker's admonition to practice kindness calls her back to her understanding that her work of helping makes her work rewarding:

Advanced Practice Nurse: I got hit in the face with that just the other day. There is a large population that comes in the emergency department, especially with managed care, that either doesn't know how to access the primary care physician or they don't care, or some of them just can't figure it out and get frustrated. We see a lot of things in the emergency room that really could be dealt with better outside the emergency room. The other day, it started out with three people like that. One woman had taken an ambulance ride because she didn't feel good. You know, she had a primary care problem. And another common problem we have is dental abscesses, people who let their teeth get so bad that they end up in the emergency room for antibiotics. Then they don't ever see the dentist, and then they're back here again—at the revolving door. The next patient had a dental abscess, had been there only two days earlier, had been given penicillin, and I had already pulled up his old sheet from that day and he supposedly had a dentist appointment. I never gave this guy a chance, I just laid into him: 'Did you go to your dentist?' 'Well, yes, I went to my dentist but he wouldn't do anything until the infection was gone.' He's trying to tell me he's a lot worse and he's sick. I wasn't listening. I had already made up my mind that...'these people' are not doing what they're supposed to do and I didn't want to deal with it. I had myself all worked up, and somewhere in there, I actually examined him. Well, I was humbled because he <u>was</u> really sick and he went from the emergency room to the OR with a big massive infection. And he had <u>done</u> everything he was supposed to do. He had taken his antibiotics but he flunked. He got really sick. I apologized to him because he was trying to tell me 'I wouldn't be here if I wasn't sick' but I'd just made up my mind... He looked like a street person, or a little step above it, and I wasn't listening. It didn't matter what he said, I wasn't going to listen. And I hate that when it happens to me. We have an emergency room technician who will always say you have to practice kindness, practice kindness, and I say 'Yes, I can do that.' But I forgot to do that and that really upsets me that I can get in that mode so easily. And that's real scary. It happens. It seems like it happens here a lot because of our clientele. It's really easy to forget kindness and compassion and that everybody deserves it, at least for a few minutes before you decide that they're bull or not. That happened just the other day and I still really worry about it. It's a personal struggle. [The interview continues and the nurse picks up her reflection about her loss of kindness, and her inability to meet the other as a person.]

Advanced Practice Nurse: You try to remember why you came to do this in the first place, some little joyful things happen. But at the same time, what I see coming out of this is the same attitude that I had: <u>These people</u>. What are <u>these people</u> doing? Why are we funding <u>these people</u>? And that, to me, was worse. To just start thinking 'this group, these people,' it doesn't matter. That is the worst to me, worse than just removing yourself from feeling [She is referring to numbing feelings, and loss of connection to people's suffering]. You can easily process feelings later, but if you've already gotten to the point where you're not seeing anybody as a person at all, then there's nothing left to do. That's it. And I mean, it's demoralizing.

Interviewer: So what will you do differently after the situation with the dental patient.

Advanced Practice Nurse: ...What I usually do is I give people a couple minutes to talk to me about every question. Just kind of hear what they have to say and to remember to always practice kindness, and that's when things are fun again. I didn't have any fun that one morning, I was already angry. I was already off on a tirade, and there was no way I was going to enjoy the day. It didn't matter how challenging a patient was until I got back to the reason I do this. Because I <u>love</u> it. And I feel that, ... it's a gift to be able to help with someone's healing. It's fun. But I'd have to [reconsider] how you think about it, that it's not 'us vs. them.' It could be me, could be you out there. And I'm going to try to treat you the way I want to be treated. So that's always a challenge. But once I changed my gears, it was a good day. Busy, but a good day. We have a tech, he's a Buddhist. He's very open, kind, and he always reminds me when I get a little edgy we need to practice kindness, and that's what I try to do.

The nurse's strategy for managing breakdown here is to return to her own practices and bolster her own ability to be in the situation in a more positive way possible. She responds to a reminder from a colleague to practice kindness. In this instance, breakdown in the form of loss of respect for the humanity of another becomes the occasion for the nurse's reflection and regrouping. The interview reveals that those who push her too far or are too different, as in "street people," may still fall outside her circle of respect and attentiveness. The reminder of the common morality of "treating others as you want to be treated" calls her not to separate people into groups of "us/them." She acknowledges that this is a personal struggle. Taking a practical stance of kindness and respect pushes back her personal alienation and helps restore her practice. Her reflection stops at the personal level and with the immediate social support of a colleague. She stops short of seeking administrative and political change, perhaps because she is so absorbed in just coping with a failing system. But reflection and change of attitude that she describes is often the condition for being able to move one's emotional energy outward to change the system in ways that make good practice possible on unit- and system-wide levels. Focusing only on one's own responsibility without taking active measures to change the system can lead to repeated cycles of victimization and failure.

We found that the practice of most nurses in this study, whether in home care, the community, acute care settings, or hospice care, was impacted by highly destablized and rapidly changing work environments. This is illustrated in the observation of advanced practice nurses in a trauma clinic:

Observational Note: Before starting the observation, I passed through the clinic waiting room and noticed that it was full of patients waiting to be seen. Upon entering the clinic, there were five to seven charts piled up on the desk signifying patients waiting to be seen. Jean was in the clinic with another trauma APN, Sue. They did not have a physician backup readily available even though a physician should have been available. Evidently, one of the physicians was still in rounds on the hospital units. Although needed earlier, he didn't show up until 12:00 noon, so they didn't have backup to see the sicker patients that needed to be seen by a physician, or where collaborative judgment was needed in the care of a patient. To exacerbate the problem, the people (secretaries) at the front desk were swamped. There was a new person who was handling situations for other clinics when she was supposed to be focusing on the trauma clinic patients. So Jean and Sue could not get patients mobilized out of the clinic and get what the trauma patients needed because the secretaries were just not available or responsive. This situation was particularly frustrating to Jean and I recognized that as soon as I saw her. So, Jean was quite serious and throughout the morning, she was not very talkative about what was going on with the patients or about her concerns, etc. Because she was so busy and stressed, Jean gave me very little information about each patient as we rounded. She just had too many other things on her mind that she was trying to keep track of, but seemed fine with me continuing the observation. So, most of the discussion in this observation involved interactions with patients. Compared to the last observation where Jean dictated her notes about the patients, the history, the physical exam, the findings, and the treatment plan immediately after she saw each patient, today Jean dictated none of the charts while I was there. The charts just continued to stack up and she would have to complete them later (Observational Note).

The observation and informal interview continues as the nurse sees patients. She discovers a repeated problem for patients from long distances with poor transportation being scheduled for one specialty service (orthopedic trauma) and not scheduled on the <u>same</u> day for needed follow-up from the surgical trauma service. The theme of being over-scheduled in a poorly staffed system continues:

Observational Note: Today the advanced practice nurse recognized that [scheduling for one specialty service while needing to see another specialty as well, and scheduling for the wrong specialty] had become a recurrent problem, and instead of just taking care of the particular situations of this day, she went ahead and began to trouble shoot in the system to identify where the problem was and began to try and resolve the problems so that patients didn't continue to get scheduled in the wrong clinic, or to one clinic only. Interestingly, Jean, despite her frustration, remained very attentive to patients, as in the past. She looked them straight in the eye when she was talking to them. She got close to them and touched them. She seemed to be undistracted by anything else when she was with patients. As soon as we left the room, however, she seemed to be very preoccupied with other matters. One of the major things I noticed (in recognizing the influence the stress was having on her in relation to patients) was that she would often go ahead and finish sentences for the patients, or she would hurry them in their discussions about, not about the reasons that they came in, but about other unrelated things, particularly with the first patient, who was giving a lot about his past history that was not particularly relevant to his illness today. In that situation, and several others, she would either try to end the conversation, change the course of conversation or she would turn away, and not look at him in the eye any longer.

This is a familiar story of work overload due to poor staffing, in this case, of other physicians, advanced nurse practitioners, and secretaries. Despite this, the advanced practice nurse maintains a high level of contact with her patients. But she is more hurried than usual and less open to listening to the patient's story. The charts pile up, and most likely are less complete than they would have been had the staffing been adequate.

In the next example in a small group interview with emergency department advanced practice nurses, the nurses describe the overload and chaos in their work setting. They describe the impact of downsizing and cross training on their own role effectiveness. Because their own roles have expanded to a breaking point, they have refused to do some things. Although they did not meet earlier to agree on limits to their work overload, setting limits to accommodating a failing system is a form of agency. Because the emergency department is the final point of access for those who cannot find healthcare in other settings, there is great pressure to do far more to meet the patient's needs than is officially mandated in descriptions of operations in the emergency department (Malone, 1995a; 1995b). This is a repetitive system failure that nurses and physicians try to compensate for on an individual level:

Nurse 2: I think that the emergency room is also going through so many changes just because of cuts in the hospital. This big cut in X-ray, so it takes longer to get patients through X-ray. Then they had all these cuts in the lab, so it takes longer to get lab tests back. There's all these nursing cuts, so they tell you 'You're the nurse, you answer the phone, you draw the blood, and you push all the patients to x-ray' and there are these physicians and medical students who tell you to do this. I mean, last night a medical student says to me 'You need to put a new diaper on so-and-so.' And I said (laughing) 'I don't do diapers. Ask someone else. That's where I draw the line.' At some point, 'No, I'm not going to do all this stuff for you.' All those things get really hard and then there's the pressures of, 'You're not moving enough patients,':—where you have to cut our patient's time down to so-and-so and 'This is what you're going to do to make that better' and you go, 'But wait a minute, how can I do that because X-ray's taking longer, and lab's taking longer, and I have to answer the phone? How can I move my patients when I'm doing all this stuff? And there's just this blur, and so I think that sometimes, when I feel rushed and I don't want to hear that someone with something like menstrual cramps took an ambulance to the hospital. When you start hearing those things, and all this other stuff is there, and today it really hits you. You know, there's no nurse, there's no tech, somebody says 'put these people in the computer' and you don't know how to do it. And then you get sudden-onset episiotomy pain from a delivery six weeks ago (laughing) came in by ambulance, it's very easy to see yourself fall into the, uh, 'I don't want to deal with this.' You know, these people have to learn that this isn't appropriate (laugh) because I can't do my job if they're doing this. And how can I move the legitimate people and do what I need to do, when, when this stuff happens? And sometimes they're very legitimate reports, or very legitimate complaints, and really important reasons for being there. But I think that is one of the reasons it happens [inappropriate dismissal of patients]. It's just all the outside stuff that's happening in health care and happening in this institution. Just because the emergency department hasn't figured out how it's going to float in the managed care world. Hospitals around have gone through these growing pains and are going through the next set of growing pains, and while our medical center is still learning how to survive. We have a whole different set of challenges, just on a daily basis.

Interviewer: So what do you do with that situation, with the entering things in the computer and no nurses?.

Advanced Practice Nurse: Oh I can't, (laughing) I can't enter things in the computer. I'd screw it all up. I say, I'll write everything in the book and then just have somebody come do it later on. I said 'I can't do that. I just can't. I just can't.' They're all going to be in the waiting room till tomorrow.' (laugh) That's what happens. And sure enough, you know, they sent a secretary back because I said 'This is where I draw the line.' I can't do the computer. I can answer the phone, I can draw the labs, I can do those things, but this is where I just can't cross over and be the secretary too... I can't do that too. And I just won't. And sure enough they can send somebody over for 30 minutes at two o'clock in the morning and put all those things in. It's not a big deal that, and sometimes you just have to enlist someone to understand that. You know, this is it. This is the point at which...and I'll do everything I can to keep all these charts straight so that someone else can do it, I just can't do this. And I've had pretty good success with that... We get people that come back because they want more pain medicine or they want something else. But there are also people that genuinely come back that say 'Something's not right here. Something's just not right.' And, like her dental person, you need to really listen and see what's going on because we miss things. I mean, it's the practice of medicine. The practice of nursing. And there's art and skill and knowledge and good decision making involved, but still a lot of it is practice and there's not a lot of hard rules, I mean, a lot of it is just judgment (Small Group Interview).

At the point of extreme pressures, these nurses refuse to do additional secretarial tasks. Setting limits to accommodate the unreasonable system is crucial for nurses who are typically the most highly skilled and most generally prepared workers. The question is whether the lines drawn are reasonable? Standing in for other roles that require less clinical judgment dilutes the effectiveness of the nurse in attending to patients. It is doubtful that having nurses answer the phone is cost-efficient. More to the point, it is not safe. The reliability and good clinical judgment that is crucial in complex healthcare settings are lost with the multiple distracting tasks.

In the following section of this same group interview, it becomes clear that there are also pressures to expand emergency department services in order to compensate for lack of patient access to other services. The interview continues with vivid descriptions of the current chaos in the system:

Advanced Practice Nurse: I think a practice in this setting is different than it would be in private practice because I don't feel that they [patients] come back very often. I feel that we only get one shot to do it. And I may get an X-ray on somebody who I probably wouldn't if I was in private practice, you know, rather than see them the next day and take a listen, I might not get it the first time I see them. Here, I'm always afraid that I might really miss something and they won't come back. They'll be out there floating, you know, to a primary care center, maybe here, maybe there. That changes the way I do things. I think that probably I order more tests and more X-rays overall than I would in another setting.

Interviewer: I'm curious as to what you see different.

Advanced Practice Nurse: I don't always, you know, if I just relied on my clinical judgment, I would probably get a lot less tests and X-rays, say for people with a cough. And, you know, generally they'll have a little bit of rhonchi, but you really know in your heart of hearts that they're not sick. But you're sort of afraid that you only get this one time to see 'em and you can miss something, and sometimes people present not sounding very bad but they end up really sick. And every once in a while, you get burned on something like that. You know, you don't get a chest X-ray. And they do come back and they say, 'Can I get admitted?' so ...I just worry about some of these people out there. Street people. I just worry about them... they just, can't get good access to care. They can do everything that we ask them to do, they'll go to the primary care center, they'll stand in line all day, five or six hours and still never get seen. And, you know, what can you say? How...would you like to take five hours out of your day to see a doctor? And just because you're poor or you only have a job that doesn't pay very much, that doesn't make it right. And that's very difficult. And it's difficult to get follow-up care especially, a person who doesn't have insurance. And it's hard. So sometimes I feel that I'm not just relying on my clinical judgment, I'm taking a little extra insurance out, and, it's not as comfortable as I'd like it to be. More expensive, and that's not necessarily going to give you any more information, but I just have to do it anyhow. I have to feel that 'I have been complete.' I don't know, maybe that'll get better.

This is a different form of accommodation, an attempt to compensate for an inadequate and unjust health care system. To rely strictly on her clinical judgment with no back-up tests in a system with no redundancy is riskier. Even in ambulatory clinics, follow-up visits and laboratory studies are frequently a trade-off in costs. It is a form of moral agency that the nurse steps in and does more than is normally required in this particular system. Patients who have no other access to care are given additional scrutiny, sometimes in the form of added tests, because no second observation is likely. If a diagnosis is missed, it is more serious because little or no follow-up is possible. Here, care and justice are needed (O'Neill, 1996; Sherman, 1997). Care, in the form of added vigilance, patches up an inadequate system rendering it less dangerous, but this care can never correct the lack of justice in access to healthcare or the injustice of requiring such extreme work overload.

Political action is required to change the system (Gordon, 1997; Gordon, Benner, & Noddings, 1996). Nurses are just beginning to become more politically active to address the issues of justice in access and equal treatment (National Academy of Sciences, 2009; Smedley, Stith, & Nelson, 2002: Commission on the Social Determinants of Health, 2008). The issue of raising action to system and community intervention will be addressed in Chapter 12 on leadership. As illustrated in the continued interview, nurses tend to act locally to make up for system failure instead of taking the problem to the next level of system correction. The small group interview with nurses continues with a discussion of follow-up:

Advanced Practice Nurse: ...On the line of follow-up, I had a patient who had what was the equivalent of boxer's fracture, but when I looked at it, it was very, very strange. He had this sharp point of bone kind of displaced and I looked at it and said: 'Well this is one I'm not going to reduce.' And I very regularly reduce boxer's fractures because I can get really good alignment and I feel very comfortable doing them... So I called the two second year orthopedic residents, and I said, 'You know, I would do this, but he's right-handed and he's a carpenter and this is a funny looking fracture. He's never going to get any more care, so if we don't do this right today, it's just not going to happen...' They said, 'You know, you're right. What's going to happen to this guy? If he doesn't have both hands functional he can't work. And this emergency room is all he has, because no insurance company is going to approve anything. They'll just leave him in this splint for six weeks and hopefully, you know as long as he doesn't have some horrible angulation, the county clinic isn't going to care. He's never going to get any specialty care.'

> So, what happened following that was, the chief who was on came down and redid—they took off the whole thing and they reinjected it and they re-x-rayed him and they ended up casting him, so that he got like the whole continuum of care right there, because, he said, 'You know, you're right. This is somebody who will never know.'

As this example highlights, the advanced practice nurse's clinical judgment and strong grasp of the situation guided her to seek consultation with orthopedic residents since the patient's fracture was on his dominant hand. Although this nurse is comfortable and confident in her skills, she realizes that the fracture is atypical in presentation, thereby prompting her to seek clinical assistance from others for the sake of the patient. The patient's livelihood depended on his being able to use his hands deftly. The nurse's agency is crucial in bridging the gaps that currently exist in healthcare.

PROVIDING HIGHLY TECHNICAL MEDICAL CARE WITHOUT ADEQUATE NURSING CARE AND SOCIAL SERVICES

There were numerous examples of the dangers and moral tensions of providing too few supportive services for patients in need of major medical care. For example, a 16-year-old girl was placed in the care of her twenty-one-year-old cousin by Child Protective Services because her house was considered unsafe. She had extensive injuries due to an automobile accident that included multiple fractures of her pelvis and of her tibia which was pinned. She was receiving coumadin daily to prevent thrombus formation in her legs. Home health care funds were running out and the cousin, who had three young children, was unable to bring the patient in for follow-up visits.

The nurse practitioner pointed out that it was dangerous to take the patient off coumadin and risk thrombus formation because the patient was still confined to a wheel chair. Likewise, it was dangerous to leave her on coumadin without adequate medical supervision. The patient missed her appointment and coumadin was discontinued. The provision of surgical repair was provided, but the supportive care needed to render that care safe was not funded. The outcome of discontinuing the coumadin was still not known at the end of our data collection. We checked back six months later to find that this 16-year-old had been "lost to the system." No one knew the outcome of her care. In this chilling example, anonymous, economic forces become the hidden agents of high risk and even possible death. Nursing advocacy is tenacious but silenced by the inability to make the system work. System manipulation and repair are abandoned because the breakdowns in the system are too pervasive to be managed by the individual nurse. What would have been considered unacceptable only five years earlier is now accepted. The nurse with great regret, but with resignation over the immutability of the system, expresses no sense of personal responsibility, only remorse over a failing system that requires her to choose between two unsafe alternatives: no treatment with risks or unsafe treatment with untenable risks. The nurse practitioner is forced to accept the "anonymous" tragedy, meaning that no one felt directly responsible, including the parents, foster parent, and the healthcare team. The moral understanding was that the tragedy was caused by outside economic forces. It is too reminiscent of Hannah Arendt's observation of the banality of evil in the Nuremberg Trials for Nazi War Crimes where people committed unspeakable crimes in the name of carrying out orders (Arendt, 1963; Bliton & Finder, 1996; Levinas, 1985). This is a dangerous separation of system and lifeworld, and it is only by the demands of those within the system that this chasm can be closed.

Another advanced practice nurse poignantly describes the moral dilemmas of the nurse and social worker confronting the absence of adequate basic care and social services:

Advanced Practice Nurse: Medicare certification manages costs through 'chronic care.' In other words, if you have somebody who's got COPD or congestive heart failure or something like that, once their condition stabilizes, <u>you're</u> supposed to get out [stop home care]. But with lots of our elderly people that are socially marginalized, have language barriers, or they've got caregivers who aren't compliant or they're not able to comply with their meds, what's keeping them stable is the nurse going in. As soon as the nurse pulls out, they get off their diet, they get off their meds, or one thing or another and then wind up hospitalized. But the MediCare rules say, 'Once they're stabilized, you're out.' If the patient gets hospitalized, that's just tough, that is just the way it is. But staff have a tremendous problem discharging people because, you know, you can tell when somebody's just going to fall on their face and be rehospitalized, and this is a tremendous struggle we're having.

The nurse in this excerpt describes predictable repetitive system failure. Care of the chronically ill in ways that prevent acute exacerbations is not provided by the system. The above description of the general problem provides the background for the nurse's next story, which describes the crisis in the care of a 43-year-old former school teacher who was suffering from early dementia due to AIDS:

Advanced Practice Nurse 1: [The above description of repeated system failure] is a long way to get around to talking about a case I consulted on today, a forty-three year old former school teacher was suffering from early dementia due to AIDS. He has a very low CD4 count but he's not had any opportunist infections. He was in the acute care hospital, then he was in the skilled nursing facility, and he's a managed care patient. He is a school teacher who has been living and teaching in [city], and then when he became symptomatic, he sold all of his furniture, sold everything, went and lived with his mother for a while, then showed back up here. And for reasons we can't discern, has no support system,—really has no friends, no one to help him out—but he is not compliant, as many people with early dementia are, and he's ambulatory. [His HMO required that] he be discharged from the skilled nursing facility today and there's no place for him to go. He's basically homeless. And it's not possible to 5150 him [place him on a psychiatric hold]. He's not a danger to self, not a danger to others. He's greatly disabled because he has no place to go, but the way they define 'greatly disabled' in [this city], is that you <u>literally</u> have to be so psychotic, essentially talking to yourself and incontinent, you know, very, very debilitated. But he's ambulatory and he can sort of pattern the right things but is unable to follow through. You give him contacts, you try to get him on the wait list here and there, nothing can happen [because he cannot follow through]. So that's what has to happen with him, because he's on managed care, and he's run out of time that he can be in the skilled nursing facility, and there's no legal way to hold on to him. On the surface, he can identify what the consequences are, but in reality, we know what's going to happen. He's going to go out; we're going to have to <u>refer</u> him to a homeless shelter, which is what we did. We said to him: 'You've got to go here. This homeless shelter...' And hope that we can just get him there in a taxi cab. <u>Hopefully</u> he'll log in there; he'll make a referral to us here so that <u>hopefully</u>, can get a nurse to chase him down, but we basically have to wait until he is like 'really, really sick,' so that he is rehospitalized and hopefully he's debilitated enough that then we have something to work with. And it's—was working with the discharge planner, who's a social worker for him—we really have no options. We know that the hand writing's on the wall here. This is where our medical system and our preoccupation with individual liberties ill serves somebody who obviously is going to be a problem. I actually went over to the skilled nursing facility campus, interviewed the guy, and he's very typical...has an intact social façade, can sort of pander a good line, but has a complete inability to follow through— and I tried to point out a consequence and he has a fast out answer like many people with early dementia do. And it's like trying to let the discharge planner know, 'You're not a bad person; it's a lousy system. He's going to have to go out and it's going to be a <u>horrible</u> experience for him, being homeless. This is a middle class high school math teacher who has no street skills, and we're going to have to put into a homeless shelter probably down close to a high drug-dealing area. He's probably not going to show up there. He's got no support system and no money; siblings won't have anything to do with him. He has a mother who is elderly back in [another state] who can't take care of him and is hoping that we can take care of him here. The AIDS Foundation for Housing, you have to go as a drop in—you know, you have to go physically and drop in and sit there and go through their sign-up list—he's unable to do that sort of thing. We wait for the inevitable train wreck to happen. It's one of those things where you just have to tell people, 'You gotta let go and let the system fail, so that when he's sick enough, the system will kick in.' And it just sort of gives everybody a real knot in the pit of their stomach. You know, it's sort of like trying to prove domestic abuse or child abuse, where suddenly it gets very gray and you don't have the support that you really should, and you know what's going to happen to somebody. You just feel lousy, your skilled intervention, your expertise is...you've crossed all the T's, you've got dotted all the I's. We have no leverage here...we have to let this guy walk out the front door, you know, knowing he probably won't even make it to the shelter...

Interviewer 1: Do you have conversations with anyone from the HMO about this—is there—have you?

Advanced Practice Nurse 1: There's nothing they can do. They are there for medical reasons. This is a social issue—he needs housing—it's not their problem. That's what HMOs do. An HMO is not going to find him a house, or a place to live, if he can't sit with you and fill out a form and follow through with it. HMOs...that's not their respon- sibility...He has no opportunistic infections. He's well hydrated, he's well nourished, he eats well, he's well groomed. I mean he looks fine, and he's not debilitated in any way because he doesn't really have any opportunistic infections... (He is), you know, like a magnet to any predatory type folks that you have in these environments. But he just doesn't have the skills for the arena he's going to be in for awhile.

Interviewer 2: —tell me more about how you consulted with the social worker?

Advanced Practice Nurse 1: Well the social worker called up, just practically on the verge of tears, and she said, you know, 'I've got a situation here; I don't know what to do.' You know, '<u>I don't know what to do</u>.' Now this is a brand new social worker who's only been in this job—oh a number of months and has just graduated from school so she's a new social worker to begin with, and then has been presented with a horrible situation. So it's not even like this is a seasoned social worker who, you know, has all sorts of ways to call people, pull strings, or—. I mean if you work with a social worker who's very good—who has been doing it for a number of years—lots of times, you know, they will know every trick in manipulating the system, checking the hoops, and, you know, one thing or another. It just so happens I'm in the position with having been in the community, that I know all the hoops and, you know, all those sorts of things to help manipulate. And, really, I looked at it and racked my brain, made some phone calls, there's just nothing. We were trapped—we were painted into a corner simply because there is <u>nothing</u> in the system that deals with <u>this</u> one particular issue—where you have someone who has a neurological deterioration and they're ambulatory and non-compliant. It's everybody's worst nightmare in home care essentially. And you have a support system and someone who's unable to accept—access anything. So it's really just reassuring the social worker that every decision, or everything has been looked at, and that the only option we have, which is inadequate and is like, 'here our one-shot chance.' Make a referral to <u>this</u> homeless shelter, which I happen to know also has medical services there and has dealt with a lot of HIV; make a referral to visiting nurses; just <u>hope</u> that we can like 'connect' and 'hook' and get <u>our</u> social worker involved so that we can then get them to start like pounding on the doors of some of these agencies to get this person triaged through more quickly on wait list, you know, as a compelling thing. But we have to get him niched into the right part of the system right now, you know, we just—we have to get him out of door and into a place where we can then work with him and hope that he'll just follow through minimally enough with that. And, and, it's sort of shepherding the social worker through her feelings with, you know. I mean this was a very distraught person because, you know, this is the first time she's had to do something like this; I've been through this before. You never feel good about it but it's—it's like the administrative physician says—his recurrent theme is that sometimes the system has to fail—So I—I —I actually spent as much time with her, soothing her, that this is what you have to do. You know...'it's not your fault. And that people are going to scream at you,' you know, 'the mother's going to call and scream at you.' The one sort of friend who wants something done but can't provide any care, is going to scream at you. You know, 'there's <u>nothing</u> you can do.' You know, 'it's a larger social systems failure, you know, it's not that you're a bad clinician; it's not that you're a bad person.'

We include this very real agonizing discussion because it points up the moral dilemmas of confronting the particular person who needs more than the system has to offer. The nurse has found a way to rationalize about the repetitive system failure and now coaches the social worker into the limits of the personal action and sphere of influence of the single practitioner. The moral agency of the nurse and social worker are weakened by the chronic and constant breakdowns in the system. This weakening disperses the power of caring practices. Instead of coaching the social worker on how to manipulate the system on behalf of this patient, the nurse accepts the untenable premise that she sometimes must "let the system fail." The patient is sent out to an almost certain injury or even death because his HMO benefits have ceased. There are no social services that can be accessed for him. The nurse expresses little or no sense that she can alter the course of this overwhelming need in the context of the few social services offered.

Discharging patients entails a fiduciary moral duty to discharge the patient to some level of safety. The nurse feels helpless and abdicates this responsibility. The nurse perceives that the patient's social safety network has been unraveled beyond repair. The endangerment and potential wrongful death of a fellow human being is covered over by the phrase "letting the system fail." Economic forces triumph over the moral and human.

Mohr and Mahon (1996, p.29) describe the moral dilemma of "dirty hands"—the problem of how to act morally in untenable situations that constrain the actor to choose between two bad alternatives:

> These situations differ from most moral dilemmas in that those commonly encountered are cases in which there is no right act open to the agent; every option is simply wrong. Dirty hands cases are those instances in which one agent is morally forced by someone else's immorality to do what is, or otherwise would be, wrong. A key element of dirty hands situations is not only the choice between two options, but also the role of immorality in creating situations that necessitate and justify acting with dirty hands.

The press for cost-savings for the sake of profit margins as large as twenty percent in privately owned healthcare systems are at the expense of safety for patients. The lack of societal vision and will to ensure that everyone has access to healthcare create immoral structures and public healthcare policy. Those asked to administer such unjust systems are left with "dirty hands." Discharging a person too ill to survive to the streets because there are no social services available occurs often in the United States. Nurses are under pressure to discharge patients according to protocols and guidelines. When patients fall outside these guidelines, then it is the nurse who must advocate for lengthier stays with the insurance companies, or else be put in the morally untenable position of discharging patients under dangerous conditions. Mohr and Mahon (1996), citing the work of Lifton (1986) who studied dehumanized behavior of doctors in the extreme circumstances of the Nazi Holocaust, described "psychological doubling" or splitting off one side of the self in order to maintain oneself in situations that conflict with one's sense of the good. They cite a nurse interview excerpt that matches the demoralization and struggle to cope with chaotic systems that we observed:

> But I was stuck, so I just went to work and did what they wanted, almost everything they wanted... It was like I was there but I wasn't. I was doing these functions, like passing [medications] and writing on charts and sitting in the team meetings, but I'm sorry to say I wasn't nursing. I stayed away from the patients as much as I could because I thought that I really didn't want to get involved (p. 33).

Logstrup (1995) draws attention to the focus on "decisional ethics," where the locus of responsibility is limited to the "decisions" made rather than the actions taken. This study uncovers the moral import of engagement, attentiveness, and being the one who takes the moral action (Weil, 1952). Distraction and work overload disrupts the possibility of seeing the human face of suffering (Halpern, 2001; Levinas,1985; Logstrup,1997; Vetleson, 1994) and ethical demands create immoral climates for the nurturing and protective work of caring for the sick and the vulnerable. The provision of highly technical medical care creates its own risks and vulnerabilities. To provide this care in the absence of the necessary social and nursing care which renders the treatments safe and bearable also creates immoral situations. This is illustrated in the case of the teenage girl who cannot be maintained on coumadin despite the medical risks of immobility and supportive metal bone implants, and the school teacher who is homeless, ill, and mentally disabled.

System failure is not benign. The patient's life is at stake. No formal avenue exists to get the help that is needed, but neither the nurse nor the social worker escape a sense of moral anguish (Reich, 1984). Such a failure-ridden system calls for all practitioners to become ethical heroes in order to do good practice. However, daily repeated heroic performance is unsustainable. This a disturbing and violent story. It is equally disturbing that the only form of activism that is discussed is "manipulating" the system. While such a failing system requires manipulation, it also demands clinical and political action (e.g. in the form of strong agency) to transform it into a more humane system. It takes courage to face up to repeated breakdowns in the system, but until system failures are faced and become a public policy issue, the system will not be changed, and we will continue to have good reasons why we cannot respond to the suffering of others.

SUMMARY

The aim of this chapter was to describe the pervasive nature of monitoring and improving quality and managing breakdown in nursing practice. The role of prevention of complications of hospitalization and promotion of patient safety has been central in nursing education and practice long before the current Institute of Medicine (IOM) focus on the massive proportions of patient safety issues in current hospitals and long term care facilities. But the IOM Reports and increased societal recognition of the problems of practice breakdown and patient safety have drawn widespread attention and a burgeoning science of patient care improvement and safety promotion.

During the first phase of the study we did not anticipate the level of strain that was to come during the development of a market-driven healthcare system. We have presented the role of moral agency in being good practitioners, i.e. living out the notions of good internal to the practice of nursing (MacIntyre, 1981). Some have suggested that, when system failure is pervasive, that caring or moral agency becomes less relevant or even irrelevant (Chambliss, 1996). We believe that organizational life has to be restructured for care and justice. However, the daily courageous moral agency to monitor quality, bridge gaps, and manage breakdown will <u>always </u>be needed, even in the most just and perfectly designed systems.

The nurses' stories in this chapter, even in the worst cases, give a glimpse of a style of practice that nurses are trying to achieve. By style we mean the way pragmatic activity is interrelated and organized with equipment, purposes, and identities (Spinosa, Flores & Dreyfus, 1997). Spinosa, Flores and Dreyfus (1997) point to the way that a style of practice is constitutive, that is, creates and shapes the way we are in situations:

> ...When people change their practices in meaningful ways, they do so on the basis of the style they already have. Style acts as the basis on which practices are conserved and also the basis on which new practices are developed. Thus style is the ground of meaning in human activity. A style, or the coordination of actions, opens a disclosive space and does so in a threefold manner: (1) by <u>coordinating</u> actions, (2) by determining how things and people <u>matter</u>, and (3) by being what is <u>transferred</u> from situation to situation. These three functions of style determine the way anything shows up and makes sense for us (p. 20).

The style of best nursing practice throughout this book is one of attentiveness and concernful comportment. Protection, nurturance, and competence are constitutive of nurses' style of practice. Spinosa, Flores and Dreyfus go on to point to <u>disharmonies</u> in style as an impetus for change. The contrast cases in this chapter are examples of strong disharmonies in practice. The instability and even crisis in current healthcare systems create an opportunity to redesign our systems to facilitate best practice. How can we design our systems for attentiveness and engagement rather than distraction and neglect? Organizations that are truly patient-focused will be designed not with just one standard patient in mind, but rather the range of diversity. Such diversity requires a diverse cadre of healthcare providers whose style of practice is to meet the other in their vulnerability as well as in their strengths and resourcefulness.

Once we acknowledge the pervasive informal nursing role of front-line quality monitoring, managing breakdown, system repair, and team building, we can build in supports and sanctions for nursing performance of these roles. In all the examples used in this chapter, notions of what constitutes good patient care shape the nurses' advocacy and direct their action. If this aspect of the nursing role were formally sanctioned with specific organizational aims supported by the administrative and medical staff less role conflict and hesitation in acting in breakdown situations would occur. These day-to-day functions could be linked with the current structures for quality monitoring and risk management.

It is important to tell stories of breakdown and stories of moral suffering because in them lie some of our most highly valued notions of good patient care. An institution that truly values patient-focused care will work to direct positive energy on immediate correction of breakdown in the situation, not on assigning responsibility and blame after the situation has progressed to major breakdown. Quality development, team building, and system design are best done by those closest to the solution of the problems (Demming, 1986; Senge, 1990). Failure-ridden systems that require daily ethical heroism in order to achieve good practice require both system and public policy level change.

Havel's (1986) ideas on the power of the powerless create a moral vision of the power of dispersed goodness that could help us overcome our collective guilt over our complicity with system failures in the daily work of bridging gaps and "making up" for system failures. However, moral outrage over being the ones who are asked to administer distant economic decisions that put patients and families at risk must be moved to personal and collective political action. The moral outrage needs to be channeled in dispersed forms of communication and action at the local, system, and societal levels. Nurses can write editorials and letters to the state and federal legislatures bearing witness to the injustices that they daily observe. Many nurses have joined a national grassroots social action movement to support a new national healthcare program. This movement received attention in newspapers when the following "Call to Action" was published in *Journal of the American Medical Association* (1997):

> We criticize market medicine not to obscure or excuse the failings of the past, but to warn that the changes afoot push nursing and medicine further from caring, fairness and efficiency. We differ on many aspect of reform, but on the following we find common ground:
>
> *1.* Medicine and nursing must not be diverted from their primary tasks; the relief of suffering, the prevention and treatment of illness, and the promotion of health. The efficient deployment of resources is critical, but must not detract from these goals.

2. Pursuit of corporate profit and personal fortune has no place in care giving.

3. Potent financial incentives that reward overcare or undercare weaken doctor-patient and nurse-patient bonds, and should be prohibited. Similarly, business arrangements that allow corporations and employers to control the care of patients should be proscribed.

4. A patient's right to a physician, nurse or other health care professional of choice must not be curtailed.

5. Access to health care must be the right of all. (Ad Hoc Committee to Defend Health Care, 1997)

> Before the values we cherish are irretrievably lost, we invite members of the health professions and the public to join in a dialogue on healthcare's future. The headlong rush to profit-driven care has occurred without the assent of patients or practitioners, through a process largely hidden from public scrutiny and above citizen participation. This must be replaced by an open and inclusive process that is not dominated by the loudest voices—those amplified by money and political influence.
>
> America's history is replete with examples of powerful social movements kindled by courageous moral voices: in the eighteenth century the Boston Tea Party; in the nineteenth, abolitionism; and in the twentieth century, civil rights and nuclear disarmament. Only a comparable public outcry can reclaim medicine.'

Other forms of action are the development of clinics and outreach programs that to serve the poor and uninsured. Nurses have also created a movement to provide healthcare through churches and religious communities, as participants in health ministries, and as parish nurses (Solari-Twadell, 1999).

The ominous finding in this study is that the tradition of informal repair of breakdown is undermined in today's market-driven healthcare where social policy prohibits basic nursing care and social services, while continuing to provide highly technical medical care. Consequently the very social fabric that renders highly technical medicine safe is being unraveled (Benner, 1997; Gordon, 1997). A language of economism has replaced the language of advocacy and moral obligations to do no harm (non-maleficence) and to do well by the patient (beneficence) (Beauchamp & Childress, 1994). Both patient's rights and the notions of good internal to the practice of nursing and medicine are undermined.

We hope that the knowledge work of front-line quality development and risk management that occupies much of the work of nurses in all settings will become more visible, publicly acknowledged, and designed into ongoing formal efforts of organizational development, thus increasing the knowledge embedded in this vital social function of nursing.

We offer the following beginning list of implications of furthering the best style of practice in monitoring and improving quality and managing breakdown.

1. Establish interdisciplinary communities of learning, where clinical knowing and expert clinical judgment are captured and made available to others. We have done this as forms of developing clinical wisdom in local settings (Benner, Tanner & Chesla, 2009; Kyriakidis & Vitello, In Progress). Narratives of experiential learning are shared and interpreted for the wisdom, notions of good, and innovation in actual practice. Sharing patient care stories with peers, particularly newer nurses, about situations where breakdown was managed well assists others in learning how to better handle difficult situations with various individuals and disciplines. This creates a way to develop cumulative wisdom in specific work units.

This wisdom can also be passed on to other units. Nurses' stories can be published locally and in the professional literature. Stories create moral imagination and provide warnings.

2. Establish formal nursing consults, so that nurses do not have the 'unentitled' feeling that they are interrupting, or stepping out of their working role boundaries to intervene in any hazardous patient situation. Rapid Response Teams can serve this purpose, but adequate training and ongoing coordination are crucial to their effectiveness. The professional notion of the community of care and responsibility needs to be nourished in addition to the moral vision of the autonomous professional.

3. Enhance nurses' ability in making a clinical case to other clinicians. Clinical knowledge is always an interpretation and requires good communication strategies to present clearly to others, both inside and outside the discipline. Situated coaching of less experienced clinicians is invaluable in developing the skill of making a strong clinical case.

4. Clinical specialists or advanced practice nurses, who provide practice and system knowledge and enable situated learning, are particularly important when many healthcare team members are new, inexperienced, or part-time, or in situations where the clinicians do not know the patient. In highly destabilized units it may become necessary to hire advanced practice nurses to staff each shift in order to provide situated coaching and direction to temporary personnel so that they do not make errors based on ignorance of the local specific knowledge which is required to function safely in the particular environment.

5. Attention must be given to ensuring that nurses with clinical expertise are scheduled to work as situated coaches (see Chapter 13) with newer nurses who may be in the early stages of developing agency. This strategy is essential for creating the vision of practice where skillful patient advocacy is expected.

6. Advanced practice nurses can also work at the system level to ensure that the reimbursement rates from insurance companies more closely match the care required by patients. Increasingly, efforts must be taken to shape the insurance companies policies of reimbursement and entitlement procedures. Also nurses can act as advocates for patients who have grievances with insurance companies. Paying attention to the particularly vulnerable populations within pools of insured people can prevent hiding the weaknesses in the system by averaging outcomes for large groups of patients.

7. In complex organizations where reliability is as crucial as efficiency, it is essential to clarify what can be delegated to lesser trained workers and what is best kept in a whole task, professional model. Hospitals have mixed models of professional practice and bureaucratic organization, and this creates a tension to move to the efficiency of the part-task model. The role of the knowledge worker must be clarified and strengthened so that effectiveness and efficiency are kept together.

8. Providing highly technical care in the absence of the necessary supportive nursing and social services is untenable, creating situations of moral anguish and conflict. Public resources for cure and care are related. Currently, medical services are sought because they are the only point of contact for assistance. Caring <u>only</u> for emergencies and critical illness creates emergencies and critical illnesses. With an aging population comes increased chronic illness, and chronic illness calls for long-term care including attentiveness to housing, nutrition, and basic public health. Letting the system fail has already occurred. It is time to infuse our systems with our lifeworld concerns. The fee for service healthcare system has been dismantled, and the market model is not working well in terms of reduced costs or quality of care. In a time of chaos and change with the promise of systematic Federal efforts at Health Care Reform lies the opportunity to create a more integrated care-oriented healthcare system where care and cure are fully integrated.

9. The Carnegie National Nursing Education Study (Benner, Sutphen, Leonard & Day, 2010) has identified a practice-education gap in nursing education and called for upgrading nursing education, increasing the natural and social sciences, and improving the trajectories of students who currently spend too long in getting through over-crowded and under-funded community college systems. In their book, the complexities of the health care provided and the complexities of current health care delivery systems require better education for all nurses. More nurses need to advance to graduate level education. To that end, The Carnegie Study recommends more A.D.N. to Master's level Programs in Nursing, and that within ten years of graduating from the entry level nursing program, all nurses complete their Master's Degree in Nursing.

10. Every newly graduated nurse should be provided a one year residency that includes a mentorship in order to learn to use in-depth clinical knowledge about selected patient populations with whom they work. In addition this clinical residency should also help the newly graduated nurse learn the local knowledge prevalent in particular health care organizations due to different patient populations, styles of practice, and patterns of care that develop in local institutions.

11. Finally, we recommend that every nursing practice setting provide more practical continuing education and situated coaching for the development of new clinical knowledge and the advancement of clinical nurses through to expert levels of practice (See Hooper-Kyriakidis & Vitello, In Progress). Education departments in every practice setting need to emphasize more than regulations, standardization, and new technologies. Though these aspects of staff development are important, they will do little to improve patient safety and quality of patient care unless nurses are coached and supported in developing their clinical expertise over time.

We believe that the style of nursing practice as presented in the narratives of nurses has something substantive to offer in the public world of market and organizational redesign. Nursing as an institution is but one public caring practice, but it embodies the cultural innovation of the compassionate stranger. We must design our organizational life to better enable nurses to continue to be compassionate strangers. Such work constitutes the very fabric of our society of kinship.

REFERENCES

Ad Hoc Committee to Defend Health Care (1997). For our patients, not for profits: A call to action. *Journal of the American medical Association, 278,* 1733–1735.

American Nurses' Association (1996a). *Nursing quality indicators: Definitions and implications.* Washington D.C.: ANA.

American Nurses' Association (1996b). *Nursing quality indicators: Guide for implementation.* Washington D.C.: ANA.

Arendt, H. (1963). *Eichman in Jerusalem.* New York, NY: Viking Press.

Beauchamp, T. L., & Childress, J. F. (1994). *Principles of biomedical ethics.* (4th ed.). New York, NY: Oxford University Press.

Benner, P., Malloch, K., Sheets V. (Eds.) (2010). *Nursing pathways for patient safety: Expert panel on practice breakdown.* Philadelphia, PA: Elsevier.

Benner, P., Sutphen, M., Leonard, V., & Day, L. (2010). *Educating nurses: A call for radical transformation.* San Francisco: Jossey-Bass and Stanford, CA. Carnegie Foundation for the Advancement of Teaching.

Benner, P. (2001). *From novice to expert: Excellence and power in clinical nursing practice.* Menlo Park, CA: Addison-Wesley.

Benner, P. (Ed.). (1994a). *Interpretive phenomenology: Embodiment, caring, and ethics in health and illness.* Thousand Oaks, CA: Sage.

Benner, P. (1997). A dialogue between virtue ethics and care ethics., *Theoretical Medicine, 18:*47–61.

Benner, P., Tanner, C. A., & Chesla, C. A. (2009). *Expertise in nursing practice: Caring, clinical judgment, and ethics.* New York, NY: Springer Publishing Company.

Benner, P., & Wrubel, J. (1989). *The primacy of caring: Stress and coping in health and illness.* Menlo Park, CA: Addison-Wesley.

Bliton, M. J. & Finder, S. G. (1996). The eclipse of the individual in policy (where is the place for justice?) *Cambridge Quarterly of Healthcare Ethics, 5,* 519–532.

Chambliss, D. F. (1996). *Beyond caring: Hospitals, nurses, and the social organization of ethics.* Chicago, IL: University of Chicago Press.

Champy, J. (1995). *Reengineering management.* New York, NY: Harper Business.

Commission on the Social Determinants of Health. (2008). *Closing the gap in a generation: Health equity through action on the social determinants of health.* Geneva: World Health Organization.

Cooper, J. B., Gaba, D. M., Liang, B., Woods, D., & Blum, L. N. (2000). The national patient safety foundation agenda for research and development in patient safety. *Medscape General Medicine, 2*(3), E38.

Cronenwett, L., Sherwood, G., Barnsteiner, J., Disch, J., Johnson, J., Mitchell, P., & Warren, J. (2007). Quality and safety education for nurses. *Nursing Outlook, 55*(3), 122–131

Demming, W. E. (1986). *Out of crisis.* Cambridge, MA: MIT Press.

Fridkin, S. K., Pear, S. M., Williamson, T. T., Galgiani, J. N. & Jarvis, J. R. (1996). The role of understaffing in central venous catheter-associated bloodstream infections. *Infection control and hospital epidemiology. 17*(3), 150–158.

Gawande, A. (2007). Annals of Medicine: The Checklist. If something so simple can transform intensive care, what else can it do? *The New Yorker,* December 10, 2007.

Gordon, S. (1997). *Life Support: Three nurses on the front lines.* New York, NY: Little, Brown.

Gordon, S., Benner, P., Noddings, N. (1996). *The care voice and beyond.* Philadelphia, PA: University of Pennsylvania Press.

Habermas, J. (1984/1987). Lifeworld and system: A critique of functionalist reason. In *The theory of communicative action* (Vol2). Boston, MA: Beacon.

Halpern, J. (2001). *From detached concern to empathy: Humanizing medical practice.* Oxford, England: Oxford University Press.

Havel, V. (1986). The power of the powerless. In J. Vladislav (Ed.), *Living the truth.* London, England: Faber and Faber.

Ihde, D. (1990). *Technology and lifeworld: From garden to earth.* Bloomington, IN: Indiana University Press.

Institute of Medicine (2000). Kohn, L. T., Corrigan, J. M., & Donaldson, M. S. (Eds). *To err is human: Building a safer health system.* Washington, DC: The National Academies Press.

Institute of Medicine. (2001). *Crossing the quality chasm: A new health system for the 21st century.* Washington, DC: The National Academies Press.

Institute of Medicine. (2003). Greiner, A. C., & Knebel E. (Eds.);, *Health professions education: A bridge to quality.* Washington, DC: The National Academies Press.

Institute of Medicine (2004). *Keeping patients safe:Transforming the work environment of nurses.* Washington, D. C.: The National Academies Press.

Kyriakidis, P. H. & Vitello, J. (in progress). *Applying Benner's research to entry level registered nurses: An investigation of development and retention.*

Leape, L. L., Lawthers, A. G., Brennan, T. A., & Johnson, W. G. (1993). Preventing medical injury. *Quality Review Bulletin, 19*(5), 144–149.

Levinas, E. (1985). *Ethics and infinity*. Pittsburgh, PA: Duquesne University Press.

Lifton, R. J, (1986). *The Nazi doctors*. London, England: MacMillan.

Logstrup, K. (1995). *Metaphysics*. (Vol. 1). Milwaukee, WI: Marquette University Press.

Logstrup, K. E. (1997). *The ethical demand*. Notre Dame, IN: University of Notre Dame.

MacIntyre, A. (1981). *After virtue: A study in moral theory*. Notre Dame, IN: University of Notre Dame Press.

Malone, R. E. (1995a). Heavy users of emergency services: Social construction of a policy problem. *Social Science and Medicine, 40*(4), 469–477.

Malone, R. E. (1995b). The almshouse revisited: Heavy users of emergency services. Doctoral dissertation, University of California at San Francisco, San Francisco, School of Nursing.

Martinsen, K.(2006) *Nurse – Philosopher Makes a Serious Case for COMPASSION as a Primary Value*, March 31, 2006 http://www.publicchristian.com/?p=423 accessed June 5, 2010.

Maslach, C. (1982). *Burnout: The costs of caring*. Englewood Cliffs, NJ: Prentice-Hall.

Mohr, W., & Mahon, M. (1996). Dirty hands: The underside of marketplace health care. *Advances in Nursing Science, 19*(1), 28–37.

National Academy of Sciences (2009). *Race, ethnicity, and language data: Standardization for health care quality improvement*. Washington, DC: The National Academies Press. Available at: http://www.nap.edu/catalog.php?record_id=12696 accessed 6-14-2010.

O'Neill, O. (1996). *Towards justice and virtue, a constructive account of practical reasoning*. Cambridge, England: Cambridge University Press.

Reich, W. T. (1984). Moral absurdities in critical-care medicing: Commentary on a parable. *American Journal of Emergency Medicine, 2*(6), 554–558.

Rubin, J. (2009). Impediments to the development of clinical knowledge and ethical judgment in critical care nursing. In P. Benner, C. A. Tanner, & C. A. Chesla (Eds.), *Expertise in nursing practice: Caring, clinical judgment, and ethics* (pp. 171–198). New York, NY: Springer Publishing Company.

Schindul-Rothschild, J. A., Berry, D., & Long-Middleton, E. (1996). Final results of the AJN survey. *American Journal of Nursing, 96*, 23–28.

Senge, P. (1990). *The fifth discipline, the art and practice of the learning organization*. New York, NY: Doubleday.

Sherman, N. (1997). *Making a necessity of virtue: Aristotle and Kant on Virtue*. Cambridge, England: Cambridge University Press.

Smedley, B., Stith, A., and Nelson, A. (2002). *Unequal treatment: Confronting racial and ethnic disparities in health care*. Institute of Medicine.

Solari-Twadell, P. A. & McDermott, M. A. (1999). *Parish nursing: Promoting whole person health within faith communities*. Thousand Oakes, CA: Sage.

Spinosa, C., Flores, F., & Dreyfus, H. L. (1997). *Disclosing new worlds, entrepreneurship, democratic action, and the cultivation of solidarity*. Cambridge, MA: MIT Press.

Vetleson, A. J. (1994). *Perception, empathy and judgment: An inquiry into the preconditions of moral performance*. University Park, PA: Pennsylvania State University Press.

Weick, K. & Sutcliffe, K. (2001). *Managing the unexpected: Assuring high performnance in an age of complexity*. San Francisco, CA: Jossey-Bass.

Weil, S. (1952) *The need for roots: Prelude to a declaration of duties toward mankind* (A. F. Wills, Trans.). London, England: Routledge & Kegan Paul.

Weiss, S. M., Malone, R. E., Merighi, J. R., & Benner, P. (2002) Economism, efficiency, and the moral ecology of good nursing practice. *Canadian Journal of Nursing Research, 34*(2), 95–119.

12

The Skilled Know-How of Clinical and Moral Leadership and the Coaching and Mentoring of Others

Strong clinical leaders are clinicians who embody the best of nursing practice based on the extensive, cumulative knowledge they have gained from experience and the sciences. Excellent practice requires strong clinical leadership. These leaders understand the local community of practice and the particular system within their hospital. Their ability to lead and to influence the reasoning of colleagues in the patient's best interest depends on skillful comportment, authoritative clinical knowledge and wisdom, the conviction to act as a moral agent despite adverse consequences, and the ability to listen and enhance others' strengths. The authoritative (meaning, "expert," not authoritarian or controlling) knowledge of these leaders arises from skilled knowledge <u>in</u> the clinical work. Because skilled knowledge includes formalized knowledge and skilled know-how, clinical leaders embody expert clinical know-how. Their authoritative clinical leadership provides vision and direction in specific clinical situations, with specific clinical patient populations, for redesigning the system of repair in clinical practice breakdown and for improving patient safety. This domain of practice focuses on the ways in which clinical leaders use their skilled know-how and authoritative knowledge with specific patient populations; with particular complex patient care situations; and with developing and articulating clinical knowledge, including the latest evidence-based practice knowledge, to assist the development of others and to improve the clinical functioning of the health care team.

Relational and clinical leadership skills enable nurses to adeptly and flexibly intervene in difficult or confusing situations on the patient's behalf. <u>Relational</u> leadership skills include teaching, coaching, and mentoring, to name a few. In this chapter, to avoid confusion and the repeated use of multiple relational terms, the word "coaching" is used to convey the multiple relational skills that assist others in their understanding, their judgment, their skilled know-how, and their openness to seeing new possibilities. Relational leadership skills are not unique to nursing; they are foundational for leadership in any practice (Bennis, 1997; Bennis, 2009; Black & Gregersen, 2008; Byham & Cox, 1997; Covey, 1992; Covey, 2004; Daly, 2009; George, 2004; Greenleaf, Spears & Covey, 2002; Wheatley, 2007). Basic relational skills, such as teaching and coaching, are the cornerstones that empower nurses to develop expert clinical leadership skills. <u>Clinical</u> leadership skills that characterize expert practice are the aspects of this domain and are listed in Table 12.1.

TABLE 12.1

**The Skilled Know-How of Clinical and Moral Leadership and the
Coaching and Mentoring of Others**

▦ Facilitating the clinical development of others

▦ Coaching others in interpreting, forecasting, and responding to patient transitions

▦ Bridging the gaps in patient care

▦ Negotiating conflict with angry and demanding patients and/or families; from control to connection and understanding

▦ Building and preserving collaborative relationships

▦ Transforming care delivery systems

Expert clinical leaders envision realistic possibilities for improvement and/or development in their own and others' performance. The aim of this chapter is to highlight how relational and clinical leadership skills are embodied by expert clinical leaders. First, clinical leaders facilitate the development of others by helping them learn to recognize the particularities in a situation, better manage an unstable patient's condition, more fully articulate a clinical perspective, and sharpen their clinical judgments. Second, clinical leaders work with others to improve their ability to recognize, interpret, and forecast early warnings of patient transitions and then provide skillful guidance about intervening. Third, when gaps arise in patient care that prevent or delay essential intervention, clinical leadership requires mobilizing necessary resources and assistance. Clinical leaders commonly recognize gaps in patient care, maneuver within the system to effect a response, and coach and teach others about how to bridge the gaps. Fourth, when patients are at risk of losing, or lose, their health, they and their families often experience extreme vulnerability. Various individuals are forced to cope with the multiple burdens that can result in extreme behaviors, depending on what's at stake. Expert clinical and moral leaders commonly negotiate the conflicts experienced and/or presented by angry and demanding patients and their families. Building and preserving collaborative relationships with others is the fifth and fundamental way of providing clinical leadership. Collective wisdom is generated through dialogue and collaborative practice and by enhancing the team's ability to make qualitative distinctions. The sixth aspect of clinical leadership focuses on transforming and/or teaching others how to transform care delivery systems so that they become more responsive, effective, efficient, safe, and flexible in meeting patient's needs.

Throughout this book, narrative accounts of actual practice illustrate how nurses' clinical judgment and skills of leading are pivotal in ensuring that the patient's needs are met safely and effectively. Without the understanding provided in the previous chapters, it would not be evident that clinical leadership is central to expert practice. Leadership skills are most often learned after a developing clinician masters the task world and realizes that good or even safe care of patients requires taking a stand on patients' behalf. This aspect of clinical leadership is often most visible when negotiating multiple clinical perspectives (see Chapter 10) and in breakdown situations (see Chapter 11) where the leader intervenes to facilitate a resolution to a difficult situation in the patients best interest. On the other hand, many stories illustrate how nurses quickly emerge into a clinical leadership role as the situation demands in order to mobilize resources or the team to respond to a patient's specific needs. This particular kind of situated clinical leadership is articulated as "experiential leadership" in "Managing a Crisis" (see Chapter 5). Situated clinical leadership is the basis for going on to develop additional leadership skills in assisting others in their development of practice and leadership. For care to consistently meet the patients' specific needs and preferences, the team must function collaboratively.

Many clinical leaders evolve by design; they are formally appointed into leadership roles, such as clinical nurse specialists, acute care nurse practitioners, and charge nurses.[1] Others, however, are in informal leadership roles. They are leaders because they are powerful in their ability to clinically influence and guide the situation and others as needed. Informal leaders include preceptors, colleagues, educators, and expert staff nurses. Whether formal or informal, nurses evolve as clinical leaders based on their authoritative knowledge rather than on their role or position. Despite one's particular clinical role, nurses in both bedside and advanced practice roles share similar ways of leading in clinical situations. For this reason, this chapter highlights clinical leadership activities that are common across roles.

Excellent leadership skills require good clinical judgment and an accurate "reading" of the developing clinician in order to best respond and intervene, whether with patients, families, other nurses, or colleagues. This kind of leadership may best be referred to as *situated leadership* because the leader's interventions are guided by the demands and possibilities of the situation. The following story which was shared by an expert, doctorally-prepared advanced practice nurse illustrates many of the relational and clinical leadership skills in this domain. The coaching and role modeling are collegial and attentive to the evolving patient situation and, simultaneously, to the developing clinician. Further, because of the physiological details he articulates, his thinking-in-action and reasoning-in-transition become visible:

Advanced Practice Nurse: A 32-year-old female was admitted into our Medical ICU with a diagnosis of primary pulmonary hypertension. She had noticed about a month earlier that she had some shortness of breath and a marked decrease in exercise tolerance. She had a really brief workup that yielded a tentative diagnosis of primary pulmonary hypertension and she was coming into the Medical ICU to receive prostacyclin to try to reduce her pulmonary artery pressures. In the morning when I first saw her, the nurse at the bedside and I were talking, and the patient was telling me how the patient was doing during the night. [The nurse] said her blood pressure and her other vital signs were fairly stable. Her blood pressure was about 132/78 and, if anything, at times dropped a little lower than that. And her heart rate was in the low 100s to like 108. One thing that we noticed after we went in the room to get some waveforms was the patient was <u>very crabby</u>.

Interviewer: Crabby?

Advanced Practice Nurse: ...when we went in to talk to her. And she was not having any trouble breathing at the time, as a matter of fact, she was laying flat. She was not orthopneic, but she was just very irritable, and so we didn't want to stay in the room too long. Looking at her readings, her pulmonary artery pressure was 106/50.

Interviewer: That's so high!

---

[1]Nurse managers and administrators are also formal leaders and commonly influence clinical practice. However, they are not included in this articulation because only clinicians involved in direct patient care were recruited into this study.

Advanced Practice Nurse: Her CVP was 29 and we got a cardiac index of 1.9. But with those numbers, there were two things that came to mind. When I looked at the waveform, right away something struck me because the nurse told me before I went in the room that the catheter was unable to wedge, and when I looked at the waveform, the reason it was unable to wedge was because it was a right ventricular waveform [the catheter tip was in the right ventricle instead of the pulmonary artery]. The pressures were really high and the reason that was important was the physicians were getting ready to start, not just prostacyclin therapy, which was one of the reasons the patient came in, but they were considering a trial of calcium channel blockers first. And since that's a negative inotrope, that was a concern with a cardiac index that low.

Interviewer: Yes, it is.

Advanced Practice Nurse: And the question the cardiologist had was, 'Was the index actually right or not?' They hadn't done a Fick [equation] and that was one of the things I needed to do that morning. But the important question—I asked, 'Well, how is she doing from an oxygenation point of view?' Anyway, so when you have a right ventricular waveform, immediately you know that the monitor won't read that correctly, and so the real pressure was not—at least from a diastolic view—as low as we thought. It actually would have been higher than that. But the key thing is a cardiac index of 1.9 was so low that they should have done a Fick equation and I get a kick out of the nurse, because she knew that I would ask for it. So as soon as she said that, I could see that she knew I was going to ask for that. But I asked her, 'Did you get an SVO_2 level' and she said, 'Not yet,' which normally we try and put fiber optic pulmonary catheters in because we can monitor the SVO_2 continuously. On this particular patient, they did not for whatever reasons, so I said, 'Go ahead and get an SVO_2, and let me know what it is as soon as you get it back.' Because when I looked at her vital signs, there wasn't anything really that unusual about them. Her pulse oximeter was running about 90% and she's on like six liters of oxygen. Like I said, she wasn't orthopneic, but the key thing is with an index that low, they should have been concerned about tissue oxygenation. And so, about 40 minutes later, when we got the SVO_2 level back, it was 36, which is so low that she has no reserve for meeting any new stressors. Also, in the meantime, I talked to the pulmonary attending and let him know that the catheter was not in the right spot. What they did was they removed the catheter, because her right heart was so large that the catheter wouldn't really stay in the right spot, particularly since they did a femoral approach. And so they changed to an internal jugular approach and put a fiber optic catheter in, and then they could monitor the SVO_2 level continuously. Now, the other thing is, they had to change their therapy based on that. Again, the pulmonologist and cardiologist both agreed that when they had an SVO_2 in the 30's, they couldn't give the calcium channel blocker, because it could drop her index even further. So they went just with the prostacyclin, instead of the trial of calcium channel blockers. By intervening, we learned two things. First of all, when we found that the catheter was in the right ventricle, it was pretty clear that the cardiac output couldn't be trusted.

Interviewer: Yes, I agree.

Advanced Practice Nurse: The theory for the cardiac output was that the SVO_2 level was so low, it changed the initial therapy. It's one of those things that you would hope that everybody would know to check for something like an SVO_2 level whenever you suspect a problem with blood flow. Cardiac outputs are not easily predicted by things like blood pressure and heart rate, and so, if you suspect there's a problem with a cardiac output or index, then you have to really check tissue oxygenation. And so, by finding one that low, it confirmed really that even if that output wasn't precisely correct, it was inadequate. And so, the goal was they had to as much as possible try and reduce the pulmonary artery pressure with a therapy such as Prostacyclin, rather than calcium channel blockers, to see if they could increase flow from the right side of the heart to left. The difficulty was, even though the house staff were there, none of the house staff picked any of that up, and it required a little bit more analysis of the situation to determine this person, even though she wasn't orthopneic, she was laying flat, she was only on six liters of oxygen, vital signs weren't unusual, that she was really in a very, very, serious stage of imbalance in terms of her oxygenation. Perhaps that's why she was so crabby (chuckling). It could be a clue. But, here we had a clear objective measure that she was <u>really</u> in difficulty, and as a matter of fact, when you look at her survival chances, they are very, very poor. The only treatment that she really has that would be successful, would be a lung transplant, and with her right heart failing, it's probably a heart-lung transplant. And even though we improved her therapy and fixed her [immediate] problem, we were not going to change her outcome. And that was really the next point. Once we found that her levels were <u>that</u> severe, I told the nurse that we really needed to start focusing on making sure she starts to adapt to an inevitable outcome. You know, make sure she and her family are switching gears a little bit [from] a curative therapy to one which is really a therapy that is supportive.

Interviewer: And what were the implications from this situation for a CNS [clinical nurse specialist]?

Advanced Practice Nurse: Well, basically what I [the CNS] did was two crucial things, or important things I should say. One, they knew they could read the monitor and that the monitor was not accurate because the waveform [didn't reflect] the numbers that the monitor was displaying. The bedside monitor can't read RV waveforms.

Interviewer: Right, it can't.

Advanced Practice Nurse: Because it takes the lowest point as diastole and in an RV waveform, that's not diastole. And so the monitor was incorrect, plus if you look at the waveform, you would know it's an RV waveform. I would hope that a staff nurse would pick that up. If not, you kind of bump [your clinical concerns] up to the next level clinician, and that's going to be the CNS level. And the other thing is, the CNS would be looking at—as soon as you see a low cardiac output, there's two things that you want to do. Verify the output is correct, and you can do a Fick equation for that, but more importantly, assess tissue oxygenation and see if that low output is a threat. That's where looking at the SVO_2 level was something that, again, you could argue, 'Should a staff nurse be doing that?' and I would actually hope so. But, [that's not always the case.] So, those are the two aspects I think are the most important. And as I said, they changed her therapy. They didn't use calcium channel blockers and they went with prostacyclin, even though they considered it in the beginning, that's not what they were going to do. The other thing is, they removed the pulmonary artery catheter and put in one that is capable of measuring SVO_2 levels. Now, several points in time during the next day, the SVO_2 was the indication that she was deteriorating at times or that things were getting better. Her SVO_2 would drop into the teens at times, and without that, you literally would not know that she was doing worse. No physical signs! She didn't change her behavior, she didn't change anything that was overt, and that's, again, where some technology is really irreplaceable.

Interviewer: Now, in your experience, is that typical, that you see the SVO_2 change that significantly over time <u>without</u> signs.

Advanced Practice Nurse: Yeah. As a matter of fact, it's probably the norm. Now you can find some people who'll start to change and you can say, 'Oh, I can see why they're anxious, and they're moving around, and their O_2 consumption is going up.' But when the cardiac output just starts to change, there are very few physical signs with that. Now, if they get hypotensive, sometimes that correlates with it, but we find many times that the blood pressure doesn't correlate at all. And, you can have a normotensive patient, like in this example, but blood flow is very low. And again, that makes sense. You would remember that basic physics tells you that pressure and flow aren't always correlated. That if you increase pressure, it doesn't mean that you increase flow. You actually can drop flow as you increase resistance. And that's where the CNS has to be able to convey those points and instruct nurses who ask the questions. Matter of fact, the question you asked is very good. I had a staff nurse ask that same thing, 'Does some other sign occur before the SVO_2 changes?' and the answer is, 'frequently not.' Because if it did, I wouldn't need the SVO_2. I could just watch for those signs. And it's one of the things where physical signs are well known to be late reflectors of changes in physiology rather than early reflectors.

Interviewer: The other thing I'm curious about—you said after you recognized that there was an RV waveform, '<u>they</u> pulled the catheter and <u>they</u> inserted a fiber optic cath.' Talk to me about how that happened and what your role may have been.

Advanced Practice Nurse: Basically what happened is, when I saw it was an RV waveform, I told the nurse that when they come around on rounds, that they needed to either try and advance the catheter, or they needed to pull it out, because it wasn't functional in it's current location. And just about that time the pulmonary attending came up and asked me how things were going and I told him the catheter was in the wrong position, and the cardiac outputs were suspect, and that we needed an SVO_2 level. He agreed with all that, and he said he'd take care of it. And so he went and talked to the house staff about it directly. Now, normally, I prefer to try and go through the staff nurse, and have them call me if they have trouble conveying a point. Otherwise, the staff won't advance. They need to be able to explain that themselves. And it's easier, if I, or the CNS would just do it. And some CNS's prefer to work that way. But the staff doesn't grow if the CNS handles all those [situations]. But some staff are very uncomfortable doing that. They're not as comfortable talking with physicians on an issue like that.

Interviewer: Is there anything else that you want to tell me about this particular episode or situation?

Advanced Practice Nurse: Well actually, most of this happened Wednesday. And on Friday we made plans to discharge her from the unit with the emphasis on trying to get her ready to go home. And she was put on the transplant list, the prostacyclin had very little effect on her heart. And the goal was to get her home and to really try not to do many more therapies, and just really hope that she gets along in the mean time. But the focus was palliative, making it very clear to her that [transplantation] was not likely to happen. It was a really unfortunate case.

In this situation, the advanced practice nurse immediately grasps the complexity and gravity of the patient's deteriorating condition. By coaching the staff nurse about the pulmonary artery catheter displacement and the unreliability of the cardiac output measurements, the advanced practice nurse helps the nurse perceive a critical transition in the patient's condition, anticipate likely medication therapies, and notify physicians. Here, the goal is twofold. The advanced practice nurse intervenes to provide excellent care for the patient while simultaneously creating the possibility for the nurse to perform the actions needed and experientially learn from the situation. This kind of coaching requires excellent judgment in recognizing when it is safe and possible to step back and facilitate the nurse's learning. The advanced practice nurse must balance between not putting the patient at risk for the sake of the nurse's learning; yet, not stepping in and taking over, which could affect the nurse's experience and confidence.

In this situation, the advanced practice nurse's leadership is multifaceted. First, the staff nurse recognizes that something is amiss but does not seem to grasp the whole clinical picture or the consequent implications. The advanced practice nurse then turns the situation into an occasion to clinically teach the nurse. His own grasp of the situation guides his assessment of the technology and coaching of others to understand the technical problem. Second, the advanced practice nurse role models collaborative practice with both the nurse and the resident. This advanced practice nurse recognizes gaps in the patient's care that developed overnight as a result of the evolving complications. He raises concerns (as a way of coaching) to various team members about the need to evaluate tissue oxygenation. The advanced practice nurse employs direct, straight forward discourse (not Doctor-Nurse game strategies) to collaborate and repair this breakdown situation. Once the SVO_2 confirms that the patient has little reserve, the advanced practice nurse engages in collaborative dialogue with the physicians to abandon the potentially dangerous trial of calcium channel blockers and proceed with prostacyclin therapy. Given the patient's poor prognosis, the advanced practice nurse makes the clinical and ethical judgment to coach the nurse to initiate a new clinical transition. There is no reasonable chance of recovery and little hope of survival until transplant; therefore, the nurse begins to work with the family toward palliative treatment and discharge to home.

Skilled know-how is based on <u>knowing what</u> to do, but also on <u>knowing how</u> and when to specifically respond in a particular context. Relational leadership skills, such as coaching and role modeling, are commonly inseparable in smooth, everyday practice. Further, narrative accounts allow the experts' skilled know-how to become more visible. The stories assist in showing how the significance and meaning of the leader's judgment and performance are context-sensitive and therefore cannot be used to develop routinized or step-wise procedural responses.

FACILITATING THE CLINICAL DEVELOPMENT OF OTHERS

Throughout nursing practice, we found that the clinical leadership skill of facilitating the development of others is a pervasive theme. Not only did expert clinical leaders help other learn but developing nurses also assisted in teaching peers. This aspect of the domain is so pervasive that passing one's clinical knowledge on to others is central in the practice of nursing. Further, the mutual sharing of experiential wisdom commonly crosses disciplines, and therefore the narrative accounts and observations reflect this multidisciplinary teaching and learning.

One of the most common ways in which expert staff nurses assist in the development of others occurs in the everyday practice of orienting new nurses. Although much of the orientation involves teaching about policies, procedures, and routines, expert nurses also point out qualitative distinctions in critical areas of practice. In the following clinical observation, an expert burn nurse coaches an orientee in the debridement of a third degree burn wound in a newly admitted patient. This is a particularly difficult area of clinical teaching because it involves providing good pain management and learning to cope with a noxious, pain-inflicting task. While they begin debridement, the charge nurse is on the patient's other side scrubbing the burned areas. The nurse points out the different appearances and significance of the burn areas, and the sensations that the patient will likely feel. The nurse coaches the orientee through the skillful performance as well as the emotional difficulty of doing a painful procedure:

> **Orientee:** Uhmm. [Nurse observes the orientee who is more timid. The patient seems unaware of the debridement due to pain medication. The orientee's face reveals that this is a painful procedure for her.]
>
> **Nurse:** Okay. All this burned skin's got to come off...Okay? This is what we call eschar, this right here [points to the charred layer on the back of the hand]
>
> **Orientee:** Hmmm!
>
> **Nurse:** ...And just so you'll know that this area here, see this brown area... [pointing out differences in burned skin]
>
> **Orientee:** Yeah?
>
> **Nurse:** ...that all needs to come off [debriding], but it's going to be very sore for him.
>
> **Orientee:** How? It will come off eventually? Or it will come off right now, with me?
>
> **Nurse:** No, it should come off now, with you.
>
> **Orientee:** Scrubbing with this?
>
> **Nurse:** Yes. And instead of big motions, you can use just little short ones. Try and get him to either—you push against him or—you want to get him nice and clean [pointing out other areas where burned skin must come off and then shows her how to scrub in short rapid, firm strokes]. This will all come off. You want to debride all that off. [Now showing her areas of skin that are charred and blistering.] So, just, go forth. Don't pass out. (Observational Interview)

In this situation, the nurse carefully observes the whole hand and wrist area and points out the qualitative differences in the appearance of the burn areas. Earlier, the nurse compares the various areas for color, texture, thickness, and the appearance of the outer skin layers. In addition to pointing out the qualitative distinctions, the nurse carefully shows the orientee how to scrub and debride each different area of the wound while simultaneously informing her about the expected sensation experienced by the patient. In this way, the nurse passes on her skilled know-how about how to carefully but thoroughly debride the wound. Teaching qualitative distinctions is best accomplished directly at the bedside so that the learner can see exactly what is being pointed out. Additionally, the expert nurse tacitly (without articulation) passes on valuable knowledge that the orientee learns through the senses as she feels, sees, hears, and perceives what the expert points at without necessarily speaking about it. The next best alternative for this direct situated coaching would include visual aids, such as CD-ROM interactive modules or DVDs.

The superiority of experiential learning in the moment, or situated learning, is that the orientee also tacitly learns the skilled know-how, learns HOW to perform in particular ways that are context-specific. The expert shows how to and where to use short rapid, but firm strokes instead of slow, long ones. The orientee can immediately see and connect (knowledge use) the process of how that produces desired outcomes. Situated learning enhances the ability to reason in transition as she is hearing the expert's reasoning as they both see the situation unfold. This is the kind of experiential learning and coaching that is sorely needed to close the gap described by Burritt & Steckel (2009) of too many non-experts at the bedside. Orientees are a small group of the developing nurses who would tremendously benefit from situated learning experiences. As great a need exists for non-expert nurses who are no longer in orientation, but are assigned to off-shifts or transfer to a new specialty where few resources are available to coach good clinical judgment and reasoning.

Signs and symptoms, skills, and interventions in one patient population do not necessarily have the same significance or meaning in another population; thus, a nurse's clinical judgment and grasp of a situation must often change when a nurse practices in a new specialty. Similarly, the skill of how to perform particular interventions must also change. For instance, a premature infant should not be covered with a blanket in the same way as a one month old baby, if rest is expected. Without the skill of knowing-how, a nurse's efforts to provide comfort or care can be futile or even harmful. As illustrated in the story below, a nurse who is new to neonatal ICU nursing learns that a neonate must be handled differently than other patients:

Nurse 1: I was in charge in the Intensive Care Nursery (ICN) and one of the physicians came to me and was very frustrated because he was taking care of a small premature infant on a ventilator. He felt that the bedside nurse was not giving the baby good care. The nurse had thought the baby needed a septic workup because he was desaturating and had an unstable temperature. The physician felt very frustrated because the baby really wasn't that sick but was symptomatic because the baby wasn't getting good nursing care. He wanted me to go and see what I thought. So I went in and the baby was lying in the isolette naked, flailed out, on his back with the bilirubin light shining down and the baby's eyes were not totally covered. The portholes on the isolette were open on either side because they'd been obviously trying to get him to oxygenate better. He was desaturating, he was cold, and the nurse was saying, 'I think the baby's really sick. He keeps desaturating; I can't get him warmed up. You know, this, this, and this.' I had to take her through the steps, 'Okay, let's start with the temperature. When did his temperature become unstable?' 'Well after two hours of hand ventilation.' 'Well, you've had the four holes open on either side, there's a lot of cross wind—the baby's cold, so let's get the baby warm.' So we got the baby under a warmer which helped his temperature but he was really flailing. I then talked to her about positioning him and getting him contained so that his arms and legs were closer to his body and so that he would have some boundaries. He would feel more secure and stop flailing around.

Interviewer: And how did you make those boundaries?

Nurse 2: You actually build a nest with linen.

Nurse 1: With linen. And now we actually have little devices that you use. The new nurse felt very strongly that the baby needed to be sedated. She wanted to give the baby ativan or pain medication and the attending was like, 'This baby does <u>not</u> need pain or any kind of medication; there's nothing wrong with this baby.'

Nurse 2: She wanted to sedate the baby because she felt the baby was sick and needed to be sedated. It would just not stop flailing around. We got the baby on his tummy, got him positioned, turned out the lights except the phototherapy light he needed— that one bright light—but we covered his eyes so he wouldn't have the light in his eyes. And within fifteen minutes the baby was fine.

Interviewer: So you advocated and coached for doing these other alternatives rather than...

Nurse 1: Right! Well, it's not really an alternative. In ICN care, it's really the first thing. It's the standard of care. But for her, she was new to the ICN... So I did my educational piece with her and then I went to the physician and he was very, very frustrated and angry that the baby had gone through all this, and he said, 'I don't understand. This is <u>basic</u> nursing care—basic, basic, basic nursing care.' He thanked me for doing it, and I said, 'There really wasn't anything wrong with her reacting this way as a new ICN nurse. The temperature was a little up, the baby was desaturating. So she went in to examine the baby. That means take the bunting away and doing a head to toe assessment. You're confusing the science, I think, of ICN nursing with the art, and the science can come easily but it's the art, I think, that takes a long long time to get to... You know for us [experienced ICN clinicians], it would be instinctive to go in and to look at the baby and say, 'There's nothing wrong with this baby that a little good nursing care won't take care of.' But it's also really understandable that any new nurse—and even an <u>expert</u> adult ICU nurse that would come in, see the baby on his back with his limbs stretched out, desaturating, and cold—would think that he could be really sick. I mean that would be an astute adult observation. But for us, we take it beyond that science and really get to the art—but I couldn't get it across to this physician that this was not really basic ICN care; it's really an art that comes from doing it for a long, long time and being able to see everything as a whole and how they interact.

The physician is outraged that the new ICN nurse is advocating for pain medication or sedation and inappropriate invasive procedures for a septic workup when all that is needed is "basic" neonatal care. His outrage stems from the ethical stance that a technological procedure or pharmacological agent should never be used as a substitute for caregiving and comfort measures. Inexperienced nurses commonly support this stance but, without experience, their under-developed skills of clinical grasp can hinder them from making this distinction in the early stages of their practice. The charge nurse works to show the new ICN nurse how to position, bundle, and nest a premature infant. These are population specific practices that the new nurse would not have been taught outside the ICN. By linking the neonate's symptoms to particular environmental factors that are initially uncontrolled, the charge nurse teaches the new nurse that the neonate's position, being cold, the bright lights, and being un-nested can lead to the clinical picture of a sick infant. By linking the symptoms with the environmental factors, the charge nurse helps the nurse begin to alter her grasp of the situation in a way that is specific to neonates. The charge nurse then skillfully teaches and coaches the new ICN nurse in developing specialty-specific skills and passes on aspects of her practical wisdom as she demonstrates how to perform each intervention. This kind of clinical leadership encourages and enables the nurse to more skillfully care for the infant, prevent the infant's uncontrollable response, and avert the harmful consequences in the future.

Developing nurses cannot always be taught or coached under calm or controlled conditions without experiencing the pressure in a crisis to perform well. Many skills are learned in the heat of crisis or in time-sensitive, high-demand situations. A calm, experienced coach, such as a preceptor, senior nurse, nurse educator, or advanced practice nurse, can nurture learning and skill acquisition during a crisis so that the developing nurse remains eager to learn and perform in future situations. This kind of smooth, imperturbable coaching is illustrated in the following story:

Advanced Practice Nurse: A memorable incident occurred on a Med-Surg unit when a cardiac arrest alarm went off, or we call it a Dr. Resus. At the time, I was the clinical nurse specialist and attended all the Dr. Resusses within the institution if I was [in-house]. So, I got to that particular unit and normally my role is to help or facilitate the nursing staff, and because there are so few people within the institution that are ACLS certified, I usually end up taking a lead role in facilitating the whole arrest. I got there and CPR had been started and the physicians had started arriving. In a community institution, <u>thousands</u> of people come, so one of the things I do is ask the excess people to leave. And then I stepped back a little bit to let the nurses take over their roles and let the main resident proceed in running the arrest. What I was finding was that there was one particular nurse standing next to me whom I could tell had not been a situation like this before, so I thought it would be a good opportunity to mentor her through it. With her by my side, I went into the role of the IV push nurse and told her, 'Why don't you do this? I'll let you do everything, but I'll be here right next to you to help get you through the situation.' And the arrest went very well, she did a great job, and the patient ended up being transferred to the Intensive Care Unit. Afterwards, it was rather rewarding because she said, 'Thank you very much for being there. This was my first code and I really appreciate you taking the time to do this with me.' So I felt rather rewarded in that situation by helping her get through that.

Interviewer: Now, you said you could tell that she had never participated before. What did you notice that lead you to understand that she had not?

Advanced Practice Nurse: Well, while the arrest was going on, before I approached her, she was standing back and just observing everything. She wasn't really taking an active role in the arrest situation. So she was an outside observer rather than being a really active participant. So, seeing her as the outside observer clued me in that maybe she hadn't experienced this a great deal.

Interviewer: I'm thinking sometimes very experienced people may stand back and observe in order to let less experienced people gain experience. Is there something about her 'standing back' that made you notice that she was not an experienced nurse?

Advanced Practice Nurse: Actually, the thing that comes to mind is that she looked so young. Too young to be experienced (laughing).

In this situation, the critical care advanced practice nurse responds to a code on another unit. Upon arriving and observing the team function, he quickly grasps that one of the nurses has little or no experience participating in a code. Because involvement in a crisis can be intimidating, he first role models involvement by taking on the medication administration role of the IV push nurse. Role modeling is very instructive for new nurses because it allows them the opportunity to see how they should perform and then imagine themselves actually performing the interventions. This kind of imaginative rehearsal opens up the possibility of actually doing it. Once the new nurse has a chance to gain a sense of what the IV medication role involves and sees that she can do it, the advanced practice nurse quickly coaxes her into the role. The advanced practice nurse allays the new nurse's fear by standing right next to her and talking her through the situation. He then serves as a safety net which enables the new nurse to perform well. The confidence provided by the fact that an experienced clinician is closely observing and will not allow the nurse to make a mistake can help learners to be less self-conscious and thus pay closer attention to what is happening and what needs to be done. The new nurse's enthusiastic appreciation reinforces for the advanced practice nurse that his judgment about the timing and the progression of her involvement was excellent and that his skill in coaching her development was deft.

If this nurse had attended an Advanced Cardiac Life Support (ACLS) course, she would have had the opportunity to learn and then practice functioning in and managing a code in a mock situation which is less stressful than an actual one. While true, not all necessary skills for an emergency can be learned in a mock situation or simulation. Further, although mock situations provide excellent preparation in terms of knowing what to do, when to do it, and help the learner develop strong habits of thought and anticipatory skills, simulations are not the same as actual emergencies. Simulations often lack the seriousness, the level of engagement, the particularity of an actual patient, the actual timing of patient responses, and the nuances of working in synchrony, or not, with a particular code team. For that reason, expert coaches are needed to assist learners in actual situations, even long after orientation is completed. Such situated coaching facilitates the development of expertise and clinical imagination.

To better understand how to assist in the development of others, the teacher/coach should ask the learner about what is helpful or review, after the incident, what aspects of the teaching were useful. Asking each learner about what is most helpful can strengthen the teacher's ability to "read" the situation and subsequently address the learner's specific needs. In the following story, the developing nurse has excellent preparation and training in performing an invasive procedure. However, she has never performed it on a human being or in an emergency. Here she describes how her partner, an expert nurse and coach, assists her in her first cricothyrotomy and describes what her partner does that is understood as helpful:

> **Nurse 1:** I thought of a situation with [Nurse 2] because, at the end of the last [research interview], we started talking about how Flight nursing is a little bit different because of the teamwork aspect of it. I remember the first time I did a surgical cricothyrotomy (cric), it was with [Nurse 2]. And that's probably one of the most invasive things that we do, and I remember I was so nervous about doing it. It was funny because I didn't shake or anything, but I was really nervous about doing it. [Nurse 2] was just on the other side of the patient. She was just really quietly saying, 'Okay, good, yeah, that's right, okay, you're doing fine.' And she just kept encouraging me really quietly (laughing) while I was doing it. And it was a hard procedure because the

patient had a stick through her throat. We got her cricothyrotomy done, we brought her in [to the hospital], we turned her over to the staff in the resuscitation room, and I walked out. I just remember I started shaking so bad afterwards, (laughs) because it was the first one I had ever done and it was really nerve-wracking for me. But to have [Nurse 2] there, being really <u>calm</u> was really helpful, and just to have her say, 'You're doing fine, okay,' and just be there. Her support, I think, made a big difference for me. And when we did our cric study later, we found out that this woman—she had a real bad head injury but she ended up going home after a <u>long</u> time in rehab....

Interviewer: You said that [Nurse 2]'s coaching was helpful. Talk about what she said. Or maybe, [Nurse 2], if you can remember what you did....

Nurse 1: I just remember it was helpful that she was just being calm and instead of saying what to do next, she would just say, 'Okay, that's good.' I made the incision and she goes, 'Okay, good, you're doing fine.' Then I had my finger in the incision, I was feeling for the membrane and she just served as my backup saying, 'You're doing great. It's okay.' So that was really encouraging.

Nurse 2: Well, thank you.

Nurse 1: But I think that's really important in our job.

Nurse 2: We have to balance each other out sometimes.

Nurse 1: Yeah.

Because the developing nurse is experienced, some aspects in the way the expert nurse coaches her are qualitatively different than in the previous story. In this situation, the developing nurse is pleased that the expert nurse did not coach her on what to do because she knew what to do, based on her training in the procedure. In contrast, the new nurse in the previous story is not informed about what to do in the code, so coaching her interventions is essential as well as helpful. Notice again in this story that the coach's calmness, close proximity to the learner and patient, attentiveness to the details of the learner's actions in performing the procedure, and consistent encouragement and support are understood as helpful. Multiple cases that are similar can teach what is helpful, but excellent judgment is required in knowing how to differentiate between what is <u>generally</u> good coaching from what may be <u>specifically</u> helpful to a particular nurse.

Even though this flight nurse knows what to do, the fact that a human life depends on her skillful actions gives the situation a seriousness that can never be experienced in a classroom, as reflected by her "shaking" afterwards. The expert coach and leader plays the vital role of "standing back while standing close" and enables the developing nurse to skillfully focus on the task at hand rather than on herself. The leader's role is clearly understood by the learner as integral, as reflected by her saying, "<u>We</u> got her cricothyrotomy done, <u>we</u> brought her in, and <u>we</u> turned her over to the staff."

There are situations where it is essential to coach the learner about what to do, even though the learner is knowledgeable about the skill to be performed. The need for this kind of coaching most commonly arises when the situation does not unfold smoothly. When learners are in complicated situations and try to perform a skill for the first time, they can become flustered and need specific guidance in order to remain focused and effective. Thus, a stressful and complex situation calls for a qualitatively different kind of coaching and leadership. Challenging patient situations often provoke a less experienced coach to step in and rescue or take over the management of the situation. However, a skillful coach and excellent leader resists the temptation in order to help the developing clinician learn, as long as the patient is not endangered. Although this is another story about a cricothyrotomy procedure, the similarity helps to illustrate the distinction in the leader's "reading" of the developing clinician and coaching that it is noteworthy:

Nurse 1: [Nurse 2] had to talk a resident through his first cricothyrotomy (cric).

Nurse 2: It was my first flight with a resident and my first year in Flight nursing, so... we got on scene, and the most memorable thing about the scene, when we were walking to the patient, there was glass <u>everywhere</u>. I mean broken glass everywhere. It's like, 'Were there 50 cars involved here or what?' We just didn't know. Well, it was a homeless person pushing a cart full of bottles across the street when a car hit him. So, they [paramedics] had nasally intubated this patient and we put a FEF[2] on so we could monitor his end-tidal CO_2 to see [if the tube was appropriately inserted]—and it was in the esophagus. So, we pulled their tube out, and when you're working with a resident, especially on their first scene call, they're not used to our protocols, so I said, 'We'll try the nasal tube again.' The patient was bleeding with pretty deep lacerations. So he goes, 'Well, I've never done an intubation.' I said, 'Well, I'll walk you through it.' So he attempted a nasal intubation twice. He entered the esophagus each time. So the next step down the algorithm is endotracheal intubation. So we [pharmacologically] relaxed the patient and he tried to visualize using the laryngoscope but we couldn't see vocal cords. I was going to give him one more chance to visualize and I was actually already moving around to the head to visualize after him, but at that point, the patient went into a severe bradycardia, probably from hypoxia. And so I said, 'We'll need to move on to a cric.' And this was a scene where the first responders [paramedics] were all just standing there, watching, maybe because I was with a resident. So at that point, we had to initiate the drugs and I had to ask them to check the IV and make sure that was okay, because it was getting pulled on. I told the resident, 'Okay, move over there, I'll be over here' to orchestrate. And the resident did an excellent job. Excellent job. The cric went very well. Very smoothly. The patient's heart responded to with medication administration. I think he bradyed down into the 20s and we gave him atropine and got him back.

Interviewer: Now you said the situation went well. Nurse 1 indicated that you coaching him through it? So talk more about that.

Nurse 2: I gave him step-by-step directions. I think he knew our technique. We have a specific technique.

Nurse 3: He'd never done one.

Interviewer: Oh, oh, I see.

Nurse 2: So the first thing he did, I said, 'Find your landmark.' He picked a landmark and it was <u>way</u> off. So I said, 'No, this is it up here. That's okay. It's up here.' 'Oh yeah. Oh yeah.' He took the scalpel, he made one incision, he kept the blade in just like you're supposed to. You don't pull the blade out, you leave the blade in. I handed him

---

[2]A device placed at the end of an endotracheal tube to visualize the level of exhaled CO_2, to evaluate if the tube is in the esophagus or in the trachea.

the tracheal hook. And the one thing that he did do, you're supposed to insert the tracheal hook and pull <u>down</u>. He inserted and pulled <u>up</u>. But it wasn't a problem, there was still a hole. And I inserted the tube, it was in place, and it all worked out fine. He followed suggestions very well. And the only problem after that was—my pet peeve is—and actually I have to get over this a little bit, but boy, once that's my airway, I don't want to leave it. There are times when you have to trust someone else to hold it because you <u>have</u> to do other things. But in this situation, that wasn't the case. We had plenty of people and I said, 'Okay, that's your airway, so stay with it.' But he kept getting diverted [didn't understand the importance of securing the airway]. He'd say, 'Oh, I'll pick up this.' 'No, [to the resident], That's your airway, you've <u>got to</u> stay with that.' And he bent down one more time and I grabbed the airway, and I looked at him and I go, 'You don't have to do <u>anything</u> else. There's lots of people. You don't have to do anything else.' And he goes, '<u>Ohhhh</u>, okay.' And he then he got it.

Although this is the nurse's first flight that involves teaching a resident, she is an experienced critical care nurse and coach. The resident informs the nurse that he has never intubated a patient just at the moment the procedure must be done. The nurse's response is calm and she reassures him that she will talk him through it. After four unsuccessful attempts to intubate, the patient's heart rate slows, which warns of an urgent need to secure an airway. As the pressure mounts because a code is imminent, the resident becomes somewhat unsettled, distracted, and unable to locate the landmark for the cricothyrotomy. The nurse remains composed and her skillful support and guidance enables the resident to regroup, concentrate, and then capably and rapidly complete the procedure. Although some may have stepped in and taken over, the coach knows that the resident must learn to adeptly perform under the pressures of the emergency when a safety net is not available.

As mentioned previously, the coach must have good judgment about when it is safe to stand back and facilitate learning versus when it is imperative to step in and take over for the patient's safety. In this situation, although the patient's bradycardia raises concern about allowing the resident to continue, the nurse further explains her reading of the situation:

Interviewer: Did [the resident] recognize how hypoxic the patient was?

Nurse: Well, at that point, there's really nothing you can do, because we <u>couldn't</u> nasally intubate him. Once we relaxed him, he became very hard to bag...So, even though he was hypoxic, you really couldn't focus on that, because there was nothing you could do about it.

Not visible is the rapidity with which each intubation was attempted. Because the nurse states that "we <u>couldn't</u> nasally intubate him" and because neither the resident nor the nurse could visualize the vocal cords for intubation, the nurse does not foresee a significant advantage at that point in taking over the patient's care.

In the field, clinicians' roles and responsibilities differ from in-hospital care. Physicians can typically leave the management of an airway to the nurse once intubation is successful when the patient is already in the hospital. In this situation, the resident initially does not grasp the difference. Consequently, he does not fully understand his responsibility in maintaining the airway because it can be easily dislodged. As such, the nurse tries to coach him about "staying with it." When he again becomes distracted by other aspects of care, the nurse instructs him more directly and explicitly to try to impress upon him the importance of the patient's airway. For both clinicians, teaching and learning in a crisis requires judgment, skill, and emotional labor.

Between clinicians within the same discipline, teaching and coaching often lead to closer working relationships and, as more clinicians become involved, it can lead to a community of learning. Although less true in some organizations, teaching, coaching, and facilitating the development of others across disciplines can also evolve into collaborative relationships. A staff nurse describes how her clinical leadership in coaching a new resident about ventilatory weaning modes began to evolve into a team or collaborative effort:

Nurse: I cared for a man this week who is on vacation from out of state. He had a medullary infarct with very serious neurologic deficits. He was in our Neuro ICU, transferred out to the floor, and had an arrest from his neurologic status. He was ruled out for an myocardial infarction (MI) in CCU and then eventually came back down to our unit and was intubated.

The night I admitted him, when he was transferred from the CCU, his neurology team was trying very hard to wean him from the ventilator, and I felt that they didn't have a full understanding of the particulars of weaning a patient who has medullary infarct. First of all, the physiology, respiratory regulation, and drive in these patients are different. They thought they could take a patient like this and wean very quickly whereas, in my practice, I have seen that this could be a month-long process. It is something that requires patience and time and we needed to keep the patient comfortable.

So I intervened. First, they [physicians] were using a ventilator mode inappropriately. They were trying to wean him on pressure support. When I questioned the resident about the kinds of orders he was writing and how he wanted to manage the patient, it came out in discussion that he didn't have a proper understanding of the mode. He thought that pressure support was the same as PEEP. In fact, they are two completely different therapies. We keep these flow sheets and every hour we report our observations of the patient, whereas the doctors make rounds two or three times a day, make an observation at that moment, and sometimes don't have the whole picture.

So, I pointed out this man's pattern and got some changes made. The doctor was a resident and new to the service, and he indicated that there were different pressures on him from the more senior residents about what they wanted to do. And he didn't really understand this ventilator mode and, from the way he talked about what the senior residents wanted to do, I didn't think they did either. So I said to him, 'If you want to understand this and present a reasonable case to your whole team, I'll have articles for you in the morning that explain the mode.' So, I pulled articles from my file, Xeroxed them, and had them ready for him in the morning and, in fact, he did study those and made an argument to his team. The patient is now being weaned properly. And I've worked with that resident each night he's been on call and discussed the kind of changes we want to make with the patient, especially in making this patient comfortable, because the worst feeling is to have air hunger and not like you are breathing properly. Making this patient comfortable has made a difference in the rest of his care. He was very withdrawn; he has some very strong physical weaknesses but he's not flaccid. He has some motor ability; he has sensation. There is definite rehab potential, but he was not doing as much as he could, and by making him comfortable and stabilizing his respiratory condition, his other activities have come along.

As the new resident begins to manage this patient, the nurse recognizes that he is unfamiliar with ventilatory weaning modes and with the specific patterns of responses in patients with a medullary infarction. Instead of "correcting" him, the nurse engages in discussion with the resident and points out how this particular patient's response patterns are qualitatively different from other neurological patients. The non-threatening way in which the nurse coaches and guides the resident's thinking and her authoritative knowledge prompt him to confide in her the pressure that he is experiencing from the senior residents. By confiding in the nurse, the resident opens up the possibility of a more collegial relationship. The nurse then has the opportunity to not only assist the resident's learning, but also to influence the senior residents' understanding and subsequently improve the care of that patient. The nurse begins to work collaboratively with the resident thereafter by making pertinent articles available to him and empowering him to successfully make a case to the senior residents about alternative interventions. Together, they were able to lead the team's thinking and interventions in the patient's care, especially in ensuring adequate comfort. This example of clinical leadership illustrates how a skillful staff nurse can create or facilitate collaborative interdisciplinary relationships by keeping the patient central in clinical dialogues and by avoiding an oppositional stance.

In expert clinical leadership, facilitating the development of others is not unidirectional. Leadership includes following the lead of others as much as it involves assisting others. Following the lead of others means discerning their needs in their terms and "reading" their responses in order to best judge how, when, and whether to intervene. In caring for acutely and critically ill patients in the home, advanced practice nurses point out how important it is to adopt openness to being taught and guided by the patient and family:

Advanced Practice Nurse: In home care, you have no control. Probably most important is teaching people what control they do or don't have. In the hospital you can control everything. But, when you go into somebody's home, you're essentially there in a consultant role, and you say, 'Here's what I think; here's my recommendations. Here's what happens if you do this or that and here are the outcomes, based on which you choose.' You've got to get comfortable with people [patients and their families] choosing things that you wouldn't choose for yourself or that you don't think is in their best interest. It's like, 'Okay, I'll mobilize around that decision as long as you know what you're in for,' and then carry through with it. And that, I think, is probably the hardest thing for clinicians in home care—it's how to teach new people that issue of, 'You don't have control.' You can't badger patients and families into things. You won't be back for several days. You have no idea what goes on those other twenty-three hours of the day or 160 hours of the week that you're not there. You go in with whatever good plans you've laid out and it's all rearranged and so you have to replan, you have to reformulate. And that's what I see as one of the big needs [in teaching new home care clinicians], it's, 'How do you get people to not think so rigidly?' and to model that for people.

Excellent clinical leaders commonly follow the lead of patients and their families, even when they disagree, if the patient and family understand the alternatives and consequences of their choices. Ignoring their preferences means that erroneous plans are designed and interventions are made that do not benefit the patient or family. At the same time, the nurse cannot blindly follow the patient's or family's lead when their preference is clearly harmful. Situated leadership is required and calls for keeping boundaries and understandings clear. This balanced perspective in working with patients and families reflects the primacy of "good" over "right" in shaping clinical judgment and skillful interventions. Consequently, this home care nurse understands herself more as a consultant to the patient and family on their terms. She also provides clinical leadership in home care by working to communicate this vision of care to others.

COACHING OTHERS IN INTERPRETING, FORECASTING, AND RESPONDING TO PATIENT TRANSITIONS

Patient transitions, or changes in the patient's condition, are articulated in every chapter in this book because they present the greatest puzzles, sources of ambiguity, and challenges in clinical practice. Multiple and nuanced patient transitions are a major source of the complexity in caring for acutely and critically ill patients. As Bourdieu (1980/1990) pointed out, the center and starting point of practical reasoning (i.e. clinical reasoning) is the recognition of the nature of the clinical situation. Because a patient's condition is ever-changing, nurses must continually recognize, interpret, forecast, and respond to these transitions. As clinicians gain expertise, they move from thinking and reasoning in an unfolding situation to having an immediate grasp and response when presented with familiar, everyday transitions. This recognitional skill characterizes an expert clinical nurse (Benner, Tanner, & Chesla, 1996). Earlier chapters provide guidance for learning to read transitions. Expert clinical leaders are adept at these same skills of interpreting, forecasting, and responding to patient transitions but, in addition, they are able to coach others in developing these skills. Clinical leaders, then, are expert clinical nurses who can: (a) characterize the patient's changing responses that they recognize; (b) clarify the interpretations of those changes; (c) articulate the anticipated or forecasted eventualities that accompany the particular transition; and (d) describe and explain the appropriate interventions in response to the patient's specific needs. Coaching others to recognize or anticipate a transition improves the learner's clinical grasp and clinical forethought. Articulating and characterizing transitions, however, is no small feat because much of what one grasps through the five bodily senses does not typically rise to the level of verbalization. Also, early changes in a patient's condition are commonly so subtly that they are difficult to describe. Thus, being the one to recognize and interpret early transitions and being able to articulate the nature of the transition is the hallmark of expert clinical leadership.

Transitions by their very nature require relational work. For this reason, patient transitions are excluded from most formal learning because textbooks typically focus on decontextualized facts and knowledge. In contrast, narrative accounts capture transitions because they contain the context of the situation and how the situation changes over time. Clinical leaders understand the role of the particular situation in coaching others through transitions and, thus, they typically teach in an evolving situation (a key educational strategy). The most common type of coaching through transitions occurs at a patient's bedside as preceptors coach orientees about a change in the patient's physiological condition. Coaching while at the patient's bedside is one of the best ways for learners to grasp the specific distinctions or alterations that are unfolding. In this excerpt from a clinical observation, a burn nurse coaches the orientee through the logic of two impending but related interventions:

Nurse: What I was doing was calling respiratory.

Orientee: Okay.

Nurse: Because we haven't done a gas in a while. He's been awake and we had a poor CO_2 before, so if they're not going to be able to put the CPAP on him right away...

Orientee: Oh, okay.

Nurse: ...then we need to do another gas. So I was calling to check that out. But she's [the respiratory therapist] going to try and come right over and put the CPAP on him.

Orientee: Oh, good. Okay.

Nurse: So, they can draw a gas after that. I didn't want to have to stick him and then have respiratory come over and then we'd have to stick him again... (Observational Interview)

Benner (1984/1999) described how beginners are typically focused on mastering the task world. In this situation, the burn nurse tries to orient the new nurse to the logic and progression of the tasks, because one intervention, the CPAP mask, will hopefully cause a physiological transition and improve the blood gases. Thus, it would be illogical to draw a blood gas first to evaluate the patient if the CPAP mask is to be started immediately. This kind of coaching about the logic of practice assists the learner to expect a transition in relation to particular interventions and helps the learner practically link the change with the kinds and timing of other interventions. Coaching the orientee through the transition in this way teaches the orientee about thinking-in-action and clinical judgment and about how the interventions are interrelated and necessarily sequenced.

When coaching new nurses, clinical leaders must focus on the physiological transitions and conditions of the patient for good reason; they are life-sustaining. Experts however often overlook their own skillful ways of interacting with patients, families, and others and, consequently, they do not think to coach new nurses about comportment or skillful involvement unless asked. Yet, new nurses can "see" that expert nurses embody compassionate, knowledgeable, and responsive ways of caring. Without those skills, some situations, especially death, elicit enormous distress, sadness, and helplessness that typically remains silent, and just under the surface, where it remains unaddressed (Kyriakidis & Vitello, in progress). Robin Watson, a strong clinical expert and leader, details how she coached a frightened nurse around death and skillful involvement, skills that most nurses have to learn on their own over years:

Nurse: Mary was a newbie with less than a year of experience. When I overheard report, I sensed she was apprehensive. She was assigned an elderly woman that was near the end of her life. When she was free, I approached her and offered my assistance if needed.

Mary explained that she had never cared for a dying patient and she was told death was near. Mary had never been around or seen a dead body before. She looked petrified like "a deer in the headlights" look. Her real concern was interacting with the family. "What could she say or do that would not give away her inexperience?" She wanted to be strong, caring and knowledgeable in this matter but felt very inadequate. This was never taught or even touched upon in nursing school. I could feel her anticipation and empathize.

Mary knew I had a great deal of experience in caring for a dying patient. She would come to see me if she needed help. I knew she'd be back because I remembered my first experience. I had only wished someone had taken me under their wing and showed me, taught me, as I intended to do for her.

It wasn't long before Mary sought me out. "I'm not sure what to look for or what to say to the family." I just finished with my patients and met Mary outside the room. As I entered, Mary had hung back. I gently guided her into the room. No family was present. Mary had a mix of fear and uncertainty of the unknown on her face. As I stood by the bedside I observed this woman. My first impression was that of a very pretty elderly woman in the final stages of her life. She reminded me of an elderly neighbor I adored. I had met her large family on a previous shift, and they appeared to be very loving, supportive and shared many memories about her with me. This woman whom I stood in front of was adored by them all.

She looked very peaceful as she lay sleeping, but I was aware of the signs of impending death. I gently touched the patient's arm, looked directly at her and spoke to her quietly as I observed and mentally noted all the signs of impending death I learned over the years. I sensed Mary's apprehension and gently guided her to my side as I began my assessment and quietly, verbally went over each one with her away from the bedside. I explained that there are many signs that would allow us to know that death was near.

First I observed that she had cheyne-stokes breathing. As I held her hand I felt the coolness and saw cyanotic changes of her skin. As we examined her, I pointed out these changes and explained the rationale for each. She had no urine output for the past twelve hours and her vital signs were changing. Her blood pressure was very low and hard to hear with a stethoscope. Her pulse was weak and she was unresponsive. Her eyes were slightly opened and we tried unsuccessfully to close them. She also had a gurgling sound and I noted a Scopolamine patch behind her ear. I told Mary the patch decreases the secretions a patient may have. Mary asked me, "What kinds of questions will a family ask? I want to know what to say in case I go into the room alone. I want to be able to answer them with some confidence and not feel awkward". Mary wanted to know everything but her primary question was, "What do you do and what do you say to the family after the patient dies?" As Mary talked, I continued my assessment and took the patients hands out from under the blanket and placed them together on her lap. I explained that families like to hold the family member's hand and this makes it easier for them to do so. I explain to Mary that I tell the family that a physician will come to pronounce the patient. I then instruct the family that they need to call the funeral home to let them know that the family member has expired and from then on most questions are directed to the funeral home. The funeral home will make all the other necessary arrangements such as clothing, services, etc., if these have not already been made in advance. Sometimes a family has a hard time dealing with this first phone call and asks me to make it. When I do I give the funeral home a name and phone number of a family contact from then on. I then ask if the family wishes to keep the jewelry such as a wedding band on the body. If they decide to keep it on the body, I tape it to the finger and document in my nursing notes whether they keep it on the body or take it home. I also document who takes the jewelry if someone does. I told Mary that some families ask what we do with the body after they leave and I explained that we clean the body and prepare for the funeral home to pick up. As we finished the assessment Sarah, the patient's daughter, entered the room.

Sarah knew that death was near and accepted the inevitable. She said that her mom had led a good life and now it was time to go and be at peace. I brought a chair to the bedside and dropped the side rail so she could be closer to her mom. Sarah placed her hand so gently into her mom's. I suggested that Sarah talk to her mom. I said, "Tell her whatever you wish to say. She can hear you even although she isn't able to speak. "She can hear you". Sarah looked at me in disbelief. I said that Mary and I would give her some privacy and would soon be back.

After a short time Mary came to me, "Should we go back and check on her?" I agreed. As we entered the room, Mary observed Sarah crying. When Mary saw Sarah crying, she looked away, then looked at me. I sensed this made Mary very uncomfortable. As I talked with Sarah, she said, "My mom squeezed my hand. I talked to her like you said and she heard me. Thank you."

Mary just looked on quietly observing. As Sarah talked, her Mom took her last breaths of life. Sarah was at peace with it all. She explained that talking to her mom was what she needed to do and that it meant so much to her. She thought that her mom wouldn't hear her and all of the things she wanted to say to her mom would be left unsaid and unheard.

As we gave her instructions on how to proceed, Sarah prepared to leave. She gave each of us a hug and thanked us for helping her and taking care of her mother. After Sarah left, Mary and I prepared the body. I went over the procedure step by step and helped transport the body to the morgue. When we were all finished Mary looked at me. "What you told her, to talk to her mom, was a tremendous gift for that daughter, you know. I wouldn't have known what to say or how to talk with the family. Preparing the body and all those signs of death you taught me that I hadn't learned before was a great gift to me." I explained to Mary that, through experience, this will all become easier for her. Mary thanked me as she felt this was a learning experience. She felt confident to deal with this situation again if and when it occurred. I said that one of the best lessons I learned long ago from my grandparents is if you always treat people as if they were your own, you can never go wrong. Mary thanked me for teaching her things that weren't written in any book and for sharing with her my knowledge through my experience. This is truly a gift I believe that only one nurse can give to another.

Robin compassionately and clearly coached Mary about each physiological sign and explained the transitions in the patient's physical presentation that were present or anticipated. Being able to "see," in the moment, and understand the meaning of each physical change enabled Mary to perceptually learn through her senses (sight, hearing, touch) about how the situation would unfold. Further, the nurse did not have to figure out what was salient; she was coached to see it and can later recognize salient aspects of similar situations. This kind of practical situated learning, also referred to as on-the-ground learning, differs from classroom teaching in that the knowledge <u>gained</u> is immediately <u>used</u> and therefore becomes embodied. This situation offers first hand experiential learning that may not be as easily accessed in the classroom, or even in a simulation that is necessarily less realistic.

Robin literally provided this new nurse the gift of practical knowledge, which enabled Mary to interpret the transition, anticipate and be prepared, emotionally, for herself and the family, and respond well during the last moments of life. More importantly for Mary, Robin shared ways of preserving/presenting the patient as person and creating a climate to provide the best opportunity for the family and patient to remain connected through the final moments. She coached skillful involvement, for Mary's interactions with the daughter and for the daughter's interactions with her mother. Knowing what to expect, what to do, what to say and how to help in the transition from life to death are the hardest challenges that new nurses (including Mary) repeatedly taught us that they face and dread (P.H. Kyriakidis, research field notes, September 23, 2007; Kyriakidis & Vitello, in progress). Robin gently transformed the fear and dread by creating a peaceful death, for the patient, for her daughter and for Mary. Strong clinical leaders know that knowledge is not the primary problem; instead, it is knowledge use. They do not "know how" to perform and that frustrates the development of and smooth performance in practice.

Burritt & Steckel (2009) define one of the most urgent problems in providing even safe care is the "growing gap" between the demand for and the availability of expert nurses. Nurse executives have not adequately supported the known and necessary development of expert practice; hence the predicament of too many non-expert nurses providing complex care that exceeds their reasoning and judgment. Robin's exemplar highlights the kind of situated learning and development that is urgently needed to address the huge gap and to "support the learning [and development] curve" from novice to expert.

Notice in the above exemplar that extended Robin's practical (clinical and moral) wisdom arises from strong ethics of care, concern, and responsibility, not just for this specific patient, but for future patients and family, and for her peers. Robin's notion of what it is to be a good nurse extends to include not only current but also future patients and colleagues. This deep seated self understanding is pervasive among strong clinical leaders as they are morally compelled to act on matters of significance.

Strong clinical leaders are not only attuned to step in and coach when needed, they seek out ways of helping known groups with similar needs. A good example was described by Tracy Hegg Davis (personal communications, March 24, 2010), who initiated "the Group Hug" in an Indianapolis ICU. Davis gathers the less experienced nurses for a 2-4 hour clinical debriefing/learning session where nurses can share anything they chose regarding patient care: concerns, burdens, fears, what they wish they had known, what to say in particular kinds of situations, what they want to know, etc. The group is strategically timed to gather 18 months after the "blast" of information from orientation, at a time when newer nurses recognize the significance of and experience their accountability for the care they provide and the lives in their hands. The rule is that everything that is shared remains confidential, enabling nurses to share their deepest fears and failures. It is here that many pearls of wisdom are passed on, for instance, about caring for the dying, what patients and families remember most, etc. Misunderstandings and misinterpretations about what happened to a patient are clarified, the failures the nurse believed s/he had in the patient's devastating outcome are corrected, how to cope with particularly hard situations is discussed, and so on. Although the Group Hug was initiated for new nurses, Davis reveals that developing nurses with 2 to 3 years of experience need and want to come, as many have unresolved concerns they continue to carry or because of the invaluable situated learning that occurs. Davis' vision was that the Group Hug would improve retention; however, what she accomplishes far exceeds that hope. Here, inexperienced nurses learn <u>how to</u> cope with failed notions of good and learn what to do differently next time. They learn <u>how to</u> come to peace with emotional burdens. They learn more skillful ways of <u>how to</u> be involved with patients and families. The types of help are innumerable, and in the end this type of support and care not only improves retention of staff nurses, it also assists in the development of practice and reduces the growing problem of disengagement (P.H. Kyriakidis, research field notes, October 1, 2007; Kyriakidis & Vitello, in progress; Rubin, 2009). Disengagement prevents nurses from developing expertise. The Group Hug or similar kinds of debriefing and support enable nurses to work through unresolved emotional burdens and fears or find healthy ways of coping, for instance, so that they remain engaged. Engagement is central to attunement and perceptual grasp and therefore good clinical judgment. The development of expertise depends on becoming engaged interpersonally and with the specific situation (Benner, Tanner & Chesla, 2009).

It is the breadth and depth of these kinds of concerns on which nursing as a profession currently depends if we are to preserve and extend the expertise (clinical wisdom, judgment, and skillful performance) gained over years of trial and error learning. It is no surprise that nurse colleagues can easily identify the strong clinical leaders, informal or formal, on their units. Because organizations are rapidly building or purchasing systems that exclude or dumb down the practical wisdom of experts in favor of systems that are, by design, simply safe and competent, expert practice is at high risk for disappearing. Chief Nursing Executives are urged to consult these clinical leaders about their perspectives as well as to help shape and guide executives' thinking, willingness to recognize covered-over problems, judgment, redesign, problem solving, and workable interventions/solutions. Systems re-engineering, the use of guidelines, protocols, and checklists cannot replace the continued need for situated thinking-in-action, clinical reasoning, and judgment. Evidence-based or best practice guidelines and protocols will significantly improve substandard and inexperienced clinical judgment. However, by their nature, these structured prompts to performance improvement and increasing patient safety are static, and cannot address the evolving complexities of unfolding clinical situations as the patient's condition changes (transitions).

Clinical leaders also commonly coach patients and families through transitions. Although nurses do have the opportunity to coach patients and families through favorable transitions, coaching is more often necessitated by a crisis when patients or families are distressed, confused, or traumatized. In the best of leadership, clinicians first and foremost listen in order to discover what matters to the patient or family, to understand their concerns, and to clarify what they perceive is at stake. By listening, being emotionally attuned to, and getting to know the patient and family, the nurse can then follow their lead and guide them in the direction of preference. If the preference is potentially harmful, the nurse can engage the patient and family in a discussion that helps them better understand the danger. In the story that follows, an advanced practice nurse in the emergency department illustrates empathetic and sensitive coaching that follows an emotionally traumatized patient's lead. At no time does the nurse pass judgment and try to manipulate the patient to act otherwise:

Advanced Practice Nurse: I do the interview and [then the physical exam.]...The whole exam—it takes four hours to do an evidentiary [rape] exam because they are very traumatized people and usually law enforcement [officers] arrive and [question them]. Sometimes it's a sexual assault detective, it just depends. If it's a rape by a stranger or a home invasion or something like that, it's one thing. If it's an acquaintance rape, date rape-type situation—a known acquaintance because they live in the same apartment complex, there's all kinds so—it just depends on what it's like, and sometimes they're very traumatic. The patient's very traumatized, and sometimes they're so scared that they will not report it and we're here to talk to them to see if they will, but sometimes they won't. There's just no way. And, my feeling is, we really need to respect that because the exam is nothing compared to testifying [referring to the emotional trauma to the patient]. Testifying is a big deal and if somebody really doesn't want to talk about it here, doesn't want to press charges, go through with giving that detective and the police what they need to know, then there's no reason for us to do the examination. And that's nothing compared to once they get the DA's [district attorney] office involved, and from there it's even [worse]. So victims have to be pretty motivated to be cooperative. If they don't want to press charges, they're not going to. And indeed sometimes it's because they're scared. And sometimes we can talk with them and they do [decide to press charges], but sometimes not.

Physician: [physician is listening and joins us] I tell law enforcement [officers] that if you have someone that's really reluctant to testify, and they truly understand, they know, if they choose not to press charges—if somebody really doesn't want to—I just can't force them.

Advanced Practice Nurse: I had a victim come in last week who we, I finished testifying at her first trial about a month ago, from the last time she was raped, and she got here and she said that this time it was someone she knew, and she just couldn't go through it again, and I just said 'I understand.' We've worked with her, and she said 'You know, we put that guy away for 26 years, and I know how hard it was with a stranger, and there's no way I'm going through it with somebody I know, there's just no way'. She said, 'If it was that hard, there's just no way.' And I said, 'I understand. It's fine! What can I do for you?' And she really wanted ovral (birth control pills)—so she wouldn't get pregnant—and wanted to be treated for sexually transmitted diseases, so we just did that and I let her go.

Interviewer: She knew?

Advanced Practice Nurse: ...she couldn't go through it again. She told me, 'This is what happened to me'. Her husband divorced her, her twins were given up for adoption, they were taken away from her, just all this stuff happened to her during this period of time, and she was just getting her life back together and she couldn't go through any more. It's like, 'Okay.'

Physician: And that's one of the horrible things. For some people, testifying helps bring some closure to the whole thing, but for most people, it tends to be months and months and months that they have to keep reliving it, and they can't put it behind them... (Observational Interview)

In this particular situation, where the patient presents after a second rape, the advanced practice nurse immediately recognizes the patient's reluctance to take legal action in this second rape and supports the patient's decision not to press charges. This experienced nurse finds it easier to respond to the patient in accord with the patient's wishes because she knows the horrendous ordeal that the patient has already endured and respects her preference not to subject herself or family to the repeated insults and emotional trauma. The nurse indicates that, in other cases, her clinical judgment may differ. She commonly talks to patients who may not initially want to press charges. In those cases, she then coaches so that patients are fully informed about the consequences of their decisions. At that point, she follows each patient's lead. Excellent coaching of patients through this kind of world-transforming transition is critical because the patient's and family's lives are forever changed. What the patient does in response to the trauma can make a difference in their well-being in the future.

Following the patient's lead is similar to Benner's (1994) understanding of "following the body's lead." Following the body's lead means that:

> the person's bodily capacities and responses are given moral worth and considered a form of personhood and intentionality that require attention, respect, and response. This ethical comportment...sets limits on dominance and control of the body that ignores bodily responses and needs...[and] preserves the status of the other as one who makes ethical claims for consideration when using therapies and care that alter the body's own adaptive and recuperative powers (p. 154).

Following the <u>patient's</u> lead differs from following the <u>body's</u> lead primarily in that patients express their wishes or preferences, implicitly or explicitly. Excellent clinical leaders give patients' and families' preferences moral worth and respect, preserve their status, and limit the healthcare providers' control.

Another way that expert nurses follow the patient's and family's lead is by tailoring their education and coaching to meet the specific needs and strengths of the patient and family. Current practice is and practice standards advise that nurses fully inform patients about the procedure itself and what to expect as they progress through the transitions. However, in a few instances, the patient does not want to be informed. In the following story, the nurse describes her grasp of the patient's preferences, how her grasp guided her clinical judgment, and how she skillfully followed his lead:

Nurse: Mr. Bard is a 69-year-old man who came in with an inferior wall MI but was not eligible for t-PA.

Interviewer: He was beyond the acute onset?

Nurse: Yes, beyond the acute phase and did not have strong symptomatology because it was a small MI. He went down to the cardiac cath[eterization lab] yesterday and they found several lesions. They are going to do a PTCA [percutaneous transluminal coronary angioplasty] on him this afternoon, but they have some concerns about him. One of the techs suggested he is the kind of patient that might crash...Since I worked with him yesterday prior to going down for his heart cath, I know he really doesn't want a lot of information. He wants only the basic information. He has seen the film and has the [teaching] pamphlet. Actually, he just simply wants it done and over with without a lot of discussion.

Interviewer: How have you been able to figure out how much information he wants?

Nurse: I used several tactics. I'm giving instruction and asking if he has any questions. I volunteered some information and, as things have come up, he has asked some questions. For example, he asked why he had to keep his leg straight. So I answered that and gave him a little additional information also. In giving him additional information, I tried not to overload him with information. But I really listened to what he was asking for. (Observational Interview)

Here, the nurse gains a general sense that the patient does not want much information, just the basics about the transitions he is to experience. From there, her judgment about what to teach is based on "really listening to what he was asking for." When he expresses a specific interest in an aspect of the transition, such as keeping his leg straight, she takes the opportunity to teach him about that aspect but limits her discussion based on the boundaries he set. At the same time, notice that educating patients holds importance in this nurse's practice. Consequently, she is attentive to issues that arise which warrant "volunteering some information." His ensuing questions validate the importance.

It is equally important to encourage families and patients to coach nurses through a patient's transition. There are aspects in a patient's care in which the family has a better understanding of the patient's responses and needs than the nurse. In those situations, clinical leaders involve the family to interpret the patient's response or anticipate what will be most helpful. In this way the family is solicited to coach the clinician through the patient's transition so that the clinician can better judge the intervention needed. A PACU nurse explains why she is adamant about having the family present and how they guide her judgment and interventions with the patient:

> **Nurse:** I have always advocated—and it's not going to happen—but I've always advocated that the family should be at the bedside with the patient, for a variety of reasons: just to protect the patient, to be there, to understand the goals for the patient, to help us with the patient... I say (to the family members), 'I want you to help me understand what this patient, this friend, your mother, or your father is like. Tell me about them,' and I might ask a specific question. Like when I asked that man [about his wife], he said, 'she is tough,' and that gave me a whole different take on what was going on with her. But if he had instead told me that the littlest thing makes her cry, that would have been a whole other story... But when he told me she was tough, I knew I needed to give her enough pain medication to last through the night. That's when I wanted to go with dilaudid or methadone. And see, there are so many little vital secrets in the care of the patient that the family has that we can never get from a narrative record. We can never get from anyone the whole gestalt of who that person is. It can only come from a significant other. So, I really think that the family should be there...that's really important. So I like to engage the whole family, even when it comes to giving the patient pain medicine, I'll say to the mom, 'Do you think your child is in pain?'

By eliciting the family's concerns and interpretations, this nurse gains a better grasp of the patient's responses. This example highlights how expert clinical leaders collaborate with others and allow them to coach the leaders to provide the best and, sometimes, most expedient care possible.

As nurses learn more specifically about how to best care for particular patients, continuity in the patient's care depends on communicating and coaching peers about those specifics. In some cases, the information can be written on a care plan for dissemination. However, effective ways of dealing with complex issues or with difficult situations can rarely be passed on in compressed and often cryptic, written form. In the excerpt below, an ICU nurse recounts how she coaches peers in caring for a retired military sergeant who has several life-threatening complications. No one wants to take care of him because he "acts out" in ways that make the nurses uncomfortable. This nurse, on the other hand, is quite comfortable caring for him because she knows how and does not hesitate to "draw the line," to which he appropriately responds:

> **Nurse:** If there were new nurses, then it would be the tug of war again. When I got to him, what had happened was that the nurses had somewhat backed away from him because of that. And, if he was up to it, he'd demand kisses or he'd pinch nurses until you drew the line with him. So nobody wanted to take care of him... I helped organize a patient care conference on him, because obviously I was not going to be there the whole time he was going to be there. It wasn't right that a lot of the staff were afraid to take care of him. I wrote down and also told the people who were present at the care conference what sort of approaches worked with him. One thing he didn't like was for people coming in and doing things with him without introducing themselves. Basic things, but people would forget. Basic things like saying who they were and what they were there for. That was extremely important to him. And that no matter what, you had to be very forceful but very firm and kind with him at the same time

when he would start acting out...I knew him. I think that was the difference. I knew him, and he knew me. As soon as I went in there, it was, 'How are you doing? I'm sorry you're in here, but hopefully, you'll get better, but the ground rules are: you don't pinch me and you don't ask for kisses because it makes me feel uncomfortable, and then I can't take care of you well. And that's what we're here for, we're here to take care of you.' And so, he knew. It was just a matter of always reinforcing that. But he tried. He tried with anybody who came in...

In this difficult situation, this nurse takes on a clinical leadership role by coaching other nurses in how to effectively work with the patient without becoming intimidated. Although she does not understand the patient's "acting out" behaviors, she is deeply concerned about his ongoing care and about the emotional well-being of her colleagues who would necessarily provide his care in her absence. Because she has discovered effective ways of modifying his offensive behaviors, she sets up a conference in which she coaches peers about what she has learned and about effective ways of setting boundaries. Setting boundaries opens up the possibility in each instance of a transition in the patient's behaviors. In this way, the nurse not only assists peers in working with this patient but also helps them develop skills they will need for similar situations in the future.

Expert clinical leaders commonly discover, sometimes by stumbling upon it, that it is plausible to create the possibility of a beneficial transition in a patient's condition, particularly the psychological or emotional aspects. The skill of creating the possibility for a transition can be difficult to coach, especially when those being coached are not open to trying new interventions or, in the next situation, a heavy workload precludes participation. In such cases, another way of teaching others is to role model the interventions or to figure out what intervention may be most beneficial and then taught. An oft-told adage that points to this is "Seeing is believing." In the following story, Jennifer Harley, an advanced practice nurse at the time, role models an intervention that she hopes will improve the patient's depression and withdrawal:

Advanced Practice Nurse: I was a CNS in Hematology Oncology. Jackson was a 5 year old boy I had been involved with since his diagnosis with AML. He was from rural Indiana where he spent most of his time "helping" his grandfather on his hog farm. AML therapy results in long hospitalizations and very little time at home between treatments.

During his second hospitalization that was lasting longer than 30 days, Jackson's usual talkativeness and active participation in unit activities was suppressed. He wanted to go home. "How much longer....I want to go back home." His blood count levels were not going to be high enough for at least a week.

I talked with his mom and aunt about what we could simulate of home life in the hospital. I offered the opportunity to visit the puppies that live in the medical building across the street. I thought that it might be a familiar experience to a child who grew up on a farm and, besides, it was the only "animal" I could think of on campus besides mice in the research lab. So I got a name from one of the hem/onc physicians and checked with the animal lab. There was a new litter of puppies. I worked with a CNS student and one of the animal lab employees to arrange for Jackson to visit the next day... [This took lots of discussion and assurances with the physician regarding infection risk and Jackson's needs.] ...I had answers to all his questions about infection risk. He agreed, reminding me about good hand washing.

The next morning Jackson decided he did not want to go. When I asked him why—he couldn't give an answer. His mother urged him but he was firm. I assumed that this was just a little too much out of the ordinary for him to feel comfortable, even with his mother coming with us. It was clear to me though that Jackson needed "air" or some outdoor time to serve as distraction, and decrease stress of long "imprisonment" in the hospital so that afternoon I proposed an alternative. I took Jackson to a park bench behind the hospital to watch the many squirrels that run around the lawn. This became a routine (with the nurse, Social Worker, and/or myself) when weather allowed for the remainder of this hospitalization and subsequent ones. Jackson could be a very talkative child; he was the oldest and had a story for about everything. During the visits to the "park", he would talk freely about home, family, and animals. Jackson could describe exactly how someone hunted squirrels and that his grandfather like to eat them. This prompted a game he invented—he drew pages full of animals while staff and I guessed what they were. I keep one of these pages in my office as a reminder of Jackson.

Although I missed in my first attempt to recreate something of normalcy for Jackson—the second (and easier) intervention was the successful one—a good lesson in having options. The intervention of taking patients off the unit for a special time has become a route for me in the CNS role. I have used the library, the play equipment in child psych, etc. as destinations, depending on the child's interest. It served as a great tool for communication, giving time for the parent away from the child and distraction from long hospitalizations. I will always remember Jackson; he was a boy after my own heart. Being sick was not what he was about. He was full of potential and found fishing, kindergarten, turtles and pigs much more interesting than cancer or hospitals.

Here, the advanced practice nurse is fully engaged, attuned to Jackson's world of concerns, and "knows" what realm of probabilities can contribute to the transition in his emotional well-being/. This is a superb example of the limits of science, where there is no protocol or best practice guideline to follow for excellent clinical judgment or the kind of intervention requisite for this child's well-being and recovery. Instead, guided by the logic of practice, Jennifer already knows what kind of intervention is needed at the moment she grasps that something needs to be done. Her keen sensibilities stems from knowing this child, from hearing stories that reflect his joy and what is meaningful to him. Getting him out of the hematology oncology unit and into a natural setting beckons him into reconnecting with the familiar world he loves and enables him to once again "dwell" in it. In his familiar world, Jackson becomes the talkative, entertaining child with a "story about everything." He is again full of life. The power of this kind of intervention has been observed in others' practices and is not to be underestimated. Renewal of the spirit and of hope can have tremendous recuperative power.

Recognizing what Jackson loves and creating a space for him in it, even though temporary, is a caring practice and, in some patients, can create the vital passage toward recovery. This recognition of patients' concerns and familiar lifeworld assists the nurse in helping the patient re-enter and re-engage in their world which can get "closed down" and inaccessible during a long illness and hospitalization. Although Jennifer proclaims that she missed the mark on the first intervention (the puppies), she grasped the essential nature (the right region) of what was needed and easily found "the park" to be a good option. The clinical judgment and skill of creating the possibility for a transition can be life-transforming and life-saving when working with chronically ill patients.

In the above situation, Jennifer does not start out coaching the nurse, although she is mentoring a CNS student to listen, follow Jackson's lead in terms of his interests, forecast what a good possibility might be, and respond by helping to create the possibility. The time constraints for Jackson's nurse do not allow for coaching throughout the time required in this kind of ambiguity; however, once Jennifer discovers a good option to which Jackson is very responsive; the nurse then follows her lead and continues this therapeutic, caring practice.

When nurses are coaching others through a transition they are typically available to guide the other person through the change as it unfolds. However, earlier discharge and same day surgeries are significantly reducing the clinician's access to the patient so that clinicians can no longer observe some of the important physiological transitions. Because some patients' conditions are not predictable, yet they must be discharged to home, coaching them through transitions that will occur at home is often challenging and troublesome. For this reason, expert clinicians detail, as much as possible, how the changes should unfold and point out adverse changes which should alert the patient to call for help. In the following excerpt, PACU nurses discuss how they coach patients through transitions that they forecast will occur post-discharge. As a safety net, these nurses call patients within a day or two to ensure that the transition(s) has gone smoothly:

> **Nurse 1:** ...every patient that goes home is called by one of our nurses. It's supposed to happen the next day, but it doesn't always. So we call them and ask a variety of systems questions and ask them about any problems they could be having, whether they are in pain...
>
> **Interviewer:** I'm awfully glad you're doing the phone calls, because how would you know whether you made a good decision [about discharging to home or admitting to the hospital on borderline cases], when the patient is out of sight, out of mind?
>
> **Nurse 2:** We trust, we don't know if we've made a good decision, but we're trusting that when we give them their home care instructions, and we give them a copy to take home with them with specific telephone numbers for them to call if they have any concerns or questions about how they're feeling, as those initials hours pass. And so we trust that they are in fact calling those numbers if they do need further assistance.
>
> **Nurse 1:** But I don't think they do, because I think a lot of them kind of expect that it's going to be this way. And they don't understand that it is their right to get optimal care. And they don't—like when I send my patients home, I say, 'This is how you should feel. You should hurt. The pain medicine should help you so that you can actually sleep. If you can't sleep, then you are not getting optimal relief and there's something wrong, and you need to call your doctor, because you should be sleeping. If you're not sleeping, something is wrong.' So you need to give them guidelines to understand, because not all people are proactive and self-directed enough to say, 'This is not right.'

The first nurse understands that patients do not know what to expect and are reluctant to call for help, so she forecasts and coaches them specifically about issues she knows they will face once they are at home. For instance, the nurse tries to characterize the kind of pain the patients may experience. She then coaches them on how to interpret their level of pain relief and recognize when they should call for help. In case there are problems that the patient either does not recognize or is hesitant to call about, the nurses follow up with phone calls in which they ask a number of questions that allow them to evaluate the patient's recovery. This form of clinical leadership takes on greater importance as healthcare changes reduce the exposure clinicians have to patients during important physiological transitions.

Clinical leaders in this study also taught us that they informally monitor health trends in the community and take an active role in alerting members of the community if problems of broad concern arise. When clinical leaders observe an unusual type or number of unexpected seasonal illnesses, they become attentive to new cases and investigate the problem, if warranted. For instance, an advanced practice nurse noticed an unusual number of patients with mushroom poisoning. Because of the life-threatening nature of the problem, a press conference is convened by the Liver Transplant Coordinator, an advanced practice nurse, to caution the public about mushroom picking, ingestion, and smoking:

Advanced Practice Nurse: [talking to the Liver Transplant Coordinator] As I was telling her [the interviewer] earlier, we have no beds.

Transplant Coordinator: Well, there's two more out there so...

Interviewer: Two more what?

Advanced Practice Nurse: Patients with mushroom poisonings.

Transplant Coordinator: We're doing a press conference.

Advanced Practice Nurse: I heard, I saw that on the news. Then why aren't they [the press] here yet?

Transplant Coordinator: I called G. yesterday and I said, 'We need you here now.' I called him on Friday. I said, 'We need to send out [a message].' We sent it out on Monday and that's when it made radio and television news last night.

Advanced Practice Nurse: I saw that, yeah.

Transplant Coordinator: But yesterday afternoon...[a number of patients came] in and now there's two more out there.

Advanced Practice Nurse: He's [pointing out a patient in ICU] is one of them. Yeah. We've had three...we've actually had five.

Transplant Coordinator: Actually there have been nine hospitalizations in [this region] in two weeks......

Interviewer: This press conference is for the media to get the word out?

Advanced Practice Nurse: Um hum. Yeah. It's amazing how many people we have here with mushroom poisoning.

Transplant Coordinator: We have not had this many in this short period of time— ever. Last year we had a family. One needed a transplant. And she's fine, but to have five patients in a week-and-a-half to two week period....

Advanced Practice Nurse: That's a lot of people.

Interviewer: Those are the people who take risks?

Advanced Practice Nurse: Yeah. He cooked the wrong mushrooms. In another case, we had a young kid, 18-year-old, he and his friends on New Year's Eve—well, they dried the mushrooms a few days before—they picked them and dried—and they were trying to get high. Anyway, he didn't need a transplant, but they were all lucky, very lucky. (Observational Interview)

In a two week period, nine patients are admitted to several regional hospitals with various kinds of mushroom poisoning. Because many poisonous mushrooms look similar to ingestible ones, too many people are mistakenly ingesting and/or smoking them. Since most varieties of poisonous mushrooms are toxic to the liver, the attentive liver transplant coordinator quickly recognizes an emerging community problem. Although she has initiated several public alerts in the previous week, patients are continuing to be admitted. She hopes that a press conference will capture more attention. This example highlights how clinical leaders act as community leaders as the situation demands.

BRIDGING THE GAPS IN PATIENT CARE

Gaps in patient care have always been problematic, but the recent and rapid changes in healthcare have escalated this already difficult problem. Although gaps may occur in the care of any patient, patients with more complex and debilitating physical or social situations require more care from multiple disciplines. Nurses are commonly the clinicians who notice the gaps in these complex patients and, in collaboration with physicians, initiate assistance from other disciplines. In the midst of responding to the urgent demands of a complex acutely or critically ill patient, secondary needs are sometimes temporarily overlooked until the patient's condition stabilizes. For instance, an ICU staff nurse described a situation where the patient could not be weaned from the ventilator until his nutritional needs were met and his respiratory muscles were strengthened. With dietary assistance and improved exercise, the patient was successfully weaned. Another instance involved a child who was rapidly deteriorating from a pneumothorax. The community hospital physician was unfamiliar with chest tube placement, so the transport ICU nurse coached him through the procedure in order to bridge the critical gap in the child's care. In yet another situation, the nurse recognized that a surgeon's plans and expectations for the care of a child after discharge were unrealistic due to an unusual family circumstance. With her information and guidance, the team was then able to devise a realistic and suitable plan that accommodated the child's and family's needs.

At times, the gaps are best bridged by expert nurses who grasp the entire complexity of the situation. For instance, in some socially desperate situations, the nurse instead of the social worker may best understand and be able to comfort and help narrow the gap, even in very constrained situations. Anne Benson, a special care nursery nurse, often finds herself caring for babies and parents with addictions who are or have been marginalized. Anne works in and contributes to building and preserving a culture where the marginalized are respected and cared for compassionately. By doing so, she creates possibility in some lives where there was little. Embedded in her exemplar is the richness created by a strong clinical and moral leader:

Nurse: I met Debbie and Skip while caring for their newborn son Brian, who was being monitored and treated for Neonatal Abstinence Syndrome (withdrawal). His parents were upfront about their ongoing battle with heroin and cocaine addictions. Debbie used both throughout her pregnancy. Brian was their first baby and born with positive screen for the opiates and cocaine.

As a team, we wanted to establish therapeutic communication—respectful, open, honest, and friendly. I needed to assess the parents' safety to be with Brian. I also wanted to provide emotional support, education about narcotic withdrawal, infant care and safety. I wanted to prepare these parents to care for Brian, in hopes that they would have him at their home, whenever it was appropriate and safe for them and him.

Our Social Worker and the Department of Social Service (DSS) worker were actively working with Debbie and Skip. They discussed treatment program options for each of them, clearly stating that a newborn would not be safe living with two actively using addicts. Skip and Debbie worried about the ongoing DSS investigation. Their home was being inspected, their support system interviewed, and their medical record reviewed. What was at stake was serious—custody of their son.

The couple came each day to take care of their newborn. Before each feeding, the nurses calculated the baby's Neonatal Abstinence (NAS) score. Brian received neonatal morphine solution with each feeding to help manage the GI symptoms caused by withdrawal. Both parents were able to see the symptoms: excessive sucking, poor feeding, regurgitation, and loose stools, as well as the milder neuro symptoms of irritability, tremors, and tight muscle tone. They tracked his scores and participated in providing comfort measures to help Brian. They talked with me about our plan to slowly wean Brian off of the morphine. The plan was his last dose of morphine would be mid-day Sunday, with probable discharge on Tuesday afternoon. The perceived obstacle for these parents was the DSS custody hearing on Monday.

That weekend, Debbie and Skip sat by Brian's bedside watching him sleep, waiting for him to awaken for his feeding. They held and rocked him gently when he cried or couldn't settle to sleep as the last of the narcotics left his system. They knew that we were watching them and charting our observations—describing their behaviors, which would reveal whether or not they were straight or seemed to be impaired, safe to be with their son, and demonstrating appropriate parenting behaviors.

Debbie and Skip thus far appeared to be "straight" each time they visited Brian. They demonstrated the usual new parent behaviors. They asked for help with formula feeding, and laughed as they struggled with diaper changing and swaddling. They looked for advice to help comfort him by adapting their approach and Brian's environment to calm his irritability. Their responses showed that they were implementing what they learned. Their small support system of friends and family came to visit.

On Saturday, Skip talked with me about the upcoming court proceedings. Although they were nervous about retaining custody, they were hopeful and fairly confident that they would bring him home. They both knew DSS was advocating for both to enter different long-term inpatient programs, followed by halfway house programs, since they had been long-term addicts. He thought what DSS wanted was "totally unrealistic" because they "really needed to be together with the baby." He and their friends felt sure that, because they had hidden nothing and put all of their issues on the table, their honesty would be rewarded....[He discussed an alternative plan they planned to present to DSS.] They seemed to be trying to convince me that their plan was not only practical, but also the best possible solution. "What do you think, Anne? Do you think that we'll be able to convince the judge that we can do this?"

Honestly, I thought as they talked that there was probably no chance that they would walk out of this hospital with that sweet little baby. The question to me was how to best answer honestly, realistically, and kindly, while not destroying their hope.

"Well," I started as I pulled up a chair, "I've honestly don't think that I have ever seen anyone, who has not been actively involved in a recovery program throughout their pregnancy, leave with their baby. Starting a program before the baby is born shows intent—a plan for recovery" I explained. "I don't want to dash your hope, because I do see how loving you are with Brian. What I am sure about, though, is that you deserve to be fully well and free of craving and of the power that the drugs and addiction have over you. Addictions are so tough to fight."

"You're right," Skip told me, "but I really think that we can beat it with day programs. I really want to do it this time—we NEED to do it now." "I'm sure it's going to work out," Debbie told me. "But, if for some crazy reason that it doesn't, I want to show you what we want for Brian."

Debbie then pulled out a bag with a light blue outfit with a fuzzy teddy bear on the front, matching socks, t-shirt, hat and sweater. There was also a little brown teddy bear that would go with him. Next she had a coordinating blue velour blanket. "No matter what," she said, "we both want him to wear this (car seat) when he leaves the hospital. He needs to be in his own car seat; it is the best one out there. We really want him to be safe. I'm sure that he will be leaving with us, but if not, we'll feel better if he's kept warm and safe with his own stuff," she said with tears running down her cheeks. "I'm here for the next three days," I told them, "I'll make sure that happens."

Debbie and Skip spent much time over the weekend with Brian. Their skills increased. We worked together with the understanding that they would need to be ready to care for Brian either sooner or later, so the time was well spent.

By Monday night, we learned that the parents did not get custody. Brian would be discharged to a foster mother. It was the right decision, for sure, but sad. Later that night, Debbie called in tears. She just couldn't bear to come in to say good-bye. Instead, she was packing her bags so she would be ready to go for care when a bed opened.

On Tuesday, the foster mother arrived. This was a first time foster experience and her family was hopeful and nervous. They lived nearby and she was well known as "a great friend and fabulous mom". We all worry about these babies and their families and feel relief when we find them going into what appears to be a good situation. The foster mother was excited. She smiled and hugged Brian, then dressed him in the outfit that the parents left for him.

I took a digital picture of him dressed up and with his little teddy bear and another one of him secured in his car seat. The unit "picture lady" came in and got a great picture of him. I gathered up his crib cards with his footprints on the back, hospital picture information, his first hospital hat that he wore, and the religious medal given to him by our chaplain, and kept them all aside. Then, I walked Brian out with his foster mom. Before I left for the day, I carefully constructed a letter to Debbie and Skip from Brian. I wrote:

Dear Mom and Dad,

I feel so handsome and loved today, as I leave the hospital. The nurses keep telling me that I am the "cutest boy ever" in my new outfit. I am hugging my teddy and thinking about you as I do. I tried to smile in the pictures to let you know that I am okay and that I love you.

I want you to feel better that the lady who came for me seems pretty nice. I also want you to know that I will keep you and your hugs close to my heart.

My car seat feels snuggly and safe. I wanted the rest of my stuff to be sent to you—the crib cards with my footprints, my first hat, medal, and of course some pretty great pictures of me. I hope that you like them all.

I'll be ready when you are. Love, hugs, and kisses,

Brian

At the end of the note, I secured the pictures. In the addressed large envelope, I placed the crib card, hat, medal, and welcome Brian sign. I sent the note and pictures to provide comfort and perhaps more incentive for recovery. I continue to be hopeful that they are well, in recovery, have a network of support, and maybe even parenting their son. I hope to never lose hope.

I shared this story since I was so touched by this family's hope, honesty, sincerity, and expressions of love for Brian and each other. Although I am sure that the court made the right decision, I felt so sad for them. They were credible. They put all of their cards on the table, and even so, their son was taken. I hope they make it!

Because of Anne's respectful view of and stance with the parents, she makes invisible the hard work that is invested in preparing, observing and working with addicted parents and the heartbreak of their addicted, withdrawing infants. This nurse is not a Pollyanna. She has clarity about how the baby is suffering, what the baby needs, and what is not possible with parents who are actively using drugs. Yet, she has a clearer vision about humanity, what is good, and her role or opportunity to create possibility for a future family. Anne holds onto hope and nurtures honest, realistic hope in the parents in a sincere way, as they have a long, arduous road to recovery. Love is powerful and Anne deeply understands its power, even in the midst of working through the pains of addiction with the newborn and parents. Anne's ethic of responsibility and care; her notions of what it is to be a good nurse; and her respectful, non-judgmental, ethical comportment are a hallmark of expert practice and are foundational for her strong moral and clinical leadership. Here, strong leadership bridges part of the emotional gap for the parents—she ensures that Brian enters the world as they wished, clothed in love and surrounded by symbols of their love and safety. Anne also bridges the gap in the parents' lives. She sends cherished memories of a lost infant to the parents in hopes of keeping them connected and inspiring them to one day be a family.

Having developed the perceptual acuity to grasp "the good" in the parents and in an otherwise regrettable situation enables Anne to make ethical judgments and provide exquisite caring practice. Although Anne's smooth practice covers over the enormous challenges in this situation, the extensive knowledge (physiological, emotional, sociocultural, legal, psychological, experiential) she has gained and flexibly uses is quite apparent in the integration of her clinical and ethical reasoning. It is however because of the integration of these large bodies of knowledge that Anne can realistically and compassionately help.

What is stunning is that Anne does not "work" at being nice or treating these parents in a special way, despite the suffering caused to their infant. Anne has developed a high degree of engagement where she can imaginatively stand where the parents stand, feel their struggles and concerns, understand how their social situation resulted in addiction, and therefore empathize. She has, over time, developed a strong moral and ethical lens and comportment so that, now, she simply embodies them as notions of good in an habitual way. Not surprisingly, she also embodies the habits presented throughout this work, of clinical grasp and forethought. Anne's care and coaching of Debbie and Skip are a lovely explication of her constant, astute and ongoing grasp of their performance as loving parents who are actively addicts and pose a safety risk and she is habitually thinking ahead about what they need next, what to prepare them for emotionally and legally, etc.

Strong clinical leaders like Anne fully grasp situations in which a gap exists and the difference they can make is not only physiological. In expert practice, the patient's and family's lifeworld deeply matter, and these expert nurses are compelled to act when needed. Often, a nurse is the only one who can act. At times, the simplest intervention, like helping a father hold his baby, is not so simple but can have lifelong significance. A simple act can be world transforming. Corinne Cyr Pryor, a neonatal ICU nurse, senses the salience of a father's emotions and fear; validates her impression; takes the risk; and skillfully acts as a strong clinical leadership to close the gap, from separation to connection:

Nurse 1: I took care of a family from Santa Domingo. You are intimately involved with the family, always. You HAVE to be. Very nice couple, very scared. I'll give you a little history. [Several years ago, they had <u>another</u> preemie born at 32 weeks who was doing well and is now 6 years old. When mom became pregnant again, she was at high risk. She somehow delivered in the US at 28 weeks. This baby is much sicker, 2 pounds, so they're petrified.]

The mother is crying. She doesn't speak much English but we forged a relationship between English, Spanish and French. At the beginning, she's really, really scared. This father is trying to be macho—but not. I can see, he's melting when he comes to see the baby. Gingerly touching the baby. And he's telling me, "I didn't really hold my son until he was almost a year." And I say, "you know, that must have been really hard! I know you want to hold this baby." "No! No, no, no, no, no!" and so the mother is standing in the background, understanding more and more English, saying, "yes, yes, yes" (motioning that he should hold the baby). In the NICU, we do skin-to-skin kangaroo care. It started in Bogota, Columbia, where they started keeping the babies next to the mother's skin because they didn't have enough isolettes and that kept the babies warm. We do it now as more of a bonding experience. But we also have the dads involved.

As the days go on, the baby got sicker and had a bleed in his brain…of course, they are devastated. Mom is crying but Dad is NOT going to cry. So I say to them, "this must be awful for you." I sat with them when they got the news. We had a family meeting in another room. The doctor tells them it's a med sized bleed. We talked about it, and then came back. As I talked I said, "you must be so scared." I got them an interpreter so mom could understand technically. So then I go with my French and her Spanish and we're trying to... I say, "I know this is really, really hard for you, and I know you want to stay and hold him." She said, "yes," but, she's standing behind her husband and she's pointing to him so I said, "you know what? (looking at dad) Today is your turn." And he goes, "no, no, no, no!" and I said, (in cheery voice) "yes. Today is your turn! I have the chair right here. Right here, and you sit down! You don't have to do anything. Just sit there. All you have to do is just sit there." "Oh, No, no, no." "Oh yes! Just sit—very comfortably." They're not comfortable, they're supposed to be comfy chairs but they're not, they're disgusting. The guys usually use the chairs and hold the TV remote. They fall asleep with their little babies on their chest. So, I sit him down, and before he even has the chance to think, I open up the isolette, I take the baby out, and I put the baby right on his chest. I tuck the baby right in his shirt, and of course, I say, "you have to breathe. It's important that you breathe!" So he's breathing, and then he starts crying and crying. So of course, I'm crying and mom's crying and you see him melt. He ended up holding his baby for an hour and a half. After that, he held him every other day. He wanted to hold him <u>every</u> time, but he couldn't because the mom wanted to hold him too. We don't usually take the baby out more than once a day when they are that little, so they had to take turns. And he thanked me and thanked me. And it was so cool. It was really neat. It was like, this is what needs to happen, you know? I did manhandle him into it, but it was what he needed. And you could just see his whole, sitting like this at first (straight back) and then the baby wiggled and found his nitch. He settled into a hole and went to sleep. And this particular man, you could just see him breathe, because I kept telling him to breathe, and then he just cried and cried. It was like... what he so needed. And what the family needed. Because the mom really... she was so happy. But, I made a difference.

Nurse 2: Did it get disseminated through the NICU?

Nurse 1: Well, the good thing is it's something that we use very frequently. Skin to skin is one of our standards of care. Pushing them doesn't always happen. So if somebody says "no," we say, "oh all right!"

Interviewer: So what was it that you noticed particularly that made you push harder and harder?

Nurse1: It was two things. You know how you can just tell—he *wanted* his hands on that baby—but he was scared to <u>death</u> of it. So when I said, because we do bring their hands in, so many of them are afraid the baby is going to break. But these babies are as tough as nails. They go through more than we could ever, ever survive and do well afterwards. But we do take their hands oftentimes and place their hands right on the baby. And say, "this is what you do." They can't handle being stroked, it's too much for the [neonates].... I put my hands on top of their hands, and I have them tuck them in. They tuck their feet in and put their hands on top of their heads... With this dad, because of the devastating news, which was just awful for them, he put his hands in by himself. And it was a key—he did it, he wanted his hand on the baby. And then I had the mother in the background (pointing vigorously at the father) pointing and shaking her head—because she knew him better than I did!

Nurse 2: That's beautiful

Nurse 1: In the end, he was there for two months. Lovely for me because I got to take care of him! The baby ended up getting better. When they left, they were very thankful. They thanked us every day.

When dad approaches his baby's bedside, Corrine immediately notices that he "melts." Being emotionally attuned, she understands that he wants to hold his baby. However, when asked, dad adamantly protests that "no," he does not. This clinical leader's keen sensibilities inform her that she has an accurate grasp, so she later makes another offer. Despite confidence in her judgment, she must negotiate the differences in language and culture that may warrant standing back and waiting. She ethically comports herself to follow his expressed wishes. However, given the devastating nature of this second premature son's situation and the multiple sources pointing to the gap in dad's life, she takes the risk, follows dad' emotional cues, and "helps" him to finally hold his baby. She makes a good and timely moral judgment. The blessings of this act were unspeakable; dad visibly melted. In the blink of an eye, the gap disappeared.

For the duration of the hospitalization, in the background, Corrine revealed her worry and preparation around a second and larger gap...how the baby will receive adequate care when he returned home. As the baby's primary nurse, she ensured that the parents were educated well to care for their baby. The baby went on to do well and went home.

As patients are discharged from hospitals earlier and sicker, boundaries between the hospital and home care are becoming much more fluid. In some situations, care from a home health agency is feasible and possible, while in others, it is not. Because some patients are discharged on life-support technologies, the family and home environment must be ready and able to support the patient's needs, and someone must anticipate, coordinate, and prepare for these. A good example of bridging the gaps in patient care was presented in Chapter 8 when an advanced practice nurse discussed preparing patients and families for home ventilation. The gaps the advanced practice nurse commonly addresses when ensuring discharge readiness include the following:

Advanced Practice Nurse: ...you've got the in-hospital teaching that needs to be coordinated, coordination with the home care agency, nursing as well as respiratory coordination with the medical equipment company, and try to pull all this together to come up with a plan that will get this patient in a readied sense for home support where all the resources and back-up are in line by the time he actually goes home. And those cases are always very special and challenging because there are just so many different aspects of care, coordinating—working with the nurses and setting up teaching schedules, techniques, teaching them dexterity, especially if you've got other care givers... I feel it's a predominantly nursing kind of plan. Because the skills are—whether it's tube feeding, or suctioning, or skin and wound care—all those things they're going to need to do at home. And the ventilator piece is really just a small part...you need to get the medical equipment company to go out to the house and do a safety assessment, make sure the electrical systems are compatible. They have to write letters to the fire and electrical companies, so they're put on a priority list. If there's an emergency or if they don't pay their electric bill, they don't get the power shut off.

In this kind of patient situation, the patient is dependent on the nurse to imaginatively consider and bridge gaps in care. The nurse must also prepare the patient and family with contingency plans in case of an emergency or oversight. In some situations, when the patient is physically capable, ventilator-dependent patients are taught to hand ventilate themselves. For chronically critically-ill patients such as this, it can take weeks to prepare everyone who will be involved in the patient's care, orchestrate the multiple home care services that will be needed, and ensure that the environment is properly equipped and safe. The clinical judgment, forethought, and skill required to bridge this particular gap are enormous and need further research.

As the advanced practice nurse points out, because the long term care of the patient predominantly involves nursing, nurses are typically the ones who are called upon to bridge the gaps. Nurses are responding to these demands, but the expert judgment and skill involved remain invisible. As the advanced practice nurses in the following excerpt emphasize, greater support and legitimization of this work are imperative to ensure that nurses are available to continue bridging the gaps in the future. These nurses talked about the kinds of gaps that they help bridge, particularly in marginalized populations:

Interviewer: I'm wondering, because you do provide this link for the patient, this connectedness and ongoing holistic care, I'm very curious whether or not it is apparent to the administrators.

Advanced Practice Nurse 1: I'm talking about my administration, and when there have been hospital cuts, our names are always brought up. And we are always put up there as offerings and every time that has happened, our attending physicians go to them and say, 'We'll quit. This program can't survive in the way it's surviving if we don't have the nurse practitioners.' So, we are very much recognized and appreciated by the medical staff that we work with, by our immediate administrative staff, but by the hospital in general, probably not. Or by hospital administration in general, probably not.

Interviewer: What is it that the physicians understand that you do that the nursing or hospital administrators often don't understand. What is the difference in their understanding?

Advanced Practice Nurse 1: Well, I don't think the administrators know what we do. If you ask them what do the nurse practitioners do, I don't think that they could tell you what we do. I think that some of them have absolutely no clue as to what we do. But the medical staff that we work with, they know and see us providing the continuity of care. They see us bringing up issues that might not have been brought up otherwise and so I think that they're much more appreciative.

As the interview continues, the advanced practice nurses again address this issue:

Advanced Practice Nurse 2: [This specialty group of patients] at this institution is the 800-pound gorilla. And at any time, 8-15% of the in-house beds are occupied by [this specialty group of] patients or spin-offs of [this specialty group of] patients. But actually on this service, we're talking 30 to 50 patients on any given day. And it's 450 beds, but it's not that big of a hospital. So, it drives a lot of the decision making for the whole institution. If <u>that</u> piece of the system gets clogged up, then everything is affected. If the [this specialty group of] patients don't move in an efficient way—and that's a lot of what we do. It's a fact that the attendings aren't seeing the readmissions that they used to. They're seeing patients discharged appropriately, in a condition where they're going to do okay, and that is important... We know the philosophy of the attendings, we know how each one of them takes care of patients. The residents that we see for the floor patients <u>don't</u> understand that, so we provide the consistency. And they'll ask us for help. And that's a really positive thing. They'll say, 'What should we do about this?' And it's just continuous teaching, not really in a formal sense, but informally, 'What should you do about this?' 'Well, this is what worked with Dr. So and So,' or 'This attending is following the patients this week. He's a 'don't feed them too early' guy or 'don't put that NG back in' because you should do this and that first. But also, think about this.' And, that's really positive because it seems very collaborative without being really oppressive.

Interviewer: You said that <u>part</u> of the attendings' support of you is because <u>their</u> readmission rates are lower.

Advanced Practice Nurse 2: I say that in a positive way because I think it provides them with a level of security. I think they trust us. And they trust us to—we're not driven by—I don't get paid more if the patients go home faster. I don't get paid less if the patients go home faster. They trust us to have the patients go home in an appropriate state. Not too long. Not too soon. We're a safety valve. I guess that's a fair way to say it.

Advanced Practice Nurse 1: Consequently there are fewer readmissions. And <u>that</u> makes <u>them</u> look good, because you have decreased complication rates.

Advanced Practice Nurse 2: [About trust] It happened the other day, Mr. H. had to go back to the unit. Almost all it took was, 'He's not looking good', and even <u>before</u> all of the things were done that would have normally been needed to affirm that he was not only not looking good and not doing well, he was...

Advanced Practice Nurse 1: The decision was already made.

Advanced Practice Nurse 2: The SI (Surgical ICU) resident was calling down saying, 'When is Mr. H. coming up?' And it's like, 'Well, we <u>were</u> going to get a chest X-ray and blood gas...' He said, 'Don't worry, just send him up.'

Advanced Practice Nurse 1: 'Don't you want to look at him first?' 'Nah, just send him. You've looked at him. If you're concerned, just send him.'

Advanced Practice Nurse 2: Yes. But that's all it took...The attendings we work with are phenomenal, they're great. I think that's a big deal... I think it relieves them to not have to worry about the details. It's not that they don't care about the [clinic] patients, but there's so many of them, they can't know them as intimately as they know the ICU patients. And it relieves them from the stress of thinking that they're responsible for the care and having to be paranoid about that because they've got the greenest [least experienced] interns in the institution taking care of their patients.

Interviewer: Yeah. So they don't have to keep track of every single detail.

Advanced Practice Nurse 2: Detail, yeah, we're out there as a safety net.

These nurse practitioners and their physician colleagues understand the multiple gaps that arise daily in patient care. Observational interviews demonstrate that these nurse practitioners follow and intervene in the physiological as well as other aspects of care that influence the patients' health and ability to recover. Because the physicians practiced in this clinic in years past, they recognize the breadth and depth of the issues that the nurse practitioners pursue and resolve in order to close the gaps in care. The physicians also recognize the vital gap that the nurse practitioners bridge when collaboratively working with the residents to care for the in-hospital patients. Because the nurse practitioners know the physicians' practice preferences, they can specifically coach the residents in their care of patients (Hooper, 1995). For most patients, these advanced practice nurses serve as a safety net in aspects of care that would otherwise be overlooked. Therefore, the physicians are adamant that the work of these clinicians is worth protecting and preserving.

The practices of advanced practice nurses in this study highlight how bridging the gaps in patient care is pervasive. Because they know the limitations of the care delivery system and the barriers that patients and families face when seeking care, they commonly extend themselves beyond their designated job responsibilities. An advanced practice nurse describes how she responds to urgent and essential comfort care that no longer receives priority for intervention in an economically driven system:

Advanced Practice Nurse: ...usually they're mothers of kids with brain tumors who, when their child's pain is out of control, when they need medicine, they don't need to wait three days, which is what it takes to get through the system. They need it right away. These mothers know that if they can get hold of me, it will be taken care of and they're <u>special</u> people who need that. They <u>can't</u> just go through the system the way it exists. It takes too long. So I noticed one mother when her child was terminal, I gave her my pager number and she just pages me. I just call and renew the prescription, and Dr. C. was really comfortable with that because <u>he</u> couldn't handle getting the calls. (Observational Interview)

To avoid agonizing and unwarranted delays in comfort care, the advanced practice nurse gives patients and family members 24-hour access to immediate intervention via her pager. The terminally ill patient and his distraught mother, in this case, would otherwise have to work through an unwieldy healthcare system to receive the needed care.

The gaps in the current healthcare system, however, extend beyond unwanted delays and unwieldy healthcare systems. Patients who are chronically yet very ill and those with complex long-term health problems struggle to receive adequate care. For these populations, the gaps are tremendous. The gaps, however, are most sorely felt by marginalized populations with complex long-term illnesses who commonly receive little or no care (Malone, 1995). The deeply embedded ethic of responsiveness further compels advanced practice nurses to return to the tradition of community health, push to extend care, and work on closing gaps by going into under-served communities. A researcher's observational notes describe the clinical judgment, skill, and leadership needed to bridge these kinds of gaps, for instance, in the care of persons with AIDS. Although persons with AIDS are often not considered seriously ill by care providers, their disease renders them seriously or critically ill at certain points in their illness. The gaps in care that they experience serve as a strong example of the societal bias toward acute, rather than chronic, care delivery (Jennings, 1996):

Interviewer Notes: We visit a young man with AIDS who lives in a very crowded and chaotic room. She [advanced practice nurse, Jean] meets the young man just about two feet outside his door. He does not seem to want to invite us in. Jean easily and quickly says, 'I know that you don't want us to come in, but just let me examine your lymph nodes. How are they doing?' She examines the nodes and a conversation begins. The patient has a kitten that he pets and kisses. Jean asks if he still wants to go on the new drugs, protease inhibitors. He says 'yes,' and she says, 'can we come in for a moment and talk?' He moves further into his room by this time. Jean follows. He lies down on the bed, Jean sits on the end of a table, and they talk. She explains that it is dangerous for him to be on protease inhibitors if he goes off the drugs and does not keep up the regime because he will develop new resistant strains [of the HIV virus]. It will not only cause him problems but possibly lead to new resistant strains that could infect other people. So it is important to be sure that he can first keep up the treatment. He denies taking drugs, and Jean later says that she is not sure about this. She tells him she will start him on combivir and another drug and see how his viral load responds, since he has never even taken combivir. If he does well on these medications, then he can progress to protease inhibitors. He states again that he wants to try these new drugs. He has had no T cells for almost a year and continues to survive. Jean later explains to me that he has had acute renal failure and acute liver failure and recovered from both. The nurse in the office tells of an incident of calling an ambulance for him because he was very distressed and disoriented. He was completely lucid by the time that the ambulance arrived and refusing to go to the hospital. Jean wants to give him a chance on the drugs if he proves himself. Later, she brings up the public health and ethical issues of giving the protease inhibitors to groups who may not continue with the treatment and therefore develop and introduce resistant strains into the population. She feels strongly that this whole population of patients (from a particular culture) should not be excluded. She wants them to be considered on a case by case basis as she is doing here. (Observational Interview)

Jean provides care in a clinic for patients with HIV, but she also makes home visits to those, for instance, living in inner city hotels, who are very fragile or too reluctant to come to the clinic. She embodies the ethic of care, but simultaneously balances the treatments provided by ensuring that medications are used wisely and responsibly to prevent exacerbating the development and spread of resistant viral strains. Bridging gaps in care for the chronically severely ill with complex complications remains a monumental challenge.

This parallels a growing move nationally to prepare patients for greater participation in their own care. Partnerships with patients are intended, in part, to bridge or prevent gaps in care. Within the growing constraints of managed care, nurses are developing innovative ways to care for patients. For instance, Walters (1997) reported at the American Heart Association Scientific Sessions that she and her critical care nurse colleagues have developed an intensive specialty home care practice to work with cardiac surgical patients who are discharged to home as early as the second post-operative day. Despite ongoing physiological problems (e.g., open wounds or pulmonary problems), if the patients are stable, can walk, know the signs and symptoms of exacerbation of their illness, and know who to call for help, they can be discharged into the care of a home health agency. The specialty home care nurses follow-up with intensive assessments and "teaching-in-action," that is, teaching patients and families about ongoing care (e.g., medications, activity) while in the home and while doing the actual daily care with the patient. Walters reported that only one in 50 patients has been readmitted to the hospital. She stated that "the key [to success] is pre-operative education" of the patient and family. It is essential, however, to also ensure family readiness. If patients and families expect and are prepared to go home two to three days after cardiac surgery, they respond, and patients are able to recover well, despite numerous co-morbid conditions.

This is one among many examples of the current transformation from patient education in the traditional sense to patient "self-management." The underlying premise of self-management is that clinicians can teach patients how to "read" their bodily responses. Patients are then taught specifically how they can assess the stability of their illness or condition (e.g., heart failure) on a daily basis and can learn how to adjust their own therapies (e.g., medications, diet). For most patients, as with many diabetics, patients can better manage their illness when they are fully attuned to their bodily responses. For example, teaching heart failure patients to use daily weights to adjust their diuretics has enabled many to manage their own care, not in isolation of clinicians, but in a truer partnership with them. Dracup (1997) reported that, in these changing times, clinicians need new skills. Patients are more successful self-managing when clinicians first listen to how the patients problem-solve issues that arise and then coach them if needed rather than first telling or teaching patients and families what they must know and do. The result, noted by Dracup, is fewer hospital readmissions. The good and ethical understanding of self-management is founded on a collaborative relationship or partnership with clinicians. Because the word management is gradually replacing our former use of the word "care," the term self-management can easily be misconstrued and taken up in the wrong way, as abandoning patients and families and leaving them to care for themselves in isolation. Self-management can also be misconstrued, as merely shifting the burden of care from the provider to the patient's family. Depending on the patient's illness, family interaction patterns, stability, and functioning can be negatively or even permanently altered. Research is needed to investigate not only the short term, but also long term, effects of these new trends before fully embracing new models of care. However, the current way in which nurses are embodying this concept propels them to work with patients in a way that empowers patients to help jointly bridge the gaps in their care.

NEGOTIATING CONFLICT WITH ANGRY AND DEMANDING PATIENTS AND/OR FAMILIES; FROM CONTROL TO CONNECTION AND UNDERSTANDING

One of the more silent areas of practice has been the extraordinary work and care that strong moral leaders have provided to the most challenging of patients and families. There is abundant literature available on policies and procedures that should be in place and "strategies" and "techniques" needed when dealing with "difficult" patients, that include document, document... and never losing one's temper. (Bryan & Childers, 2004; Haas, Leiser, Magill, & Sanyer, 2005). Many resources exist regarding how to reign in aggressive behaviors and to manage or get control over the behaviors, which include setting limits and using one's authority as foundational for managing them (Manos & Braun, 2006; Morrison, Ramsey & Synder, 2000). But few of those resources really address how to help or comfort the patient or family. Control of the behaviors seems to trump care of the person. On the contrary, expert nurse have taught us very significant perspectives and provided a different means to a substantially improved outcome. Narratives from these strong moral leaders in everyday practice point to how to they empathize, negotiate conflict and intervene in meaningful ways with patients or families in emotionally charged interactions to dissipate anger, aggression, and lack of cooperation (P.H. Kyriakidis, research field notes, May 4, 2007).

One of the clinical and moral leaders is Julie Chappo, a nurse on a medical unit, who was sought out by colleagues to care for the "undesirables." Halpern (2007b) states that "there is virtually no literature in medicine [or nursing] about HOW physicians [or nurses] can empathize with their patients during conflicts that evoke their own anger or other negative emotions" (pg. 696). Expert nurses, on the other hand, provide rich accounts that stir moral imagination about how to empathize in the midst of highly charged situations:

Nurse: I cared for Sandy over the past three years. She was dying of AIDS. She had the label of being a very difficult patient. She had a co-dependent relationship with her family. Sandy was abusive with her mother and felt it was okay because "She is my mom." She adored her father and wanted him to do everything for her.

It difficult to be her nurse because Sandy was in her late 20's and she was dying from a horrible disease. During my first encounter with Sandy, she had horrible diarrhea and couldn't help that she had accidents. I helped her wash up and, on weekends without housekeeping, I cleaned the floor myself. I convinced Sandy that a bedside commode was a good idea. Sandy was protective of others and insisted they use gloves. She didn't want to spread AIDS.

As Sandy's disease progressed she was in the hospital frequently. Recently she was unable to care for herself and was very demanding. At first I crossed my fingers and hoped that she would not be my patient. Nurses wrote on the schedule "Not Sandy." She did not ask, she ordered. She used foul language when I cared for her. She said, "You're mean, you don't know what you are doing!" when being turned. Sandy's bottom and heels were broken down with stage II ulcers and were very sore. She did not want to turn or have her bottom cleaned. Sandy was a challenging, both physically and emotionally. Whenever caring for Sandy, I needed a lot of patience and a caring attitude.

[She had multiple near-death emergencies but bounced back each time.] She was not ready to give up on life. Over time we developed a good relationship. She learned to trust me. She'd say, "I'm glad you're my nurse today." When I had to change her frequently, she still cussed and called out names. I knew her yelling was not personal. Some nurses argued with her and then refused to care for her. I realized she was angry at her disease and the fact that she was dying. She was fighting for some control over her life. I knew I was not going to change the personality she had grown up with. When she cussed and yelled, I told her I didn't appreciate it and I did what I had to do for her. I tried to anticipate her needs for ice, food and pain medication so she wasn't on the light constantly. I involved her family in her care as they were frequently at her bedside.

Sandy talked to her parents about the headstone for her grave and her preferred area of the cemetery. This was hard for me to hear, but it was important for Sandy to discuss. Her parents were not ready for her death. Sandy was to be released home and she fought hard for this. She did not want to go to a nursing home. I knew I was going to be off when she was released. At the end of my shift I said goodbye. I hugged and kissed Sandy on the cheek. Sandy had been particularly abusive that day. I think I surprised her. She looked at me and said, "I don't know how you can care about someone like me, the way I treat you. I guess that's why you are a nurse." I got teary eyed because with Sandy you never knew if this was going to be her last admission. She did make it home one last time for only a few days before she died.

I think caring for Sandy over the last three years has made me a better nurse. I'm able to look past the tasks of constant bed changes and look into the mind and soul of a patient in need of a caring heart. I was able to see past the social labels and see Sandy as a person.

Although there is no literature about how to empathize with a patient who is cursing and verbally abusive, the clinical wisdom is embedded in the practice of expert nurses, easily visible, and can be described. Central to empathetic care is Julie's understanding that Sandy is desperate and in despair. She is dying and she is not ready. This fiercely independent young woman is totally dependent, is unable to control her most basic bodily functions, is humiliated that a nurse is repeatedly cleaning the floor, and releases her rage about her situation to anyone close by. Despite the hostile and abusive manifestations of Sandy's pain, suffering and "fight", Julie deeply understands the very nature of the behavior. The rage is about the disease, not her personally. The maturity and wisdom to make the distinction enable Julie to compassionately care for one she sees is helpless and struggling. Being a strong moral leader, however, does not make the nurse immune to the exhaustion and the emotional effort required to negotiate conflict, particularly when it is unceasing. However, they find renewal (some of which is in the good they accomplish with the patient him/herself) to return, having developed the ability to "look into the mind and soul of patient in need of a caring heart," They have learned, how to look at the person and not just their anger. They understand the patient/family anger and distress as a manifestation of suffering and of as a defense against helplessness and powerlessness.

In a few of these accounts, the moral leader finds that setting a few limits or boundaries are helpful, both for the patient and the nurse. There are situations in which limit setting is called for, but the way in which moral leaders set limits stands in stark contrast to how many enforce limits as a primary strategy to "control" the patient or family and their behaviors or as a way of exerting power and authority. Here, Julie clearly but kindly clarifies with Sandy that swearing at her is not appreciated. Notice Julie is firm but respectful rather than angry, demanding, or dictatorial. Unlike the escalation of the patient's aggressive responses that limit setting often incites, these moral leaders are commonly successful at shifting potential anger toward more amicable interactions. Consequently, moral leaders raise expectations, not only within the healthcare team, but also with patients and families.

What is remarkable is that strong moral leaders consistently describe how they are better nurses for seeing past the labels given to patients, uncovering the fears, and responding to the person with care. It is a moral triumph, and they recognize it as such. Although it is not clear how nurses typically develop this moral compass, we have numerous accounts of how some nurses, at various stages of development, stumble upon or discover that vulnerability, fear, or helplessness as the source of so many angry and demanding behaviors. Katherine Cameron, a telemetry nurse, shares her discovery in the following paradigm case:

Nurse: George was admitted with chest pain, CHF and shortness of breath. He was overweight at 300+ lbs, his hair was disheveled, and his clothes were dirty. He was unkempt, argumentative and angry. He was a diabetic and had a prior heart attack, but his weight indicated that he was not adhering to a diabetic or heart-healthy diet. He refused to answer questions regarding his medical history, and kept yelling, "I am leaving here tomorrow! I am not staying here after tonight!" His wife and daughter were at his bedside, trying to calm him with little effect. He looked a mess but also uncooperative and disgruntled with the staff; the model "difficult" patient.

George arrived arguing. For example, he did not want the aide to tend to him. He did not want to answer questions and deferred them to family. George and his wife were "simple" people, uneducated and unsophisticated. His wife had to answer a lot of the medical questions for me, and it was very difficult. I tried to make him comfortable and asked, "If this is a bad time, should I come back later? "He yelled, "No!" I continued asking medical questions and he would cut me off saying, "I don't know!" Being a diabetic, I thought maybe he was irritable because his blood sugar may be low or he may be hungry, so I asked, "Would you like to eat dinner first, and I can come back later?" to which he again yelled "No!" I decided to move on and ask what medications he took at home, and he barked back "I don't know!" [no matter how he was asked, he yelled back] Looking at his medical history, I knew he had to be on medications. It is my job to make sure that all of his medications from home were ordered, but he refused to cooperate. I could tell that he did not want me there, but also did not want me to come back later, just did not want to answer questions.

[Similarly, George repeatedly refused to have his blood drawn, even after detailed explanation.] After yet another outburst, George was wearing on my patience. After caring for several of "this kind" of patient, I assumed George was one of the same. I thought he was angry at me and my efforts were futile. As he kept refusing one procedure after another, I decided that the most diplomatic thing to do was to tell him, "It's okay if you don't want to have these tests done. You don't have to stay." I offered him the AMA form, and explained politely the many reasons why he should remain in the hospital, but that it was his choice. He only answered me with a grunt, but did not sign out. His wife and daughter came to me at the desk, begging me, "Can't you make him stay?" I explained to them that if he does not want to be helped, I cannot force him to stay. I can try my best to encourage him and teach him, as I have been, but this is not a jail. They were visibly upset that he was going to leave, and I understood.

Not long after talking with his family, they left. George rang his call light. I did not want to answer it. I felt sure he was going to fight with me. When I went into his room he said, "I want to tell you I'm sorry." I was shocked, but accepted his apology. He followed his apology with an emphatic "But I have to be out of here tomorrow!" I thought if he had changed his mind about staying one night, that maybe he would be flexible about staying until he completed all his tests. I replied, "We'll do our best to get you home tomorrow, but let's take it one day at a time and see how you feel..." He cut me off stating again "I have to be out of here tomorrow!" I wondered why he was so insistent on leaving the very next day. What he told me was much unexpected and quite sad. He recently started a new job at a gas station. He had already been out of work for a few weeks due to diabetic complications and could not miss any more. He was at risk for losing his job completely. I offered to write a note to his boss on hospital letter head stating that he was here, but George would not receive pay for any more missed days, and he could not afford to miss a day's income. I researched the Family Medical Leave Act. A company must grant you time off for illness, but it can be unpaid. So unfair. Here was a man who was legitimately sick and needed to stay in the hospital, and yet could not afford to. His family was in a lot of financial difficulty and he absolutely had to get to work the next day. This was why he had been fighting with me. At first George's behavior made me feel frustrated, angry and annoyed, but when I found out why he had been behaving that way, I felt embarrassed.

I redirected my care with him for the night. I flooded the man with information on CHF. I found every pamphlet on heart disease and diabetes and photocopied it for George, his wife and daughter. They had never been told about his CHF and therefore did not know how to avoid the exacerbations. Teaching patients is one of the joys of nursing, and I delight in being able to show patients that they can control their heart disease. I worked diligently to teach George, his wife and daughter all that I could in that short time... [She covered every detail of every teaching point about diabetes, heart failure, heart disease, etc.] ....I overwhelmed George with educational materials that night, but knowing this was my only opportunity to teach him, I did not want to spare a second. I told him if he followed the diet, he would stay out of the hospital. He left the next morning, and I have not seen him since. I hope that my teaching stayed with him, and that he is able to stay healthy and provide for his family.

As a new nurse, I thought that I could change every difficult patient, but I was slapped down by it. Most difficult patients come in argumentative, and leave AMA argumentative. But my experience with George taught me to be different. He changed how I will treat and think of "difficult" patients from now on. Maybe they are just hard working fathers, needing care and education about their disease. I find myself being more patient with "difficult" people now. I take the time to investigate why they are anxious or argumentative and try to calm the anger and work with them. George was certainly not the first difficult patient I took care of, but the first that I saw change. In return he changed my practice, and changed my attitude.

Katherine's open and honest thoughts give insight about how we are socialized to deal with "uncooperative" patients who appear to show no interest in improving their plight or preserving their health. George maked it impossible for Katherine to provide care safely, as he refused to even tell her what medications he was taking. It was terribly frustrating and time consuming, but George forever changed her moral imagination about "difficult" patients. There was so much more at stake for George than was initially imagined. Given what he was trying to cope with (yet another major medical problem, huge financial burdens, the threat of losing his livelihood, etc), does one's diet really matter? His worries were enormous, so answering the same set of medical questions yet again (the same as those answered in the ER) was relatively unimportant. Katherine, full of good intentions, represented the constraint and therefore stressor placed on him to be hospitalized; hence, the conflict. Katherine tries many times to negotiate what she initially perceived the issue to be—the timing—without success.

This exemplar is excellent in that it uncovers what is salient about HOW expert nurses skillfully interact with distressed patients, which is distinctly different from "managing" them or their behaviors (P.H. Kyriakidis, research field notes, May 4, 2007). The turning point is when Katherine <u>fully emotionally engaged</u> and became emotionally attuned to what George was conveying as HIS concern—she recognized that there was more. She heard him but was not clear about the significance because of the emotional nature of his concern. The second important act was that she heard him, his emotional concern, and <u>empathized in a particular way</u>, what Halpern (2001, 2003, 2007b) called clinical empathy; that is, emotional attunement that compels one to become <u>curious</u> about another distinct perspective or, in this case, what is actually troubling the patient. The curiosity to find out more is what we refer to as engaged clinical problem solving and reasoning in an unfolding situation (Chapter 2). Gaining the individual skills detailed throughout this book will not assure the development of expertise unless the clinician fully and emotionally engages in the specific patient and patient situation to guide perceptual acuity, thinking, reasoning, judgment and action. What is revealing is that when Katherine fully engages and is genuinely curious, George senses, not sympathy, but one who is concerned and standing alongside. She has shown herself to be <u>worthy of trust</u>. He recognizes one he can trust and then discloses his <u>fears and helplessness</u>. Notice that this in no way resembles the typical power discourse that predictably and regrettably spirals out of control without strong moral leadership. Notice also that she does "apply" a strategy or technique but instead is genuinely interested, guided by his concerns, and that enables her to become skillfully involved in the situation.

Once George's fear, loss of his job, is disclosed, Katherine responds with every available resource, including herself, to ensure his health and personal needs are met and within his time constraints. What was at one moment an emotionally charged conflict with very difficult, noncompliant, and uncooperative patient in an untenable situation was the next moment a nurse-patient team working feverishly to ensure the patient's physical and social well-being. The above narrative exemplifies that understanding is inextricably linked to, it directs, good clinical and moral judgment and therefore interventions. At times, when very empathetic nurses persistently reach out to patients who are already troubled or marginalized in their lives and society, it is can be much tougher to alter the patient's angry response, even if the clinician's intentions and efforts are silently understood. For a while, it may seem that compassionate efforts go unnoticed and unwelcomed; yet, Sally Kerchner, a hematology oncology clinic nurse, demonstrates how strong persistent moral leadership soothed the patient's fear and eventually opened up a space for connection which was completely missing in Jack's young life. Sally unobtrusively refused to accept his continued alienation:

Nurse: Jack was a 15 year old young man undergoing treatment for osteosarcoma of the leg. He lived in a group home for delinquent teens after being in and out of trouble with the law. His family was not involved at all. He was supposedly involved with a gang.

Jack was big, muscular, and had attitude. It was not a "hard, don't mess with me 'cause I'm bad" attitude but was a "leave me alone, I don't need anyone and I certainly don't trust anyone" attitude. It was the kind of attitude you expect in a teenager who thought he had no family, no friends, and now no future. He came to each clinic visit with a new caregiver as he was moved from group home to foster home, always a new home. The only real consistency he now had in his life was his visits to clinic and admissions to the hospital.

Over several months Jack warmed up at times and talked about sports or school but kept his distance emotionally. He answered questions about his health, such as "was he nauseated? Was he having pain? Had he had any fevers, fatigue?" But he only ever shrugged his head when asked any questions about how he felt about his cancer. When he caught himself letting down his guard too much, he quickly closed down, became quiet, and was unwilling to make eye contact. If I got a smile from him it was a great day. He had an awesome smile and I told him so. He just shrugged it off.

One day, Jack was getting 2 units of PRBCs. At the end of the day, I took over for the early shift nurses. I would finish up Jack's transfusion and send him home. He was on his second unit and the nurse reported that all was well. She had just taken his 15 minute vitals, the pump was set, and Jack was sitting in the dark playing Nintendo. His foster mother would be back in awhile as she had gone to get another child from school. The curtain was pulled around Jack's cubicle. There were no other patients and the only sound came from the video game. I walked over to his cubicle, opened the curtain a bit and said, "It's you and me, Jack. Let me know if you need anything." He never looked up or acknowledged me. I started to clean up the infusion room and do my end of the day tasks.

I heard Jack cough and a few minutes later cough again. Hmmm…. Another minute or so and another cough. I called to him, "Hey Jack, where did you get that cough?" No answer. I walked in to the cubicle, pulled back the curtain and asked him again, but more directly. "Jack, did you have a cough when you came in today?" He said, "No!" He coughed some more. "Are you feeling alright, are you having any difficulty breathing?" "Yeah, I think so. You're trying to kill me is what you're doing!" I reached over, stopped the pump, and turned on the light at the same time. Jack had red, puffy eyes and now was beginning to scratch his arms. "What are you doing to me?" He was getting very agitated. As I grabbed a stethoscope and listened to his lungs, I said, "Jack, I am not trying to kill you. You are having a reaction to the blood transfusion. Just take a deep breath if you can." Jack's breath sounds were okay and he was not coughing any more but not any less either. I hooked him up to the pulse ox and his Sats were 94%. "Okay Jack, your lungs sound okay, your oxygen saturation level is okay so I know you are breathing okay. I'm going to step over to the phone and page the doctor. We need to give you some medicines for this. You're going to be okay." "Yeah, sure!" he said. "Really Jack, you can trust me on this. You are in good hands."

I paged the doctor, grabbed a bag of saline with new tubing, and some Benedryl and Hydrocortisone. I hung the saline and, as I was drawing up the doses of drugs, the doctor arrived. "Jack is having a reaction to his second unit of blood. He has hives, red puffy eyes, and a dry cough. His airway is clear, no wheezing." The doctor agreed and we gave him Benedryl and Hydrocortisone along with the saline and within the hour he was back to normal.

During that hour, Jack and I talked, really talked. He said again, "Man, you were trying to kill me or something." I said, "I bet it felt like that to you. When you have a reaction like that your airway closes a bit and you can feel like you can't breath." "Yeah, why did you do that to me?" "Well, I didn't do it to you. Your body just reacted to that unit of blood. What I did do is stop the blood and give you the treatment that would help you get over the reaction. I did the best thing for you. Remember when I said to you earlier, it's you and me Jack? I meant it. You and me, we're a team and it's all about getting you well." He looked up at me and smiled. "Okay, as long as you don't try to kill me again." I smiled back at him and said, "Fair enough."

Jack and I broke through a barrier that night. He left that night able to trust someone in a time of need. He also left knowing he had a friend, someone he could trust and would understand that he was just kidding every time he came to clinic and said, "There's the nurse who tried to kill me one night."

Wise moral leaders like Sally draw on their vast practical knowledge from life; it is not limited to their clinical knowledge. Knowing what an abandoned and delinquent teen faces, experiences, and must cope with shapes Sally's understanding of and skillful involvement with Jack. Notice that she does not need patience to "manage" or "deal" with Jack. She is, from the first, emotionally attuned and empathetic with how hard his life has been, to the point that she discerns the difference in his attitude as isolation and vulnerability rather than aggression. Notice she too embodies the requisite curiosity to delicately discover how he is coping and to understand the world from his eyes. His unresponsiveness does not equate with an inability to sense her persistent care and concern. Although their interaction was initially limited, Sally is an expert clinician who is fully engaged and therefore is constantly peripherally aware of cues like a cough while busy doing other things. Engagement and attunement are central to recognizing early warning signals of a complication, in this case, a life-threatening reaction (Benner, Tanner, & Chesla, 2009). Sally's empathy, respectful comportment, her authenticity, and skillful interactions stand in stark contrast to accounts where conflict dominates, where the clinicians' negative emotions (dislike, frustration, anger, detachment, aversion) cloud or impede their attentiveness, judgment and response. Even when Jack repeats "Were you trying to kill me?", Sally hears the fear and responds to his concern rather than the potentially inflammatory words and accusation spoken. She is fully attuned to his meaning and doesn't get distracted by his delivery. It is an outstanding example of what we mean by expert ethical comportment.

For Sally, caring for a challenging patient is very familiar. Her experience has enabled her to refine her skills of attunement, her ability to "read" the patient's verbal and nonverbal cues, and her ability to smoothly interact in negative emotion-laden situations. Sally understands Jack's nonverbal communications (his avoidance, tone, attitude, etc.) as hints that he is not ready to disclose what concerns him. In response, she continues to provide verbal and nonverbal communication that she is concerned and they are a team.

It is important for developing nurses, educators, preceptors, and coaches of all sorts to be cognizant that empathy, curiosity, and skillful involvement are all skills that can be taught and learned. Practice, such as role playing or group dialogue, based on actual situations can be invaluable for skill rehearsal. Coaching in the moment or during the care of angry patients or families can teach context based responsiveness and enable the development of flexible styles and interactions. Reflection and debriefing after situations can greatly enhance learning when the nurse is most engaged.

We have intentionally included the extensive situational details from strong moral leaders' narratives so that the reader can imaginatively enter the situation and, as much as possible, be challenged by the nuances and ambiguity, and understand in context how the expert nurse skillfully interacted and responded, and how the patient's fears and helplessness were allayed so that, for Jack, "attitude" and avoidance were no longer the norm. Each of the narratives can serve as a source of learning, reflection, and group dialogue for students and for nurses in practice. The voice of the strong moral leader differs from much of the literature because it is from an engaged or situated stance of being in the situation and guided by moral reasoning, judgment, and interaction. Knowing additional safety measures is important as a backup (rather than first line) if all else fails or if the situation turns violent; however, it is astonishing that strong moral leaders do not have those kinds of situations arise in their practice, unless they enter in the midst of one. In the care of this particular group, clinical wisdom is a better educational guide than the current "science" which focuses on strategies; techniques; guidelines; and methods of psychological, pharmacological, and physical control.

When caring for angry and aggressive patients or families, as when caring for any person, strong leaders flexibly interact with varying styles and comportment that are authentic but also attuned to the patient's receptivity. At times, the expert nurse has only a vague idea HOW to interact upon first meeting a particular patient but makes an attempt. What we know is that a clinician's emotional engagement engenders more trust (Frankel, 1995; Halpern 2001, 2003, 2007b), improves communications, decreases the patient's angst, and leads to better outcomes (Halpern, 2007b; Ptacek & Eberhardt, 1996). This is exemplified in the following narrative in which Amanda Savage, a strong moral leader on a medical-surgical unit, receives an all-too-familiar report about a gruff, difficult patient:

> **Nurse:** I cared for a very challenging patient who required a lot of thought, physical care as well as mental care, but Mr. K gave me a great gift.
>
> Carly, a newer nurse, took the call and told me I was getting a transfer from the step down unit. The reporting nurse told Carly that the patient was non-compliant, dirty and just not going to do what he needs to do. I asked Carly what else was said in report and she stated, "his sugars are high, had a stroke, blood pressure is high and he told them downstairs that, as soon as he gets out, he doesn't care, he is going to do what he wants." I told her "there is probably more to the story." I asked what they were doing for his high blood pressure and what was his last value? She "did not remember to ask nor was it reported." I asked what his last sugars were. She did not know.
>
> When Mr. K arrived on the floor, he was a large man, heavy in the middle. He had not shaved in quite some time, had not had his hair cut in a long while and generally looked unkempt. He looked pale, tired, and sad but he also looked embarrassed. I introduced myself, did my welcome to "club med" (medical unit). A gentleman accompanied Mr. K to our unit. I explained to Mr. K that I would do a quick physical assessment, take his vital signs and then go take off his orders. I did and then went out to find his chart. As I reviewed his chart there was more to the story. In fact, Mr. K was a 72 y/o, admitted with a blood sugar of 500 + mg/dl, and a new stroke. His past medical history was hazy as he "does not like to go to doctors" but he may have a "touch of the blood pressure." His blood pressures ran in the 170's/90's consistently.

Of course, I could see that this man looked like he did because he felt awful. [In further discussion with Carly] I said, "would you feel like taking care of yourself if your sugar was 500 and your blood pressure was very high, not to mention you were having a stroke?" I must have turned a wonderful shade of purple because for the first time Carly looked at me and said, "Are you mad?" I said, "No, I am not mad at you. I am mad at less-than-sensitive people."

I went back into Mr. K's room. There was something about him that "called" to me. He looked like I felt. I walked in and said hello again. I sat on the bed and said to him, "you have had a tough couple of weeks." He said, "yes." Then he asked how long he had to stay at the hospital. I told him [jokingly], "that depends on how interesting you are." I said, "I am taking care of an interesting man across the hall and I want him to stay, so if you are not interesting, you will get to go home soon." He and his friend laughed. He asked me what made that other man interesting. I said, "I will tell you what I can if you tell me something about yourself." His friend said, "Mr. K has been my sponsor for 10 years." I asked Mr. K how long he had been sober and he told me 40 years. I then said, "okay. That does it. You have to stay. You qualify as interesting." They both laughed. I congratulated both of them on their sobriety. Mr. K and his friend went on to talk about how they sponsor at least 3-4 people at a time and how fulfilling it is. Mr. K asked if he would be able to continue to do that and I said, "sure, you just need some fine tuning." Mr. K looked skeptical. Carly had walked into the room and stayed to listen to the conversation. I found out that Mr. K served in the Army and was stationed at Fort Dix during the 1960's. He talked about how he liked to go and do things but had not felt well enough. Finally he said, "you never told me what made that other man so interesting." I said, "I can tell you this. He served in the South Pacific during WWII, participated in the battle of Iwo Jima, and just missed Okinawa because the ship he was on had problems running. But that was not the most interesting thing." So then Mr. K says, " ok, I'll bite." I said, "he is a nice man and likes to talk to me." Mr. K says, "you're never going to let me leave, are you?" I said, "yes I will, but until you do, we can have a conversation?" It was the end of our shift so I told Mr. K I would see him tomorrow. Carly walked out of the room with me. I looked at her and asked her what she thought. She said, "he seems nice enough."

The next morning Mr. K was lying in bed again looking sad. I asked if there was anything he needed and he said, "I would love a shower." I said, "come and stand up with me. Let me see how stable you are." He attempted to stand independently but was very unstable; however, once he was up he was okay. I worried about fatigue in the shower so I told him he could shower but I needed to set up a shower with a chair. I went to the shower stall with chair access and found the showerhead broken. I then went across the hall and tried to fit the shower chair in those 2 stalls and that was not happening. I was uncomfortable bringing him into the shower but knew he wanted one so badly. So, I went back and I told him that I was going to wheel him to the shower and then would assistance getting him into the stall but that I had to stay. He agreed. So, I wheeled him over to the shower, took off his 1 liter of oxygen and, with help from a peer, got him into the shower. It was an iffy thing but between Mr. K and I, we managed to wash his hair, his body and gave him just a few minutes to stand underneath the warm spray. I then pulled on the cord, enlisted my peer to help me get him out of the shower, dried off and into the wheelchair. Graceful we were not and all of us found the humor in it. I was drenched but it was worth it. I then wheeled him to the room and asked him if he was fond of that beard. He said he hated it but was too sick to shave. So, I spend 30 minutes and 5 razors to give him a clean shave. After the shave, I asked him about his hair, as I had combed it and it was long. He said he hadn't felt well enough to go the barber but he normally wore it short. I asked, "do you trust me?" He paused and said, "well yeah, maybe." I said, " when my eldest son was 2-3 years old, I wanted to save money so I tried to cut his hair. Let's just say, I have not cut any hair since then nor am I allowed to have scissors in my hand when in close proximity to hair, but for you....I think I'll try again." He laughed and said, "why not, if worse comes to worse, you can just shave it off." So, I trimmed his hair and, if I do say so myself, it was not too bad. When I was done cleaning up all the hair and I looked over at him, there were tears in his eyes. Before he said anything, I said, "thank you for letting me take care of you today. You really made my day." His tears never fell, nor did mine, he nodded his head and said, "I understand my diabetes and blood pressure are bad." I said, "yup! Are you ready for some speed education?" He said, "yeah, I am." I sat on the bed and Mr. K and I had a conversation about diabetes, high blood pressure and stroke. I told him the dietitian would come in and talk with him and help him understand the diet. Also she would give pamphlets. I then told him that, by following the diabetic diet, he would be helping his high blood pressure and decrease his risk for stroke. He said, "they are related?" I said, "yup" and proceeded to tell him how and gave the stroke handbook which included blood pressure management. I asked him if he thought he could follow the diet, do the insulin and take his medications. He said, "if you asked me yesterday, I would have said no. But today I feel more human. So, yes, I think I can." I then nodded my head.

Mr. K was discharged the next day; all consults completed, home services set up to provide PT and nursing services. I went in to say good-bye and let him know he had resources so that he could continue to be a resource for others.

I saw Carly and just kept thinking, "please God, one day let her have a Mr. K and truly appreciate them." I did make a point of telling Carly that "report is a wonderful thing but sometimes things are not as they appear to be. This man was not non-compliant, dirty, etc. He was scared, he was embarrassed at how he looked and he was ill. Mr. K was ready to listen when he felt 'human.' Remember that when you get another report like the one you got on Mr. K."

Not every nurse has or needs Amanda's style, humor or comportment, but this exemplar enriches one's thinking, clinical and moral imagination, and understanding about what is possible with humor, kindness, connection and understanding about the patient's feelings and coping. The nurse is honest, and respectful. She does not engage in placation or manipulation. One does not need well refined humor, but an emotionally intelligent "read" of the situation with a patient-specific kind of witty response can often lower the defenses after the patient recognizes good intentions. Humor is not used to avoid the issue; humor enables the initial connection. Mr. K has no trouble sensing Amanda's notion of good. She comes in, sits on his bed, looks right at him while chatting and appears to have nothing more important in the world to do other than get to know him. Her moral judgment, comportment and action are so contrary to the alienation he experienced prior to transfer that he is enticed to engage. Sincere interest in Mr. K, his commitments, and accomplishments, coupled with an honest acknowledgement of rough his hospitalization has been, help him reenter the world and ask for a shower. For Mr. K, the shower signals the end of his immobilization, his incapacitation to do anything. Amanda capitalizes on this turn to cut his beard and hair which Mr. K experienced as a rebirth. This strong clinical leader empowers Mr. K to once again participate in his own care with hopes of continuing his life's work.

The most significant lesson Amanda points to is that recognition practices, or the moral commitment to see another as a person, however we find them, can restore a world almost lost. Mr. K had disengaged from the world, withdrawn into hopelessness, dwelled in despair, and resisted the constant intrusion of care providers "telling" him what he must do and having things "done to him" with seemingly little concern about what was happening to him, the person. Being recognized as a worthy soul can rescue the patient from the depths, not for the purpose of having the patient simply act nicer to staff, but because preserving personhood is a good that is worth preserving, physically and mentally. Patients who are sick and, even temporarily, lose their independence and therefore identity, at times, feel and are quite vulnerable. Being recognized as a person, rather than an illness or "issue," is liberating and creates possibility. This narrative is a stunning example of the primacy of caring and how transformative caring practices can be when patients and families appear angry, gruff, and cantankerous. Compassionate and honest recognition of the pain and suffering, the loss, and sometimes embarrassment allows a patient to see someone willing to "stand alongside" and sincerely help rather than force therapies and impose change in their already burdened lives. As is apparent, time is sometimes needed to personalize care, particularly for those who feel so outcast. However, managers should understand that it is far more efficient, effective, and humane to support the time infrequently needed to care for angry and demanding patients in ways similar to Amanda's exemplar than the enormous time and resources consumed by dealing with angrier patients when their situations spiral out of control.

The experiential and moral wisdom gained from learning that "there is probably more to the story" provokes outrage after Amanda easily finds out why the patient feels so awful and refuses to do much. The information is right there in the chart. So, she additionally acts as a moral leader, compelled to shape the experience, understanding, and thinking of newer, impressionable nurses. This kind of leadership, coached and extended into the practices of others, holds the promise that future patients who display stressed behaviors will have their fears and helplessness discovered and resolved. Strong moral leadership further averts the possibility that the nurses she mentors will disengage from angry or demanding patients, abandoning them emotionally and exacerbating the fears that are manifested. Instead, she role models hearing the patient, responding to their concerns (in this situation with humor), engages the patient in the "fun," generates curiosity, cares for the physical body to rehumanize the man, revives his spirit (and her own), and creates reentry into a world of concern where he can care and learn to care for himself. This transformation is not as easy as the exemplar may indicate, but it is not as hard as many imagine. Courage, commitment, care, and empathy are all skills that are needed and can be learned. Narratives such as this are excellent sources for reflection, group dialogue, and creating a culture and ethic of care and responsibility. For these patients, it often just takes one nurse to begin a change.

In the hectic pace of care settings today, it is easy to overlook that there is often another side to a story. In the next exemplar, Robin Watson, a medical-surgical nurse, finds herself morally outraged after several incidents where not knowing the whole story leads to insensitivity and becomes debilitating to the team and patient. Halpern (2007b) described how clinicians' negative emotions toward a patient are sensed, have contagious effects for everyone, and can escalate conflict and fuel a highly charged situation. This strong moral agent and leader repeatedly takes a stand for Kate, a patient whose disease has taken control of her life, to at the very least treat the patient with respect and dignity:

Nurse: Kate has Huntington's chorea. She was admitted to our floor after being homeless and acting out. The ER unsuccessfully tried to get her into a psychiatric facility. Huntington's chorea is a hereditary disease that affects the nervous system. It causes mental degenerative changes, emotional disturbances, loss of self control and severe behavioral issues. There is no cure and only medication helps with the behaviors.

One day, Kate was upset because she wanted a cigarette. She had no concept of time or the limits the unit was trying to set with her. She didn't care. She wanted a cigarette and now. The staff explained that she could go in a half an hour. Her behavior began to escalate, she threw coffee at a nurse and a "code white" was called…Kate was restrained and medicated as a result of her behavior. My first meeting with Kate was at the "code white". [Kate needed a 1:1 sitter every one of the 35 days of her stay, with no discharge in site.]

Through conversations with Kate, I found that she was finishing her studies to become a professor. She was in her early fifty's and her Mom and brother both died of Huntington's chorea. She saw firsthand the devastation it creates and was concerned for her son since it is a hereditary disease. She expressed her anger of the disease because Kate knew firsthand what was in store for her, there was no escaping this disease, and her future was bleak. When Kate was calm she was intelligent and very pleasant. When she was not, she was assaultive and verbally abusive. My frustration in taking care of Kate was not Kate. It was with certain events that occurred. One in particular was when Kate refused one day to come back from outside after having three cigarettes. I went to the code white that was called and we assembled around her. I was talking to her trying to deescalate her and I overheard a security guard say, "Let's just restrain her and get it over with". I turned and said, "Excuse me. That comment was uncalled for." After we got her to her room, I spoke to the Nursing supervisor and also conveyed my concerns to our Associate Chief Nursing Officer. I was appalled at the guard's lack of empathy and, if she had heard, his comments would have made the situation much more difficult for us to handle.

Over the course of weeks, Kate continued to decline, becoming more assaultive and verbally abusive. One day another code white was called. As we gathered near her room, Kate was melodically singing the staffs' names and using profanities in a rhyme. The more they asked her to stop the louder she became. As we waited for some medication to take effect, several coworkers were talking about Kate. [what they wished they could do to her]. Another nurse agreed and they continued voicing anger at having to deal with Kate. My first reaction [thinking to myself] was, "I can't believe these nurses, my coworkers and friends, would be so unsympathetic. She can't control this disease. I could only think to myself with each encounter with Kate 'Thank God above this is not me or anyone I know or love.' How could my coworkers be so cruel? She can't help how she is." I looked at them both and said nicely "Obviously you have no idea what the disease Huntington's chorea is or you would not be talking like that. I suggest you go and research it some more. She can't help it". They both looked at me and didn't say anymore. Nothing more was said about this incident but I did notice since these staff nurses have been more patient and there has been less verbal anger voiced to other staff nurses about Kate.

> I believe as a nurse it is our duty to treat all patients with dignity and respect despite their disease. [A major frustration was having a psychiatric patient on a med-surg unit where nurses were poorly prepared for multiple behavioral issues. The nurse was also frustrated that staff was completely unsympathetic to her and her disease process.] I spoke to the psych nurse liaison and discussed with her my frustrations and concerns on how to deal with the patient but also my coworkers reactions to this patient. She talked with as many staff members as she could to educate them about this disease and more importantly the behavioral issues which were hard to deal with. Why was she so behaved with me and not them? As time went on I noticed a very positive change in my coworkers and how they were dealing with Kate.
>
> My frustration was that I felt my coworkers were missing Kate as a person. I felt they overlooked that fact and were treating the disease, not her as a human being, a person with a disease she had no control over. We as a staff and team were beginning to learn together how to care for Kate more effectively. I am proud to be among my coworkers to have had this experience and feel it has made us all better nurses but also better care givers.

Robin's anger with team members prompts her to take strong moral action, to address higher expectations, and to ensure moral behavior on the team's part. In extreme situations like this, with no end in sight and without requisite skills to care or cope well, emotional tension and frustration are human. However, deterioration into a power discourse with and open rejection of a patient, particularly one who is not mentally competent, is intolerable and threatening. A power struggle will predictably exacerbate the patient's fear that no one cares or can be trusted, reinforcing the helplessness and the need to fight and fight hard for what they need. Anyone who has been a recipient of care may wholly understand the uneven playing field, fear, and worry when a caring intent is missing. Control predictably elicits many of the behaviors labeled as "difficult," "challenging," or "angry."

Robin brokers the misunderstanding by the staff about Kate's behavior by marshalling a knowledgeable resource to educate the staff about a horrible, fatal disease. It is a moral judgment, not simply a clinical one. Kate is hopeless and terrified by this unbearable disease that has already destroyed her social and emotional life. Robin's empathy is exactly what she expresses to her team members and presses them to imagine the same. She raises consciousness and raises expectations about the unit's culture of care and for their performance. There are professional boundaries just as there are behavioral boundaries. Both had been violated. They all learn and create a more positive caring environment for Kate. This kind of experiential learning at the individual and team levels makes a self-improving practice possible.

There are, on occasion, clinicians who are especially challenged by angry, manipulative, or hostile patients and families, given their own personal backgrounds. They may find themselves unable to provide the needed kind of care because they actually fear the anger, making it very hard for that nurse to see anger as a manifestation of fear, hopelessness, or helplessness. These clinicians may look to colleagues for assistance as they work to develop the skills needed to care in helpful ways for diverse populations.

In more extreme situations of breakdown (see Chapter 11), where the situation does not go well, despite how courageously the moral leader skillfully acts, the patient's or family's trust may have become irreparable and even understandably destroyed so that only consistent, intense, and persistent compassionate interaction is accepted. Although extreme, this kind of situation is unfortunately not unfamiliar. In the last exemplar, Robin became morally outraged about the undignified treatment of a vulnerable and mentally incapacitated patient. One can therefore imaginatively enter the next exemplar as Toby's grandmother (family) to understand how much more fiercely protective she was after Toby was harmed from a medication error. Laura Alter, who was a neonatal ICU nurse, shares one of her many stories about caring for difficult patients and families. Even though her colleagues try to establish better interactions with the grandmother, nothing short of expertise was successful in this situation:

Nurse: Dee, my best friend, called me at home asking a favor. She wanted my help on the team to care for our new baby. This was a complex family situation and our manager wanted to establish a care team as soon as possible and Dee was to be his primary. Toby was transferred from NICU. His family was kicked out of the Ronald McDonald house because his father had allegedly stolen a large screen TV and other items. Grandmother, Barbara, the main caregiver, had also had an altercation in newborn ICU (NBICU) with a respiratory therapist. Security was called. Now, Grandma was at the bedside 24 hours a day. Deep down I was a little nervous but up for the challenge and agreed with a yes and a quick prayer.

On Friday, I met Toby for the first time. He had multiple congenital defects including clubfeet and congenital heart defects (double outlet right ventricle). He already had many surgeries including a BT shunt, a tracheotomy and a G-tube. He needed more heart surgeries and was unable to weaned off the ventilator at this time. From report, he was ready to go home from NBICU on CPAP and was in the midst of training when he had a bad "code" and thus rebought himself the ventilator. The altercation in NBICU happened after the code and apparently Grandma and Mom were not happy at all. The night nurse told me that Grandma had been appropriate but that she was now awake and pacing nervously because Toby had a fever.

My approach with Grandma was my normal approach with a new family. I am upfront, open, and honest. I informed her of everything I was doing, asked her input on what Toby's norm was, and how she liked him to be cared for. I always try to see the good in each person and form my own opinions. I recalled how I had been pleasantly surprised in the past when "nightmare" families often turned out to be simply "scared/anxious." I learned over the years not to prejudge. With this in mind, I walked in to the room and introduced myself. Barbara was in her late 30's, not much older than myself, and greeted me with her hands on her hips. She was worried about Toby's fever and wanted to know what I would do about it. Toby was a chubby little 5-month-old with an Afro almost as big as he was. He resembled Don King. He had a little scrunched up face and a crooked little scowl. I couldn't tell who looked angrier, he or his grandma. I spoke to Barbara about what was normal for Toby and had she noticed any other signs that he was getting sick? "Toby is new to us and you know him best. Anything you can tell me that would be helpful to get to know him, please let me know." I told her what I was assessing as I checked him and that, although his temp was up (39°C), he was pink, his O2 sats were good, he was not working hard to breathe, etc. I explained that "his heart rate might be elevated because of the fever, but I will keep an eye on him and let the physicians know. When I let the resident know about the fever, he might want to do some lab work, etc, to rule out an infection." Barbara seemed pleased and I could see her visibly relax a little. I asked Barbara if she would like to stay in the room while I drew the labs. She said yes; she would help me hold him. She asked if I was any good and I told her that if I could not get it after one or two sticks I would ask someone else, but that I usually had good luck.

After labs were sent, Toby received some Tylenol and his temperature stabilized. The remainder of the day went well and Barbara remained friendly. I stopped in frequently to check in on both Toby and Barbara to make sure that they were both okay. Later that day I attended the Employee Assistance meeting with my co-workers. Although I felt I had already taken their philosophy of building trust and approaching in a respectful manner, I thought the meeting was beneficial to our staff.

With that began a relationship that for many on the unit pushed their patience to the limit and made them question if they wanted to still be a nurse. Interestingly enough it was one of my most rewarding patient and family experiences. Looking back I have to admit that one had to have a great deal of patience working with Barbara. She was at times demanding, aggravating, and sometimes just plain mean to our staff. Each and every nurse had a nickname (although I never heard mine nor would it have changed the way I felt about her) and every little thing became a fight. For example, Dee had suctioned blood-tinged secretions from Toby's trach and thus became "the Bleeder". The dietician who faithfully measured Toby on a length board every other week became known as the "Board Lady". The list continued. Many of the staff felt resentment and many battles occurred over whose turn it was to take care of him. Even Dee had enough and called me to take over as his primary. She was very intimidated by Barbara's behavior. I agreed because I got along well with Barbara and Toby was no trouble at all. I saw something that my co-workers could not seem to see.

First of all, I put up with Barbara's idiosyncrasies because I saw how much she loved her grandson and she was only trying to advocate for him. No one could care for him up to her standards, and I could see that she kept him meticulously clean, did all of his care well, and asked appropriate questions. Thus, I respected her and I think the feeling was mutual. You just had to see beyond the theatrics of her verbal outbursts such as "this is trifling'" to see that she was really there for Toby and, bottom line, that was what mattered. She had heart deep down inside. She respected and demanded people to be upfront and honest with her.

My co-workers almost seemed to avoid the room affectionately known as "the cave", because they didn't know how to please Barbara. Barbara liked to sleep in late and had Toby on her own schedule. This was different as a majority of the staff are generally "used" to being in control. People seemed to pick battles with Barbara on little things, such as how to warm up his formula, how she liked his diapers changed. I allowed her the control in these situations, because deep down with Toby being so sick, that was the only thing she could control. I attempted to bring staff along with my thinking but they disliked her so much they could not. She and I became a team and, although she never left his bedside and she was always protective of him, we worked together.

I remember asking if I could hold and rock him one afternoon, because normally she or her daughter Amber were the only ones who did. She was very protective and rarely handed him over. She told me she was pleased that I had asked and I rocked him while she took a short break. I brought my camera in for photo sessions, such as Easter, when he got a new outfit, or when his hair was braided. Grandma and Mom delighted in dressing up their little man.

Amber often visited in the evenings along with Toby's dad. Toby's dad was a gentle giant. He had a hair-do similar to Toby's and I could see the resemblance. They were involved but not like Barbara. She was definitely the main caregiver and the one in control. It was interesting to watch the family dynamics between Barbara and

Amber, because they picked at each other, but it was a strong family of women. Barbara talked about her mother often and said that none of the women took any lip in her family. Every once in awhile she would get me on the phone to talk to great grandma who seemed as spunky as Barbara.

Barbara and I spent hours talking as we cared for Toby. One day she finally told me about the event in NBICU. Although Toby had plenty of issues prior to the code, he had weaned off the ventilator and was close to going home. One day a nurse in NBICU gave Toby a potassium overdose and he coded. She was made aware of the mistake but felt people were not completely honest with her about what happened. She decided from that point forward she would not leave his side and would watch everything people did. I told her I understood why it was hard for her to trust leaving Toby in anyone else's care and that he was so lucky to have someone like her for a grand-mother. And I truly meant it.

I could tell that Barbara's trust in me had grown as that conversation revealed a lot to me of what her "toughness/attitude" was truly about. I knew that she trusted me because of her willingness to share with me her feelings…..Resentment among the staff continued to fester. I found that I was soon under attack because people [assumed I had to be] undermining them. It made me very sad that there were only a couple of people who saw the true Barbara. Barbara learned early on that I played no part in to her making fun of or belittling my co-workers. She stopped. If she did start, I just gave her a look and she would say, "I know, I know, I'll be quiet". I reassured my co-workers that I was supportive of the team.

I was honored that, one weekend, Barbara asked if I was working dayshift and actually left and went home for the day. She said, "you can spoil him all you want. I know he is in good hands."… I was pleased that she had actually gone home for the first time.

A few months later, Toby was finally ready to go home. Barbara and Amber packed him up in his wagon ventilator in tow and rolled out to the outside world. I was happy that the day had finally arrived for the family. The staff on my unit was more relieved that they were just gone. Shortly after, I was not surprised that Barbara fired her home nursing agency and they were caring for Toby on their own. However, I reassured the physicians and staff that Barbara would take excellent care of him. And she did. [Barbara called Laura during each clinic visit and they stayed in touch. Sadly, Toby was not able to endure the eventual critical surgeries. Laura continued to be a major support for the family until after Toby's death.]

Laura has most evidently become expert in caring for angry, demanding and formi-dable patients and families. She, like other expert moral leaders, was willing to care for these patients, so her peers routinely "turfed" these patients to her, missing the opportunity to learn. Because Laura has vast experience caring for so many diverse "difficult" patients, she has developed expertise in doing so. Laura has developed a genuine curiosity when car-ing for patients and families which is reinforced by her keen perception of the family's meticulous care of the baby. It's hard to have an aversion to a person who loves so deeply and is so strongly committed to a loved one. Her empathy sets her up to notice the heart and soul of Barbara, for Barbara to recognize her respect and admiration, and for a strong con-nection to develop.

Laura's moral stance with Barbara calls for reflection. In a unit where no other clini-cian was welcomed or trusted in Toby's room, despite their good intentions, what made the care Laura provided distinctly different? Laura reveals, in the way she respected and negotiated with Barbara, that she was a guest in Barbara and Toby's home. This moral leader understood and enabled Barbara to have the control she needed to provide care for Toby herself, as if she were in her own home caring for him. Laura doesn't even attempt to hold Toby without politely requesting permission. Laura recognized and conveyed the authoritative knowledge Barbara had gained and therefore the position she had earned in deciding exactly how to care for Toby's routine needs. Her recognition of Barbara's significance in Toby's life was key.

The development of expertise in working with angry, hostile, or difficult people has been stifled, if not derailed, in part by the nursing diagnosis or label of "ineffective coping." Ineffective misleads developing nurses to imagine that the issue is primarily a behavior problem. In response, nurses are taught to help the patient identify their own strengths, examine their attitudes about required lifestyle changes, help them set goals, point out maladaptive behaviors, and the like. How could one possibly imagine that Barbara, in the above exemplar, was <u>ineffectively</u> coping when she was fiercely protecting Toby from further debilitating harm after a trusted care provider overdosed him with potassium and caused him to code? Accident or not, recognizing what Barbara was trying to cope with, amidst the air of deception and Toby's complications, is more than understandable. She, like many patients and families, are forced to cope with the multiple burdens that can result in extreme behaviors when additionally threatened. She is fighting for a beloved's life. The "cave" helps paint a clearer picture of what Barbara was coping with and should help enlighten new perspectives, redefine this "difficult patient" problem, and spur new ways of intervening. A more accurate diagnosis may be "coping with overwhelming fear/stress, excessive burden or extreme vulnerability." The language itself reframes and redirects thinking, judgment, and interventions in a productive and more accurate way. Not every situation can be negotiated well or favorably, but the conflict with a majority of "difficult" (overwhelmingly stressed, excessively burdened, fearful, or extremely vulnerability) patients and families can be remedied.

Halpern (2009) agreed that extreme behaviors can understandably evoke the desire to flee, to transfer the patient to another's care, or, at least, tame the situation. Many of these patients cause some degree of distress. However, when clinicians have an aversion toward the patient, their dislike actually reinforces the problematic aggressive behaviors (Degnin, 2009; Halpern, 2009). For some clinicians, it is far too difficult to empathize with patients during a heated conflict. It is however likely that clinicians can learn to empathize and "can cultivate an ongoing practice of engaged curiosity" (Halpern, 2007, p. 698) in normal everyday care so that empathy becomes more of an embodied response, a habit, that can be expressed during conflict.

Challenging patients do not always present with anger, obstinance, and aggression. There are patients with particular types of psychiatric disorders that frustrate clinicians because of their manipulative, dependent, anxious, or delusional behaviors. Each is accompanied by different kinds of emotional and clinical demands on the clinician. Rosemary Melton, an oncology clinic nurse, shares her challenge with one of the most complex patients she ever cared for:

Nurse: I cared for a 70 year old lung cancer patient. The experience was extraordinary and memorable. Mary and her husband John were a long-term couple, childless, had limited contact with other people, and had no support except each other. Mary came to the [oncology] clinic when they found multiple nodules on her lungs, which made her condition grave. During the consulting interview, Mary shared with the doctor and me that she had obsessive compulsive disorder (OCD). She said that she does "not leave her house except for doctors' appointments." When she returns home, "I have to change all my clothing and wash myself entirely. This is just exhausting for me, but I just have to do it."…

The doctor outlined her chemotherapy treatment plan. She expressed concern about the outcome, but I could see that she was as concerned about the impact her OCD would have on her ability to get through the treatment. She feared that the [exhausting] treatment "wouldn't do any good anyway." Her husband John understood her concerns and told Mary that he would stay with her, "as he always does," to provide help with her OCD needs, if she agreed to try. At this point I knew that John had to be part of Mary's treatment. I told Mary that John could stay with her "even if all the treatment stations were taken." I was now committed to allowing John to stay in the treatment room despite the very tight space. She accepted that the treatments were the only way to extend her life with some quality. The doctor left, telling her she could start treatments whenever it was convenient.

As we walked out to set up an appointment, I began to understand the major challenge I faced to keep Mary committed to treatment. To care for the whole patient, I would have to anticipate many of her extraordinary needs; otherwise, she would fail to complete treatment. Because Mary adamantly refused any outside help [coupled with] having seen the way they looked at each other, I knew that Mary and John's relationship would be critical to successful implementation of her treatment plan. I also realized that I had to do more research on OCD to better understand how to help Mary and John.

Days prior to her visit I spent time researching OCD. My research gave me a fuller understanding of the special anxiety Mary experienced and that would intensify with treatment as she became part of the cancer community. Anticipating Mary's first treatment appointment, I began to plan her visit. I knew I needed to provide a way for her husband to stay with her for emotional and physical support. Because she could not touch anything others had touched, I knew I had to make her treatment chair a "contact-free" place for her to sit. The chair needed to be entirely covered with fresh linen; otherwise, Mary would not sit. I knew she would eat lunch during treatment and need to go the bathroom. Each problem presented unique challenges. I elicited suggestions from Mary about how she could use the bathroom. I experienced anxiety because I knew that if I could not meet these challenges, Mary would likely reject treatment, and her chances of surviving beyond a few weeks or months would not be very good.

As we walked down the hall for Mary's first treatment, I reviewed what to expect. I was somewhat anxious myself, but satisfied that I had anticipated and planned for problems we would face. Mary expressed her OCD-driven concerns: "I can't sit in the chair. I can't use the bathroom. I can't eat off the plates or use the utensils." I asked another nurse to <u>completely</u> cover the treatment chair before Mary's arrival, but the foot rest, understandably, was uncovered. Mary became upset again and repeated her distressed list of concerns. I soon learned that whenever her boundaries were threatened, she said, "You know I can't do that." I was to hear this phrase frequently during the coming weeks.

"How about if I put fresh linen over the whole chair? Will that be okay?" I asked. She responded, "It was just washed, right?" I assured her that we would never reuse the linen. She accepted my suggestion and carefully sat down in the chair. Before we began treatment, she needed to go to the bathroom, which tested our plan for bathroom visits. We had discussed how she would go without sitting on the seat and how we would take care of her hygiene needs, but didn't anticipate her not pushing the IV pole. "You know I can't do that," she said. To involve her husband, I asked him to push the pole and open the door. Once inside, Mary used the toilet but could not touch the toilet paper, so I tended to hygienic needs. Visits to the bathroom soon became routine. Our lack of understanding surfaced again, when her lunch arrived without the disposable plates and utensils I requested. A quick trip to the cafeteria took care of the problem.

Finally, actual treatment began. Starting the IV was less of a problem than I anticipated. After showing Mary the kit with all disposable materials and gloves I needed to put on, she was comfortable. I was greatly relieved that she had "great veins" (for IV infusion). Mary needed blood pressure and lung checks during her infusion. When I explained this to her, she sought the support of her husband, "What am I going to do, John?" Throughout, John's response was to smile and say, "You know, Mary, you have to let her do it." I suggested and she agreed that a blood pressure cuff on top of her sleeve and stethoscope outside of her jersey back was okay. During her treatment, I heard Mary's OCD reaction, "You know I can't do that," repeated many more times, but I knew that I always had to think of a way that we could.

We successfully completed the first and second treatments following this same pattern of behaviors. But during our third session, we experienced an amazing breakthrough. After a time, John said, "I think I'll sit in the hall for a while. Is that okay, Honey?" Mary responded, "I guess so." Mary let her husband leave the room and allow me to care for her alone. I felt that I had moved a mountain. I was awed by the amount of trust she had placed in me. I was so honored.

Mary completed her chemotherapy treatments....A month later, Mary and John came back for a monthly check up. When I saw Mary, I greeted her, "Mary it's good to see you." As I spoke, I moved to hug her, and, surprisingly, Mary's hands rose to return the hug. She actually touched me with her hands before she stopped herself and said, of course, "You know I can't do that." I said, "I know." John thanked me. I am not certain whether any of us completely understood, but I felt that I had experienced something remarkable. When I think about that moment, I think how things might have turned out differently if I had been judgmental about Mary's condition... I also realize how important this experience is to me. Patients challenge us with their individuality and unique needs [and to accommodate]. Mary is one of the most complex individuals that I have cared for. She gave me a new understanding of OCD and its ramifications. Unlike with other illnesses that become secondary when cancer is diagnosed, I learned that OCD can remain the primary illness.

Some of the most trying challenges that leave the patient feeling helpless are situations in which the illness' has taken control over the patient's emotional, social, and physical life. In this case, the patient is not belligerent; yet, there is no possibility of reasoning through a problem with her. Mary is simply rendered incapable for managing their fears which are of such magnitude that she is shut in from society all together. In situations like this, the hardest part of caring for the patient has little to do with the reason for current treatment. Instead, Rosemary's constant and consuming challenge is to anticipate everything that Mary will need, prepare everything so that Mary does not have to touch anything "dirty", and keep Mary comfortable in her surroundings so that she will return and complete treatment. When problems arise, the test is of Rosemary's ingenuity and imperturbability, not necessarily negotiation of conflict.

We include many of the details described by Rosemary so that the reader or learner can imaginatively experience the challenges, accommodations, and puzzles Rosemary had to solve or make. This and all the narratives here provide rich sources for "rehearsal" for developing clinicians. One could imagine different settings and how procedures or care might be provided for patients with particular disorders so that the patient could feel known and cared about and subsequently interact more openly and amicably with care providers.

The clinical and moral leaders highlighted in this section, most of whom are or were staff nurses, do not misunderstand themselves to be heroes or saints. They are, however, astute clinical learners who have such strong notions of good and ethics of care and responsibility. They have learned how to stay engaged and curious, and continue to develop their skills at working with persons who are weathering difficult times. They have been morally compelled to learn, figure out, or notice the significance and meaning of the angry, threatened and threatening, and demanding behaviors. The discovery each nurse made of the patient's/family's vulnerability, terror, and alienation that can be incapacitating helped the nurses recognize the true nature of the conflicts. These nurses then understood themselves in a new light and they understood that these human beings sorely needed support, comfort, problems solved and a trustworthy partner in care.

The clinical wisdom embedded within each story provides a rich account for reflection and learning. These narratives are not intended to be prescriptive; instead, they offer ways of individualizing care and concern for a specific person in a particular situation. Together, however, the narratives give insight into what is pervasive in the expert practices of nurses caring for "fearful, stressed, burdened, or vulnerable" patients and their families who have recognized and welcomed honest, genuine, trustworthy, and compassionate care and concern. There is no one best way to work through the conflicts; there are many. Central in each of the ways, however, are meeting of other as a worthy person, a human being; genuine respect; a grasp that fear or helplessness are common; engaged empathy; listening coupled with curiosity that can provide understanding and insight; and understanding that guides a caring response. Strong clinical and moral leadership can be transformative.

Understanding is a great gift in the midst of times of transition, confusion and loss. Understanding can be transformative, as each of these strong moral leaders have demonstrated. In turn, from the patient's or family's perspective, being understood makes the person feel known and recognized in their new circumstance, and opens up new situated possibilities. After all, it is the confusion and isolation that occur during a rejected, fearful transition that prevents the person from seeing what is now possible rather than only experiencing the "no longer possible" or the impossible (Benner & Wrubel, 1989).

BUILDING AND PRESERVING COLLABORATIVE RELATIONSHIPS

An ethic of responsiveness is internal to excellent nursing practices, as discussed in previous chapters and by Benner, Tanner, and Chesla (1996). Collective wisdom typically exceeds that of any one individual. Consequently, engaging in dialogue and assisting in the development of others to do the same facilitates the evolution of collective wisdom (Hooper, 1995). As Covey (2004) explains, a habit of excellent leaders is that they consistently embrace and facilitate interdependence, for they understand the significance of the synergy that evolves from diversity. Hence, as they develop expertise, clinical leaders come to understand themselves as a part of a team, not necessarily as the team leader, even though their knowledge and experiential wisdom often influences the direction of the team. In addition, expert clinical leaders are compelled to do what is good on behalf of the patient. The best of practice, therefore, is characterized by collaboration and the facilitation of collaboration with and among others.

In the following story, the advanced practice nurse recognizes that, although the appropriate mechanism for collaboration (daily rounds) is in place, the staff nurses' important contributions and concerns are receiving limited consideration because their ability to articulate their thoughts is under-developed. Without the nurses' contributions, the best care for the infants is not possible:

Advanced Practice Nurse: I work in a neonatal ICU. We have work rounds everyday with our fellows, residents, and attendings. About a year after I started here, I noticed that many of the nurses had great ideas for patient care but their articulation was [vague], like, 'The baby doesn't look right.' They would always be questioned, 'Well, what do you mean by that?' and sometimes the nurses would get angry, 'I'm tired of you saying, 'What do you mean by that?' So, I did a project where we developed teams of nurses who followed patients and just by grouping them in teams, they gained expert power just because they knew every detail about the patient. So they actually could say, 'I know the patient. This is specifically what is different about the patient. Every day at 3:00 he gets mottled. That's just how he is and we don't need another septic work up.' So I mentored them for about a year, going with them to pre-round and saying, 'What's your plan for today?' and they went through everything about the baby, and I said, 'So why do you want to give the baby blood today?' 'Well, I have the answer for that,' and they would start to articulate, 'The hematocrit is this and my baby is symptomatic with this.' Before, they were never able to do that. But the crescendo for me was when I was on rounds and I'd hear them articulate their plan, and the physician's like, 'Well that's a really good idea, and that's great,' and they really were better able to articulate. It took a year to get them there. It took them a year to get the confidence to do it. It took them a year of looking at the X-rays to get ready for rounds and to change their level of practice. That's what I actually did with this program. Their level of practice is now way above some of the residents and now, instead of looking at the numbers, the residents look at the nurse, 'What do we need to do today?' And we actually were able to show a decrease in costs because the physicians no longer work up these babies just out of fear that they are going to miss something. They trust the nurses and their assessments, and before, I think they didn't trust them because the nurses didn't articulate findings as well. 'The baby didn't look right.' That was a really common statement in our unit, but the nurses couldn't say exactly why. So I think as the nurses at the bedside became better able to work with physicians and my role was really mentoring them. At first they were concerned about 'The physicians are going to yell at me, or I'm not going to be part of the team' and so I would work with them. Pretty soon I started hearing better articulation, which has really made them better nurses, the babies got better care, and it was much more cooperative. Now the physicians respect the nurse for her 12 hours a day at the bedside and I think that's been really powerful for us... I think the nurses are more ready to prepare the families better. I think they're interacting with families at a different level than they were when they were just information-givers. I think they are seen as a higher level of practitioner as a result of their ability to assess and articulate what they're seeing to the medical team, social workers, and respiratory therapists...It's bridged the gap to move on to other things.

This advanced practice nurse chooses one of a number of ways to help staff nurses really "know" the babies they are caring for. By knowing the infant, the nurse is better positioned to notice specific changes, nuances, and qualitative distinctions that can then be articulated to others to convey and support their concerns and intervention preferences. Further, the advanced practice nurse rehearses with and role models for the staff so that they can learn what kinds of details and distinctions are meaningful and they can "safely" gain experience articulating their views to their peers. Within a year, the staff nurses form better collaborative relationships with all team members. Raising the nurses to an equal or partnership level with other team members is a notable accomplishment. However, the two most significant and powerful interventions by the advanced practice nurse are first, getting the nurses to know the infants which facilitated the development of their clinical expertise and second, validating and rehearsing their observations and perspectives which gave greater authoritative voice to their expertise.

Another feature of excellent clinical leadership is the generous and respectful promotion or sponsorship of others whenever possible. This clinical leader as coach and mentor withdraws to the sidelines as the developing clinicians and young leaders emerge. The advanced practice nurse expresses great satisfaction upon hearing these budding leaders articulate their perspectives in daily rounds. She delights in "working herself out of a job" so that they, as a team, can move on to "other things." Such team development is central to strong clinical leadership. Since the aim is to improve the quality of care, there is no end to the number of "bigger things" that require attention and change, consequently the leadership roles of the staff and advanced practice nurse continue to evolve.

In many healthcare settings, collaboration is not yet the norm and there may not be a formal clinical leader to assist in the more global changes needed to support collaborative practice. However, staff nurse leaders commonly evolve and take a stand when patients are high risk for complications and when what is at stake for the patient demands the voice of experiential knowledge. The following excerpt is a continuation from the story above about the ventilator patient with a medullary infarction. In the previous excerpt, the Neuro ICU nurse described coaching the intern (first-year resident) about differences in ventilatory support and he, in turn, made a case to senior residents about choosing a particular ventilator mode over the one they preferred. In the following excerpt, as a few problems continue, this developing nurse leader collaborates with peers and the respiratory therapist to ensure that mistakes in this fragile patient's weaning are minimized:

Nurse: As we altered his ventilator settings, we would explain to the patient the changes we were making, 'Now we are decreasing the amount of support so you are going to really have to work harder, and if it gets to be too much, let us know, but do expect to have to work a little harder these next couple of hours. Or I realize you're in trouble; we're going to turn your ventilator support back up for the night so you are going to feel more rested.' But it took a few days for us to get everyone trained about what ventilator mode was what and how it worked. And each day, I would care for him on night shift and the other nurse would have him on day shift. We had made a very specific agreement among all of us about how strict we would be with the residents. We would refuse incorrect ventilator orders and if they insisted on changing something, we would call a respiratory therapist up to the unit right away and have a discussion before any changes were be made. We really concentrated our efforts on making his weaning go as smoothly as possible. Our main thing was to psychologically keep him boosted enough so that he could go through the weaning process.

Interviewer: It sounds like you had a lot of background understanding of what patients with this particular kind of infarct need in terms of coming off a ventilator. How did you acquire that background?

Nurse: Just through my work experience. I worked in a neuro unit before and we can watch a respiratory waveform on our monitors. If the rates or patterns vary, we can pick up if for some reason they are not having auto regulation from the brain. Just looking at his clinical picture, knowing where all his injuries were, it's like expecting something from a patient. Looking at his injury, we expect this deficit or we expect a problem here. We had reasons to believe that there would be problems in certain areas. As far as weaning, I have worked with other patients that way, and I think the medical team had an expectation that weaning would go very quickly. But I had seen in previous experience that it could even be a month-long process, and it wouldn't hurt anyone to have a little patience.

This developing nurse leader recognizes the need to act in order to protect the patient physiologically and psychologically from small but devastating setbacks caused by weaning to quickly or inappropriate ventilator changes. That requires attentiveness and collaboration from the "experienced" members on the team who "know to expect particular deficits" and problems in patients with this kind of neurological injury. In this situation, gaining support from peers and the respiratory therapist is possible and encourages each member to take a leadership role in the care of this patient.

Collaborative relationships are most easily formed when team members (a) are knowledgeable about the specific patient, (b) can articulate their perspectives in an understandable and logical way, and (c) in the best interests of the patient, are open to the contributions and perspectives of others. These three skills are foundational, whether developing collaborative relationships or collaborating with well-established allies. The advanced practice nurse continues the first story presented in this chapter about the patient with primary pulmonary hypertension. Here the advanced practice nurse explains further:

Advanced Practice Nurse: The importance [of a previous story] is how often a Clinical Nurse Specialist can help guide decisions and guide interactions with physicians.

Interviewer: Now, what I'm not clear about is, what would <u>not</u> have happened had you not been there? Because once you started talking to the Fellow about the patient getting intubated and the blood gases didn't look good, then you started talking about 'We. We did this, and we did that.' So it wasn't clear to me what role you had.

Advanced Practice Nurse: Basically, what we did was done upon my suggestion. In other words, the fellow and I would discuss ideas of what might work. And then the ideas that we tried would be the ones that we both agreed would probably work. The reasons my suggestions were done was because I could discuss <u>why</u> I wanted to do them, [physiologically]. And not just because I thought they would work, or I've seen them work before, but the <u>physiological</u> rationale behind [my thoughts] was solid. So, for example, one of the first things that we did was put capnography on the patient. So, the end tidal CO_2 was telling us if our therapies were working and if we were effective in ventilating or not. So we'd make a change, increase inspiratory flow and increase inspiratory time. We could tell immediately if that was working.

This advanced practice nurse is able to assist the Fellow in reasoning through the patient's physiological changes and understanding, in physiological detail, the benefits of the suggested interventions. Further, he highlights how that particular intervention assists in immediately evaluating the patient's responses to therapeutic changes. The nurse's scientific and experiential knowledge enable him to be recognized as an authoritative or reliable clinical leader. His collaborative style coaches and teaches others while respectfully acknowledging their clinical background, experiential knowledge, and disciplinary perspectives, and maintaining equal positions. In some situations, it may be more appropriate to move into a teacher-learner relationship. But, in situations such as this, where both clinicians have a good background knowledge of the sciences, a collaborative dialogue and plan are possible.

The interviewer clarifies the specific influences on treatment changes instigated by the advanced practice nurse because he told the story in terms of "I." However, once the clarification is made, the nurse quickly moves back into the dialogue of "we." The disappearance of "I" in favor of "we" reflects his self-understanding as part of a team. But his reference to "we" is markedly different from the anonymous use of "we" seen in the discourse of clinicians preferring anonymity or invisibility. He is clear about his contributions and clear about his preference for collaboration.

Not all collaborative efforts involve teaching. At times, team members consult a trusted colleague to confirm their clinical reasoning, judgment, or the necessity of an intervention. This kind of collaboration ranges from extensive dialogue to the simple nod of the head, depending on the colleague's presence and/or understanding of the situation. This is illustrated in the example below in which two flight nurses together describe an unexpected situation:

Nurse 1: I remember the cric[othyrotomy] that you did in the south area on that one patient—a man, remember?

Nurse 2: Yeah, the one I gave to you?

Nurse 1: No, I think we both kind of ended up doing [the procedure] at the end. But he, when you incised his neck, there was a pretty good amount of bleeding.

Nurse 2: A lot! It wasn't a little bit, it was a lot.

Nurse 1: It wasn't arterial, though. But we hit the vein. There's a vein that goes right across the cricothyroid membrane. For some people it's there, and in some people it's not. We'd always been warned that we might do that, and obviously this man had it and it just looked like a faucet. And [Nurse 2] looked at that and I think you were just stunned for a minute....

Nurse 2: I was. I looked at [Nurse 2] and I went, 'Oh my God!' [Nurse 2] said, 'Well, you have to do it anyway.'

Nurse 1: Yeah, this is work, you've just got to go for it. And the bleeding stopped as soon as we packed it with 4x4s. And we got his airway.

Nurse 2: We just wanted to get back to the hospital.

Nurse 1: But it was really disconcerting at first to see that. Because sometimes cricothyrotomies are not bloody at all. I've seen some that were very, very clean and then others that were very, very bloody. And that one, that was surprising.

Nurse 2: Yes.

Nurse 1: And I think once again we just bantered back and forth and talked about it, and I said, 'Well, we just—we have to do it. You can't stop because he's bleeding.'

Nurse 2: I just remember being surprised there was so much blood and looking up at [Nurse 1] and I said, 'What do you think we should do?' and [Nurse 1] said, 'Well, we still have to do the cric, even if he's bleeding.' And I said, 'Well, that's true,' and we just talked about it for about three seconds.

Nurse 1: I think we just verified with each that this is normal and this is natural and now we have to move on. Sometimes it's just good to hear somebody else say that, 'Yeah, this is okay, this is how it is sometimes.'

Nurse 2: Yeah.

Nurse 1: I mean in this profession, you see a lot of things for the first time that you've never seen in your life and it's helpful if you're with somebody that's already seen it, has maybe been there before.

This situation can be interpreted in two different ways. First, if Nurse 1 was less experienced than her colleague, the brief moment of reassurance was enough to give her the confidence to adeptly complete the procedure and secure the airway. Second, for two experienced nurses, this example highlights how collaboration is bidirectional, each supporting the other to do what at first seems difficult or risky. Although collaboration can take time, there are many instances in everyday practice when it occurs instantaneously.

The leadership literature often encourages celebrating the contributions of others. We did find that strong clinical leaders who actively work to build a collaborative team take the extra effort to recognize the performance of colleagues within and across disciplines. In an exemplar presented in the "Managing a Crisis" (see Chapter 5), the pilot (Nan) on a flight crew was vital in assisting the nurses to perform life-saving procedures involving multiple burn victims. For her team efforts and response beyond the call of duty, the two nurses nominated the pilot for an award:

Nurse 1: She won an award for that...

Nurse 2: Yeah. Rita and I nominated her for an award, which she won.

The nurses convey great pride in the pilot's award and describe how she often accompanies them to the scene in case extra help is needed. These extra efforts to recognize colleagues extend beyond rewarding extraordinary efforts. They build a strong collaborative culture that can exist beyond the tenure of the people who built it.

TRANSFORMING CARE DELIVERY SYSTEMS

As illustrated throughout this book, whenever problems arose in everyday practice, nurses would respond to resolve the issues in the particular situation. Less visible are the attentiveness and skillful intervention needed to detect problems that recur as a result of a systems problem. A systems problem, for instance, is one that causes a disturbance or disrupts smooth functioning in other parts of the system. For example, if a busy unit's supplies are restocked during the afternoon, yet the majority of procedures are done in the morning, then there is a greater likelihood that staff will find depleted shelves when procedure kits and other equipment are needed. Another growing systems problem is the implementation of some types of electronic records which, by design, force redundant data entry, fails to follow the prevailing logic of practice, consumes inordinate amounts of time, places heavy demand on clinicians who have limited access to too few computers, and completion of data entry is mandated within a predetermined time following admission. Clinical leaders are attentive to the repetition of problems and collaborate with others to bring the problem to the fore for resolution.

Since hospitals house the practice of multiple health care practitioners, they play a crucial role in ensuring that the organizational practices, systems, and infrastructures are "fit" to house good nursing, medical, pharmaceutical, social work, et cetera, practices. A practice is a socially organized body of knowledge and community of practitioners who have notions of good that are internal to their practice (MacIntyre, 1984; Weiss, Malone, Merighi, Benner, 2002). As emphasized in this book, institutions house socially embedded knowledge and notions of good practices, as well as playing a role in forming and sustaining good practices. Good systems engineering and effective information systems are *critical but not sufficient* to ensure good practice…including all the practices housed by the institution of hospitals, health care centers, outpatient surgery, and ambulatory care.

Similar to the growing but erroneous belief that clinical protocols and guidelines can replace expert, or even safe, clinical thinking and judgment, managerialism cannot replace good leadership judgment. Instead of good judgment, managerialism involves the application of <u>generic</u> skills, techniques, solutions, rules and personnel to all organizations as "if one size fits all". Again, experience and practical knowledge are assumed to offer little value. Unfortunately, managerialism, no matter how it increases efficiency, cannot supplant the need for on-the-ground practice knowledge (Sullivan & Benner. 2005). Hospitals are mixed organizations in that they have to accommodate professional, bureaucratic and even crisis modes of organizational structures, processes, and content (Benner, 1973). Yet, bureaucratic organizations are always tempted to substitute structures and processes for the ends or notions of good practice (Merton, 1968; Weber, 2008). This is why Chief Nursing Officers have to seek out their expert nurse clinicians and strong clinical leaders to guide them on organizational design and structural impediments to good practice.

Chief Nursing Executives also need to identify and look to expert clinical nurse leaders in their organizations in order to keep the institution on its essential goals of quality patient care, patient safety, and cost-effectiveness. Poor clinical nursing care is exorbitantly costly in terms of patients' lives and costs of delivering care. Quality really is job number one in the hospital industry, even more so than in the automobile industry that initiated this slogan.

One of the ways in which clinical leaders are working to transform systems is by developing critical pathways, practice guidelines, best practices, evidence-based practices, and the like in specific patient populations and evaluating patient outcomes to improve the quality of care while controlling the costs (AHCPR, 2010, Wojner, 1996). These pathways, guidelines or practices and the tracking of patient outcomes, over time, can inform and guide clinicians to marshal essential resources and can assist in determining likely clinical trajectories and appropriate clinical interventions in similar types of situations.

There is, however, a subtle but critical distinction in understanding the use and limitations of a pathway, practice guideline, standard, or evidence-based practice and outcomes data. Although guidelines or outcomes data may support or prompt the clinician's judgment to initiate intervention, they do not instruct clinicians about <u>how</u> to intervene and comport themselves in specific situations, particularly when the patient's condition deviates from the predicted norm. The nurse's style and interventions require skilled know-how that can only be gained through experience. In clinical practice, it is the clinicians' reasoning about the pathway, guidelines and outcome data, their reasoning about the issues and risks in the particular situation, and their leadership in working with others that improve care while managing costs. It is the excellent clinical leader's engagement in dialogue with the data and guidelines and the use of data and evidence-based practices as supports that lead to the best interventions for particular patients.

Although pathways, guidelines and evidence-based practices and outcomes data are best used to make clinicians more attentive to early changes in the patient's situation and <u>assist</u> clinicians to make better decisions regarding interventions, they should never <u>replace</u> clinical wisdom. A standard of practice, guidelines, pathway, or outcomes management can improve substandard care but these "technolog[ies] of patient experiences" (Ellwood, 1988, p. 1549) do not weigh the issues involved in the care of a specific patient and thus cannot best or even appropriately meet the needs of all patients in every situation (Bliton & Finder, 1996; Frankford, 1994; Halpern, 1995). Expert reasoning and judgment are required for best practice. "Already, there are potential safety and quality risks to patients and organizations with nonexperts at the besdside (Burritt & Steckel, 2009, p. 479), particularly when nonexperts are exactly the clinicians who depend on guidelines to serve AS judgment until theirs is further developed. Knowledge from the outcome data can alert staff nurses to consult a clinician who is expert in a particular patient population about an emerging problem; however, it is the skilled judgment and interventions of the expert nurse, not the standard or data that can exceed minimal expectations, and standards in the care of a patient or family member. For example, in excellent practice that is innovative and has patient outcomes that exceed patient standards, or patient outcome standards, then, following guidelines to achieve standards will actually diminish the excellent practice. However in situations that fall below standard expectations, implementing standards can raise the level of patient care.

Leaders and clinicians commonly misunderstand the limitations of practice guidelines and evidence-based practice and outcome data. The danger is to replace thinking and reasoning with predefined interventions specified by the pathways, guidelines or protocols. Mindless reliance on outcome data or pathways and guidelines can create poorer patient outcomes and eventually lead to deskilling of clinicians. Guidelines and pathways should never be implemented to serve as prescriptions for care or replace thinking and judgment in particular situations. Good and wise use of clinical guidelines and evidence-based practices requires that staff be taught how and when to best integrate them into practice; thus, the value of these patient technologies, as with any technology, lies in the clinicians' skillfulness in employing their use rather than in the technology itself. Greater emphasis needs to be placed on how the clinician's wisdom and expertise are central in the intelligent use of "technologies." As Wojner (1996) stressed, the success of these patient care technologies lies in the expertise of the clinical leaders using them and teaching their use. Information systems and patient care guidelines need to prompt and augment health professional's decision making and knowledge use, rather than mistakenly being understood as a replacement for good clinical reasoning and situated judgment.

Although recurring problems in specific patient populations are more likely to receive attention, clinical leaders tend to notice a single incident that is of critical significance, particularly when a patient suffers an unnecessary or potentially preventable complication. In the story below, a staff nurse describes how she recognized a breakdown in a patient's care.

Although only one incident occurred, she realizes that the team's current skills will predictably lead to repeated breakdown. Hence, she works with the team to educate everyone about emergency procedures, equipment, and mobilizing high risk patients early:

Nurse 1: The next day, after the code, we were talking—I have really good rapport with the attending in cardiology and the patient was one of our patients in the ICU the next day after the code. I was just rehashing what had happened and why this patient had the torsades—a run of ventricular tachycardia. Was there anything that was going on during the day that could have clued us in that this was going to happen. We were just trying to see what we could do for future patients to prevent any codes on the floor if at all possible. And we found out a lot of information by going through the whole situation. Apparently the patient had runs of torsades all day long. The patient should have been transferred into the ICU in the morning at 7:30 when he had his <u>first</u> run. It was investigated and later discussed at a joint session with nursing and the attending. So a lot of things came out of this incident.

Nurse 2: Did he just convert on his own earlier in the day?

Nurse 1: He did. He did. He went into short runs and would come out of it and…

Interviewer: So he was on a telemetry unit?

Nurse 1: He was on the telemetry unit. The previous day he was on the defibrillation pads on the telemetry unit, and somehow they got taken off during the night. But really, he should have been transferred to the ICU in the morning. Not at 6:00 at night when he coded, so…

Interviewer: So how did this evolve into a system change? Are you looking at standardized practice?

Nurse 1: Well, the [Clinical Nurse Specialist], a couple of other ICU nurses, and I are going to do classes with CEU credit for the telemetry unit nurses on cardioversion, defibrillation, and code situations, just to get them more familiar with the equipment and assisting them in a code. In the ICU, we're also going to develop equipment check lists, so to speak, for the staff so that we are all up to par as far as our comfort level with the equipment. The code team is being looked at to determine whether Intensive Care Unit nurses should respond to codes in house. So there's a lot that is happening as a result.

Interviewer: And how did you get recruited into this education?

Nurse 1: I volunteered. I brought my concerns to [the Clinical Nurse Specialist].

In this situation, the patient experiences several "near-codes" throughout the day. However, no one providing his immediate care understands the runs of torsades de pointes (a type of ventricular tachycardia) as an ominous sign of impending danger, so he is not moved into the ICU where he can be closely monitored and instantaneous intervention is possible. This patient's course of events raise concern, so the nurse reviews the situation in detail with other team members, hoping to discover a way to prevent similar incidents in the future. During the course of the problem search, a number of generalized issues that could and did lead to breakdown are detected. In response, the nurse recruits colleagues and they work with the clinical nurse specialist to define and implement interventions that will change how clinicians care for high risk patients.

Similar serious problems are being created in the current healthcare climate in which skilled nurses are being systematically replaced by under-skilled and/or ill-prepared assistive personnel. Managers and executives are often removed from an engaged clinical practice; consequently, they overlook the skills required to perform "tasks" and interpret data. When skilled clinical knowledge is overlooked, all that shows up as work are the procedural tasks in isolation from the essential thinking and reasoning. Tasks then appear as if they can simply be delegated to under-skilled or unprepared "thinkers." Depending on what is delegated, this move can unwittingly create a systems error that can have devastating consequences in patients, especially when it is imperative to think about the data collected in relation to the specific patient. An advanced practice nurse highlights this growing problem in an example from her practice and then points to her role as a clinical leader in working to repair the systems problem:

Advanced Practice Nurse: We had a patient with an intracoronary stent who was doing well, had gone to the telemetry floor, and was recovering there. Several things happened, but not all were positive. But there was some positive learning that came out of it. The patient was being cared for by a nurse as his primary care giver, but also nursing assistants (CNAs), who would assist with things like vital signs. And I happened to be on the night shift this particular night, and I remember very clearly that I heard a Code Blue call to this telemetry floor. It was one of my units, and off I go. Actually, I got there two to three minutes after the code was called. I was doing something I had to complete at the time. I got up there and one of our cardiologists had intubated the patient, and people were very settled in the room. I asked if they needed further assistance from me. Our ICU nurses were there and said, 'No, we'll be okay. Why don't you go make sure there's a bed ready in the ICU.' 'Fine.' So I go back down, I tell the nurse who will be admitting this patient—who has about two years of experience in critical care, a fine nurse, but there are always things to learn—that he would be receiving the patient. 30, 40, 45 minutes, almost an hour goes by. Patient hasn't come. No call. That's concerning! So I go up to see what the delay is, and the physician meets me coming out of the room...he tells me what had occurred. It turns out this was his patient, and he happened to be in the emergency room. He wanted me to look at the chart with him. We looked at the chart, and in looking at the vital signs graphic record, we see that there had been a <u>huge</u> change in vital signs that very much reflected a shock state. Well, that was concerning, and it was just at the time of shift change. My first thought was, 'I bet CNAs did the vital signs and the nurse had not had a chance to review the vital signs on the record, so they hadn't noticed the change.' In going back and looking at his record, we found there were situations where this patient had continued to complain of pain in the groin site and had a lot of pain. The physician came to see him once, but then the patient continued to have increased pain medication requirements. Bottom line, the patient had a retroperitoneal bleed, was in very bad condition, entered the critical care unit, and was intubated. He was literally on 11 different drug infusions of some form or another. Another nurse and I were caring for the patient and that almost wasn't enough...This patient did pass away about 48 hours later. They did go to surgery at one point, but the patient wasn't able to recover....

On certain patients with increased risks, CNAs don't take vital signs on the patients any more on the Telemetry floor. Also trend reports of vital signs and special parameters are now done with those patients. It certainly presented a very big educational opportunity for many, many people. The fact is that it potentially could occur in any of the three critical care areas. Not only was it like a learning [experience]—it wasn't like a hand-slapping experience—it was more like, 'These are things that can occur and this is why you use the nurse or the coordinator to care for a patient. This is why nurses have responsibilities in knowing what the CNAs are doing. We now teach the CNAs, 'You have to know that 100/60 blood pressure is not normal for everyone. This patient's normal pressure ran 150 to 170 over 80-90, and for him, 100/60 was way too low and way too different,' and it was very obvious to me on the first glance. And so, there are many things learned from that but there were good things that came out of it hopefully for other patients. But you know, that's where it starts getting pretty scary sometimes when you start working with assistive personnel.

In the above story, the advanced practice nurse details a disastrous situation that evolved because the "routine" patient data were not interpreted by a skilled clinician. From outside the situation, one may criticize the nurse responsible for that patient for not reviewing the graphics record in a timely manner. From inside the situation, particularly at change of shift, fewer skilled clinicians are struggling to manage increased workloads with sicker patients. For this reason alone, clinical aspects of systems must not be developed or changed without understanding the practice, the kind of thinking involved, and the kind of access that nurses must have to patients. In the story above, upon reviewing the work structures, the advanced practice nurse recognizes that degrees of clinical judgment and thinking had been delegated to unskilled CNAs along with the vital signs. The advanced practice nurse and others take a closer look at the design of the clinical system and transform it to give the nurses better access to vital information in a timely manner. Staff are then better educated about their roles and responsibilities in working together. As systems are being designed or changed, great care must be taken not to delegate clinical judgment and thinking along with the tasks. Nursing care is not a sequence of tasks. Nursing care involves a constellation of clinical judgment, thinking-in-action, and skillful interventions. Patient care is endangered if this multifaceted practice is reduced to isolated tasks that are delegated to under-skilled assistive personnel.

In this second edition of this book, because the economic climate is forcing the use of under-skilled assistants, the above story has repeated itself over and over. In response to this known and planned systems risk, a strong clinical leader in oncology nursing from Massachusetts, Clara Reagan, for example, negotiated teaching time to carefully prepare new assistive personnel about their vital role in collecting and recording patient data. They were educated about how clinicians depend on their discernment and judgment when patient data are out of the patient's normal range and the imperative of reporting those "red flags" to the patient's nurse. This effort has reduced the patients' risks and, secondarily, improved the team's collaboration.

In contrast to the problems that are evolving from changes in healthcare today, there are many more improvements in patient care that stem from thoughtful redesign in care delivery. Beneficial changes are no less easy for staff to adjust to, but many changes improve the care that patients receive. An advanced practice nurse shared an example of a transformation in care delivery:

Interviewer: Why is a 3-day-old patient coming <u>here</u> (Pediatric ICU)?

Advanced Practice Nurse: All the post-op cardiac surgery patients [with congenital malformations] come to this unit, regardless of their age. We get all the adults with congenital heart defects. So pre-term infants, adults, and everything in between.

Interviewer: I've always thought that it might be very challenging to work here, to be able to know your parameters and then the difference in physiology of the pre-term versus an elderly guy or a young adult.

Advanced Practice Nurse: It is challenging. It's been extremely tricky in terms of education and in terms of support from the staff, because they don't want to take care of adults. They're not in the Pediatric ICU to take care of adults, so there was a tremendous amount of resistance, and they expressed it in terms of not knowing what to do or how to take care of them. But after doing a lot of assessment and information gathering, I found out that they really <u>did</u> know how to take care of them. Because they're the experts in these kinds of patients post-operatively. They're the absolute experts. Physiologically they're not that different than the kids that we get. The defects are the same, the repairs are the same, the post-op complications are the same, and once those are all resolved, they leave the ICU. But what I found out, really, where the stress was, it was just how to communicate with adults and how to emotionally and psychologically work with them. They are just used to working with parents, not spouses, and they didn't know how to handle them or talk to them or work with them. So we did a lot of education around that, and it's been better since then. (Observational Interview)

As the advanced practice nurse describes, it was a difficult transition for the pediatric ICU nurses—to care for adults as well as children. However, the advanced practice nurse worked closely with the staff to educate them about the similarities and differences in caring for adults and their families. By transforming the system according to the logic of practice, the patients receive care from nurses who have the clinical judgment and knowledge specific to this particular patient population.

The larger systems changes in healthcare are challenging clinicians, patients, and families to adapt to and manage higher acuity conditions outside hospitals. In some cases, this includes the chronically critically ill. Nurses in home care are continually transforming their practices and systems to care for sicker patients at home. In some cases, the patients are discharged directly from the ICU to home. Although many of the new patient care skills are learned by nurses while trying to provide care for a patient, the patients themselves are making this transformation possible:

Advanced Practice Nurse: Many, many years ago I actually supervised an ICU and an ER, and patients, 10 or 15 years ago, that we actually used to have in ICU and in the ER, we now have in the home, especially where HIV care is concerned. And we are actually seeing—from my perspective in home care—the envelope just keeps getting pushed more and more. And we had a patient that came out of the hospital 2 years ago. He had no opportunistic infections. He had a T-cell count around 600, but he had a cardiomyopathy secondary to his HIV disease and he was in heart failure. I walked in, and, name a cardiac drug, any drug and he was on it. I mean he was on <u>every one imaginable</u> and he was on a milrinone drip in the ICU and they sent him home with the milrinone drip. So we really had assumed that he would have a very limited and short prognosis. And, of course, we had never done milrinone in the home; it was always in ICU drug. We got him home and got that set up, and did the patient teaching. The first day I walked in, he was lying in bed; he had cyanotic fingertips and mouth; he had conversational shortness of breath; he was still fluid overloaded by about 35 pounds at that point—and I increased the milrinone. And to make it a long story short, I white-knuckled my way through 2 weeks of this, just, every day thinking, 'I don't know what I'm doing.' And I made multiple phone calls to pharmacists, to the physicians, and everybody was hyper-scrutinizing this. This guy has been on several cruises now. He goes out of town to Reno periodically. And he periodically goes back into heart failure, hops back into the CCU, gets tuned up, and comes back out. But he literally went from looking like he had a prognosis of, it could have been just days, to becoming independent again. And we've gone up and down and up and down with his milrinone. He's learned to titrate it himself. Yeah, I call him Lazarus because he has been at the point of death probably four times. Then we've had to keep upping and upping and upping the milrinone dose, and now we're way beyond any of the normal limits of that. He still has about 500 T-cells, no opportunistic infections, and he's one of those outliers that we've dealt with, and he's pretty <u>amazing</u>. But it's <u>that</u> level of nursing that we're actually doing in the home now. And when I was a supervisor around here, it reached the point where we needed to have virtual ICU level or ER level type of skills for the amount of high tech interventions that we were doing in the home with our HIV patients. When it gets very complicated, we get these very highly skilled nurses who are used to working with technologies.

This patient situation from the research highlights the quality and outcome of care that can be achieved when the patient is able to learn how to manage his care jointly with the clinician. In this situation, the patient learns to read his bodily responses as the nurse titrates his milrinone. Because he learned well, he is able to take over the titration of the milrinone himself, achieve physiological stability most of the time, and improve the quality and quantity of his life. Since the first edition of this book, nurses are now starting to teach a few patients how to manage their chronic and barely stable heart failure on multiple vasoactive drugs, like milrinone with dobutamine. Without adequate studies, it is still untested and unclear how far such intensive therapies should be pursued in the home. Judgment is required every step of the way. It would be dangerous to create guidelines for all patients based upon this individual's success. However, this is an example of developing new clinical knowledge based on changing patterns and structures of care.

SUMMARY

Effective clinical leaders share a number of essential commonalities. They are first authoritative knowledge workers, based on their knowledge of the sciences and their extensive knowledge in the practice itself. For this reason, the best of practice is embodied in expert clinical leaders. Second, expert clinical leaders have developed relational leadership skills, such as teaching and coaching, that enable them to assist in the strong and lasting development of others. This ensures the preservation and continuing development of good practice. Further, clinical leaders influence the care of individuals, groups, and the community. Finally, when executives and administrators recognize the significance and capabilities of strong clinical leaders to close the growing gap between the demand for expert nurses and their limited availability, the necessary emphasis and an unyielding support can be invested in the development of practice in the less experienced clinicians, something schools of nursing can begin but never primarily provide. Hospitals spend a great deal of time educating nurses about new procedures, technology and regulation. However, a disproportionately scarce amount of resources and time are invested in staff development (Frenk et al., 2010), on ongoing clinical practice development and articulating new clinical knowledge that is developed in particular patient care units. With increasing pressure from nursing studies and professional nursing organizations to upgrade nursing education and provide clinical residencies, or new graduate transition programs (Benner, et al., 2009), clinical practice development and the making of experiential learning in practice needs to be at the forefront of nursing education departments in practice settings. All practice settings are complex learning organizations where professional knowledge workers (nurses and physicians) work to daily develop new clinical knowledge about and insights into clinical practice. That clinical experiential knowledge development on the part of clinicians needs to be articulated, made public and examined so that it can be tested, and become cumulative. To paraphrase Anne Benson in her exemplar, with recognition of and guidance from our strong clinical and moral leaders, we have to "hope to never lose hope."

REFERENCES

Agency for Healthcare Research and Quality (2010). *Evidence-based practices*. Retrieved from http://www.ahrq.gov/clinic. Accessed, March 20, 2010.

Benner, P. (1984/1999). *From novice to expert: Excellence and power in clinical nursing practice*. Menlo Park, CA: Addison-Wesley.

Benner, P. (Ed.). (1994). *Interpretive phenomenology: Embodiment, caring, and ethics in health and illness*. Thousand Oaks, CA: Sage.

Benner, P., Tanner, C. A., & Chesla, C. A. (2009). *Expertise in nursing practice: Caring, clinical judgment, and ethics*. New York, NY: Springer Publishing Company.

Bennis, W. (2009). *On becoming a leader*. New York, NY: Basic Books

Bennis, W. (1997) *Why leaders can't lead: The unconscious conspiracy continues*. San Francisco, CA: Jossey-Bass.

Black, J.S. & Gregersen, H. (2008). *It starts with one: Changing individuals changes organizations* (2nd ed.) Upper Saddle River, NJ: Wharton School Publishing

Bliton, M. J., & Finder, S. G. (1996). The eclipse of the individual in policy (where is the place for justice?). *Cambridge Quarterly of Healthcare Ethics, 5*, 519–532.

Bordieu, P. (1980/1990). *The logic of practice*. (R. Nice, trans.). Stanford, CA: Stanford University Press.

Byham, W. & Cox, J. (1997). *Zapp! The lightening of empowerment*. New York, NY: Ballantine Publishing Group,

Bryan, R. & Childers, L. (2004). *Handling difficult patients: A nurse manager's guide*. Marblehead, MA: HCPro Inc.

Covey, S. (1992). *Principle centered leadership*. New York, NY: Simon & Schuster.

Covey, S. (2004). *The seven habits of highly effective people: Restoring the character ethic*. New York, NY: Simon & Schuster.

Daly, L. A. (2009). *Humans Being: Creating your life from the inside out*. Bloomington, IN: AuthorHouse.

Degnin, F. D. (2009). Difficult patients, overmedication, and groupthink. *Journal of Clinical Ethics, 20*(1), 70–74.

Dracup, K. (1997, November). *Preventing readmission: Integrating complex medical therapies in the outpatient setting*. Paper presented at the American Heart Association's 70th Scientific Sessions, Orlando, FL.

Ellwood, P. (1988). Outcomes management: A technology of patient experience. *New England Journal of Medicine, 318*, 1549–1556.

Frankel, R. M. (1995). Emotion and the physician-patient relationship. *Motiv Emotion, 19*, 163–173.

Frankford, D. M. (1994). Scientism and economism in the regulation of health care. *Journal of Politics, Policy and Law, 19*(4), 773–799.

Frenk, J., Chen, L., Bhutta, Z., Cohen, J., Crisp, N., Evans, T., . . . Zurayk, H. (2010). Health professionals for a new century: Transforming education to strengthen health systems in an interdependent world. *The Lancet, 376*, 1923–1958.

George, B. (2004). *Authentic leadership: Rediscovering the secrets to creating lasting value* (J-B Warren Bennis Series). San Francisco, CA: Jossey-Bass.

Greenleaf, R. K., Spears, L. C., & Covey, S. R. (2002). *Servant leadership: A journey into the nature of legitimate power and greatness.* New York, NY: Paulist Press.

Haas, L., Leiser, J., Magill, M., & Sanyer, O. (2005). Management of the difficult patient. *American Family Physician, 72*(10), 2063–2068.

Halpern, J. (1995). Can the development of practice guidelines safeguard patient values? *Journal of Law, Medicine & Ethics, 23*(1), 75–81.

Halpern, J. (2001). *From detached concern to empathy: Humanizing medical practice.* New York, NY: Oxford University Press.

Halpern, J. (2003). What is clinical empathy? *Journal of General Internal Medicine, 18*(8): 670–674.

Halpern, J. (2007b). Empathy and patient-physician conflicts. *Journal of General Internal Medicine, 22*(5): 696–700.

Halpern, J. (2009). Groupthink and caregivers' projections: addressing barriers to empathy. *Journal of Clinical Ethics, 20*(1), 75–78.

Hegg Davis, T. (personal communication. March 24, 2010)

Hooper, P. L. (1995). *Expert titration of multiple vasoactive drugs in post-cardiac surgical patients: An interpretive study of clinical judgment and perceptual acuity.* Doctoral dissertation, University of California at San Francisco, San Francisco. School of Nursing

Kyriakidis, P. H. (research field notes, May 4, 2007)

Kyriakidis, P. H. (research field notes. September 23, 2007)

Kyriakidis, P. H. (research field notes. October 1, 2007)

Kyriakidis, P. H. & Vitello, J. (in progress). *Applying Benner's research to entry level registered nurses: An investigation of development and retention.* (Unpublished research, Nashville, TN. & Boston, MA.)

MacIntyre, A. (1984). *After virtue.* (Second edition). Notre Dame, IN: University of Notre Dame Press.

Malloch, K., Benner, P., Weeks, V. (2010). *Nursing Pathways to Patient Safety.* National Council of State Boards of Nursing, Elsevier International Press.

Manos, P. & Braun, J. (2006). *Care of the difficult patient: A nurse's guide.* New York, NY: Routledge.

Merton, R. K. (1968). *Social Theory and Social Structure.* New York: The Free Press.

Morrison, E. F., Ramsey, A., & Synder, B. A. (2000). Managing the care of complex, difficult paitents in the medical-surgical setting. *Medsurg Nursing, 9*(1), 21–26.

Ptacek, J. T. & Eberhardt, T. L. (1996). Breaking bad news: A review of the literature. *Journal of the American Medical Association, 276*(6), 496–502.

Sullivan, W. & Benner, P. (2005). Challenges to professionalism: Work integrity and the call to renew and strengthen the social contract of the professions. *American Journal of Critical Care, 14*(1), 78–84.

Walters, J. (1997, November). *Post-discharge follow-up: Home health critical path.* Paper presented at the American Heart Association's 70th Scientific Sessions, Orlando, FL.

Weber, M. (2008). *The Protestant ethic and the spirit of capitalism.* New York, NY: BN Publisher/ BNpublisher.net

Weick, K. E. (2009). *Making sense of the organization: Volume 2: The impermanent organization.* Chichester, West Sussex, Wiltshire, England: John Wiley & Sons, Ltd.

Weick, K. E., & Sutcliffe, K. M. (2007). *Managing the unexpected: Resilient performance in an age of uncertainty.* San Francisco, CA: Jossey-Bass.

Weiss, S. M., Malone, R. E., Merighi, J. R., & Benner, P. (2002). Economism, efficiency, and the moral ecology of good nursing practice. *Canadian Journal of Nursing Research, 34*(2), 95–119.

Wheatley, M. (2007). *Finding our way: Leadership for an uncertain time.* San Francisco, CA: Berrett-Koehler Publishers.

Wojner, A. (1996). Outcomes management: An interdisciplinary search for best practices. *AACN Clinical Issues, 7*(1), 133–145.

13

Educational Strategies and Implications

*I*n a practice, the point of life-saving and life-preserving knowledge is the ability to use it, in every way and at the moment it is needed, not simply to have it. For education in a human practice to be effective, the most important teaching and learning for clinicians enable them to provide good care (to perform with embodied intelligence) for groups, but also for specific patients and families. Skillfully performing in an intelligent and ethical way requires the acquisition and development of: knowledge (natural, nursing and social sciences, humanities, etc.) and the ability to use that knowledge, engaged clinical and moral reasoning, clinical imagination, clinical judgment, skillful interventions and ethical comportment (Benner, Sutphen, Leonard, & Day, 2010; Sullivan, 2004). Knowledge use requires situated embodied cognition (Gallagher, 2009; Lave & Wenger, 1991); that is, the productive thinking and knowledge retrieval which is relevant to the situation at hand.

Most tacit and experiential knowledge are best elicited by situations that call for or demand the knowledge as used in similar past experiences. Similarly, scientific and theoretical knowledge or information are also brought to mind when the situation demands their use, either through questions or the nature of the situation. For example, after achieving Advanced Cardiac Life Saving (ACLS) certification, the extreme situations of cardiac arrest or apnea just call forth the use of ACLS knowledge and skillful embodied performance. Embodied performance is distinctly different from the cognitive searching by the inexperienced clinicians for what is best to do, focally having to think about it, and then intentionally deciding on which algorithm to follow. Instead, in skillful embodied performance, one's body fluidly nonreflectively responds, doing what has been learned, repeatedly rehearsed, and has been successful. Problems with wound healing call forth knowledge already acquired. Without experiential knowledge, which is gained through one's own actual experience or may be gained from learning through experiences shared by others, unfamiliar problems stimulate a cognitive search for best practices from the literature or in collaboration with others.

THE CHALLENGE OF EDUCATING NURSES FOR INTELLIGENT, SKILLFUL AND ETHICAL PRACTICE

Good everyday practice is so much wider, deeper and more complex than the weighty cognitive emphasis stressed by universities and colleges (Sullivan, 2005). Without the fundamental integration and assimilation of knowledge acquisition and situated knowledge use, a clinician cannot provide excellent, and possibly not safe, patient care. In organizations today, there is a soaring number of clinicians who have been in practice for many years but have not become fully competent and have arrested in their development (Kyriakidis, research field notes, October 1, 2007). The rigorous academic years of learning scientific facts and cutting edge knowledge did not prepare these underdeveloped clinicians to <u>use</u> that knowledge or use it appropriately in practice. Further, although some of these nurses continue to seek new knowledge, can site the latest science, and technically perform competently, they have not independently discovered or been coached on how to recognize the nature of the situation by drawing on past similar and different situations in order to learn to practically use the knowledge gained in a competent way (Kyriakidis, research field notes, October 1, 2007). Observations and findings in hospital settings unfortunately mirror the outcomes (Burritt & Steckel, 2009) of the perpetuated problems in nursing education that are detailed by Benner, Sutphen, Leonard, and Day (2010); that is, nurses today enter practice without the ability to skillfully use the extensive knowledge they acquired, so that the gap between the clinical reasoning and judgment needed, and the availability of expertise among nurses to provide good care continues to widen.

Often a major source of the problem for the clinician is a lack of developing a sense of salience so that clinical situations do not stimulate the nurse's use or search for relevant knowledge. The emphasis on memorization and knowledge acquisition without developing situated knowledge use and a sense of salience remain the norm in educational and practice settings. Clinicians who go on to become expert, and even virtuoso skilled clinical knowledge users, do learn from their clinical experience, often coached (tacitly or explicitly) by strong colleagues, and continue to be active situated learners in everyday practice and in seeking ongoing continuing education in their field.

Researchers who have studied practice and practice development have made strong cases for transforming the way practitioners (one engaged in a practice) are taught, based on how adults best learn (Benner, 2000; Benner, Tanner & Chesla, 2009; Benner, Hooper-Kyriakidis & Stannard, 1999; Benner, Sutphen, Leonard & Day, 2010; Brown, Collins & Duguid, 1989; Hooper, 1995; Kyriakidis & Vitello, in progress; Lave & Wenger, 1991). Most learning opportunities, even IN practice settings, are removed to a classroom where abstract knowledge (scientific facts, decontextualized information, protocols, etc) is presented out of context of required clinical performance and clinicians are expected to simply know how and when to cognitively access and <u>use</u> that knowledge whenever needed in the midst of an unfolding situation. In contrast, learning is most astute when knowledge addresses the clinician's concerns, is needed to think through and solve a problem, is gained as one uses it to intervene in a changing situation, etc; that is, when it is embedded in one's activity (or practical activity) in a specific context. Experiential or on-the-ground learning is "the way that clinicians use knowledge as they think and act in ever-changing situations" (Benner, Sutphen, Leonard & Day, 2010, p. 13) and is referred to as <u>situated learning</u> (Lave & Wenger, 1991) and thinking-in-action. When knowledge becomes integrated so that the clinician can function well in a situation, that knowledge becomes embodied, easily accessible, and enables the clinician to continue to develop expertise. The challenge confronting educators, preceptors, coaches, and mentors is how to teach knowledge for performance. Similarly, the charge for administrators and managers is how to redefine educator roles and solidly support their transformation into situated coaches (see situated learning strategies to follow). An educator or staff development instructor cannot prepare developing nurses for knowledge use if they are routinely tied up in a classroom presenting policies, regulatory information, orientation, annual competencies, etc. The ability to document that knowledge was presented is not the same as ensuring that the knowledge was learned or is used or even that it is related to clinical reasoning and performance in actual clinical situations.

With higher demands and dwindling resources, we can no longer teach in impoverished ways, place unprepared clinicians in positions of responsibility that have high stakes but exceed their abilities, and wait for them to learn through trial and error. Therefore, this chapter is intended to be practical. The goal of this work is to bring effective situated clinical learning (learning in context) and everyday clinical inquiry in from the margins and into planned educational endeavors and programs. Developing clinicians need their educational preparation and continued learning aligned with the way that adults learn best and perform daily, which necessarily includes the way they are confronted by ambiguous situations, use knowledge, anticipate eventualities, think and reason in unfolding situations, flexibly perform based on the patient's responses to interventions, learn by reflecting on particular situations, and develop ethical comportment from formation in everyday learning (Benner, Sutphen, Leonard & Day, 2010). Consequently, the purpose of this chapter is to present some of the educational strategies and implications of integrative teaching and learning. These strategies illustrate how to integrate classroom and clinical teaching, integrate knowledge acquisition with knowledge use, teach clinical reasoning in transitions in unfolding clinical situations over time with the accompanying changing relevance of assessment data and interventions, stimulate clinical and moral imagination around eventualities and skillful involvement, and demonstrate situated judgment and action.

We describe two major types of integrative strategies that follow the logic of practice in this chapter (Bourdieu 1980/1990). Because the logic of practice (which directs how good clinicians organize their practice and their work) is aligned with the everyday engaged reasoning, judgment, and performance of expert nurses, it is preferable over the logic of science where disengaged, analytical reasoning is the norm. First, multiple examples of how to coach *situated learning* in actual practice, that have proven successful in developing embodied knowledge and skillful, intelligent performance, are detailed. In addition to these, we embedded an extensive number of situated learning examples and recommendations in each chapter. Situating those recommendations in the context of a particular narrative enables the best understanding of how to coach the specific aspect of skilled know-how. Second, a Thinking-In-Action approach to integrating classroom with clinical teaching exemplifies *how to teach learners to use* extensive scientific, technological, and theoretical knowledge in the context of an unfolding patient situation (using a narrative account) that changes over time, while imaginatively responding to the patient's multiple needs and other demands in the situation. For first year nursing student novices, the learning goals using this approach can focus on simpler aspects of complex clinical situations and then increased sophistication and complexity can be added as learners gain integrated classroom and clinical knowledge. In order to be effective clinicians, the student and developing nurse must progress to grasping the nature of whole clinical situations, developing an experience-based sense of salience and using multiple frames of reference that encompass patient and family-focused care (Benner, 2000).

SITUATED LEARNING: LEARNING IN THE MIDST OF CARING FOR PATIENTS AND FAMILIES

Pockets of situated teaching and learning have always existed in practice. Examples were captured in our research during observational interviews when expert nurses were precepting orientees or collaborating with developing nurses. However, the growing lack of expert development in current practice has raised important concerns about administrative decisions to shift support from, or eliminate altogether, nurses who are skillful coaches (educators, clinical nurse specialists, overloaded experienced staff nurses, etc.). Instead of coaching clinical reasoning and judgment in actual practice, educators have instead been pressed to classrooms to repetitively teach policies, orientation, general information and the like. Presenting knowledge does not ensure that it transferred, accessible or even relevant to most clinical situations. The mass of educators presenting PowerPoint presentations with "canned" lectures, therefore, are not counted as beneficial coaches to new and developing nurses who must learn how to clinically reason and <u>clinically use</u> the extensive knowledge they have acquired. Thus, the gap between the experts needed and those developed has deepened and widened to the point that the majority of nurses have not gone on to become expert in practice. In addition, an alarming number of nurses have not developed the most fundamental aspect of practice: engagement with the problem or the patient as a person. Engagement requires learning (or being taught) how to emotionally connect in critical ways that set up and then guide a good clinician's grasp, thinking, reasoning, judgment, interventions, and interactions. Without engagement in a situation, the clinician simply fails to notice meaningful and important cues, changes, and occurrences and, therefore, is crippled in trying to adequately care for the patient.

So, how is engagement learned or taught? Not surprisingly, engagement is most visible and best learned in an authentic context where the expert nurses' notions of good and ethics of care are pervasive and order thinking, judgment, interactions and interventions. Situated learning in actual patient situations is superior to other methods of teaching because it provide the rich opportunity for simultaneously learning multiple aspects of skilled know-how, knowledge use, and formation of how the layperson takes up being a nurse. Martina Skibola, a senior student nurse, reveals the strongest, most enduring way that engagement and formation occur, which is IN ordinary, everyday practice. Her story captures the incredible transformation of the layperson into the nurse and illustrates what is otherwise hard to explain:

> **Student:** The phrase "nurses treat the whole patient" could not have rung truer than it did today. I was privileged to witness the remarkable work of all of the nurses involved in this special case...A woman was coming from the neuro ICU as a withdrawal of care and organ donation. She arrived [in pre-op], accompanied by her neuro ICU nurse, respiratory [therapist], and the Organ Bank coordinator who was essentially running the transplant operation. After extubation, the monitor was closely watched and respirations were carefully counted. The patient remained in ventricular tachycardia for a long time, and it became doubtful that she would pass before the one hour cut-off, when her kidneys would become unviable. Sam, the ICU nurse, used great discretion when measuring the patient's discomfort, which could only be assessed by her respirations. He explained the fine line between keeping the patient comfortable with just enough morphine while refraining from unethically speeding up her dying process with too much morphine. We stood there for what seemed like an eternity, waiting....so she could give someone a new chance at a kidney, while we simultaneously consoled the family who stood at her side saying their final goodbyes. Minutes before the hour mark, our patient took her final breaths, and we rushed to the OR.
>
> After removal, parts of the kidneys were measured and evaluated for size, shape and color. As the kidneys were put into a special pump to keep them fresh until implantation, the Organ Bank coordinator explained that it takes hours of testing before they know if the kidneys can even be transplanted. I could not help but think that all of this strife could have been in vain and this woman's body could have been

left in peace. We could only hope that her will to help another life was so strong that, even after death, a part of her would heroically pull through.

As we got ready to close, we were informed that two special family members did not get to see the patient before she passed. Because she would later be cremated, they would not have the opportunity to see her unless we brought her back to pre-op after the surgery was over. This is where I witnessed some of the most beautiful nursing care, and I was reminded (as I am over and over again) why this profession is so special. The same nurses who were working diligently during surgery were the same who were left there in the end. Suddenly the unified goal was to make this patient look presentable for her family. We worked to scrub the blood out of her hair and off of her body, dressed her in a clean [gown], wrapped her in blankets, and fussed over the angles her head and hands should be in. One nurse said a prayer and thanked the patient for being willing to go through this to help another life. As I stepped back to analyze this situation, I noticed that only nurses remained, some whose shift had already ended, all willing to give as much love and time as necessary to care for this patient even after her passing.

As myself and the OR nurses wheeled her back into the pre-op slot where she had taken her last breaths, there was a somberness in the air. There was news that this woman had been a pediatric nurse practitioner for 35 years. Suddenly there was a feeling that she was not only a wonderful person for being willing to make this sacrifice for another, but also that she was one of us. To prepare for the family members' arrival, we placed heated blankets on the patient's hands so they would be warm to the touch when the family held them to say goodbye. When the family arrived, we were moved to find that it was the patient's friend and her daughter, a blind and deaf young woman who had been treated by the nurse practitioner for many years. We all stood around them, tears in our eyes, offering warmth and consolation.

This special day I was able to see the heart of nursing revealed in so many ways—beginning with the patient, a nurse herself, who was willing make sacrifices to help the sick even after her death; the ICU nurse who thoughtfully assessed the patient's discomfort down to her last moments; the OR nurses who went beyond their OR duties to present the patient to her family, who would otherwise have never had the chance to see her again; the pre-op nurse who made sure the slot was ready and chairs were present for when they arrived—and the way they all acted as a support group as the women grieved over their beloved. All of the nurses present today have different roles at the [hospital]. Some of them may have never even met. But the remarkable quality of care given to this patient and her family is what unifies them. The selfless tasks that they carried out come from the ingrained compassion for others that those in the nursing profession all seem to possess. As I graduate nursing school in 3 days, and the confusion of job applications and NCLEX studying clouds my life, I am certain of one thing. People like those I described make me so proud to become a nurse.

Without the nurses intentionally coaching her, Martina actively engages in being formed as a good nurse through first hand experiential learning; that is, learning the socially embedded notions of good and ethics of care that she sees in the ethical comportment of the nurses. She recognizes that each nurse has been formed, or shaped, by the traditions and understandings held sacred within the culture and community of nurses. She sees that each nurse shares a common self-understanding of what it is to be a nurse, respectfully and reverently in the presence of one who has passed, and particularly with another dedicated nurse. Martina is also struck by each nurse knowing what and how to collectively create a space for family and each other to honor this life spent in devoted service to others. Martina learns early in the day about engagement in the problem of successfully harvesting the desperately needed life-saving organs from a generous patient whose death could have been more peaceful. Later, she learns a deeper level of engagement with the patient as a deserving, beneficent, and beloved human being and is more strongly formed by the pains-taking care the expert nurses invest in the presentation of the body, even after death. These are emotionally ladened lessons that become embodied in the learner's ethics, self-understanding, commitments, concerns, and agency. In this situation, engagement, ethical comportment and formation are tacitly passed on, nonverbally. Embedded in the situation, Martina readily grasps and embodies some of the most important yet fundamental knowledge and skilled know-how of her career. Learning in the midst of excellent nurses inspires and shows learners how to become more than they originally imagined.

Not every nurse requires this kind of situation to learn engagement, ethical comportment, or to be formed in such a powerful way in a single incident. More commonly, learners are involved in multiple situations where excellent nurses, coaches or faculty demonstrate similar ethical comportment. Learning is enhanced when developing nurses or students are coached to notice and subsequently become attuned to the ethical comportment of others. Ethics is embedded in the everyday practice of nurses, as in other professional practices like medicine, teaching, or ministering. The notions of good are socially embedded in these practices and student and developing clinicians learn to take up a new identity as a professional with new capacities, to see and act. Practice-based ethics cannot be reduced to formal principles used to adjudicate and make decisions about practice breakdown or just to ensure patient and professional rights. Practice-based ethics requires that the clinician learn how to instantiate notions of good in actual, everyday practice situations. Students and developing clinicians seek to be formed as an attuned, compassionate nurse. There will inevitably be situations where ethical comportment is missing. Dialogue about differences in comportment from specific contexts can provide strong instances of learning, because instances of what is missing can point out exactly what is so important.

For students and developing nurses, this particular narrative can be used to teach engagement and formation and, additionally, notions of good (those of the patient and the nurses), ethical comportment, weighing competing goods when using morphine at the end of life, withdrawal of life-sustaining technologies in the family's presence, skillful involvement with the family, responding to the unexpected, presenting the "person" to the family after death", and moral agency, to name a few. Kyriakidis and Vitello (in progress) found that dialogue with new nurses about similar narratives that described strong ethical comportment, engagement, and expert caring practices not only influenced the engagement and formation of beginners but also significantly improved their skillful performance earlier in practice than previous research described. We prefer the terms formation and ethical comportment over the term "socialization" because these terms refer not to just the role messages and pressures of the social community of practitioners and patients, but also to the clinician's active engagement with being formed as a good nurse in particular situations (Benner, Sutphen, Leonard & Day, 2010). For developing nurses who are early in practice and have not yet learned to emotionally engage, similar narratives with questions that coach the learner to imaginatively engage in the situation can be helpful. Educators should be aware that for clinicians who are later in practice and did not learned to or were not taught how to emotionally engage, their self-understanding is still formed, but it is dissimilar from that of excellent nurses. Teaching with the same narrative may have little to no effect on the nurse's learning after a certain point in formation. The nurse may notice what others are doing, but it commonly does not alter the nurse's willingness or ability to engage and it may not alter or transform the nurse's formed self-understanding and judgments. For nurses who are later in their practice, situated coaching for attunement and involvement can be helpful.

In addition to engagement and formation, most aspects of skillful performance which depend on the intelligent use of knowledge are best learned in the midst of an unfolding situation. To point out coaching strategies for situated learning and to recognize how specific situations call forth acquired knowledge, the reader is invited to imaginatively enter the following exemplar as the nurse, Mary Nottingham, who shared this story, and envision oneself as an educator, preceptor, or teacher who is coaching a less experienced nurse as s/he is caring for this baby and family. By imaginatively being present, one can experience the urgency, the baby's rapidly approaching end of life, the imperative to act on the parents' behalf, the intrusion of a policy that does not apply, the distress of withdrawing life support and the joy of holding Paul's twin. One can also experience the high stakes demands, Mary's constant reasoning in the ever changing situation, and complex judgments to intervene in the face of ambiguity, risks, and time constraints. The story is presented in parts so that one can reflect on how to coach a less experienced nurse as the situation changes over time:

Nurse: Paul was 2 months old and had a twin brother, Peter, and 2 year-old sister, Mary. Paul's mom had put him down on the couch after his 4 am feeding. Unfortunately, Paul was a belly sleeper. Paul's mom went to check on him 3 hours later and he wasn't breathing. What a nightmare for anyone, especially a mom, to ever experience! They called 911 and they were able to revive him. However, no one really knew how long he had been down. He was brought directly to the PICU around noon, his parents arriving shortly thereafter. A CT scan showed significant anoxic injury. Even if Paul survived, his quality of life would be minimal. Throughout that 1st day, Paul was put on maximal support. It was evident that Paul was not going to survive this traumatic injury. I cared for Paul and his family on the second day. He had been in the PICU for around 20 hours. I listened to report about the drips (he was maxed out on dopamine, dobutamine and on the same path with the levophed), blood products (we were ordering 20 cc/kg of FFP and PRBCs) and neuro status (his pupils were fixed and dilated).

Immediately following report, the coach may question the learner which engages the learner in thinking and reasoning about the situation and calls for situated cognition. This kind of learning is distinctly different from telling the learner what they should be thinking or what knowledge is needed. Depending on the learner's level of experience, questions may vary in specificity. Questions that elicit connection, understanding, thinking, hunches, anticipations, and judgment, which keep the learner in an engaged stance with the situation, are superior to analytic questions about "why" which elicit factual information but tend to throw the learner into a disengaged, objectified view of the situation. Good questions that stimulate excellent dialogue and learning include: What are your concerns in this situation? What stood out as salient to you in this situation? Talk about your concerns for the parents. How might you interaction with them? What might you say or do when they arrive? Thinking ahead serves as a dress rehearsal for one of the more challenging interactions that newer nurses experience (Kyriakidis & Vitello, in progress). Talk about the meaning of "significant anoxic injury." How is that linked to the quality of his life? What is the meaning and significance of fixed and dilated pupils? What kinds of interventions will you prioritize in this situation? What are you expecting to happen with this baby? How soon? What are we going to be watching out for? What is needed before the baby deteriorates? What particular parental needs are you anticipating and want to plan for? What are those plans? Good coaches are consistently cognizant that learning is the goal rather than quick and correct answers. One of the most important questions to the learner is: What questions do you have?

Embedded in these questions are coaching for engagement, involvement, grasp, clinical forethought, clinical reasoning, and clinical judgment. More experienced learners may not require this level of detailed coaching but instead may have specific aspects of practice they want help with. For instance, nurses at 1 to 2 years of practice may not have learned how to interact with parents who are close to losing a child. What do you say? What do you do to be helpful? What is comforting? Good coaches gage the kind of coaching they do in accordance with what the learner needs. One must follow the learner's lead which is understood from listening and observing what they already know how to do well. For very timid learners, making suggestions about what to do or how to do something can be most helpful. Anxious learners may benefit from having various aspects of practice role modeled. The coach needs to get a sense of what is needed, and then step back to enable the learner to take over at the earliest possible time.

Good coaches learn that "telling" the learner the "answers" never ensures learning or sustainable practice. Seeing something that another points out is not the same skill as recognizing it in the first instance. The challenge is recognizing the nature of the problem, recognizing what is salient or not, and making sense of all the data and findings, some of which are abnormal but do not factor into the big picture.

Not immediately in this urgent situation, but good questions that situate learning in later discussions may include: Talk about the use of each of the three vasoactive drugs? What is the meaning and benefit of using these drugs in combination if they all have similar actions? What other neuro assessments would you or did you find that were congruent with fixed and dilated pupils? with severe anoxic brain injury? With prolonged use of simultaneous vasoactive drug infusion that are all maxed out? Talk about the indications and use of blood products for this particular baby. Talk about the risk of an infant that belly sleeps. In response to all the questions suggested, an excellent coach will primarily listen and further coach with more questions that help the learner draw forth related and needed knowledge. Dialogue is another excellent source of learning when the learner is unclear in their reasoning and knowledge use. Questions that stimulate strong instances of learning require sensitivity so as not to put the learner on the spot or create a "test" atmosphere. Questions should stay true to the situation in the way that expert clinicians think about clinical situations that then guide the care they provide.

As the coach enters the room with the learner, an important question is, "how will you interact with the baby? " Questions, asked repeatedly over time in different patient situations set up the learner's habits of thinking, reasoning, and forethought or habits of expert clinicians. To continue with Mary's story, she left report thinking:

Nurse: But the whole time [during report] I knew that my focus was going to be on giving the family as much quality time with their son as possible.

I went into the room to meet Paul. He was beautiful, despite the oversized c-collar, puffy eyes and swollen tongue. My first thought was "how can I make him look more like the baby that came into this hospital yesterday?" I immediately went out to ask if we could get an x-ray, to clear his c-spine so we could remove the c-collar. I knew that if we could remove it, [it would reduce] some of the fluid in his eyes and tongue. I knew how important it would be for his parents to look into his precious blue eyes one last time. Unfortunately, the resident said that we were unable to take off the collar, as it was impossible to get the appropriate film to clear his c-spine. I immediately sought out the attending down the hall and asked the same question. She, also, said that we could not remove it. I knew that they had to follow protocol, but it was obvious this little guy was not going to make it. I was not going to give up on this!

Good situated coaching may include but is not limited to the following questions and dialogues: Given the situation and what is expected, what is your first priority right now? As sick as Paul is, talk about the first priority of making Paul look more like himself. What do you anticipate the most important thing will be for the parents? Talk about what you anticipate is most important even though you have not yet met them or talked with them? Talk about how you make a case with the physician about removing the c-collar? Talk about the reasoning for going over the resident's head to ask the attending the same question? What was the nature of the problem of not getting the x-ray and removing the c-collar? What were you feeling while you were talking with the physicians about removing the c-collar? What influences may shape that dialogue in turning out differently? The protocol ensures safe practice, so talk about the clinical wisdom of breaking away from protocol. Talk about the ethics of breaking from protocol? What is the need for strong agency in this situation, what is at stake? What will stronger agency need to look like? How can you make a stronger case, and should you?

These coaching questions assist the learner to stay engaged with the specific patient situation and reasoning through the changes that need to occur. Rehearsal with a coach is enormously helpful prior to what is typically an anxiety provoking interaction. A good coach will know the physicians and be able to best prepare the learner for what is to come. In some specialties where physicians may not be particularly collaborative, the nurse may need to develop the habit of multiple attempts with mounting evidence. Making a case and acting as a strong agent for the patient and family is particularly challenging for inexperienced learners. It's hard to act in strong ways when there is little experiential wisdom or confidence that are essential prior to acting in strong ways, and, especially difficult when one must act independently. This is one of the key areas of practice where a concerned charge nurse, a trusted peer, or a coach is needed as a safety net for the clinical judgment and rehearsal for making a case. It is also an area of practice that typically develops later and a more experienced colleague or coach may need to demonstrate how to negotiate conflicting perspectives. Because making a case and negotiating with physicians is commonly experienced as very demanding and anxiety provoking, interactive sessions (dress rehearsal, role playing, conflict management) can be incredibly helpful to learn embodied skills and responses that enable the newer nurse to more effectively negotiate. In each situation, the coach should prepare the learner on how the "leave the door open" for future dialogue with even the most difficult of colleagues. Learning how to build trust and earn trust are important lessons for collaboration.

Again, given the urgency of the Paul's situation, there are questions that are better suited for later discussion. These include: What was the concern about Paul's c-spine? What was you looking for on an x-ray? What were you expecting to see the x-ray? How could removal of the c-collar reduce fluid in Paul's eyes and tongue?

Returning to Mary's story:

> **Nurse:** Shortly after, Paul's parents came into the room—sleep-deprived, tearful, wearing the same clothes that they had on when they put young Paul to bed that fateful early morning. I introduced myself and updated them on Paul's condition. Mom was holding it together (as mom's often do), asking questions and dad was up talking to Paul, telling him how much he loved him and that he was missing him so much. I asked them if they would like to hold Paul. This was rather risky as it could create a rapid shift in his hemodynamics while moving him from his bed, but I felt that they needed this time with him. They were very surprised at this offer, with their son in such critical condition, but said yes. Deep down, they knew that it would only be a short while before the medications would not keep his blood pressure up. I went out to talk to the physicians and told them that I wanted to allow Paul's parents to hold him. I knew that I needed some leeway with titrating drips to keep Paul's pressure up while they held him until they made a decision to make him a DNR or withdraw support. I didn't want the physicians to talk to them yet. I wanted them to have a little hope while they held Paul—to talk to him and love him. Mom and dad each had time to hold him and talk to him. Mom, telling him that he was her brave little soldier. Dad, begging Paul to come back to him. What a desperate situation! I wanted so badly to snap my fingers and make him all better. When we put him back in bed, I could see that they needed a break. Dad was pacing. I suggested that they get something to eat. I sent them downstairs with one of our low-frequency phones and told them that I would call them if anything changed. I also gave them my number and told them to call me if they wanted.

The parents' arrival adds new complexity to the new or developing nurse's demands for attention, thinking, judgment and performance. What is not visible in this particular narrative account, yet so apparent in the actual situation, is the continuous physiological and pharmacological interventions necessary to manage Paul's multiple organ systems failure. The coach will easily recognize the competing demands on the less skillful learner—the priority of the parents ability to be as close to Paul for as long as possible versus maintaining Paul's failing stability until crucial issues are addressed. Either priority for the inexperienced learner can be totalizing. How one coaches may necessarily change to enable the learner to best perform, yet simultaneously learn. Depending on what the learner needs most, two distinctly different lines of questions can stimulate situated learning. Questions that would be helpful in learning to interact with the parents and clinically reason in the changing, tenuous situation, either at the time or later, include: With the parents' arrival, what are you noticing? Be as specific as possible. What are you expecting? Have your concerns changed? To what? What actions are you going to take, based on your current grasp of how the parents are doing? What cues are you getting from the parents about what they need? What do the parents understand about Paul's situation and possibilities? What are you thinking about in terms of the parents in this situation now? What are you feeling as you care for the baby? As you care for the parents? What are you hoping to be able to do for this family? Talk about wanting to give the parents time with Paul before they make a DNR decision. What did you notice that signaled dad's changing needs? How might you ensure that dad gets the break he needs, yet maintains a close connection in case something happens sooner than expected? This line of inquiry focuses on the central concern overall in this situation but must be weighed in terms of care of the baby.

It is uncommon for situated learning to focus on only one aspect of development at a time because the complexity in each situation simply requires multiple aspects of situated cognition, skilled know-how, and ethical comportment, often simultaneously. Many aspects of skillful performance are linked in specific situations even though they may not typically be linked in every situation. Here, interacting with the parents is linked to grasp, engagement, reasoning over time, judgment, interventions and forethought. Thus, it is clear to see why there is no rule or guideline that enables developing clinicians to skillfully perform. They must learn how to think in action and flexibly respond in ever-changing, ever-different situations.

The second line of inquiry focuses on Paul's physiological support until an anguishing decision can be made and the parents have some time as a family and may include: What is Paul's current physiological status? What responses are you noticing from Paul? How is Paul responding to the interventions you are making? What risks are you encountering by acting in this situation? When you move Paul from the bed to let his parents hold him, what are you watching out for? How do these risks compare to others you have taken? What are you expecting and what interventions do you anticipate needing to make? How are you going to make a case to the physician for titrating the drips, if needed, when you move Paul? What drips are you going to preferentially titrate? The point of coaching by using inquiry and questioning is to have learners think, learn to use knowledge in a particular context, puzzle solve, make cognitive links, and learn in habitual ways that enable them to perform like good clinicians do in everyday practice. They will take up inquiry as a form of thinking and reflecting which sets them up as lifelong learners.

If or when the new or developing nurse becomes stressed, overwhelmed, needs to more narrowly focus, stops learning due to the demands of the situation, or compromised by trying to manage/intervene in too many ways simultaneously, role modeling as a way of situated learning is very helpful. Also, in a rapidly changing situation, when a developing nurse requires more time than available to reason through the situation, the coach can help by offering requested suggestions, instructions, and answers. All count as experiential, just-in-time learning in a context.

In Mary's clinical story, the parents had some time to hold Paul without the burden of an impending DNR or withdrawal decision. They decided to leave the unit for a time to get something to eat:

Nurse: As soon as [the parents] left, I spoke to the physicians about Paul's condition. In the last hour and a half, I had titrated the levophed from 200 to 750 nanos. We were approaching the end point and I feared that we would have to code him soon if we didn't get a DNR. The physicians said that they would speak to the parents as soon as they got back upstairs. I wanted this to be a very controlled situation. I didn't want to have to talk about this while Paul's pressure was dipping dangerously low. I wanted them to feel that they had time to make a good decision. Because of the circumstances that [resulted in Paul's admission], I wanted them to have no regrets about this decision. As soon as they came back up I went to get the physicians. They said they would be in after they finished rounding on another patient. I waited and waited. A watched pot never boils. I finally went out after 10 minutes. "They were sorry, they forgot." "What!" I thought to myself. "How can they forget when a babies' life is dependent on this next 5-minute discussion?" I reminded them that we were very close to having to "pound on this precious baby's chest" and that they had better talk with this family now. I realize that this sounded harsh, but I was desperate to have this family attended to.

The physicians came in and spoke with the family. Mom and dad wanted to talk about it before they made their decision of whether to withdraw support or just make him a DNR and let nature take its course. I left them alone to talk and followed the resident out to ask again about the c-collar. She was still uncomfortable removing it without getting an okay from the coroner. This was a somewhat complex situation, as a '310' had been filed due to the "questionable" circumstances surrounding Paul's injury. Anytime there is a question regarding the mechanism of injury in a child that could *potentially* be non-accidental, Child Welfare becomes involved and a '310' is filed. If the child dies, he immediately becomes a coroner's case. The resident was afraid that removing the c-collar might alter the coroner's assessment. It was obvious in this situation that this was a purely accidental injury, but the resident did not want to bend the rules. I then asked the attending the same question and she finally conceded!

As Paul's condition deteriorates and the complexity of the situation grows, a good coach nudges the learner to continuously reason through the multiple declining transitions in order to anticipate what is needed, be prepared, and flexibly respond to Paul and his parents. The urgency and complexity calls for attunement, modus operandi thinking, reasoning in an unfolding situation, clinical judgment, caring practices, the role of emotion, and agency so the coaches questions can guide the learner in developing those aspects of practice. Questions can include: Talk about how you titrated the levophed and the baby's response to tremendous increase. What are you noticing that indicates that Paul may code soon. Have your concerns changed, and if so, what are they? What are you going to talk with the physicians about? What are your notions of what is good to do for Paul in this situation? What are you hoping for when the physicians talk with Paul's parents? How are you feeling and what are you thinking while waiting for the physicians to come and talk with Paul's parents? When you went to get the physicians, after they didn't come in 10 minutes, talk about the way you experienced time during those 10 minutes. You expressed outrage about the physicians forgetting to come…talk about that. What was at stake when you felt desperate to have the family attended to? What did you notice about the situation that the resident did not see that made you comfortable about Paul's injury being accidental? What did you say to the attending or what happened that made the difference in removing the c-collar?

At this point in the situation, it is doubtful that the learner as clinician would have even a moment to respond to or think about actual questions. The urgency and demands to provide the needed care would consume the attention of most learners. However, the coaching questions may fuel substantive dialogue later in a debriefing session or in reflection on the situation. Whether student or practicing clinician, nurses must learn to reflect on their practice to develop expertise and become adept in articulating what they are learning from their direct clinical experiential learning. No clinician ever gets beyond the need to learn directly from practice, since clinical inquiry and knowledge development is required in all clinical practice.

As we re-enter the situation with Mary, the parents have been sitting and determining what is best for Paul:

Nurse: I went back into the room to see if mom and dad had any questions. We went over the scenarios of withdrawing support. I gave them multiple options: weaning drips, completely turning off drips, and extubating. I knew he would not last long either way, but I wanted the family's perception to be that he went as peacefully as possible. I removed the c-collar and handed him to his mother. Shortly thereafter, when the family was ready, we did a terminal wean on the drips, gave him some morphine and then extubated him. He passed within minutes. I left mom and dad to hold him. When they were ready for a break, I started getting things ready to give him his bath. Dad stepped out with the chaplain so I asked mom if she would like to help. I left to get warm water for his bath. When I returned, dad was back. I asked if he would like to help us. Tears welled up in his eyes. He said that he had never been able to give him a bath. This would be his first.

We spent the next 30 minutes talking about Paul and Peter's birth, how they were different, how they were the same. They showed me pictures of the boys "holding hands" in the crib while they were in the NICU....a picture "set-up" by the NICU nurse one night.

Child Life [services] arrived to redo a couple of the plaster casts of Paul's feet that were made the night before but had not turned out. Mom really wanted one of each hand and foot. She said she would take *any* piece of him that she could have. She wanted to place them next to the casket so everyone could see them. I knew it was very important to make sure they had whatever we could give them. Unfortunately the plaster takes awhile to cure. I knew they wouldn't be ready by the time the family was ready to go. So, before the family left, I took their number from the patient info sheet so I could make arrangements with them to drop those little feet off before the funeral.

As they left, mom and dad came up to thank me and each gave me a hug. They said that I was able to make a very hard time for them a little more bearable. It is so hard to accept the gratitude and gratefulness from families in a situation like this. But, what they didn't know was that in only 6 hours, they had made a significant impact in my life as well. I in turn thanked them for allowing me to share in Paul's life. When I went to their house to drop off those precious little feet, I got a special surprise. I got to hold Paul's twin brother, Peter, who now has a special angel in heaven with precious little feet!

In this short 6 hours, the new or developing nurse has experienced incredible challenge. There is a need for debriefing, but the coach must gage what, when, and how much was helpful. Inexperienced nurses commonly talk about going home and crying alone. In contrast, expert nurses who shared tragic situations with colleagues often talked and cried together. Because clinicians vary in how they best cope, the coach needs to read each situation and determine what might be most helpful. At some point after the incident, it may be beneficial to reflect on the following questions: Talk about the withdrawal options that you need to discuss with Paul's parents. If they ask what you suggest, what will you tell them? When they ask what to expect once support has been withdrawn, what will you explain to them? When you give Paul morphine after withdrawal, how will you gage how much to give him? How do you feel about that? Tell me how you situated the baby for the terminal wean... at what point did the parents hold him? Talk more about inviting the parents to help give Paul a bath. How did "talking about Paul and Peter's birth" come up? How did you feel about the experience of being with Paul's parents after his death? Contrast for me the professional boundaries you've learned about with taking Paul's precious little feet to his parents' home. Can you talk about some of the ways you are learning to cope with the death of young patients? Are there things or support you need to assist you in coping?

At the end of each situation that one coaches, a good coach commonly asks a few additional questions to create the habit of reflection which is a habit of continuous learning. These questions include: Is there anything you would do differently if you had it to do over again? What was most demanding about this situation? What was most satisfying? Are there any suggestions you would give another nurse in this same situation? Talk about what was most "critical or important or memorable" to you in this situation. Was there anything particular you learned from this situation, the patient, or from the family? The questions posed for situated learning can be raised by the learner in dialogue with oneself, though far from ideal, or raised in collaboration with a colleague. The extent of the effectiveness has not been studied, but learning is possible when clinical reasoning and situated cognition are developed.

As mentioned, our goal in presenting situated learning as a key strategy to teach in an integrative way is to provide examples of situated coaching and learning. These few and situation-specific questions only begin to scratch the surface of the possibilities which are called forth in various situations. Lines of inquiry can be broader and simpler when the learner is very inexperienced and become more focused when coaching higher levels of development and specific aspects of skillful performance and situated cognition. The teacher introduces new levels of complexity as the student progresses from novice to expert (Benner, 2000). The goal of situated learning is that the new or developing clinician learns to engage in situated cognition and think-in-action in real clinical situations. We have tried to illustrate that, as one actually or imaginatively works through an authentic situation, the diversity and extent of knowledge called forth by the situation becomes apparent. It exemplifies how clinicians must draw on and use the vast knowledge they acquire and how the situations often necessitates acquiring further specialized knowledge that was not needed prior. Situated learning typifies the clinical reasoning and situated cognition of everyday practice; yet, it has not been a common or recognized method of teaching clinicians. If educators, administrators, and nurses hope to narrow the growing gap between beginner and expert, then clinicians must have the sufficient coaching and support to learn to use knowledge as it is used in everyday excellent practice.

A THINKING-IN-ACTION APPROACH: INTEGRATING CLASSROOM AND CLINICAL EDUCATION

We piloted the "Thinking-In-Action" approach in a class of critical care and trauma master's students who were enrolled in a monitoring and management course[1]. Although this was a higher level course, a similar but less complex situation can be employed for undergraduate programs. At the beginning of the course, attention was paid to explaining to students how to imaginatively enter or "walk around" in a clinical narrative. Because we ultimately wanted students to reflect on their own practice and generate and share their own clinical incidents with their peers, we stressed the importance of the inside-out or engaged (first-person) stance that is required for respectful listening and understanding. For each class session, students were given one or two relevant narratives to situate and bound the discussion and clinical problem solving. We selected two habits of thought, two (of the many) domains of practice, and one pervasive thread to which we pointed to throughout the discussions, which included: clinical grasp and clinical inquiry; clinical forethought; diagnosing and managing life-sustaining physiologic functions; communicating and negotiating multiple perspectives; and the thread of skilled know-how, technical finesse, and craft.

---

[1]The description of this class was adapted from Benner, P., Stannard, D., & Hooper, P. (1996). A "thinking-in-action" approach to teaching clinical judgment: A classroom innovation for acute care advanced practice nurses. *Advanced Practice Nursing Quarterly, 1*(4), 70–77.

Students read each assigned narrative prior to class. Additionally, each class session had a set of required and recommended readings on the science and research studies relevant to the assigned narrative(s). Study questions, generated by content experts, were designed to set up a dialogue between the skilled clinical knowledge from the narratives and the scientific principles presented in the readings (Benner, Stannard & Hooper, 1996). Therefore, prior to class, students began to engage in thinking, use the knowledge acquired, puzzle solving, and imaginatively rehearsing for intervention the practical way that a clinician performs in actual practice.

In class, each narrative was read aloud in portions by student volunteers, with each portion followed by class discussion. Class discussion was located in the narrative as it unfolded. To closely mimic clinical thinking-in-action, students were directed to imaginatively enter the clinical situation and to tailor their discussion to the issues and risks at hand in the clinical narrative in order to discourage them from offering unrelated content (from a disengaged stance) they had gleaned from their readings or from practice. In other words, it was not enough to simply state decontextualized facts; discussion was centered on information relevant to the situation at hand, as illustrated in the narrative. Students could speculate about different interpretations and courses of action, but, in order to simulate engaged thinking, these had to relate to the situation itself (Benner, Stannard & Hooper, 1996). The narratives served to situate the discussion and required students to select and use relevant science and theory. The narratives also illustrated ambiguities and missing information in practice. Students would sometimes reflect on their anxieties about ambiguities and under-determined clinical situations. This naturally occurring anxiety in the classroom was used to focus on how clinicians cope with and reason through indeterminate data and under-determined and open-ended clinical situations. The narratives also opened the possibility of discussing problem identification and issues of salience (e.g. why one problem might be more relevant than others). Ways of coping with information overload, high time demand, high stakes, and indeterminate data became a part of the reflection on practice and a point of experiential clinical learning. In addition, situations of breakdown, where things did not go well, were included for students to reflect on what clinical and moral actions they may take, how, and with whom as a way of exploring and experientially learning ethical comportment.

To foster active and engaged clinical reasoning, students were encouraged to make connections between the narrative at hand and examples from their own practice. They were asked to compare and contrast the situations, just as expert clinicians do in actual everyday practice and learning. This link is central to practical reasoning and to ongoing reflection on practice. Students had to identify with and consider the risks, possibilities, and opportunities of the clinicians in the narrative. They had to imagine that they might soon be in that clinician's situation. This teaching-learning strategy provided a level of engagement for the students that we hypothesized (though did not test in this pilot course) would increase the students' ability to remember the issues in clinical and ethical reasoning. The learning principle we were calling on is that emotional engagement with the situation is closely linked with present and future perception and identification of similar clinical problems and distinctions (Benner, Tanner & Chesla, 2009; Damasio, 1994). Since the first edition, Kyriakidis & Vitello (in progress) have shown that, not only did beginning nurses learn from the issues in others' clinical and ethical reasoning, but also they learned what actions to take on those issues and what strong ethical comportment was needed. Without prior experience, new graduate nurses actually took appropriate action in their own first real patient situation (based on experiential learning from a shared narrative), felt morally compelled to do so despite high anxiety, and they used essential scientific knowledge to substantiate their actions.

In each class, a clinical content expert co-facilitated with a member of the teaching team who primarily encouraged engaged reasoning, dialogue about the domains of skillful performance, ethical comportment, and an inside-out discussion. Because this was a monitoring and management course with a strong pathophysiological focus, content experts and students discussed the scientific rationale behind nurses' monitoring and management interventions in the narratives, and facilitated, often through questions, the students' integration of the required readings into the class discussions.

Students were evaluated by their preparedness and participation in class based upon their readings, by the quality of their classroom participation, and by their thoughtful responses on three evaluative tools we called response sheets. Each of the three evaluative methods required the student's integration of knowledge, skilled know-how, and ethical comportment. Each response sheet referred the student back to an exemplar that was presented in class and required engaged reasoning. Students were asked to discuss the critical points or junctures that occurred in the chosen exemplar and to describe the major monitoring and management issues in the situation. This encouraged thinking, reasoning and judgment about patients' transitions. It was expected that students would integrate their readings into their responses and create succinct and scholarly responses to the questions posed. Additionally, students were asked to provide a two to five page exemplar from their own practice that they contrasted and compared to the chosen exemplar. Students were not required to "match" a pulmonary exemplar with an exemplar that, for instance, described a patient with pulmonary problems; rather, students were encouraged to think about how the situation unfolded and to link a clinical incident from their own practice to the chosen exemplar. Based upon the chosen exemplar and the student-authored exemplar, two additional questions were asked. First, based on one of the two exemplars, students were asked how they would respond to the situation now, given their style of practice, newly acquired scientific and experiential knowledge, and skill related to the content within the exemplar. This question encouraged students to habitually and actively reflect on their practice. Secondly, we asked students to discuss the major points of clinical judgment and/or excellent caring practices evident in one of the two exemplars, as well as to identify what they would have done if they had been an advanced practice nurse in the situation (the role they were preparing for in the masters program). Finally, we asked students to discuss the implications for change and/or for extending the practice arising from one of the two exemplars. This question was to encourage rehearsal and role-play relative to their future roles as advanced practice nurses.

By asking students to generate their own narratives from practice on each of the three response sheets, we encouraged students to make connections between the classroom discussion and their own practice. Additionally, the students' narratives formed the basis for a dialogue with the faculty on the student's practice. With the mutual consent of the student and faculty, the students' narratives became a student-generated text on clinical experiential learning and wisdom.

Because this was a pilot approach, we did not formally evaluate this teaching-learning method. However, based on student evaluations and the growth many students demonstrated in their class discussion and response sheets as the course proceeded, we believe this innovative strategy succeeds in teaching clinical judgment and science in a way that closely resembles the way in which expert nurses actually think and reason in patient situations as they unfold. Learning from an engaged stance with the narratives allowed students to safely, yet realistically and imaginatively experience high stakes clinical and ethical issues. It also encouraged students to dialogue with their practice and with their peers in order to learn from everyday practice. Finally, by using the logic of practice to guide the development and implementation of the course, we succeeded in fusing both process and content. Because one's understanding of an actual patient's condition is always situated, students were taught to think from within a situation, with all its ambiguities and contingencies, while integrating the best of science.

REFLECTION ON PRACTICE

Questions that elicit clinical thinking and reasoning about a particular situation are an excellent way of encouraging learning from practice. Response sheets, described above, were used as a learning tool with students. Response sheets for clinical learning can be developed following the nine aspects of clinical learning, habits of thought and action, and the domains described in this book. Learners can use the nine aspects of clinical judgment to make their own clinical and ethical reasoning more apparent: 1) developing a sense of salience; 2) situated learning and integrating knowledge acquisition and knowledge use; 3) engaged reasoning-in-transition; 4) skilled know-how; 5) response-based practice; 6) agency; 7) perceptual acuity and interpersonal engagement with patients; 8) integrating clinical and ethical reasoning; and finally, 9) developing clinical imagination. Habits of thought and action—clinical grasp and clinical forethought—are useful both for planning a clinical assignment and for reflecting on it after the clinical assignment. For example, students can identify their clinical forethought and the ways that they prepared the environment for likely clinical eventualities, as well as their own expectations based upon theory and clinical literature. They can then ask clinicians who have taken care of the patient or who are expert with similar patients what they anticipate during the next 4 to 8 hours and what they expect within the next 2 days. Comparing one's own expectations with others makes clinical learning more visible and initiates a learning habit that expert nurses develop; that is, learning through communities of colleagues.

Reasoning-in-transition and clinical grasp can be enhanced by asking students via the response sheet to identify past and present patient transitions. Patient transitions can be evaluated for how the transition was recognized or not recognized by the clinicians caring for the patient. Comfort level with skills can be assessed and practice can be arranged for areas where the student has little or no habitual skilled know-how. Distinctions can be made between skilled know-how and the use of thinking-in-action required to adapt technical interventions for particular patients. While beginning students cannot be expected to adjust their interventions based upon patient responses, response-based practice can be pointed out to them, and they can note the development of gauging and changing their interventions based upon patient responses to therapy such as pain medication or activity tolerance.

Students can reflect on their own and others' level and kind of clinical agency in the clinical situation. Questions posed on the response sheet, such as what made connecting with this patient and family easy or difficult, can reveal aspects of the student's coping and style of engagement. It is useful to have students assess their own family styles of engagement and compare these with patients and families. What are signs they recognize of over-involvement and identification with the patient's plight? What are signs that they recognize for under-involvement?

Questions can elicit early reflections on how notions of good influence clinical reasoning can enhance an early understanding and expectation that ethical and clinical reasoning will be linked in practice. Students can reflect on the development of their own moral compass as ethical dilemmas and ethical breaches in practice are encountered. This will enable students to see the development of their own ethical and clinical agency as the level of their practice changes.

Identifying the major concerns in the clinical situation and how these concerns order interventions and attentiveness should improve the student's thinking-in-action. Understanding the practical logic of how one's understanding of the clinical situation shapes the nurse-patient-family relationship, strategies for problem identification and problem solving should assist in the development of clinical grasp and the recognition of situations when grasp is lacking. Initially, students will not have sufficient experience to identify the nature of clinical situations as sources of problem identification and problem solving, but understanding the situatedness of clinical judgment and thinking-in-action should enhance the students' recognition of the nature of clinical situations (strong situations such as managing a crisis, caring for the family, or monitoring and managing hemodynamically unstable patients). The goal is to help the student develop their ability to recognize similar and dissimilar situations in order to improve their clinical grasp.

GUIDELINES FOR WRITING NURSING NARRATIVES

Using clinical narratives for teaching is based upon two major premises. First, there are two kinds of knowledge involved in human expertise: practical knowledge (or "knowing how") and formal or theoretical knowledge (or "knowing that"). While these two forms of knowledge are related, the relationship is not unidirectional or linear. "Knowing how" may precede "knowing that." Indeed, much of "knowing how" may be so contextual and situational that it does not lend itself to be captured in formal theoretical terms.

The practical world is always more complex than can ever be captured by a formal theoretical model. This does not mean that the practical world is completely random, capricious, or chaotic. Even chaotic and random events quickly become patterned due to human responses to those events. Because the practical everyday world is made up of habits, skills, practices, common meanings, cultures, and customs, there are always patterns. Human expertise is characterized by the ability to read situations and to recognize and understand patterns. Unlike formal expert systems, human experts can read fuzzy resemblances and patterns. Because there are always human variations in patients' response patterns, good clinical reasoning will continue to be central in expert practice.

Second, when a person becomes competent in the practical world of whatever enterprise, the situation is seen as patterns full of risks and opportunities. The world becomes more differentiated. When the person becomes proficient (according to the Dreyfus Model of Skill Acquisition), situations are read in terms of past whole situations (Benner, 1984; Dreyfus & Dreyfus, 1986). Experience, as it is used in this perspective, always means a turning around of preconceptions or an adding of nuances to a former understanding of a situation; it never means the mere passing of time. Instead of understanding performance as it is often idealized (namely, cool, rational, distant, and unemotional), performance is linked to emotional investment in good outcomes and in avoiding bad outcomes. Once performers become competent, they realize that they must choose a plan or perspective and that by choosing one plan or perspective, they preclude others. Risk and opportunity are involved and the performer is invested in the outcome. Good outcomes are deeply satisfying and poor outcomes cause disappointment (Benner et al., 1996).

So, how does one capture "practical knowledge", everyday understanding, or "know how"? It is best captured in narrative or "story" form that includes all the feelings of risk, opportunity, concerns, meaning, chronology, and changing relevance, complete with puzzles. This way, "know how" can be charted, even though "knowing that" or theoretical knowledge may be incomplete or even non-existent. Thus, narratives encourage the storyteller to give a first person account of the critical incident (exemplar) that include her or his concerns, hunches, dialogue, changing understanding over time, interventions, and puzzles. The storyteller should be encouraged to give the story complete with fears, risks, opportunities, and satisfactions in order to uncover the storyteller's practical knowledge and her or his read of the situation.

Selecting an Exemplar

Actually, the exemplar selects the storyteller or narrator in a way. A particular situation stands out in one's mind because it is laden with significance. It expresses important knowledge or meanings or expresses one's notion of excellent practice or breakdown. The best exemplars will select themselves, because they are the situations the storyteller thinks of over and over again. Typically, the narrator does not remember the outstanding situations through generalizations or labels, but directly as a memorable instance, a valued time, or with a sense of pride and pleasure over outcomes. Phrases that may jog the storyteller's memory include:

- A situation that stands out as the quintessence of good nursing
- A situation that taught you something new, opened up new ways of helping, new lines of inquiry, or made you notice something new
- A memorable exchange or encounter that taught you something new
- A situation where you clearly made a difference
- A situation of breakdown, error, or moral dilemma, and the situation is memorable because of the issues and problems it raised for you as a clinician.

It is usually easier to think of particular situations rather than categories or types of situations. You can trust that a situation stands out because it was meaningful in a variety of ways and on a number of different levels.

Writing the Exemplar

The exemplar should be presented as a narrative account. The storyteller may use the typical abbreviated and condensed "clinical" voice (as in shift report) describing the clinical situation, but it should be a story with a first person reporting style. Actually, the narrator may find it helpful to "tell" her or his story first into a tape recorder and transcribe the tape and edit it, tightening it and filling in any needed details. Oral reporting of the exemplar may be helpful because the oral tradition is less linear than writing, and it is more natural to include passing thoughts, and associated feelings and concerns in the oral tradition. While length of the exemplar is a consideration, it is best to tell the complete story first and then edit it down to the essential narrative account, preferably to four or five double-spaced, typewritten pages.

There are a few things the storyteller should note when editing her or his exemplar. Avoid summary statements or general phrases that do not communicate what actually occurred. For example, avoid phrases such as: "I analyzed the possible losses and took action to minimize them." Instead, tell the reader how you recognized the possible losses, how you minimized them, and when possible, describe the actual outcomes. Another example is: "I comforted the patient." Instead, provide details about what you did with or for the patient and how the patient responded. Include dialogue, when possible, to give the reader a first-hand account of the situation as it unfolded. Include your concerns or what you were anticipating when you took a particular action because that gives a window to your judgment. You may change the organization, hospital, department, or other identifying information to protect confidentiality. It would be helpful if the situation you chose as an exemplar could be shared publicly with others in the class or in a gathering.

EVALUATING NARRATIVES

Nursing narratives open up the possibility of demonstrating clinical inquiry in practice. For example, the faculty and students may want to do a thematic analysis of the narratives presented in a particular class. The clinical and ethical concerns that shape the story can be identified, along with the nursing knowledge, skills, and knowledge gaps evident in the story. Rich stories containing clinical knowledge that may not be well articulated in the nursing literature can be shared and reflecting on practice can be demonstrated both by the faculty and the students.

First person, experience-near narratives (written about the situation as it unfolded) require risk taking and trust on the part of the student and the teacher. The student has a right to demand that the teacher respect the experiential learning presented by the student. Therefore, criteria for evaluating nursing narratives, either in journals or in written exemplars, include: candor; veracity; vividness of description; clarity and coherence; and good use of narrative writing style, such as dialogue and first person statements. A well told and reflective story of error and breakdown can receive an "A" based on these criteria, whereas an exemplar that points to flawless practice in a vague and non-reflective fashion should be evaluated more carefully. The goal is to encourage honest exploration.

Narrators almost always reveal more than they are aware of or intend to in the telling of a story. Consequently, students should have the opportunity to reflect on their narrative account. The student should separate the first person, experience-near narration from the reflective commentary that follows the narrative. Allowing some time to lapse between the telling and writing of the actual story and writing reflections on the story later can be helpful. A teacher must be respectful of the student's self-revelation (students do not typically experience "why didn't you…" questions as respectful) and enter into a dialogue that relates to the student's understanding of the situation. Questions often extend the student's reflection.

Not everything, however, is best taught in this form of exploration and reflection. This teaching-learning strategy works best for experiential learning. Information giving and clarification of factual information is best gained from texts and interactive learning guides. A climate of trust and respect is essential to the success of such reflective classroom exercises. But it is a rewarding experience to make the knowledge evident in excellent practice more visible.

THE CALL FOR INTEGRATIVE CLASSROOM AND CLINICAL LEARNING IN ACADEMICS

Since the first edition of *Clinical Wisdom*, Dr. Patricia Benner led the Carnegie National Nursing Education program of research for the Carnegie Foundation for the Advancement of Teaching. Nursing is one of five key professions (along with engineering, clergy, law, and medicine) in a large program of research to study professional education. One of the overarching frameworks was that all professional education required at least three professional apprenticeships. The term "apprenticeship" was used as a metaphor for learning a practice, rather than as a model of work organization. All professional education requires situated cognition (that is, knowing exists, inseparable from context, people, activity, culture) (Lave & Wenger, 1991), coaching, and guidance in how to take up the practice, in addition to the knowledge and science required by the professional practice. The three apprenticeships central to all professional education include:

- The cognitive apprenticeship, which refers to learning how to use the science, theory and humanities education required to think like a nurse. For instance, a knowledgeable coach describes her thoughts as the coach and student work together to care for a patient, as a way of teaching to make thinking, reasoning, and inquiry visible.
- The practice apprenticeship, where the professional learns to effectively practice the discipline, for example, skilled know-how, practical or clinical reasoning, situated cognition and the use of knowledge in complex under-determined situations as well as the structured use of technology.
- The ethical comportment (formation) apprenticeship, where the professional learns to perceive and practice the notions of good, and the best practices in actual situations.

These three apprenticeships are discussed in *Educating Nurses: A Call for Radical Transformation* (Benner, Sutphen, Leonard, & Day, 2010). The call for a radical transformation to educate students and nurses, as well as physicians (Frenk et al., 2010), for practice presents the greatest challenge to educators who have long taught according to the logic of science, as expected and rewarded in academic settings for decades. That is, they have taught the sciences, humanities, etc. in their purer forms and from the objective or disengaged scientific stance. Integration of the three apprenticeships calls for teaching from the engaged stance of practice, where learning to clinically reason and make context-specific judgments follows the logic of practice and, consequently, prepares the learner for situated cognition by developing the habits of knowledge use and skillful performance of good clinicians. As a result, the clinician learns to think, be, and act like an excellent knowledge worker and care provider. All knowledge work requires knowledge use, and engaged emotional attunement to the problem, to interpersonal concerns, and to the stakes in the situation as it unfolds. This is an engaged, practical or clinical form of reasoning, rather than a formal criterial reasoning. Our hope is to assist educators in making the transformation by describing methods that are successful and inspiring innovative pedagogical strategies that integrate knowledge acquisition, knowledge use, and engaged attuned reasoning as the situation changes across time.

Benner, Sutphen, Leonard & Day (2010) describe ways of integrating the three apprenticeships in academics and suggest teaching for a sense of salience—helping students identify what stands out as most and least important in actual clinical situations. Educators will find these integrative strategies very helpful when rethinking the curriculum. This second edition of *Clinical Wisdom* repeatedly illustrates expert nurses' sense of salience in clinical situations by demonstrating their clinical grasp and clinical forethought in particular clinical situations. The clinical exemplars in this book can be integrated into classroom teaching in numerous ways to illustrate how clinical grasp and forethought, as well as the many other aspects of clinical knowledge are used in everyday clinical situations, and to provide rich clinical learning through dialogue along with the imaginative use of the considerable knowledge called forth by each narrative.

Individually and collectively, the narratives point out and set up expectations for professional practice as both demands and aspirations surpass what can be learned using a theoretical teaching approach. Narratives of expert patient and family care simultaneously provide a vision of excellent practice which strongly influences the formation of both students and developing nurses in shaping their understanding of what it is and how to be an excellent nurse. Practicing nurses need to be educated using methods that integrate the three professional apprenticeships (cognitive, theory and science, practical skilled knowhow with clinical reasoning, and ethical comportment) *whenever possible*. The kinds of teaching strategies we have detailed offer integrated approaches, and our hope is to stimulate additional novel strategies that integrate the three apprenticeships to enable students and developing nurses to intelligently and skillfully use the appropriate knowledge called for at the moment needed when caring for patients and their families.

SUMMARY

We end with a note of profound gratitude to the nurses who have so generously shared their stories from their practice. We hope that their stories inspire teaching and learning in authentic contexts so that we may not only preserve but also extend the expertise disclosed in each story into the practices of developing nurses and students. We trust that students and developing clinicians, clinical and academic educators, experienced nurses who coach others, and managers alike will read these stories and enlarge their clinical and moral imagination on the extraordinary human possibilities embedded in nursing practice.

REFERENCES

Benner, P. (2000). *From novice to expert: Excellence and power in clinical nursing practice.* Menlo Park, CA: Addison-Wesley.

Benner, P., Stannard, D., & Hooper, P. L. (1996). A "thinking-in-action" approach to teaching clinical judgment: A classroom innovation for acute care advanced practice nurses. *Advanced Practice Nursing Quarterly, 1*(4), 70–77.

Benner, P., Sutphen, M., Leonard, V., & Day, L. (2010). *Educating nurses: A Call for radical transformation.* San Francisco: Jossey-Bass and Carnegie Foundation for the Advancement of Teaching.

Benner, P., Tanner, C. A., & Chesla, C. A. (2009). *Expertise in nursing practice: Caring, clinical judgment, and ethics* (Second Edition) New York, NY: Springer Publishing Company.

Berkow, S., Virkstis, K., Stewart, J. & Conway, L. (2008). Assessing new graduate nurse performance. *Journal of Nursing Administration, 38*(11): 468–474.

Bourdieu, P. (1980/1990). *The logic of practice.* (R. Nice, trans.). Stanford, CA: Stanford University Press.

Collins, A., Brown, J. & Holum, A. (1991). Cognitive apprenticeship: Making thinking visible. *American Educator,* Winter; 1991, pp. 1–18.

Damasio, A. R. (1994). *Descartes' error: Emotion, reason, and the human brain.* New York, NY: Avon.

Dreyfus, H. L., & Dreyfus, S. E. (1986). *Mind over machine: The power of human intuition and expertise in the era of the computer.* New York, NY: Free Press.

Frenk, J., Chen, L., Bhutta, Z., Cohen, J., Crisp, N., Evans, T., . . . Zurayk, H. (2010). Health professionals for a new century: Transforming education to strengthen health systems in an interdependent world. *The Lancet, 376,* 1923–1958.

Gallagher, S. (2009). Philosophical antecedents of situated cognition. In P. Robbins & M. Aydede (Eds.), *The Cambridge Handbook of situated cognition* (pp. 35-52). Cambridge, England: Cambridge University Press.

Kyriakidis, P.H. (2007). Research field notes, Social and Environmental Conditions that Support or Impede the Development of Expertise, September 2, 2007.

Kyriakidis, P. H., & Vitello, J. (in progress). *Applying Benner's research to entry level registered nurses: An investigation of development and retention.*

Lave, J., & Wenger, E. (1991). *Situated learning: Legitimate peripheral participation.* New York, NY: Cambridge University Press.

Montgomery, K . (2006). *How doctors think: Clinical judgment and the practice of medicine.* New York, NY: Oxford University Press.

Sullivan, W. M. (2004). *Work and integrity: The crisis and promise of professionalism in America* (2nd ed.). San Francisco, CA: Jossey-Bass.

Sullivan, W.M. (2005). Markets vs. professions: value added? *Daedalus, 134*(3), 19–26.

Appendix

DESCRIPTION OF RESEARCH DESIGN AND DATA ANALYSIS

The design of this two-phase study was descriptive, interpretive, and naturalistic. Phase 1 data were collected from 1990 to 1991 and included small group interviews with 130 critical care nurses from eight different hospitals and observations and individual interviews with a subsample of 48 of these nurses. Phase 2 data were collected from 1996 to 1997 and extended the phase 1 data to include other critical care areas, as well as to enlarge our sample of advanced practice nurses. For this second edition of *Clinical Wisdom*, 271 narrative accounts were collected with written consent from each contributor. Narratives were contributed from 2004 to 2010 and included small group interviews and written exemplars from 104 nurses in 16 different hospitals. Because this second edition was enlarged to include acute care practices, we collected 81.2% of the narratives from acute care specialties to include staff nurses, advanced practice nurses, and nurse anesthetists from across all specialties in both inpatient and outpatient settings, The three samples are summarized in Tables 1.2, 1.3, 1.4, and 1.5 in Chapter 1. The Phase 1 data were collected and analyzed with two major goals: 1) to describe skill acquisition and clinical judgment in critical care and 2) to articulate the content of critical care practice in relation to therapeutic interventions and clinical and ethical reasoning. The book, *Expertise in Nursing Practice: Caring, Clinical Judgment, and Ethics* (Benner, Tanner, & Chesla, 1996/2009), which is based on Phase 1 data, presents some of the major findings pertaining to clinical judgment and the development of expertise. The focus of the first edition of *Clinical Wisdom* (based on Phase 1 and Phase 2 data) was aimed at articulating the nature of critical care nursing practice. The aim of this second edition of *Clinical Wisdom* is similar to the first, but expands the articulation of nursing practice to include specialties across acute and critical care.

Subject Populations

In Phase 1, we deliberately sampled four groups of nurses: 1) nurses whose practice was considered expert by their peers and supervisors and who had practiced for 5 or more years. We asked peers and supervisors to select nurses to whom they would go for advice in solving a clinical problem and who were considered excellent preceptors; 2) nurses who had 2 to 3 years of experience and were considered to be good nurses; 3) nurses with less than 1.5 years of nursing experience; 4) nurses with 5 or more years of experience but who were not usually selected to be preceptors nor considered to be outstanding clinicians. This categorization yielded four classes for small group interviews at each hospital. Regardless of group assignment, however, the narratives were evaluated for level of skill acquisition.

A snowball approach was used for purposive sample selection in Phase 2. The research participants were sampled as follows: Group 1 was comprised of experienced clinical nurses who were considered to have a high level of clinical expertise by their peers and supervisors; Group 2 was comprised of nurses who were experienced in their clinical specialty and in their advanced practice nursing role. Like Group 1, Group 2 participants were considered to have a high level of clinical expertise by their peers and/or supervisors. This categorization yielded two classes for small group interviews at each site. For inclusion in Phase 2 of the study, clinical nurses had to be engaged primarily in direct patient care and advanced practice nurses had to have a master's degree in nursing and have patient care responsibilities. Group 3 was comprised of nurse who were experienced in their specialties and roles and whose developmental stage of practice were consensually validated by an interpretive team. To be included in Group 3, nurses had patient care responsibilities, as direct care providers, as strong clinical leaders who simultaneously cared for patients, or as situated coaches.

PROCEDURES

Research participants in Phase 1 and Phase 2 of the study gave written consent and participated in at least one, and no more than three, 1-hour small group interviews (see Table A.1 for interview protocol). Care was taken to make the tone of the interview informal with each

TABLE A.1
Interview Questions and Probes: Memorable Clinical Situations

- In working with patients, can you describe a recent patient care situation where you made a difference?
- Can you give a brief patient history to familiarize me/us with the patient?
- Describe the context of the incident (shift, time of day, available resources).
- Describe what happened in detail, including as much dialogue as possible.
- Why was the situation critical to you?
- What were your concerns at the time? What were the conflicts?
- What were you thinking about as the situation was unfolding?
- What were you watching out for in this situation?
- What were you feeling during and after the incident?
- What were the hunches you had about this patient/family?
- What were your priorities at the time?
- Did your priorities change during the situation? How?
- Did anything take you by surprise during the situation?
- Have you worked with similar patients before?
- Did any particular case come to mind while you were working with this patient/family?
- What was the primary source of your learning about managing this particular situation?
- Were there things you learned from books/lectures that guided you in this situation?
- What guidelines would you give other nurses for managing this situation?
- Would that change if you were talking to an inexperienced nurse? An expert nurse?
- What did you find most satisfying about the situation?
- Can you describe a clinical situation that changed the way you deal with patients and/or their families (use preceding probes)?

Adapted from Patricia Benner.

participant engaging in active listening. There were two interviewers present at each small group interview to ensure that active listening and follow-up probes were consistent and of good quality. Participants were encouraged to ask for clarification and to talk directly to their peers rather than to the interviewers who may have been more or less familiar with the specialty at hand. Using everyday language, participants were asked to tell stories from their practice that were memorable for any reason (Benner et al., 1996/2009, Appendix A).

Using the original ethnographic classification from the study published in *Expertise in Nursing Practice* (Benner et al., 1996/2009), we analyzed all Phase 1 interview data classified under the categories of diagnostic and treatment interventions, which had not been previously analyzed. We also analyzed all written narratives about diagnosis and intervention submitted by participants in Phase 1 of the study, as well as all observations related to interventions, skilled know-how, and reasoning-in-transitions. We were specifically seeking to articulate major domains of therapeutic interventions in critical care nursing and to describe how these interventions were related to ethical and clinical reasoning in particular clinical situations. In Phase 2 and in the narratives and interviews collected for this second edition of *Clinical Wisdom*, interviews were guided by early thematic findings from the Phase 1 diagnostic and therapeutic interpretations. This analysis was completely separate from the analysis completed for other published works from Phase 1 (Benner, Tanner, & Chesla, 1992; Benner et al., 1996/2009; Tanner, Benner, Chesla, & Gordon, 1993).

Patricia Benner was the only overlapping member on the two research teams. Some of the same textual data were extracted in this analysis that were abstracted in the earlier studies. In both studies, we edited the text so that the oral language could be more easily accessed as written language. We sought to edit as lightly as possible for clarity and readability. Similarly, we made minor editorial changes to improve clarity and readability in the newly collected narratives without altering the contributor's intent, concerns, meanings, or content. Because the editing was done separately and without reference to earlier publications, there may be slight editorial differences between earlier publications and this one. There are, however, no substantive differences. We have tried to reference all instances where we have used the same interview material in earlier publications. The narratives are multivocal and, because the perspective of this study was not on the level of skill acquisition, but on articulating the content of the practice itself in relation to therapeutic interventions and ethical and clinical reasoning, the interpretation of the text in this work has a different focus. We do not believe that there are any contradictory interpretations, only different interpretations related to focusing on different aspects of the text. We sought to explicate the practical logic used in the everyday practice of clinical nurses and advanced practice nurses as evident in the small group interviews and in the observational interviews.

Based on the Phase 1 data, we had already identified the habits of thought and action—clinical forethought and clinical grasp—and the nine domains of practice articulated here. These were the broad themes for coding the data collected in Phase 2 of the study. Each author revised and refined the aspects in each of the major classifications. These were further refined when we extended the work to include acute care practices. When there was overlap and redundancy between the broad categories, we discussed and reached consensus on the interpretation of the narratives and which domain of practice they best fit. Because the narratives are complex, they do not fall into mutually excluded categories, and are thus classified according to the major organizing concern in the narrative.

In both Phase 1 and Phase 2, a subsample of participants' practices were observed at least once, and no more than three times, for 1 to 2 hours (see Table A.2 for observation protocol). These were called *observational interviews* because the responses to questions about

TABLE A.2

Questions and Probes for Clinical Observations

- What are your concerns about this patient?
- What are you noticing in this situation?
- What is going on at this point?
- What hunches do you have about this patient?
- What do you anticipate with this patient?
- What are your priorities at this time?
- What did you learn from shift report that helped you care for the patient?
- I noticed that you did _____. Tell me about this.
- How is this situation similar to other situations you have experienced?
- How is it different?
- Is this situation familiar to you? In what ways?
- What are you thinking about in this situation?
- What are you watching out for in this situation?
- What are you feeling about this situation?
- Is the situation going as you expected?
- What would you prefer to see happen?
- What are the typical interventions for patients like this?
- What interventions do you anticipate needing for this patient?
- In this situation, what do you expect this intervention to do for this patient?
- Have your priorities changed during this situation? How?
- What was your primary source of learning about interventions like this?
- Were there things you learned from books/lectures that guided you with this problem?
- What guidelines would you give other nurses for managing this situation?
- What did you find most satisfying about the situation?
- If you had to do it over again, would you do anything differently?
- (Observe change of shift report for skilled knowledge that is passed on).

the nurse's actions on the spot were tape recorded and transcribed verbatim. In addition, nurses were interviewed immediately following an observation to clarify any questions the interviewer had about the observation. Field notes were also made about what the interviewer observed. The aim of observing nurses in everyday practice was to further articulate the practices that nurses described in the small group interviews (Benner et al., 1996/2009, Appendix A). All observational interviews and small group interview transcripts were reviewed by the researcher involved to ensure accuracy of the transcripts.

DATA ANALYSIS

The aim of interpretive phenomenology is to understand patterns of meaning and action in the lives of those studied, taking into account the context, their history, and their concerns (Chesla, Martinson, & Muwaswes, 1994). This is achieved by studying persons, events, and practices in their own terms (Benner, 1994). In an interpretive study, data analysis begins with the initial data collection and continues through the writing process. Interpretive phenomenology is, thus, dialogical in nature. The data analysis associated with this method comprises three interrelated interpretive strategies: paradigm cases, thematic analysis, and analysis of exemplars (Benner, 1994). For a more detailed discussion of the data analysis and evaluation associated with this method, please refer to Appendix A in Benner et al. (1996/2009).

REFERENCES

Benner, P., Tanner, C., & Chesla, C. (1992). From beginner to expert: Gaining a differentiated clinical world in critical care nursing. *Advances in Nursing Science, 14*(3), 13–28.

Benner, P., Tanner, C. A., & Chesla, C. A. (1996/2009). *Expertise in nursing practice: Caring, clinical judgment, and ethics.* New York, NY: Springer Publishing Company.

Chesla, C., Martinson, I., & Muwaswes, M. (1994). Continuities and discontinuities in family members' relationships with Alzheimer's patients. *Family Relations, 43*(1), 3–9.

Tanner, C. A., Benner, P., Chesla, C., & Gordon, D. R. (1993). The phenomenology of knowing the patient. *Image, 25*(4), 273–280.

Glossary

Agency: one's sense of responsibility and ability to act so as to influence the situation based on understanding what is needed and one's capacity to act. This includes, but is not limited to, decision making.

Attunement: emotionally engaged and connected in a way that enables accurate perception of nonverbal and verbal concerns or needs from the patient and family, including their plight. Attunement is evident when a good grasp and good understanding between nurse–patient or nurse–family exist and enables a responsive relationship.

Breakdown: a situation in which things do *not* go smoothly or optimally.

Changing relevance: turning points, transitions, and changes in a clinical situation that alter the meaning of the clinical data and/or therapeutic goals. For example, if the patient and family decide to forego further curative therapy or it is determined that the patient is dying, the relevance of clinical data and interventions change.

Clinical and moral imagination: refers to one's ability to envision being in a patient's situation, being confronted by the patient's physiologic and human needs, recognizing the challenge of competing goods, feeling the risks and uncertainty, and feeling the constraints or possibilities inherent in the context of an unfolding situation. Clinical and moral imagination provide the nurse with appropriate actions and strategies in open-ended and underdetermined clinical situations. One develops clinical and moral imagination over time from experiential learning directly from patients, families, and other practitioners.

Clinical inquiry: the formal and informal processes of problem search and problem identification or extending clinical understanding, which often results in new knowledge development.

Comportment: refers to style, intents, and manner of acting and interacting, which includes gestures, posture, and stance; thoughts and feelings that are fused with physical presence and action: includes one's ways of being with patients and families, such as tone of voice, touch, accessibility, tact, and staying open and curious in clinical situations.

Concern: a way of being involved in situations and with people; a form of directed attention and engagement. Concerns are the way a person is oriented meaningfully in the situation and constitute what matters to the person. In narrative, one's concerns and notions of good organize the story.

Deliberative rationality: may be contrasted with rational calculation, in which situations are broken down into their smallest elements. Deliberative rationality entails using whole interpretations and intuitions, stepping back and reflecting on one's understanding of a situation, and deliberately evaluating other possible understandings and perspectives. Stepping out of a current understanding can prevent tunnel vision. Considering relevance and adequacy of past experiences for the current situation can prevent inappropriate rote responses.

Domain of practice: an orienting cluster of clinical concerns and interventions that can be thought of as strong situations that order actions, thought, and practical logic.

Embodiment: the ways in which meanings, expectations, skillfulness, styles, and habits are expressed and experienced in the body through comportment. Skilled know-how in a practice domain is embodied and situated.

Engagement: refers to emotional involvement or connection with a person, problem, and/ or the situation.

Ethical comportment: embodied, skilled know-how of relating to others in ways that are respectful, responsive, and supportive of their concerns; develops experientially and is guided by situated understanding of particular human concerns in particular contexts and transitions.

Ethic of responsiveness: responding to the concerns, needs, preferences, and tendencies of the patient and/or family within a timely manner.

Ethos: the characteristic spirit or attitude of a person, group, community, or culture that reflects moral worth (e.g., notions of good and that which is harmful; that which is sacred and that which is profane).

Exemplar: a narrative or clinical story from one's practice that conveys concerns, meanings, knowledge, and skills common to the practice. An exemplar is a single clinical situation that illustrates clinical issues or patterns. Exemplars illustrate the context for qualitative distinctions and narrative understanding.

Experience: refers to being turned around, adding nuance, and amending or changing preconceived notions or perceptions of a situation; occurs when one encounters a practical situation in such a way that one's understanding of the situation is altered.

Experiential learning: clinical learning that is accomplished by being open to having one's expectations refined, challenged, or disconfirmed by the unfolding situation.

Formal criterial (or snapshot) reasoning: spells out all the relevant criteria and essential characteristics at one discrete point in time. This can be contrasted to the knowledge or understanding that is gained or lost by an agent moving through transitions in understanding of a situation.

Formalism: the perspective and practice of making elements and attributes of a situation explicit so that formal properties or mathematical formulas are spelled out, as in algorithms. Habits of thought and action; styles of practice, thought, and action that constitute typical approaches or modus operandi.

Formation: how a professional is morally and ethically shaped and takes up becoming and being a nurse; how one learns to instantiate the notions of good in actual everyday practice and in the skills of involvement with patients, families, and colleagues.

Intuition: the direct understanding of the meaning and particulars in a situation without conscious deliberation, awareness, or articulation. Intuitive grasp is based on an experiential background of similar and dissimilar situations. It does not refer to extrasensory perception or intrapsychic skills.

Making a case: presenting relevant clinical information to a clinician, patient, or family member, highlighting the salient local and specific aspects of the situation in such a way that he or she grasps the proposed clinical perspective and rationale for any proposed interventions.

Maxim: a brief characterization of skilled performance or "rules of thumb" that can benefit one who has enough skill to recognize the implications of the instructions. For example, many expert nurses have learned to make only one change at a time in a critically ill patient's therapeutics so that they can keep track of the patient's responses to specific interventions.

Modus operandi thinking: a kind of engaged reasoning where sequencing of events matter and sources of influence in a chain of events are uncertain and must be deduced; similar to detective work thinking.

Paradigm case: a clinical episode that alters one's way of understanding and perceiving future clinical situations; an instance of strong or significant learning. A paradigm case opens up new understandings and possibilities in clinical practice. Paradigm cases make public patterns of practice, skilled know-how, taken-for-granted meanings, and notions of the good.

Perceptual awareness: refers to the skill of "seeing," which requires skillful engagement both with problems and persons. Skills of recognition, visual discrimination, and comparative distinctions are implied.

Practical knowledge: knowledge gained through directly practicing skills and taking up cultural practices. It is "knowing how" to dwell in and act in a local, specific human world such as clinical nursing practice. In excellent practice, one may "know how" without "knowing that," which is associated with theoretical or formal knowledge. Likewise, one may know theoretical knowledge without knowing how or when to use it. Knowing how may go beyond current theoretical formulations, but it should not lag behind theoretical developments.

Practical reasoning: is "historical" reasoning over time. It is particular and contextual. It takes into account trends and trajectories in a patient's condition and recovery. Clinical reasoning is a form of practical reasoning, that is, reasoning across time about changes in the patient's condition and/or changes in the clinician's understanding of the patient's condition.

Practical technology assessment: weighing the risks and benefits of a given technological intervention with a particular patient by assessing the actual and potential side effects and possible sequelae.

Practice: a socially embedded, historically situated, and shared activity with notions of good internal to the practice itself. For example, nursing, medicine, and law are a few among many such practices.

Qualitative distinctions: meaningful differences that can only be made in particular, contextual, or historical situations. Recognizing a qualitative distinction relies on one's understanding of the situation. For example, familiarity and expertise with certain patient populations can enable nurses to distinguish between levels of consciousness, sleepiness and arousal, and states of confusion with particular patients in specific contexts.

Reasoning-in-transition, clinical reasoning, practical reasoning: refers to practical reasoning where a clinician takes account of gains and losses in understanding a situation as transitions occur. A nurse recovering a patient who is emerging from general anesthesia might realize, for example, that the patient's high blood pressure is related to pain and not to hypothermia or emergence from the anesthetic gases. This is reflected in her statement, "I thought his hypertension was related to his anesthesia, and then I thought it was because he was cold and vasoconstricted. Now, after successfully treating his blood pressure with some morphine, I think it must have been pain-related."

Salience: the condition where certain aspects stand out as more or less important in a situation.

Set: a predisposition to understand and act in certain ways in particular situations. For example, nurses who are familiar and skilled at caring for patients who sustain traumatic injuries can foresee the need to transfuse large volumes of fluid and/or blood products.

Situated cognition: productive thinking and knowledge retrieval which is called forth by and relevant to particular, concrete circumstances in the continuously changing situation at hand. Situated cognition relies on embodied skilled know-how as well as formal knowledge and is based on recognition of the nature of the situation.

Situated learning: learning while engaged in an actual situation or context; learning to use knowledge while thinking and acting in an ever-changing situation

Situation: the relevant concerns, issues, constraints, and resources at a given time or place as experienced by particular person(s). Naming or understanding the nature of a situation is a starting point for thinking-in-action and practical reasoning.

Skill of involvement: refers to the interpersonal interactions or relational connection between the nurse and the patient and/or family. Skills of involvement are experientially learned over time, as well as being formally taught. Skills of interpersonal and problem engagement allow for paying attention, noticing, and understanding the nature of the clinical situation. Skills of involvement vary in different professional practices, such as, teaching, law, and medicine. Skills of interpersonal and problem engagement are the positive project that goes beyond the remedial skills of "boundary" work where one sorts out issues of self and not self or other.

Skilled know-how: refers to skilled performance or embodied intelligence. It is not only knowing what to do and when to do it; it is knowing how to do what is needed. It requires skillful embodied responses and capacities.

Stance: the habits, practices, concerns, and skills one brings to the situation. The orienting perspective of a clinician in a particular situation is an example of stance.

Strong situation: a prevailing understanding of the nature of a situation (e.g., acutely injured patient with hemorrhage) so that understanding directs and prioritizes interventions and concerns.

Thick description: an anthropologic term coined by Clifford Geertz to refer to descriptions that include meanings as they are understood contextually. Such an account is more than a strategic or process account; it includes significance of actions, events, or signs in their context.

Thinking-in-action: the patterns and habits of thought and action that are directly tied to responding to patients and families and the demands of a changing situation and for noticing when clinical assumptions and expectations are not met.

Index